Retinal Imaging

Retinal Imaging

David Huang, MD, PhD
Associate Professor of Ophthalmology
University of Southern California
Doheny Eye Institute
Los Angeles, California

Peter K. Kaiser, MD
Director, Retinal Clinical Research Center
Director, Digital Optical Coherence Tomography Reading Center (DOCTR)
Cole Eye Institute
Cleveland Clinic Foundation
Cleveland, Ohio

Careen Y. Lowder, MD, PhD
Full Professional Staff
Cole Eye Institute
Cleveland Clinic Foundation
Cleveland, Ohio

Elias I. Traboulsi, MD
Professor of Ophthalmology
Cole Eye Institute
Cleveland Clinic Lerner College of Medicine
Director, Pediatric Ophthalmology and Strabismus
Chairman, Department of Graduate Medical Education
Cleveland Clinic Foundation
Cleveland, Ohio

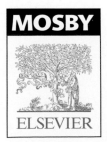

MOSBY

ELSEVIER

MOSBY
ELSEVIER

1600 John F. Kennedy Blvd.
Ste 1800
Philadelphia, PA 19103-2899

RETINAL IMAGING
Copyright © 2006, by Elsevier Inc.

ISBN 13: 978-0-323-02346-7
ISBN 10: 0-323-02346-0

NOTICE

Knowledge and best practice in this field are constantly changing. As new research and experience broaden our knowledge, changes in practice, treatment and drug therapy may become necessary or appropriate. Readers are advised to check the most current information provided (i) on procedures featured or (ii) by the manufacturer of each product to be administered, to verify the recommended dose or formula, the method and duration of administration, and contraindications. It is the responsibility of the practitioner, relying on his or her own experience and knowledge of the patient, to make diagnoses, to determine dosages and the best treatment for each individual patient, and to take all appropriate safety precautions. To the fullest extent of the law, neither the Publisher nor the Editors assume any liability for any injury and/or damage to persons or property arising from or related to any use of the material contained in this book.

The Publisher

ISBN 13: 978-0-323-02346-7
ISBN 10: 0-323-02346-0

Acquisitions Editor: Paul Fam
Developmental Editor: Heather Krehling
Project Manager: Cecelia Bayruns
Design Direction: Gene Harris
Marketing Mananger: Lisa D'Amico

Printed in China

Last digit is the print number: 9 8 7 6 5 4 3 2 1

Working together to grow
libraries in developing countries

www.elsevier.com | www.bookaid.org | www.sabre.org

ELSEVIER | BOOK AID International | Sabre Foundation

Foreword

It is a special honor to be invited to write the Foreword to the first edition of what I predict will be an important new text, *Retinal Imaging*.

For decades, clinicians and basic scientists alike have marveled at both the simplicity of the retinal structure and the complexity of its function. The intimacy of the relationship between retinal structure and function is one of the wonders of biology. However, until the second half of the twentieth century, the retina could be examined only by visual inspection. The first approaches to retinal imaging by fluorescein angiography have allowed us to assess retinal structure and function and better understand retinal diseases, thereby enabling us to diagnose retinal diseases more accurately, and treat patients more effectively.

During the past two decades, ophthalmologists and engineers have devoted enormous efforts to the development of noninvasive imaging techniques. As a consequence, in addition to conventional fluorescein angiography, we now have a broad array of such techniques available, including optical coherence tomography, indocyanine green angiography, scanning laser ophthalmoscopy, ultrasonography, and many others. Consider, for example, how the care of patients with choroidal neovascularization, diabetic retinopathy, and many other diseases have been facilitated by these techniques.

By applying a number of noninvasive imaging techniques, modern ophthalmologists can now better assess vitreoretinal structure. These techniques can provide the information required for developing a rational therapeutic plan.

In this new book, the editors from the Cole Eye Institute of the Cleveland Clinic Foundation worked with a group of talented authors to provide an elegant analysis of the most important retinal diagnostic imaging techniques currently available. It will provide medical students, residents, ophthalmologists, and vitreoretinal specialists with information on theoretical background, clinical utility, and relative values and limitations of each of these imaging techniques. The first section of the book includes clear presentations of the goals and quantitative and perceptual aspects of retinal imaging; subsequent sections emphasize specific diseases.

The editors deserve congratulations for preparing a timely book that will benefit ophthalmologists, regardless of subspecialty, who bear responsibility for and who have a deep interest in patients with retinal diseases, as well as the serious student who seeks to acquire the most up-to-date information on retinal imaging.

Hilel Lewis, MD
Chairman, Division of Ophthalmology
Director, Cole Eye Institute

Cleveland, Ohio

Preface

The diagnosis of ophthalmic disease is primarily based on visual impressions, and ophthalmologists are blessed with a great variety of imaging methods to aid in our "pattern recognition." We have at our disposal a vast array of imaging modalities to supplement our clinical exam, including wide-field color photography, fluorescein angiography, optical coherence tomography (OCT), indocyanine green (ICG) angiography, scanning laser ophthalmoscopy and its derivatives (tomography, polarimetry), ultrasonography, and the retinal thickness analyzer. With the recent advances and proliferation in imaging modalities comes a need for a comprehensive text to summarize our current understanding and utilization of these diagnostic tools.

This book on retinal imaging is designed for all ophthalmologists, even those without a particular expertise in retina, who use these imaging modalities and want to improve their ability to diagnose posterior segment diseases. To make it easy to find a given diagnosis, the book is disease-oriented and organized by pathophysiology and anatomy. Each chapter presents a variety of disease-specific images using the full arsenal of imaging modalities that help a clinician to recognize disease states. Not all imaging modalities are useful in any given disease, and the best choices for each diagnosis are discussed in the chapters. The images are accompanied by succinct legends to help with clinical interpretation. The chapters are set up to correspond to the ones found in Dr. Stephen Ryan's excellent treatise, simply titled *Retina* (Elsevier, 2005). Thus if readers are interested in a more in-depth discussion of a certain disease, its management, and an extensive bibliography, we heartily suggest using the Ryan text as a companion resource.

In Section I of *Retinal Imaging*, the fundamental principles and basic interpretation of the various imaging modalities are introduced by their inventors and preeminent practitioners. The most important imaging methods for macular and retinal vascular diseases remain fluorescein and ICG angiography. The principles of angiography are discussed with clues to interpretation of the images. Optical coherence tomography (OCT) can provide detailed cross-sectional retinal images, and its use in the diagnosis and management of macular diseases and glaucoma has grown rapidly over recent years. We introduce the principles of OCT and illustrate anatomic correlation using recently available ultra-high–resolution (3-micron) images. Examples of images from the various generations of commercially available OCT systems are compared. Throughout the book, we predominantly use images from the newest, high-resolution, Stratus OCT system. Although OCT has a higher resolution, ultrasound has better ocular penetration and is necessary for the diagnosis of ocular tumors. The principles of ultrasound and basic echographic features of ocular pathologies are introduced in Section I. Scanning laser ophthalmoscopy (SLO) has found specialized applications with several technological extensions. Here we concentrate on two extensions that have made strides in glaucoma diagnosis: tomography and polarimetry. The retinal thickness analyzer, which is capable of rapidly mapping retinal thickness of the posterior pole using a scanning-slit laser beam, is described in detail. Finally, we introduce experimental technologies and applications such as combined OCT-SLO, adaptive optics, and blood-flow imaging.

In the subsequent sections of the text, the various imaging modalities are used to highlight disease states. Section II explores the world of macular disease with particular emphasis on entities that lead to choroidal neovascular membranes, including age-related macular degeneration, pathologic myopia, and angioid streaks. Epiretinal membranes and macular holes are also described. Section III looks at retinal vascular diseases, including diabetic retinopathy, retinal vascular occlusions, retinopathy of prematurity, and other less-common diseases. Section IV explores inflammatory diseases with particular attention to the white dot syndromes, viral retinitis, and endophthalmitis. Hereditary chorioretinal and retinal degenerations and drug toxicity are covered in Section V. Section VI concentrates on posterior segment tumors, with particular emphasis on retinoblastoma, melanoma, metastasis, and lymphoma. Finally, Section VII looks at disorders of the optic nerve, with a large section on glaucoma.

The 72 chapters in this text are authored by internationally recognized experts in retina, glaucoma, and imaging techniques and provide a complete review of our current understanding of posterior segment imaging. However, since the field is so vast and is constantly changing, this text cannot be comprehensive. Instead it is meant to serve as an expanded atlas. We did not attempt to address etiology or management of these diseases, which are already covered by a number of excellent books. Moreover, textbooks for the individual imaging modalities are available, but none that covers all modalities like this text. Finally, the field of retinal imaging is constantly improving. The information contained in this text is current at the time of printing; however, research continues to provide better ways to image the posterior segment, and improve our ability to diagnose disease.

We intended to have this expanded atlas serve both as a text and as a reference. It is brief enough to read as a primer on ophthalmic imaging, yet comprehensive enough to refer to when a clinician encounters an unusual clinical picture and wants examples to examine.

We hope we have achieved our goal of producing a definitive text on retinal imaging.

David Huang, MD, PhD

Peter K. Kaiser, MD

Careen Y. Lowder, MD, PhD

Elias I. Traboulsi, MD

Contributors

Nicholas G. Anderson, MD
Southeastern Retina Associates
Knoxville, Tennessee

Lourdes Arellanes-García, MD
Associate Professor, Medicine Faculty
Universidad Autónoma de México
Director, Inflammatory Eye Diseases Clinic
Asociacion para Evitar la Ceguera en México
México, D.F., México

J. Fernando Arevalo, MD, FACS
Director, Department of Retina and Vitreous
Clinica Oftalmologica Centro Caracas
Caracas, Venezuela

Sanjay Asrani, MD
Assistant Professor of Ophthalmology
Department of Glaucoma Service
Duke University Eye Center
Durham, North Carolina

Neal H. Atebara, MD
Assistant Professor, Department of Surgery
John A. Burns School of Medicine
University of Hawaii
Surgeon, The Queens Medical Center
Honolulu, Hawaii

Harmohina Bagga, MD
Research Associate, Department of Ophthalmology
Bascom Palmer Eye Institute
University of Miami School of Medicine
Palm Beach Gardens, Florida

Sophie J. Bakri, MD
Assistant Professor of Ophthalmology
Department of Vitreoretinal Diseases and Surgery
College of Medicine
Mayo Clinic
Rochester, Minnesota

Rubens Belfort, Jr., MD, PhD
Head Professor, Vision Institute
Federal University of São Paulo
São Paulo, Brazil

Audina M. Berrocal, MD
Assistant Professor, Department of Ophthalmology
Bascom Palmer Eye Institute
University of Miami School of Medicine
Miami, Florida

Mark Borchert, MD
Associate Professor, Department of Ophthalmology
University of Southern California Keck School of
    Medicine
Division Head, Ophthalmology
Children's Hospital Los Angeles
Los Angeles, California

Miguel N. Burnier, Jr., MD, PhD, FRCS(C)
Professor and Krayna and Thomas Hecht Chair
Department of Ophthalmology
Ophthalmologist in Chief
McGill University Health Center
Jewish General Hospital
Director, Henry C. Witelson Ocular Pathology
    Laboratory
Montreal, Quebec, Canada

Mark T. Cahill, FRCSI (Ophth), FRCO
Duke University Department of Ophthalmology
Durham, North Carolina

Joseph Carroll, PhD
Center for Visual Science
University of Rochester
Rochester, New York

Sai H. Chavala, MD
Division of Ophthalmology
Cole Eye Institute
Cleveland Clinic Foundation
Cleveland, Ohio

Diane Chialant, RN, RDMS, ROUB
Chief Technologist, Ophthalmic Diagnostics
Department of Ophthalmology
University of Ottawa Eye Institute
Ottawa Hospital
Ottawa, Ontario, Canada

Louis J. Chorich III, MD
Clinical Assistant Professor of Ophthalmology
Department of Ophthalmology
Ohio State University College of Medicine
Ohio State University Medical Center
Columbus, Ohio

Antonio P. Ciardella, MD
Assistant Professor, Department of Ophthalmology
Rocky Mountain Lions Eye Institute
University of Colorado Health Sciences Center
Chief of Ophthalmology
Denver Health Hospital Authority
Denver, Colorado

S. Yves Cohen, MD, PhD
Responsible, AMD Clinic
Department of Ophthalmology
Hôpital Lariboisière
Paris, France

Gabriel Coscas, MD
Emeritus Professor and Chairman
Department of Ophthalmology
University of Paris-XII
Hospital of Créteil
Créteil, France

Janet L. Davis, MD
Professor, Department of Ophthalmology
Bascom Palmer Eye Institute
University of Miami School of Medicine
Anne Bates Leach Eye Hospital
Miami, Florida

Johannes F. de Boer, PhD
Associate Professor, Wellman Center for Photomedicine
Massachusetts General Hospital
Harvard Medical School
Boston, Massachusetts

Haroldo Vieira de Moraes, Jr., MD, PhD
Professor, Department of Ophthalmology
Federal University of Rio de Janeiro
Rio de Janeiro, Brazil

Jean Deschênes, MD, FRCS(C)
Professor, Department of Ophthalmology
McGill University Health Center
Department Head, Uveitis and Ocular Immunology Unit
Royal Victoria Hospital
Montreal, Quebec, Canada

Cathy W. DiBernardo, RN, RDMS, ROUB
Associate Professor, Department of Ophthalmology
Wilmer Eye Institute
Johns Hopkins University
Baltimore, Maryland

Emilio M. Dodds, MD
Vitreoretinal Diseases and Uveitis
Consultores Oftalmologicos
Buenos Aires, Argentina

Wolfgang Drexler, PhD
Medical University of Vienna
Christian Doppler Laboratory
Institute of Medical Physics
Vienna, Austria

Shane Dunne, PhD
Vice President, Research and Development
Ophthalmic Technologies Inc.
Toronto, Ontario, Canada

Chiara M. Eandi, MD
Retina Fellow, Eye Clinic
Department of Clinical Physiopathology
University of Torino
Torino, Italy
Manhattan Eye, Ear, and Throat Hospital
New York, New York

Fiona J. Ehlies, BSC (HONS), RDMS
Director, Department of Echography
Bascom Palmer Eye Institute
University of Miami School of Medicine
Miami, Florida

Ali Erginay, MD
Praticien Hospitalier, Hôpital Lariboisière
Service d'Ophtalmologie
Paris, France

Sharon Fekrat, MD
Associate Professor
Department of Ophthalmology
Duke University Medical Center
Durham, North Carolina

Carlos F. Fernández, MD
Clinica Oftalmologica Centro Caracas
Fundacion Arevalo-Coutinho para la Investigacion en
    Oftalmologia
Caracas, Venezuela

Harry W. Flynn, Jr., MD
Professor, Department of Ophthalmology
Bascom Palmer Eye Institute
University of Miami
Miami, Florida

William R. Freeman, MD
Director, Joan and Irwin Jacobs Retina Center
Shiley Eye Center
Department of Ophthalmology
University of California, San Diego, School of Medicine
La Jolla, California

James G. Fujimoto, PhD
Professor of Electrical Engineering
Department of Electrical Engineering and Computer
  Science
Research Laboratory of Electronics
Massachusetts Institute of Technology
Cambridge, Massachusetts

Anat Galor, MD
Division of Ophthalmology
Cole Eye Institute
Cleveland Clinic Foundation
Cleveland, Ohio

Patricia M.T. Garcia, MD
Assistant Professor, Department of Ophthalmology
New York Medical College
Valhalla, New York
Research Associate, Department of Ophthalmology
The New York Eye and Ear Infirmary
New York, New York

Sunir J. Garg, MD
Assistant Professor, Department of Ophthalmology
  and Visual Sciences
Barnes Retina Institute
Washington University School of Medicine
St. Louis, Missouri

Alain Gaudric, MD
Department of Opthalmology
Hôpital Lariboisière, Assistance Publique Hôpitaux
  de Paris
Paris, France

Nicola G. Ghazi, MD
Department of Ophthalmology
University of Virginia Health System
Charlottesville, Virginia

Debra A. Goldstein, MD, FRCSC
Associate Professor, Department of Ophthalmology
University of Illinois at Chicago College of Medicine
Chicago, Illinois

Evangelos S. Gragoudas, MD
Professor, Department of Ophthalmology
Harvard Medical School
Director, Retina Service
Massachusetts Eye and Ear Infirmary
Boston, Massachusetts

David S. Greenfield, MD
Associate Professor, Department of Ophthalmology
Bascom Palmer Eye Institute
University of Miami
Palm Beach Gardens, Florida

Alon Harris, MS, PhD
Letzter Endowed Professor of Ophthalmology
Professor of Physiology and Biophysics
Department of Ophthalmology
Indiana University School of Medicine
Indianapolis, Indiana

Charles Hejny, MD
Clinical Instructor, Department of Ophthalmology
  and Visual Sciences
University of Wisconsin Medical School
Madison, Wisconsin

Toshio Hisatomi, MD, PhD
Research Associate, Department of Ophthalmology
Graduate School of Medical Sciences
Kyushu University
Fukuoka, Japan

Allen C. Ho, MD
Professor of Ophthalmology
Department of Retina Service
Thomas Jefferson University
Attending Surgeon
Department of Retina Service
Wills Eye Hospital
Philadelphia, Pennsylvania

Heidi J. Hofer, PhD
Assistant Professor
University of Houston College of Optometry
Houston, Texas

Peter G. Hovland, MD, PhD
Department of Ophthalmology and Visual Sciences
University of Wisconsin Medical School
Madison Wisconsin

Lily Im, MD
Department of Glaucoma
Duke University Eye Center
Durham, North Carolina

Michael S. Ip, MD
Assistant Professor, Department of Ophthalmology
  and Visual Sciences
University of Wisconsin Medical School
University of Wisconsin Hospitals and Clinics
Madison, Wisconsin

Reza Iranmanesh, MD
Department of Ophthalmology
Rocky Mountain Lions Eye Institute
University of Colorado Health Sciences Center
Aurora, Colorado

Tatsuro Ishibashi, MD, PhD
Professor, Department of Ophthalmology
Graduate School of Medical Sciences
Kyushu University
Fukuoka, Japan

Glenn J. Jaffe, MD
Professor, Department of Ophthalmology
Duke University Medical Center
Durham, North Carolina

Larry Kagemann, MS, BME
Assistant Director, Glaucoma Research
Department of Ophthalmology
Indiana University School of Medicine
Indianapolis, Indiana

Motohiro Kamei, MD
Assistant Professor, Department of Ophthalmology
Osaka University Medical School
Suita, Osaka, Japan

Ivana K. Kim, MD
Instructor, Department of Ophthalmology
Harvard Medical School
Assistant in Ophthalmology
Department of Retina Service
Massachusetts Eye and Ear Infirmary
Boston, Massachusetts

Christina M. Klais, MD
LuEsther T. Mertz Retinal Research Center
Department of Ophthalmology
Manhattan Eye, Ear, and Throat Hospital
New York, New York

Brian R. Kosobucki, MD
Shiley Eye Center
Department of Ophthalmology
University of California, San Diego, School of Medicine
San Diego, California
Associate, Carolina Retina and Vitreous Consultants, PA
Charlotte, North Carolina

Andrzej Kowalczyk, PhD
Institute of Physics
Nicolaus Copernicus University
Torun, KujPom, Poland

Ferenc Kuhn, MD, PhD
Associate Professor of Clinical Ophthalmology
Department of Ophthalmology
University of Alabama at Birmingham
Director of Clinical Research
Helen Keller Foundation for Research and Education
President, American Society of Ocular Trauma
Birmingham, Alabama
Professor, Department of Ophthalmology
University of Pecs
Pecs, Hungary

Wico W. Lai, MD, FACS
Assistant Professor, Department of Ophthalmology
University of Illinois at Chicago College of Medicine
Chicago, Illinois

Raymond P. LeBlanc, MD, FRCSC
Professor, Department of Ophthalmology
Dalhousie University Faculty of Medicine
Halifax, Nova Scotia, Canada

Leonid E. Lerner, MD, PhD
Division of Ophthalmology
Cole Eye Institute
Cleveland Clinic Foundation
Cleveland, Ohio

Anita Leys, MD, PhD
Hooed Docent
Associate Professor, Ophthalmology Section
Katholicke Universiteit
Kliniek Hooed
University Hospitals Leuven
Leuven, Belgium

Naresh Mandava, MD
Assistant Professor, Department of Ophthalmology
Rocky Mountain Lions Eye Institute
University of Colorado Health Sciences Center
Denver, Colorado

Elias C. Mavrofrides, MD
Department of Ophthalmology
Bascom Palmer Eye Institute
University of Miami School of Medicine
Miami, Florida

Craig A. McKeown, MD
Associate Professor of Clinical Ophthalmology
Bascom Palmer Eye Institute
University of Miami School of Medicine
Miami, Florida

Alex Melamud, MA, MD
Resident, Division of Ophthalmology
Cole Eye Institute
Cleveland Clinic Foundation
Cleveland, Ohio

Aristides J. Mendoza, MD
Department of Retina and Vitreous
Clinica Oftalmologica Centro Caracas and Fundacion
   Arevalo-Coutinho para la Investigacion en
   Oftalmologia
Caracas, Venezuela

William F. Mieler, MD
Professor and Chairman, Department of Visual Science
University of Chicago Pritzker School of Medicine
Chicago, Illinois

Robert A. Mittra, MD
Vitreoretinal Surgery—Minneapolis Center
Minneapolis, Minnesota

Cristina Muccioli, MD, MBA
Professor, Department of Ophthalmology
Federal University of São Paulo-Paulista School of
  Medicine (UNIFESP/EPM)
Director of Uveitis/AIDS Section and Clinical Trials
  Section
Department of Ophthalmology
Hospital São Paulo
Department of Ophthalmology
Hospital Santa Cruz
São Paulo, Brazil

Timothy G. Murray, MD
Professor, Department of Ophthalmology
Bascom Palmer Eye Institute
University of Miami
Miami, Florida

Jeffrey L. Olson, MD
Department of Ophthalmology
Rocky Mountain Lions Eye Institute
University of Colorado
Aurora, Colorado

David L. Parver, MD
Attending Physician, Department of Ophthalmology
Washington Hospital Center
Washington, DC
Surburban Hospital
Bethesda, Maryland
Associate, Department of Diseases and Surgery of the
  Retina and Vitreous
Retina Consultants, P.C.
Washington, DC

Victor L. Perez, MD
Principal Investigator, Laboratory of Ocular
  Immunology and Transplantation
Cole Eye Institute
Associate Staff, Division of Ophthalmology-Cornea
  and Uveitis
Cleveland Clinic Foundation
Cleveland, Ohio

Dante J. Pieramici, MD
California Retina Research Foundation
Cottage Eye Hospital
Santa Barbara, California

Adrian Podoleanu, PhD
Professor of Biomedical Optics
School of Physical Sciences
University of Kent
Canterbury, Kent, United Kingdom

Ranjan Rajendram, MBBS, MRCOphth
Department of Ocular Immunology and Pathology
Doheny Eye Institute
University of Southern California Keck School of
  Medicine
Los Angeles, California

Narsing A. Rao, MD
Professor of Ophthalmology and Pathology
Department of Ophthalmology
Doheny Eye Institute
University of Southern California
Physician, Department of Ophthalmology
USC University Hospital
Los Angeles, California

Carl D. Regillo, MD
Professor, Department of Ophthalmology
Thomas Jefferson University
Director, Clinical Retina Research
Wills Eye Hospital
Philadelphia, Pennsylvania

Adam H. Rogers, MD
Assistant Professor, Department of Ophthalmology
New England Eye Center
Tufts University
Boston, Massachusetts

Fernando Romero-Borja, Dr. rer. nat.
Senior Research Scientist
College of Optometry
University of Houston
Houston, Texas

Austin Roorda, PhD
Associate Professor
College of Optometry
University of Houston
Houston, Texas

Richard B. Rosen, MD, FACS
Associate Professor of Clinical Ophthalmology
Department of Ophthalmology
New York Medical College
Valhalla, New York
Surgeon Director and Residency Program Director
Department of Ophthalmology
Director of Research
The Advanced Retinal Imaging Laboratory
The Retina Center
The New York Eye and Ear Infirmary
New York, New York

Matilde Ruiz-Cruz, MD
Ophthalmologist, Hospital General "Manuel Gea
    Gonzalez"
Ophthalmologist, Center of Research in Infectious
    Diseases
Instituto Nacional de Enfermedades Respiratorias
    (I.N.E.R.)
México, D.F., México

Andrew P. Schachat, MD
Karl Hagen Professor of Ophthalmology
Wilmer Eye Institute
Johns Hopkins University
Baltimore, Maryland

Joel S. Schuman, MD
Professor and Chairman of Bioengineering
Department of Ophthalmology
University of Pittsburgh School of Medicine
Chairman of Ophthalmology and Director
UPMC Eye Center
University of Pittsburgh Medical Center
Pittsburgh, Pennsylvania

Stephen G. Schwartz, MD
Assistant Professor of Clinical Ophtalmology
Bascom Palmer Eye Institute
University of Miami School of Medicine
Miami, Florida
Medical Director and Division Chief
Bascom Palmer Eye Institute
Retina Center at Naples
University of Miami
Naples, Florida

Ingrid U. Scott, MD, MPH
Professor of Ophthalmology and Health Evaluation
    Sciences
Department of Health Evaluation Sciences
Pennsylvania State University College of Medicine
Hershey, Pennsylvania

Jonathan Sears, MD
Associate Staff, Department of Cell Biology
    and Division of Ophthalmology
Cole Eye Institute
Cleveland Clinic Foundation
Cleveland, Ohio

Robert F. See, MD
Department of Ophthalmology
Doheny Eye Institute
University of Southern California
Physician, Department of Ophthalmology
USC University Hospital
Los Angeles, California

Carol L. Shields, MD
Professor of Ophthalmology
Thomas Jefferson University
Co-Director, Oncology Service
Wills Eye Hospital
Philadelphia, Pennsylvania

Jerry A. Shields, MD
Professor of Ophthalmology
Thomas Jefferson University
Co-Director, Oncology Service
Wills Eye Hospital
Philadelphia, Pennsylvania

Brent A. Siesky, PhD
Department of Ophthalmology
Indiana University School of Medicine
Indianapolis, Indiana

Arun D. Singh, MD
Director, Department of Ophthalmic Oncology
Cole Eye Institute
Cleveland Clinic Foundation
Cleveland, Ohio

Jason S. Slakter, MD
Clinical Professor, Department of Ophthalmology
New York University School of Medicine
Surgeon Director, Department of Ophthalmology
Director, Digital Angiography Reading Center (DARC)
Manhattan Eye, Ear, and Throat Hospital
New York, New York

Adael S. Soares, MD
Department of Ophthalmology
Dalhousie University Faculty of Medicine
Halifax, Nova Scotia, Canada
Ophthalmologist
Federal University of São Paulo
São Paulo, Brazil

Gisèle Soubrane, MD, PhD, FEBO
Chairman MD, Department of Ophthalmology
University of Paris XII
Créteil, France

Richard F. Spaide, MD
Clinical Associate Professor, Department of
    Ophthalmology
New York University School of Medicine
Vitreous, Retina, Macula Consultants of New York
New York, New York

Sunil K. Srivastava, MD
Assistant Professor, Department of Ophthalmology
Emory Eye Center
Emory University
Atlanta, Georgia

Daniel M. Stein, BA
Visting Scholar, Department of Ophthalmology
UPMC Eye Center
University of Pittsburgh Medical Center
Pittsburgh, Pennsylvania

Jay M. Stewart, MD
Clinical Instructor, Doheny Retina Institute
Doheny Eye Institute
University of Southern California
Los Angeles, California

Ou Tan, PhD
Department of Ophthalmology
University of Southern California
Los Angeles, California

Yasuo Tano, MD
Chairman, Department of Ophthalmology
Osaka University Medical School
Suita, Osaka, Japan

Howard H. Tessler, MD
Professor, Department of Ophthalmology
University of Illinois at Chicago College of Medicine
Chicago, Illinois

Rafael L. Ufret-Vincenty, MD
Vitreoretinal Surgery Department
Cole Eye Institute
Cleveland Clinic Foundation
Cleveland, Ohio

Krishnakumar Venkateswaran, PhD
University of Houston College of Optometry
Houston, Texas

Raul N. G. Vianna, MD, PhD
Associate Professor, Department of Ophthalmology
Fluminense Federal University
Head, Retina and Vitreous Unit
Antonio Pedro University Hospital
Niteroi, Rio de Janeiro, Brazil

Qing Wang, PhD
Associate Professor, Department of Molecular Medicine
Cleveland Clinic Lerner College of Medicine
Case Western Reserve University
Director, Center for Cardiovascular Genetics
Cleveland Clinic Foundation
Cleveland, Ohio

David R. Williams, PhD
Director, Center for Visual Science
University of Rochester
Rochester, New York

Andre Witkin, BS
Department of Ophthalmology
New England Eye Center
Tufts University
Boston, Massachusetts

Maciej Wojtkowski, PhD
Assistant Professor, Institute of Physics
Nicolaus Copernicus University
Torun, KujPom, Poland

Gadi Wollstein, MD
Assistant Professor, Department of Ophthalmology
University of Pittsburgh School of Medicine
UPMC Eye Center
Pittsburgh, Pennsylvania

Howard S. Ying, MD, PhD
Assistant Professor, Department of Ophthalmology
Wilmer Eye Institute
Johns Hopkins University
Baltimore, Maryland

Ran Zeimer, PhD
Morton F. Goldberg Professor of Ophthalmology
Wilmer Eye Institute
Johns Hopkins University
Baltimore, Maryland

Contents

CONTENTS

CONTENTS

Imaging Modalities: Basic Principles and Interpretation

Chapter 1

Fluorescein Angiography

JEFFREY L. OLSON, MD • NARESH MANDAVA, MD

1.1 Physical Principles

1.1.1 PROPERTIES OF SODIUM FLUORESCEIN DYE

Sodium fluorescein, first synthesized by von Baeyer in 1871, is a hydrocarbon that is yellow-red in color. It has a molecular weight of 376.67. It is available as 2 to 3 mL of 25% concentration or 5 mL of 10% sodium fluorescein in a sterile aqueous solution. After injection into the bloodstream, approximately 80% of fluorescein dye is bound to plasma proteins, primarily albumin. The dye undergoes both hepatic and renal metabolism and within 24 to 36 hours is eliminated in the urine.

Fluorescence occurs when a molecule or atom is excited by a photon of a specific wavelength, which raises an electron to a higher energy level and then a longer-wavelength photon is emitted as the electron returns to its original state. Fluorescein is stimulated by blue light (465 to 490 nm) and emits at a green wavelength (520 to 530 nm). Fluorescein angiography requires the use of two filters, an exciter filter that transmits the blue light and a barrier filter that transmits the emitted green light.

1.1.2 SIDE EFFECTS AND COMPLICATIONS

Fluorescein dye injection is a relatively safe procedure, with an overall risk of anaphylactic reaction of less than 1 in 100,000.[9] Patients should be forewarned that they will experience a transient yellowing of the skin and conjunctiva lasting 8 to 12 hours and an orange discoloration of the urine lasting 24 to 30 hours. Adverse reactions to intravenous fluorescein angiography can be either local or systemic and range from mild to severe.[8,9]

Local complications result from extravasation of dye at the injection site and include local skin irritation, sloughing of skin, and thrombophlebitis. Cold compresses should be applied to the injection site when extravasation occurs.

The most common systemic reaction is nausea, which usually occurs after a rapid injection, and is seen in 3% to 15% of patients. Vomiting occurs in less than 7% of patients and can be prevented by restricting food intake 2 to 3 hours before angiography. A generalized pruritus occurs in less than 5% of patients and is usually mild and transient.

Moderate adverse reactions typically resolve with medical intervention and include urticaria, syncope, pyrexia, and nerve palsy. Patients with a history of hay fever, asthma, or allergies may benefit from prophylactic administration of antihistamines.

Severe adverse reactions are rare but include laryngeal edema, bronchospasm, anaphylaxis, shock, myocardial infarction, seizures, and death.[9]

Vasovagal attacks can occur during fluorescein angiography and are usually caused by patient anxiety rather than by the actual dye injection. Smelling salts can help reverse the vasovagal episode if the symptoms are noted early, and care should be taken to prevent the patient from suffering a fall injury.

Relative contraindications to fluorescein angiography include pregnancy in the first trimester,[4] a previous history of severe reactions to fluorescein, or a history of multiple allergies. Lower dosages of fluorescein are advisable for patients with renal compromise. In children, the recommended dosage is 0.1 mL/kg.

1.1.3 EQUIPMENT

Fluorescein angiography is a technical endeavor that requires the following equipment:

1. Fundus camera, including illuminating light, focusing lenses, flash unit, and powerpack

2. Matched filters

3. Film and film development equipment for analog setup

4. Computer, software, and memory space for digital photography

5. Sodium fluorescein dye

6. 21-gauge butterfly needles

7. 5-mL syringe

8. Tourniquet

9. Cotton swabs

10. Emesis basin

11. Arm rest for injection

12. Emergency equipment

1.1.4 PHOTOGRAPHIC PROCEDURE

Patient cooperation is essential for adequate imaging with fluorescein angiography. This begins with a thorough discussion of the procedure, including side effects and chronology of events. Maximal pupillary dilation is necessary for adequate visualization of the fundus. The patient should be seated comfortably at the headrest and chin rest and supplied with a fixation target.

The camera should be adjusted to the photographer's refractive error by using the crosshairs built into one of the oculars. The crosshairs are brought into focus using the fogging technique to neutralize any operator accommodation. A sharply focused photograph depends on the operator viewing both the crosshairs and the fundus details in sharp focus simultaneously.

Before injection of fluorescein, red-free monochromatic fundus photographs, which highlight the superficial retina and retinal vessels, are taken. Stereoscopic photographs are produced by taking pictures of the same area of retina at either lateral extreme of the pupil. As distance between these two photographs becomes longer, the stereo effect becomes greater.

Misalignment of the camera can cause artifacts, which appear as either peripheral or central blurring or shadows in the images. Slight lateral movement of the camera joystick can be used to eliminate artifacts and produce even illumination of the image.

After injection of fluorescein, fundus photographs are taken at 2 to 3 seconds, and then at 1- to 2-second intervals during the early transit and mid-transit stages of the involved eye. Fundus photographs during late transit are taken 10 to 15 minutes after injection. The overall photographic strategy will depend upon the disease in question.

1.2 Technology Development

1.2.1 HISTORICAL PERSPECTIVE

The first attempt to perform fundus photography was carried out by Henry Noyes more than 100 years ago in rabbits[2] and met with limited success. It was not until the production of the first reliable fundus camera by Zeiss and Nordensen that fundus photography was possible. In 1955, Zeiss' introduction of the electronic flash heralded the advent of modern fundus photography. In 1960, MacLean and Maumenee were the first to use intravenous fluorescein to study choroidal hemangiomas using a slit lamp and a cobalt blue filter to stimulate the dye.[5] In 1961, Novotony and Alvis[6] combined this technique with a fundus camera in human subjects, resulting in the first successful photographic fluorescein angiography.

1.2.2 DIGITAL ANGIOGRAPHY

Digital angiography allows for the production of instant fundus images that can be altered with computer software, thus enhancing rapid diagnosis and management or vitreoretinal disorders by allowing treatment mapping and overlays.

Although the initial costs for the camera, software, and associated hardware can be substantial, the dividends are seen in increased clinical efficiency and patient convenience. However, some practitioners feel that the resolution obtained with digital images is not the same quality as that obtained with film. Further, stereoscopic viewing is often greater with images obtained on film.

1.3 Image Interpretation

1.3.1 ANATOMIC CONSIDERATIONS

The retina has a dual blood supply, as well as an inner and outer blood-retinal barrier. The retinal circulation, provided by the central retinal artery, serves the inner half of the retina, and the tight junctions formed by endothelial cells comprise the inner blood-retinal barrier. Neither bound nor unbound fluorescein molecules can pass through this barrier under normal conditions.

The choroidal circulation serves the outer half of the retina, and the retinal pigment endothelial (RPE) cells comprise the outer blood-retinal barrier. Unbound fluorescein molecules can diffuse freely through the fenestrated walls of the choriocapillaris into the extravascular space and through Bruch's membrane, but under normal conditions are unable to pass through the RPE.

An understanding the anatomy of the macula is essential for interpretation of fluorescein angiographic results. The macula is centered between the temporal vascular arcades and measures approximately 6 mm or 4 disc diameters in width. Histologically, it is defined as the area of the posterior retina that has two or more layers of ganglion cells and contains xanthophyll pigment. It is the high concentration of this pigment, in conjunction with the increased density of RPE cells that causes the relative hypofluorescence of the macula seen on fluorescein angiography. The center of the macula is the fovea, which is approximately 1.5 mm or 1 disc diameter in width. The foveal avascular zone, which is more readily apparent during fluorescein angiography, is an area approximately 0.5 mm or $1/3$ disc diameter in width centered within the fovea.

1.3.2 NORMAL FLUORESCEIN ANGIOGRAPHY

The time interval between injection of dye into the bloodstream and its subsequent appearance in the retina is variable and depends on several factors, including the patient's age and cardiovascular status, as well as the rate of dye injection. The transit time usually ranges from 10 to 15 seconds but can be as short as 5 or as long as 30 seconds.[1,4,7]

The injected dye reaches the eye by way of the ophthalmic artery and then enters either the retinal circulation through the central retinal artery or the choroidal circulation through the short posterior ciliary arteries. Because of the shorter anatomic course of the choroidal circulation, dye generally reaches it 1 second before it reaches the retinal circulation. Approximately 10% to 15% of subjects will have a cilioretinal artery, which arises from the choroidal circulation and will fill before the other retinal vessels, in concert with choroidal filling.

Choroidal filling is characterized by a patchy choroidal flush (**Figure 1–1**). The lobules of the choriocapillaris can be seen to fill sequentially on angiography, with a variable mottling of fluorescence attributable to blockage by the RPE.

The arterial phase follows the choroidal phase by approximately 1 second and begins with the appearance of dye within the retinal arteries (**Figure 1–2**).

The early arteriovenous phase, also called the capillary phase, is manifest by complete retinal artery, arteriole, and capillary filling (**Figure 1–3**).

The late arteriovenous phase is characterized early by laminar venous filling (**Figure 1–3**) and fluorescence of retinal capillaries as well as by the appearance of dye filling the retinal veins (**Figure 1–4**). This phase is also

referred to as the peak phase, during which the detail of the juxtafoveal capillary network is highlighted against the dark background of the macula.

The recirculation phase begins within the first minute after dye injection and is characterized by gradually declining fluorescence (**Figure 1–5**).

The late stages of the angiogram are characterized by staining of the choroid, Bruch's membrane, and sclera (**Figure 1–6**). Larger choroidal vessels can be seen as black shadows against the deeper background fluorescence from the sclera and deeper choroid.

1.3.3 TERMINOLOGY

Hyperfluoresence is an increased or abnormal fluorescence.

Hypofluorescence is a reduction or absence of normal fluorescence.

Autofluorescence is seen in preinjection photographs and is caused by highly reflective substances such as optic disk drusen and astrocytic hamartomas.

Pseudofluorescence occurs when there is overlap between the spectra of light transmitted by the barrier filter and the exciter filter.

Blocking defects can be seen in areas in which the normal underlying fluorescence is blocked by a barrier to light, such as blood, pigment, or exudate.

Filling defects denote areas of hypofluorescence due to ischemia or occlusion of normal blood flow.

Pooling refers to the accumulation of fluorescein dye in an anatomic space.

Leakage is manifest as hyperfluorescence that increases in either intensity or size from the early to the late

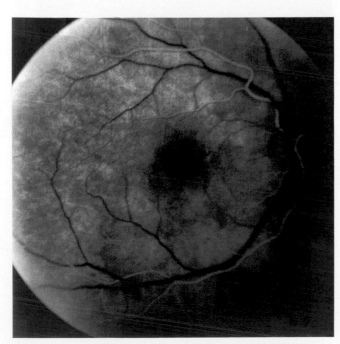

Figure 1–1 Normal fluorescein angiography. Choroidal filling is characterized by patchy hyperfluorescence.

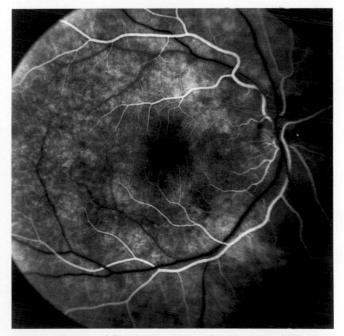

Figure 1–2 Normal fluorescein angiography. One second later the arterial phase begins. Note the increased choroidal filling as well.

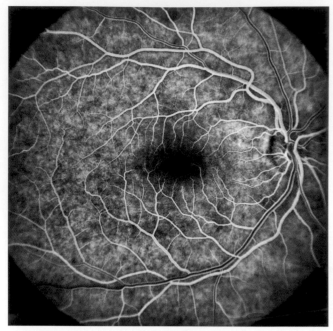

Figure 1–3 Normal fluorescein angiography. The arteriovenous phase is evident by the appearance of dye in a laminar pattern in the retinal veins.

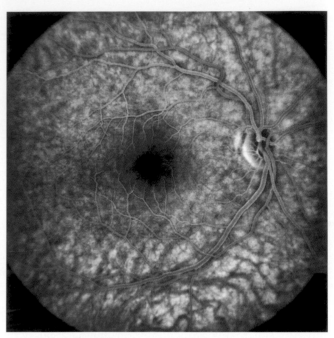

Figure 1–5 Normal fluorescein angiography. The recirculation phase demonstrates declining fluorescence throughout.

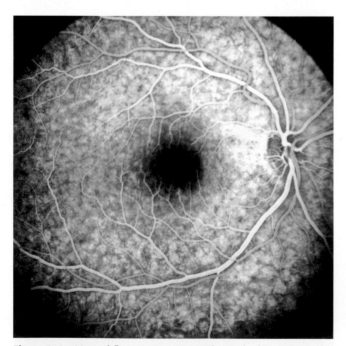

Figure 1–4 Normal fluorescein angiography. In the late venous phases, fluorescein is most evident in the veins.

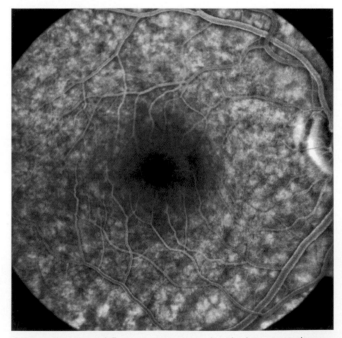

Figure 1–6 Normal fluorescein angiography. The late stages show staining of the disc, choroid, and Bruch's membrane. Note the large-caliber choroidal vessels seen in relief against the staining of the sclera and deep choroid.

phase of the angiogram. In the later phases of the angiogram, the borders of an area of leakage generally become indistinct. Use of the term *leakage* denotes a breakdown in the blood-retinal barrier, either the inner barrier at the level of the retinal capillary or the outer barrier at the RPE.

Staining occurs when dye leaks into tissues and is typically seen as a late hyperfluorescence.

A *transmission* or *window defect* is caused by absence or atrophy of the RPE, which in its normal state causes blockage of the underlying choroidal fluorescence. The intensity of fluorescence seen through a window defect parallels the flow and concentration of dye through the choroid. That is, it will be seen as an area of hyperfluorescence early, which progressively fades throughout the angiogram, but maintains well-defined edges throughout.

1.4 Clinical Applications

1.4.1 CONDITIONS CAUSING HYPOFLUORESCENCE

Hypofluorescence is caused by either a blocking defect or a vascular filling defect. In the former, any opacity that masks or diminishes the visualization of the retinal circulation is considered a blocking defect. Media opacities in the cornea, lens, or vitreous can cause a global reduction in fluorescence.

Blocking defects can provide clues as to the level of the blocking substance (vitreal, retinal, and subretinal) based on the fluorescence that is blocked. For example, the hemorrhage in **Figure 1–7** blocks both retinal and choroidal circulations, so it must be preretinal. In contrast, the hemorrhage in **Figure 1–8** blocks the choroidal circulation, but not the retinal circulation, indicating that it has a subretinal location. Blocking can occur with other substances including melanin, lipid, fibrin, lipofuscin, and inflammatory material.

A distinctive type of blocking defect is seen in Stargardt's disease and fundus flavimaculatus (**Figure 1–9**). An abnormally high concentration of lipofuscin in the RPE causes a relative blocking of choroidal fluorescence, giving the distinctive "silent choroid" as seen on angiography. The pinpoint flecks of hyper-

fluorescence are focal accumulations of subretinal lipofuscin.

Vascular filling defects, the second category of conditions responsible for hypofluorescence, occur due to reduced or absent perfusion of ocular tissues. Artery occlusions, both branch and central, will demonstrate

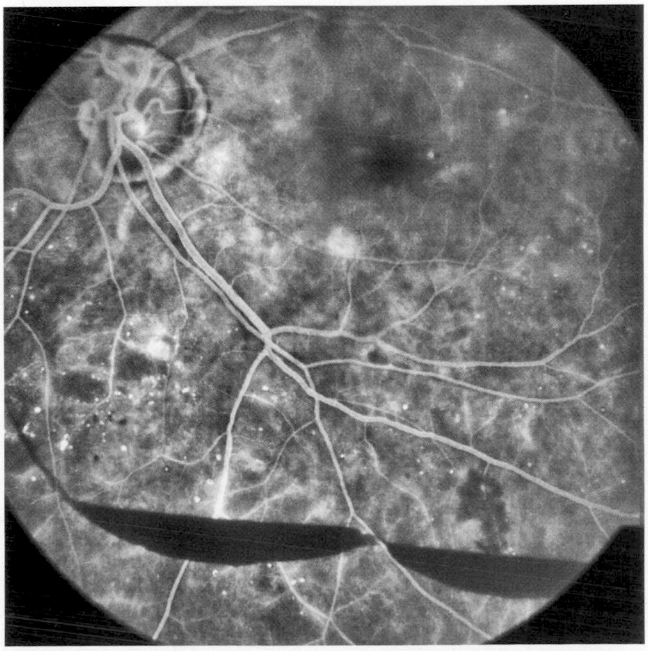

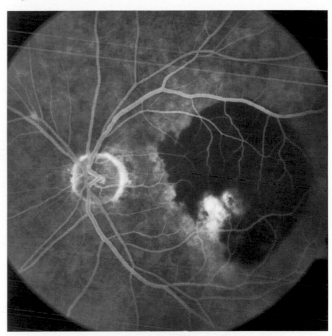

Figure 1–8 Blocking defect. The subretinal blood seen in this patient with exudative macular degeneration blocks the choroidal circulation, but not the overlying retinal vessels.

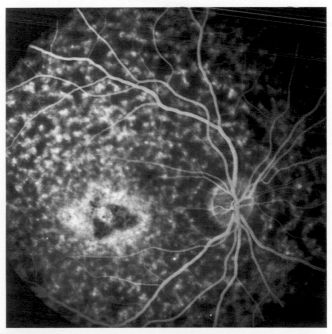

Figure 1–9 Blocking defect. In this patient with fundus flavimaculatus the choroidal fluorescence is blocked by the lipofuscin-rich RPE. The focal areas of hyperfluorescence correspond to subretinal accumulations of lipofuscin. Centrally, a window defect due to RPE atrophy is seen.

Figure 1–7 Blocking defect. Preretinal blood, seen here inferiorly in a patient with diabetic retinopathy, blocks both retinal and choroidal circulations.

hypofluorescence following the distribution of the involved arterial tree (**Figures 1–10** and **1–11**).

Capillary nonperfusion is a type of vascular filling defect seen commonly in diabetes, vein occlusion, and radiation retinopathy. Zones of hypofluorescence can be seen, such as those in **Figure 1–12,** corresponding to the area of ischemia.

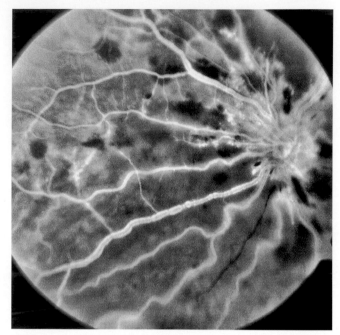

Figure 1–12 Vascular filling defect. Widespread areas of capillary nonperfusion are evident in this patient with a central retinal vein occlusion.

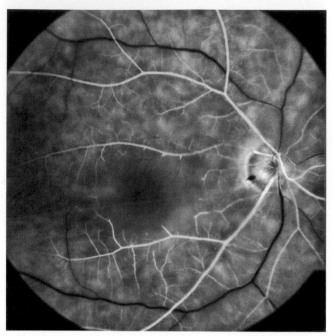

Figure 1–10 Vascular filling defect. In this patient with a central retinal artery occlusion there is irregular filling of the arterial tree.

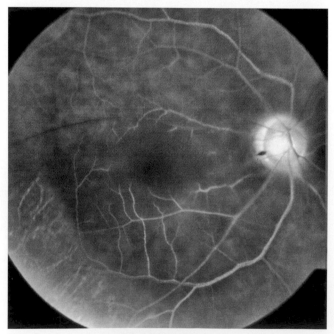

Figure 1–11 Vascular filling defect. Same patient as previous image, late phase of angiogram demonstrates markedly delayed and reduced filling of the retinal vasculature.

Choroidal vascular filling defects can occur with conditions such as malignant hypertension, lupus choroidopathy, and toxemia of pregnancy. When larger-caliber choroidal vessels are involved, the occlusion will manifest as a sectoral, wedge-shaped area of hypofluorescence.

Atrophic degeneration of the choriocapillaris is seen in choroideremia and may be involved in the angiographic appearance of acute posterior multifocal placoid pigment epitheliopathy.

Vascular filling defects of the optic nerve head can be visualized using fluorescein angiography as well. Ischemic optic neuropathy will exhibit peripapillary sectoral or complete hypofluorescence. Congenital anomalies, including optic nerve head colobomas, optic nerve hypoplasia, and optic pits may also present with hypofluorescence.

1.4.2 CONDITIONS CAUSING HYPERFLUORESCENCE

Pseudofluorescence occurs when there is overlap between the exciter and barrier filters, causing highly reflective fundus lesions to appear fluorescent. This can be eliminated by proper selection of filters with no overlap in their absorption curves.

Autofluorescence is created by highly reflective fundus structures when viewed through both the exciter blue and barrier green filters and is seen in preinjection photographs. This is commonly seen with optic nerve head drusen, astrocytic hamartomas, and large deposits of lipofuscin.

A transmission window defect is a type of hyperfluorescence seen in areas in which there is a decrease or atrophy of the RPE. This acts as a window through which the choroidal fluorescence can be seen directly and may occur focally, such as in macular degeneration (**Figures 1–13** to **1–15**), or be more widespread, such as in cone dystrophy (**Figure 1–16**). Transmitted fluorescence is seen in common disease entities such as the atrophic form of age-related macular degeneration, full-thickness macular holes, chorioretinal atrophic scars, and drusen.

Hyperfluorescence can also occur in association with abnormal retinal vasculature in conditions such as retinal artery macroaneurysm (**Figures 1–17** and **1–18**), retinal capillary hemangiomas, arterial venous malformations, Coat's disease, cavernous hemangioma,

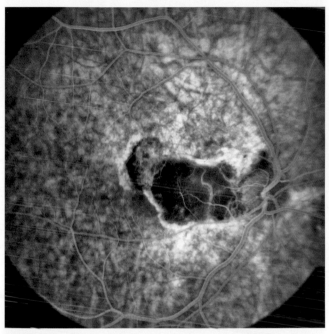

Figure 1–13 Window defect. Focal defect in patient with large macular RPE defect after laser therapy for choroidal neovascularization.

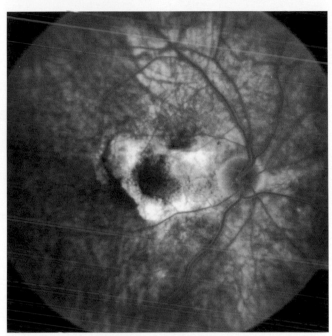

Figure 1–15 Window defect. Same patient as previous image. The window defect transmits the underlying scleral staining.

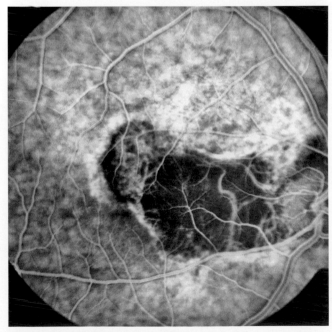

Figure 1–14 Window defect. Mid-phase angiogram in same patient as previous image, note that the larger choroidal vessels can be seen through the window defect.

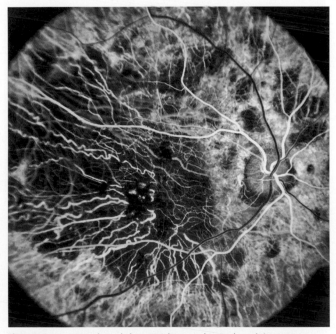

Figure 1–16 Window defect. Widespread atrophy of the RPE in a patient with cone dystrophy allows for visualization of choroidal circulation. Note the loss of choriocapillaris.

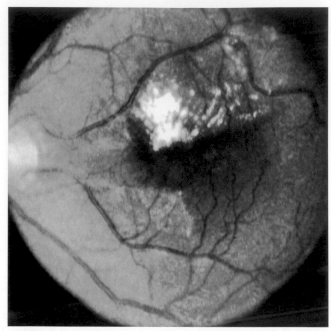

Figure 1–17 Leakage of dye. Red-free photograph of a patient with retinal artery macroaneurysm, demonstrating lipid exudates in the macula.

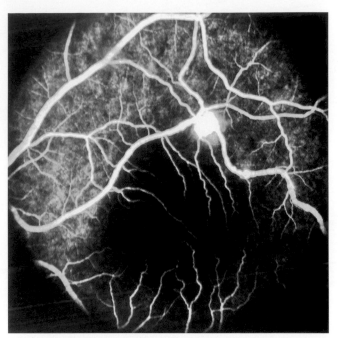

Figure 1–18 Leakage of dye. Late-phase angiogram of the same patient demonstrates leakage of dye from a retinal artery macroaneurysm. Note multiple areas of vessel dilation along the course of the superotemporal arcade.

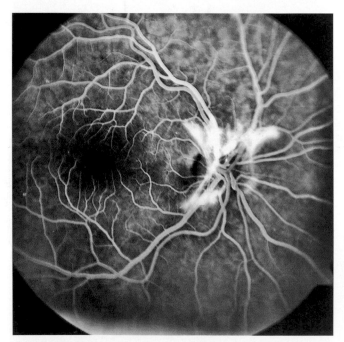

Figure 1–19 Leakage of dye. In this diabetic patient with neovascularization of the disc, the abnormal vessels hyperfluoresce early.

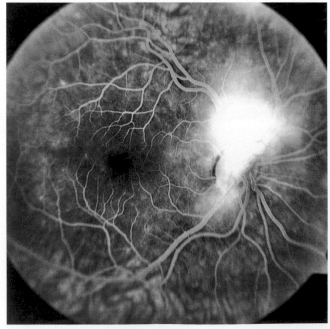

Figure 1–20 Leakage of dye. In the same patient, the abnormal disc vessels leak late.

Wyburn-Mason disease, and combined hamartoma of the retina and RPE. The most common retinal vascular abnormality encountered is neovascularization (**Figures 1–19** and **1–20**), which will manifest as early hyperfluorescence with late leakage of dye. Often the neovascularization will be located adjacent to an area of capillary nonperfusion.

Hyperfluorescence is a feature of abnormal choroidal vasculature as well. Choroidal hemangiomas have a distinctive angiographic appearance (**Figures 1–21** and

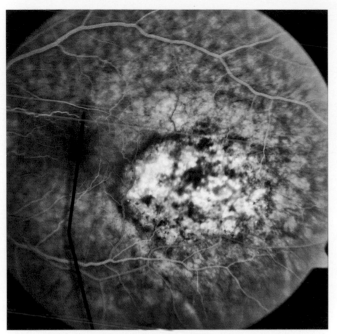

Figure 1–21 Choroidal hemangioma. Circumscribed choroidal hemangiomas are highly vascular lesions that will typically have lacy hyperfluorescence early.

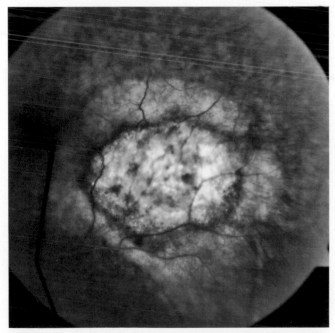

Figure 1–22 Choroidal hemangioma. Late phases often demonstrate intense and widespread hyperfluorescence. On B scan ultrasonography the lesion demonstrated high internal reflectivity.

1–22) as do choroidal melanomas (**Figures 1–23** and **1–24**). The exudative form of age-related macular degeneration will often demonstrate early hyperfluorescence and late leakage of choroidal neovascular membranes (**Figures 1–25** to **1–28**).

Leakage of fluorescein dye causes a hyperfluorescence that generally increases in the later frames of angiography. Vasculitis causes an increased permeability of the retinal vessels, causing leakage of dye into the retina and vitreous. Macular edema is the most common cause of intraretinal leakage and can be seen with a variety of disorders including diabetes and inflammatory conditions and in postsurgical patients. **Figures 1–29** and **1–30** show a typical picture of diabetic retinopathy with significant macular edema. Cystoid macular edema (**Figure 1–31**) occurs most commonly after cataract surgery and appears as leakage of fluorescein in the macula in a petaloid pattern. It is caused by a breakdown of the inner blood-retinal barrier, resulting in the accumulation of extracellular fluid in the outer plexiform layer.

Leakage of dye is often seen near the optic nerve head in normal subjects from the adjacent choroidal capillaries. Optic nerve pathologic conditions such as papilledema and ischemic optic neuropathy will often produce a more pronounced and widespread leakage of fluorescein (**Figures 1–32** and **1–33**). Neuroretinitis may also demonstrate leakage from the optic nerve head (**Figures 1–34** and **1–35**).

Hyperfluorescence is also seen in pooling, which refers to the accumulation of dye within an anatomic space. For example, central serous chorioretinopathy (CSC) is seen clinically as a central neurosensory detachment, which can produce a distinctive angiographic pattern (**Figures 1–36** to **1–39**), due to leakage of dye through small pinpoint areas in the RPE. In contrast, RPE detachments are indicative of more widespread RPE pathologic conditions and are characterized angiographically by a more diffuse and rapid filling of the anatomic space (**Figures 1–40** to **1–43**).

Staining produces hyperfluorescence and is characterized by deposition of fluorescein dye into tissues. This can occur in normal subjects and is commonly seen in the optic disc and the sclera. Staining of the sclera is more common and more readily seen in high myopia and in those patients with lightly pigmented fundi (**Figure 1–44**). Scar tissue from previous trauma or involuted choroidal neovascular membranes will often stain (**Figure 1–45**).

Angioid streaks are breaks in Bruch's membrane and will demonstrate hyperfluorescence on angiography (**Figure 1–46**). The streaks are seen ophthalmoscopically as reddish, irregular lines radiating from the optic nerve head and may be associated with adjacent degenerative changes in the RPE. Patients with angioid streaks can develop serous detachments of the neurosensory retina or choroidal neovascularization.

Fluorescein angiography can be useful in the diagnosis of disorders of the retinal pigment epithelium and choroid such as birdshot choroidopathy, acute macular neuroretinopathy, sympathetic ophthalmia, multiple evanescent white dot syndrome, and infectious choroidopathies.

Sympathetic ophthalmia is a clinical diagnosis that can be aided by fluorescein angiography, which will typically show multiple hyperfluorescent dots at the level of the RPE (**Figures 1–47** to **1–49**).

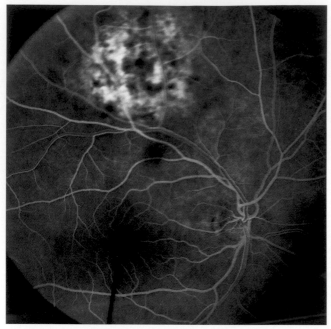

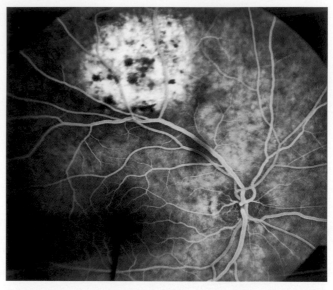

Figure 1–24   Choroidal melanoma. Late phase shows increased dye accumulation. B scan ultrasonography showed low internal reflectivity with choroidal excavation.

Figure 1–23   Choroidal melanoma. In the arteriovenous phase there is irregular and patchy fluorescence of the lesion. The hypopigmented areas are caused by blocking from overlying orange pigment.

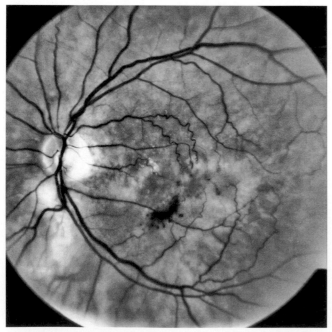

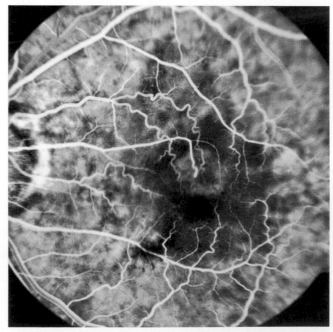

Figure 1–25   Choroidal neovascularization (CNV). In this patient with macular degeneration, the red-free photograph demonstrates hemorrhage and exudates in the macula.

Figure 1–26   CNV. Same eye as Figure 1–25. The arteriovenous phase reveals a classic neovascular membrane that hyperfluoresces in a lacy cartwheel pattern early.

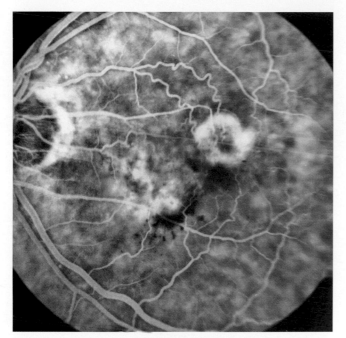

Figure 1–27 CNV. Same eye as Figures 1–25 and 1–26. Note increased leakage in mid-phase and the retinochoroidal anastomosis with a right angle retinal vessel.

Multiple evanescent white dot syndrome is an inflammatory disease affecting the photoreceptors and RPE usually seen in young, otherwise healthy, females. Angiography will sometimes demonstrate small areas of hyperfluorescence in a wreath-like pattern (**Figures 1–50 to 1–52**).

Fluorescein angiography can also be helpful in the diagnosis and management of newly emerging diseases, such as West Nile virus infection. Ocular involvement can be evident by anterior and posterior uveitis and by choroiditis with a distinctive angiographic pattern (**Figures 1–53** to **1–55**).

1.5 Strengths and Limitations

1.5.1 STRENGTHS

Fluorescein angiography has greatly increased our fund of knowledge of retinal and choroidal physiology and pathology. It allows us to assess both the anatomy and function of the retinal and choroidal vasculature in a minimally invasive manner.

Fluorescein angiography has been an indispensable clinical and research tool for the retinal specialist. Over the past half century, it has become a vital component in the diagnosis, treatment, and management of vitreoretinal disorders.

By allowing the ophthalmologist to precisely define the location of pathologic changes, such as those in choroidal neovascular membranes, treatment can be initiated for the pathologic condition while the unaffected areas are preserved.

1.5.2 LIMITATIONS

The major limitation of fluorescein angiography is its inability to precisely image the choroidal circulation. However, newer diagnostic techniques such as indocyanine green angiography have become complimentary

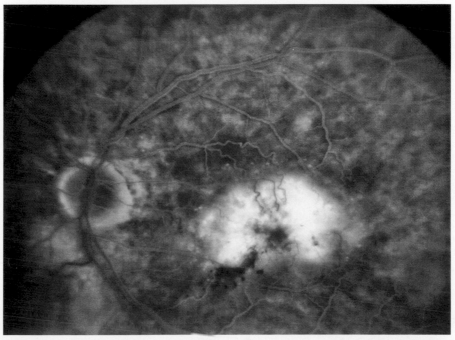

Figure 1–28 CNV. Same eye as Figures 1–25 through 1–27. The late phase is manifest by marked leakage.

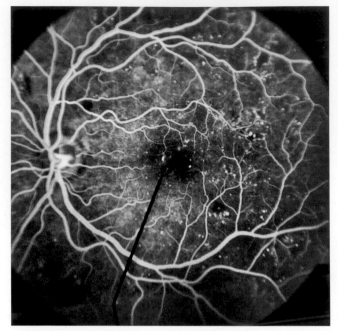

Figure 1–29 Leakage of dye. In this patient with diabetic retinopathy, the arteriovenous phase demonstrates multiple microaneurysms seen as pinpoint areas of hyperfluorescence.

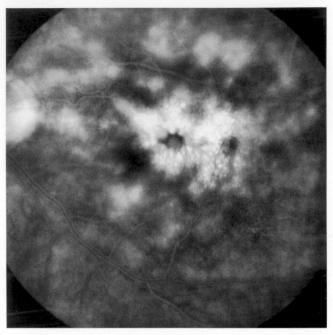

Figure 1–31 Leakage of dye. This patient has cystoid macular edema, with a classic petaloid appearance, due to posterior uveitis.

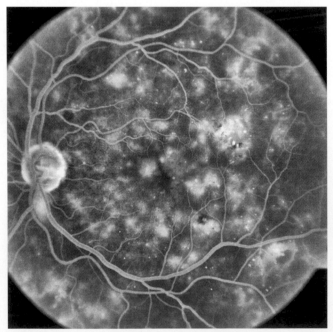

Figure 1–30 Leakage of dye. Same patient as Figure 1–29, later phases of the angiogram demonstrate leakage from microaneurysms causing macular edema.

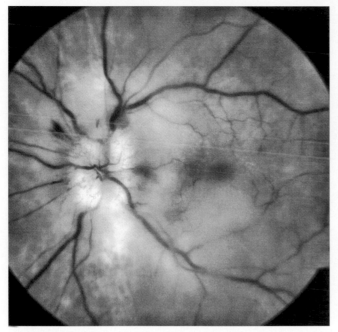

Figure 1–32   Optic nerve leakage of dye. Red-free photograph of a patient with ischemic optic neuropathy and marked optic nerve head swelling and hyperemia.

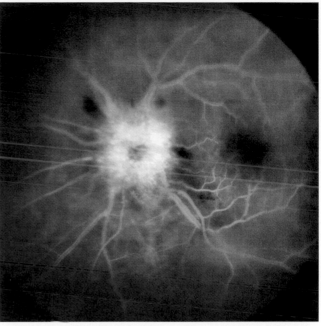

Figure 1–33   Optic nerve leakage of dye. In the same patient as Figure 1–32, the mid-transit phase of angiogram shows marked optic nerve head hyperemia and leakage. The somewhat hazy view is due to cataract.

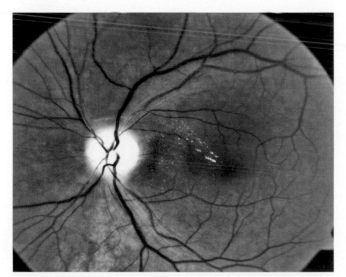

Figure 1–34   Optic nerve leakage of dye. Red-free photograph of a patient with *Bartonella* neuroretinitis; notice the partial macular star.

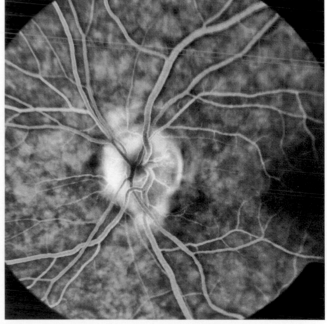

Figure 1–35   Optic nerve leakage of dye. Same patient as Figure 1–34, recirculation phase of angiogram demonstrates leakage of dye from the optic nerve head.

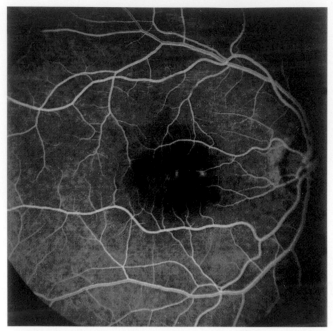

Figure 1–36 Pooling of dye. Central serous chorioretinopathy (CSC) in this patient has a classic angiographic appearance. Early phases show two pinpoint spots of hyperfluorescence.

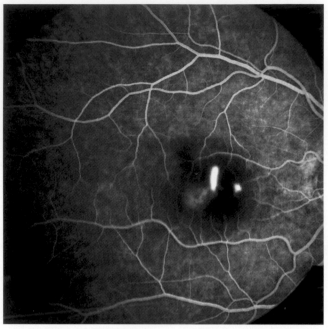

Figure 1–37 Pooling of dye. Same eye with CSC as Figure 1–36, mid phase. Earlier pinpoint hyperfluorescence has progressed to a "smokestack" pattern.

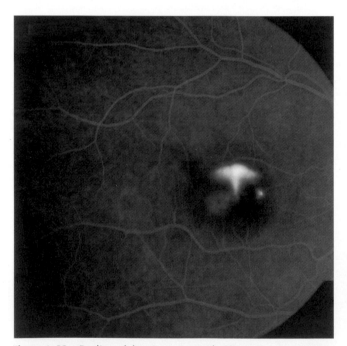

Figure 1–38 Pooling of dye. Same eye with CSC as Figures 1–36 and 1–37, late phase.

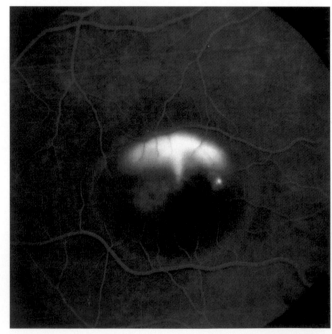

Figure 1–39 Pooling of dye. Same eye with CSC as Figures 1–36 through 1–38, recirculation phase. Pooling of dye is seen in the sub-neurosensory space.

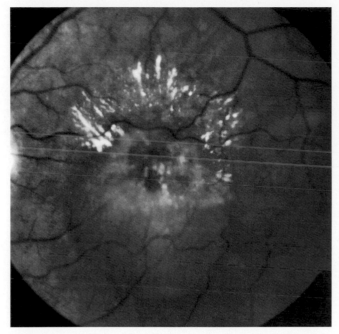

Figure 1–40   Pooling of dye. Red-free photograph demonstrates the extent of a retinal pigment epithelial detachment (RPED) with adjacent exudate.

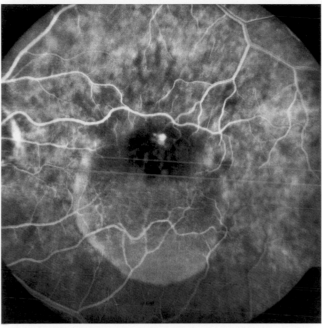

Figure 1–41   Pooling of dye. RPED, which demonstrates rapid and progressive hyperfluorescence.

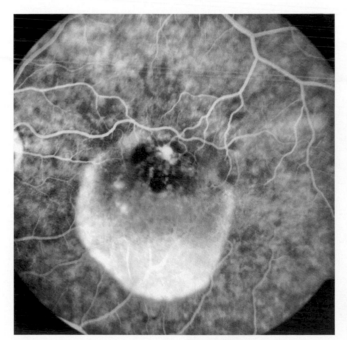

Figure 1–42   Pooling of dye. RPED, late phase.

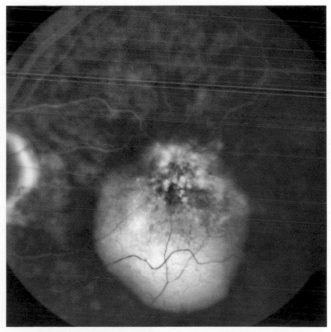

Figure 1–43   Pooling of dye. RPED, recirculation phase.

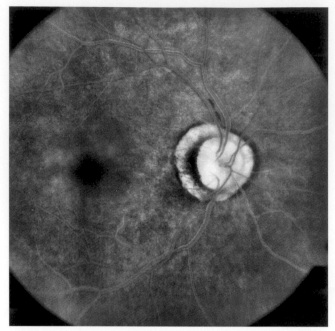

Figure 1–44 Staining. In this patient with high myopia, there is an encircling ring of hyperfluorescence around the optic nerve in the late frames from scleral staining.

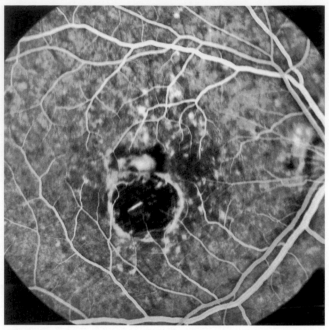

Figure 1–45 Staining. This eye has involuted CNV from punctate inner choroidopathy. The recirculation phase of the angiogram demonstrates a rim of hyperfluorescence from the staining of scar tissue.

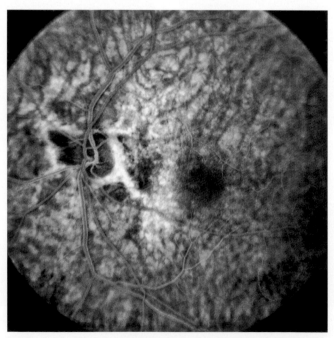

Figure 1–46 Staining. In a patient with pseudoxanthoma elasticum, angioid streaks can be seen emanating from the optic nerve head.

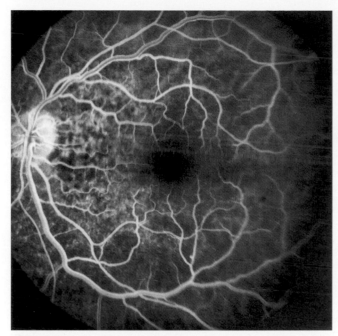

Figure 1–47 Sympathetic ophthalmia. After trauma to the exciting eye, a fluorescein angiogram of a patient's sympathizing eye demonstrates multiple pinpoint hyperfluorescent lesions at the level of the RPE in the early arteriovenous phase.

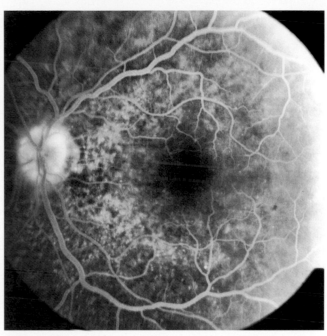

Figure 1–48 Sympathetic ophthalmia. Mid-phase angiogram reveals increased hyperfluorescence of the pinpoint lesions.

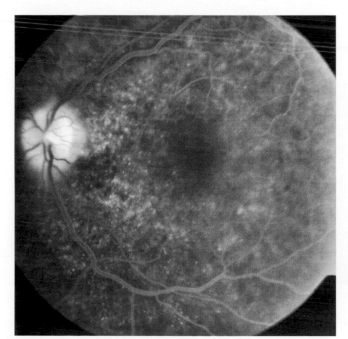

Figure 1–49 Sympathetic ophthalmia. Late-phase angiogram shows multiple pinpoint areas of hyperfluorescence concentrated in the posterior pole.

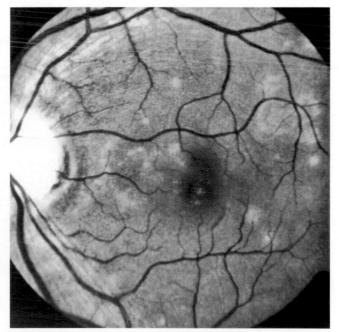

Figure 1–50 Multiple evanescent white dot syndrome (MEWDS). This red-free photograph shows multiple circular lesions deep to the retina.

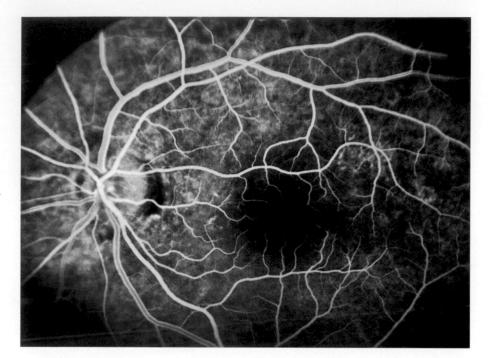

Figure 1–51 MEWDS. Early-phase angiogram shows areas of hyperfluorescence in a wreath-like pattern.

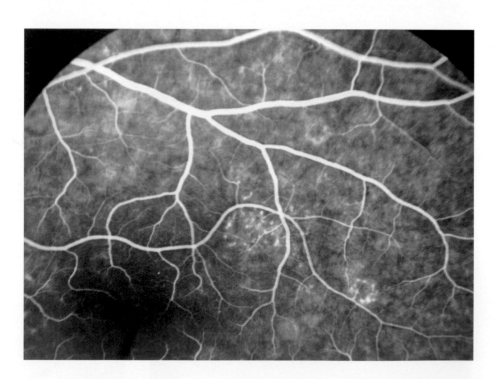

Figure 1–52 MEWDS. Peak-phase angiogram of the same patient as Figure 1–51 demonstrates increased hyperfluorescence of the lesions.

in the evaluation of choroidal diseases. Another limitation of fluorescein angiography is the fact that it is a technically involved procedure, requiring precise photographic equipment in addition to a well-trained photographer to produce quality results. The delay in diagnosis and treatment due to the interval between performing fluorescein angiography, processing the film, and interpreting the results is a limitation that digital angiography has, for the most part, eliminated. Quantification of macular edema is not possible with fluorescein angiography and to a large extent, it has been replaced with ocular coherence tomography in the management of certain diseases such as diffuse diabetic macular edema, uveitic macular edema, and the Irvine-Gass syndrome.

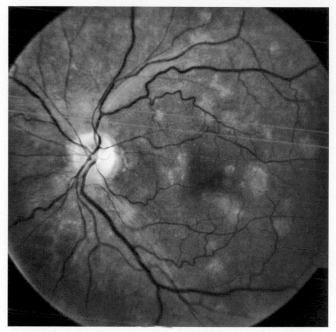

Figure 1–53 West Nile virus choroiditis. The red-free photograph demonstrates multiple nummular choroidal infiltrates concentrated in the posterior pole.

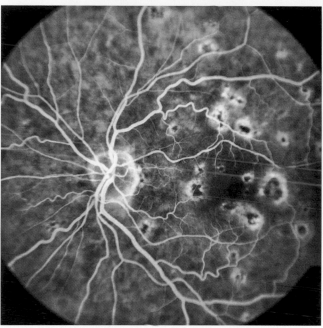

Figure 1–55 West Nile virus choroiditis. Peak phase shows an intense rim of hyperfluorescence surrounding the central hypofluorescence. The etiology could be an infiltrate or scar rather than focal choroidal ischemia.

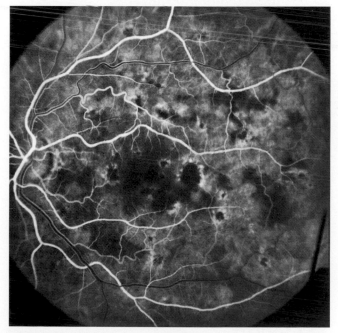

Figure 1–54 West Nile virus choroiditis. Arteriovenous phase of the angiogram shows areas of choroidal hypofluorescence surrounded by a halo of hyperfluorescence.

ACKNOWLEDGMENT

The authors would like to acknowledge Barry Broswick and C. J. Barnett for their outstanding ophthalmic photography.

REFERENCES

1. Gass JDM. Stereoscopic Atlas of Macular Diseases: Diagnosis and Treatment. 4th ed. St Louis, Mo: Mosby-Year Book; 1997.
2. Guyer DR, Yannuzzi LA, Chang S, et al. Retina, Vitreous, Macula. Philadelphia, Pa: WB Saunders Co; 1999.
3. Halperin LS, Olk J, Soubrane G, Coscas G. Safety of fluorescein angiography during pregnancy. Am J Ophthalmol. 1990;109:563–566.
4. Jalkh AE, Celorio JM, Arzabe CW. Atlas of Fluorescein Angiography. Philadelphia, Pa: WB Saunders Co; 1992.
5. MacLean AL, Maumenee AE. Hemangioma of the choroid. Am J Ophthalmol. 1960;50:3–11.
6. Novotny HR, Alvis DL: A method of photographing fluorescence in circulation blood in the human retina. Circulation. 1961;24:82–86.
7. Stein MR, Parker CW. Reactions following intravenous fluorescein. Am J Ophthalmol. 1971;72:861–868.
8. Ryan SJ, ed. Retina. 3rd ed. St. Louis, Mo: Mosby; 2001
9. Yannuzzi LA, Rohrer MA, Tindel LJ, et al: Fluorescein angiography complication survey. Ophthalmology. 1986;93:611–617.

Chapter 2

Indocyanine Green Angiography

ANTONIO P. CIARDELLA, MD • CHRISTINA M. KLAIS, MD •
CHIARA M. EANDI, MD • JASON S. SLAKTER, MD

2.1 Physical Principles

2.1.1. CHEMICAL PROPERTIES

Indocyanine green (ICG) is a sterile, water-soluble tricarbocyanine dye. Chemically it is an anhdyro-3,3,3′,3′-tetramethyl-1-1′-di-(4-sulfobutyl)-4,5,4′,5-dibenzoindotricarbocyanine hydroxide sodium salt with the empirical formula $C_{43}H_{47}N_2NaO_6S_2$ and a molecular mass of 775 daltons.[24] It is supplied with an aqueous solvent, and its pH when dissolved with this solvent is between 5.5 and 6.5. ICG is formulated with a complex synthetic process.

2.1.2 OPTICAL PROPERTIES

ICG absorbs and fluoresces in the near-infrared range between 790 and 805 nm.[4] Because of its longer operating wavelength, there is less blockage by normal eye pigments than with fluorescein, which allows enhanced imaging of the choroid and its associated abnormality. Geeraets and Berry[10] have reported that the retinal pigment epithelium (RPE) and choroid absorb 59% to 75% of blue-green (500 nm) light, but only 21% to 38% of near-infrared (800 nm) light. The activity of ICG in the near-infrared range also allows visualization of pathologic conditions through overlying hemorrhage (**Figures 2–1** and **2–2**) serous fluid, lipid, and pigment that may block the blue light exciting fluorescein dye. This property allows enhanced imaging of occult choroidal neovascularization (CNV) and pigment epithelium detachment (PED).[38]

2.2 Pharmacologic Properties

ICG dye is administered intravenously for ophthalmic angiography. It is highly protein bound (98%). Although it was thought that ICG is primarily bound to albumin in the serum,[4] it is known that 80% of ICG in the blood is actually bound to globulins, such as A1-lipoproteins. Therefore, less dye escapes from the choroidal vasculature, allowing for enhanced imaging of choroidal vessels. This is in sharp contrast to fluorescein, which extravasates rapidly from the choriocapillaris and fluoresces in the extracellular space, thus preventing delineation of the choroidal anatomy.

2.2.1 PHARMACOKINETICS

The liver excretes ICG into the bile. The dye does not cross into the cerebrospinal fluid and placenta.[4,26] Excretion by the kidney does not occur. These properties are probably a result of its strong binding to plasma proteins.

2.2.2 TOXICITY

ICG is a relatively safe dye, with only a few reported side effects.[2] In our experience, it is safer than sodium fluorescein. Unlike with fluorescein angiography (FA), nausea and vomiting are extremely uncommon during ICG angiography. However, we have observed two serious vasovagal-type reactions during ICG angiography. In one study that reported on ICG angiography performed on 1226 consecutive patients, there were three (0.15%)

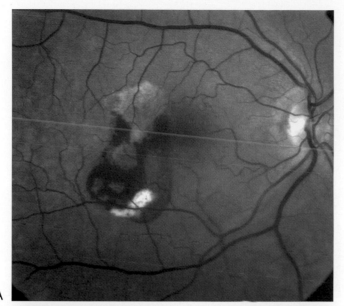

A

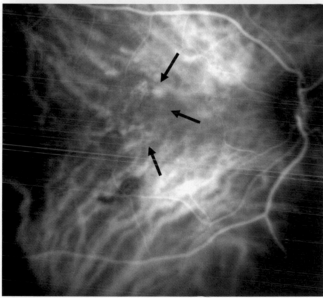

B

Figure 2–1 ICG angiography allows visualization of pathologic conditions through overlying hemorrhages (*B*) as visible in this patient with polypoidal choroidal vasculopathy (*A*). The arrows indicate the polypoidal lesions.

and Hochheimer performed intravenous absorption ICG angiography for the first time in a human[8]; however, the infrared film was not sensitive enough to adequately capture the low-intensity ICG fluorescence. The resolution of ICG angiography was improved in the mid-1980s by Hayashi and DeLaey,[15] who developed improved filter combinations and described ICG videoangiography. In 1989 Scheider and Schroedel[28] reported on the use of the scanning laser ophthalmoscope for ICG video-angiography. In 1992, Yannuzzi and associates[38] introduced the use of a 1024-line digital imaging system to produce high-resolution ICG angiography, which made it clinically practical.

2.4 Technology Development

2.4.1 DIGITAL IMAGING SYSTEMS

The coupling of a digital imaging system with an ICG camera enables production of enhanced high-resolution (1024-line) images necessary for ICG angiography. This combined system produces instantaneous images, decreasing patient waiting time and expediting possible laser photocoagulation treatment. Digital imaging systems allow image archiving, hard-copy generation, and direct qualitative comparison between fluorescein and ICG angiography findings. In addition, these systems are useful for planning laser treatment strategies and monitoring the adequacy of treatment postoperatively.

Digital imaging systems contain electronic still and video cameras with special antireflective coatings as well as appropriate excitatory and barrier filters. A video camera is mounted in the camera viewfinder and is connected to a video monitor. The photographer selects the image and activates a trigger, which sends the image to the video adapter. The charge-coupling device (CCD) camera (mega-plus camera) then captures the images digitally and transmits them to a computer. Flash synchronization allows high-resolution image capture; images are captured at 1 frame per second, stored in buffer memory, and displayed on a high-contrast, high-resolution video monitor. CD-ROMs or DVDs are used to store images after editing. Finally, digital imaging allows remote telemedicine consultation via satellite and other telecommunication routes.

2.4.2 NEW TECHNIQUES

Advanced features in ICG angiography include real-time angiography, wide-angle angiography,[32] digital subtraction ICG angiography,[33] and high-speed ICG videoangiography.[28]

Real-time ICG angiography uses a modified fundus camera with a diode laser illumination system that has an output at 805 nm, produces images at 30 frames/sec, and allows continuous recording. The images can be acquired either as a videotape or as a single image at a frequency of 30 images per second. To make printed copies of these images, single frames are digitized, but the resolution is currently limited to 640 × 480 pixels.

mild adverse reactions, four (0.2%) moderate adverse reactions, and one (0.05%) severe adverse reaction. There were no deaths.[16] ICG angiography should not be performed on patients who are allergic to iodide, who are uremic, or who have liver disease. Appropriate emergency equipment should be readily available, as with FA.

2.3 Historical Perspectives

The first ICG angiogram in a human was performed by David[5] during carotid angiography. In 1972 Flower

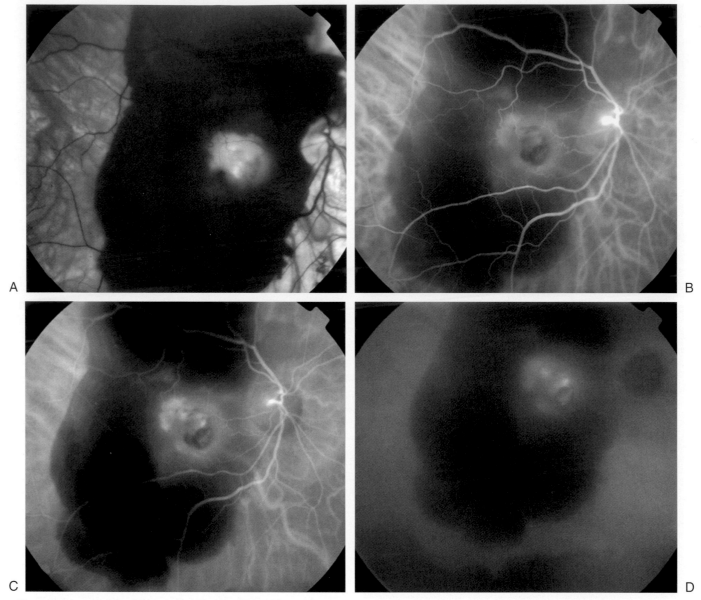

Figure 2–2 *A:* Red-free photograph of large subretinal hemorrhage surrounding fibrovascular scar. *B, C,* and *D:* ICG angiography is able to penetrate through a substantial hemorrhage as seen in this patient with neovascular age-related macular degeneration.

Wide-angle images of the fundus can be obtained by performing ICG angiography with the aid of wide-angle contact lenses. Because the image formed by these lenses lies about 1 cm in front of the lens, the fundus camera is set on "A" or "+" so that the camera is focused on the image plane of the contact lens. This technique allows instantaneous imaging of a large area of the fundus, up to 160 degrees of field of view (**Figure 2–3**).

Digital subtraction ICG angiography (DS-ICGA) uses digital subtraction of sequentially acquired ICG angiographic frames to image the progression of the dye front within the choroidal circulation (**Figure 2–4**). Pseudocolor imaging of the choroid allows differentiation and identification of choroidal arteries and veins. DS-ICGA allows imaging of occult CNV with greater

detail and in a shorter period of time than with conventional ICG angiography.

A fundamental problem for fundus imaging is reflection from the interfaces of the ocular optical media. Confocal scanning laser ophthalmoscopy (SLO) eliminates these out-of-focus reflections by a confocal filter in the imaging (collection) light path that is conjugate to the focus of illuminating beam. SLO improves imaging contrast and speed, making high-speed ICG videoangiography[35] possible. SLO also facilitates multimode imaging, acquiring FA images using an argon laser (488-nm wavelength), ICG images using an infrared diode laser (795 nm), simultaneous FA and ICG images, autofluorescence images, normal fundus reflectance images with green light (514 nm), and images of the

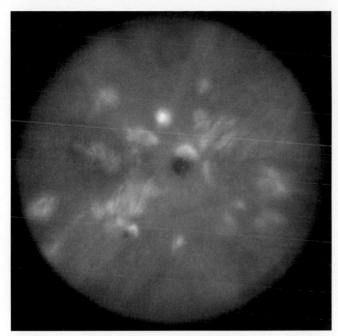

Figure 2–3 The wide-angle ICG angiogram of a patient with central serous chorioretinopathy illustrates multifocal hyperpermeable areas of a presumed "occult" PEDs that extend far beyond the posterior pole.

nerve fiber with infrared light (830 nm). Barrier filters at 500 and 810 nm are added to provide a higher efficiency of fluorescence light detection. Single images can be acquired, as well as image sequences with a frame rate up to 20 images per second. Images are digitized in real time in frames of 256×256 or 512×512 pixels with 8-bit intensity resolution.

2.4.3 TECHNIQUE OF INJECTION

ICG videoangiography can be performed immediately before or after FA. A dose of 25 to 50 mg of ICG (IC-Green; Akorn, Inc., Buffalo Grove, IL), diluted in the manufacturer-supplied aqueous solvent is injected intravenously. Rapid injection is essential. The injection may be immediately followed by a 5-mL normal saline flush. For wide-angle angiography, the dosage is increased to 75 mg.

2.5 Image Interpretation

2.5.1 INTERPRETATION OF ICG ANGIOGRAPHY FINDINGS IN AGE-RELATED MACULAR DEGENERATION

Definitions

The terminology used to describe the angiographic manifestations of age-related macular degeneration (AMD) corresponds, with certain exceptions described below, to definitions previously reported by the Macular Photocoagulation Study Group (MPS).[23] Most relevant

to the interpretation of ICG angiography in AMD are the definitions of serous PED, vascularized PED, classic CNV, and occult CNV.[8,15,28,38]

Serous PED

Serous PED is an ovoid or circular detachment of the RPE. ICG angiography reveals a variable, minimal blockage of normal choroidal vessels, more evident in the mid-phase of the angiogram (**Figure 2–5**). In comparison to FA, on the ICG study, a serous PED is dark (hypofluorescent). This difference is caused by the fact that the ICG molecules are larger and almost completely bound to plasma proteins and are prevented from free passage through the fenestrated choriocapillaris into the sub-RPE space.

CNV

CNV is defined as a choroidal capillary proliferation through a break in the outer aspect of Bruch's membrane under the RPE and the neurosensory retina. CNV is divided into classic and occult types based on the FA appearance.

Classic CNV

Classic CNV represents an area of bright hyperfluorescence, which is usually not delineated as well as in a FA study (**Figures 2–6** and **2–7**).

Occult CNV

Occult CNV is characterized as either a fibrovascular PED consisting of irregular elevation of the RPE or late leakage of undetermined source. There are two main types of occult CNV that are recognized by ICG angiography.

Without serous PED. The first type of occult CNV is caused by sub-RPE CNV that is not associated with a serous PED. The ICG angiogram reveals early vascular hyperfluorescence and late staining of the abnormal vessels (**Figure 2–8**). The image with distinct margins is considered to be a well-defined CNV on ICG angiography.

With serous PED. The second type of occult CNV is associated with a serous PED of at least 1 disc diameter in size (**Figure 2–9**). The combination of CNV and serous PED is called a vascularized PED (V-PED) (**Figure 2–10**). This lesion is the result of sub-RPE neovascularization associated with a serous detachment of the RPE. ICG angiography reveals early vascular hyperfluorescence and late staining of the CNV. ICG angiography is more helpful than FA in differentiating between a serous PED and a V-PED. It also permits better identification of the vascularized and serous component of V-PEDs. The serous component of a PED is hypofluorescent and the vascularized component is hyperfluorescent.[33]

Occult CNV is also subdivided further into two types, one with a solitary area of well-defined focal

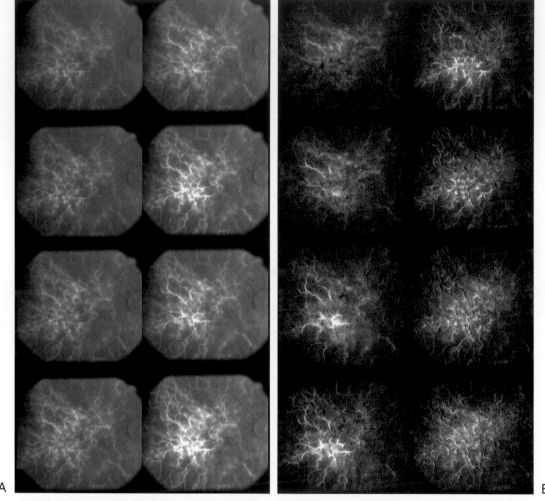

Figure 2–4 Sequential subtraction of ICG angiogram images from the eye of a normal young man, acquired at 30 images per second using fundus camera optics. *A*: The original angiogram (read from top to bottom). *B*: The resultant subtracted images; the first image resulted from subtracting the first original image from the second, the second image resulted from subtracting the second image from the third, etc. (Courtesy of Robert Flower.)

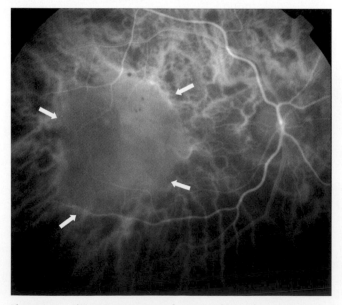

Figure 2–5 The ICG angiogram of a serous PED (*white arrows*) demonstrates a minimal blockage of normal choroidal vessels.

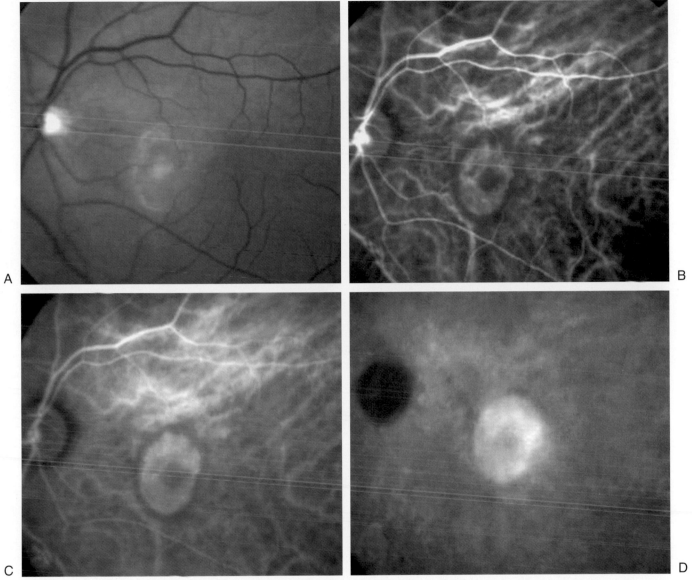

Figure 2–6   *A:* Red-free photograph of a patient with classic CNV. *B:* The early-phase ICG angiogram reveals hyperfluorescence of the CNV. Mid-phase (*C*) and late-phase ICG angiograms (*D*) show staining of the hyperfluorescent CNV.

neovascularization (hot spot) and the other with a larger, delineated area of neovascularization (plaque).

Hot spot (*focal* CNV). Focal CNV or a "hot spot" is an area of occult CNV that is well delineated and no more than 1 disc diameter in size on ICG angiography. In addition, a hot spot represents an area of actively proliferating and more highly permeable regions of neovascularization (active occult CNV). Retinal angiomatous proliferation (RAP), focal occult CNV (**Figure 2–11**), and polypoidal-type CNV may represent subgroups of hot spots.

Plaque. A plaque is an area of occult CNV larger than 1 disc diameter in size. A plaque is often formed by late-staining vessels, which are more likely to be quiescent areas of neovascularization that are not associated with appreciable leakage (inactive occult CNV). Plaques of

occult CNV seem to grow slowly in dimension with time. Both well-defined and ill-defined plaques are recognized on an ICG angiography study. A well-defined plaque has distinct borders throughout the study, allowing the assessment of the full extent of the lesion (**Figure 2–12**). An ill-defined plaque has indistinct margins (**Figure 2–13**) or may be the one in which any part of the neovascularization is blocked by the blood.

In a review of 1000 patients with occult CNV diagnosed by FA and imaged by ICG angiography, three morphologic types of occult CNV were noted: focal CNV (hot spots), plaques (well-defined and ill-defined), and combination lesions, with both hot spots and plaques. The relative frequency of these lesions was hot spots 29%, plaques 61%, and combination lesions 8%. Combination lesions were further subdivided into *marginal*

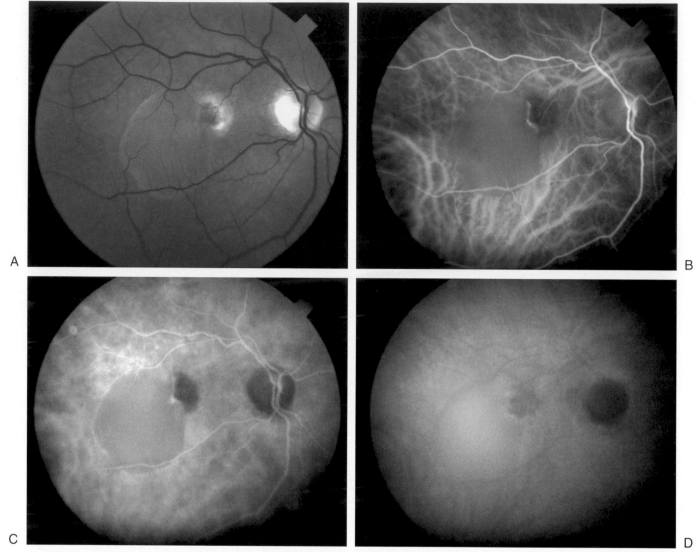

A B

C D

Figure 2–7 *A:* Red-free photograph shows a large PED in a patient who underwent focal thermal laser treatment for classic CNV. *b, c,* and *d:* There is a well-defined hyperfluorescent area in the early ICG study (*B*) representing a recurrent CNV at the edge of the treated area which stains in the mid-phase (*C*) and late-phase (*D*) phase of the study. The serous PED remains hypofluorescent throughout the study.

spots (hot spots at the edge of plaques of neovascularization), *overlying spots* (hot spots on top of plaques of neovascularization), and *remote spots* (hot spots not in contiguity with plaques of neovascularization) (**Figure 2–14**).[14]

Two other forms of occult CNV are identified by ICG angiography: polypoidal choroidal vasculopathy (PCV) and RAP.

Polypoidal choroidal vasculopathy. PCV is a primary abnormality of the choroidal circulation characterized by an inner choroidal vascular network of vessels ending in an aneurysmal bulge or outward projection, visible clinically as a reddish-orange, spheroid, polyp-like structure. The disorder is associated with multiple, recurrent, serosanguineous detachments of the RPE and neurosensory retina due to leakage and bleeding from the peculiar choroidal vascular abnormality.[35] ICG angiography has been used to detect and characterize the PCV abnormality with enhanced sensitivity and specificity.[14,36,39] In the initial phases of the ICG study, a distinct network of vessels within the choroid becomes visible. In patients with juxtapapillary involvement, the vascular channels extend in a radial, arching pattern and are interconnected with the smaller spanning branches that become more evident and more numerous at the edge of the PCV lesion. Early in the course of the ICG study, the larger vessels of the PCV network start to fill before the retinal vessels. The area within and surrounding the network is relatively hypofluorescent compared with the uninvolved choroid. The vessels of the network appear to fill at a slower rate than the retinal vessels. Shortly after the network can be identified on the ICG angiogram, small hyperfluorescent "polyps" become visible within the choroids (**Figure 2–15**). These polypoidal structures correspond to the reddish-orange choroidal excrescence seen on the clinical examination.

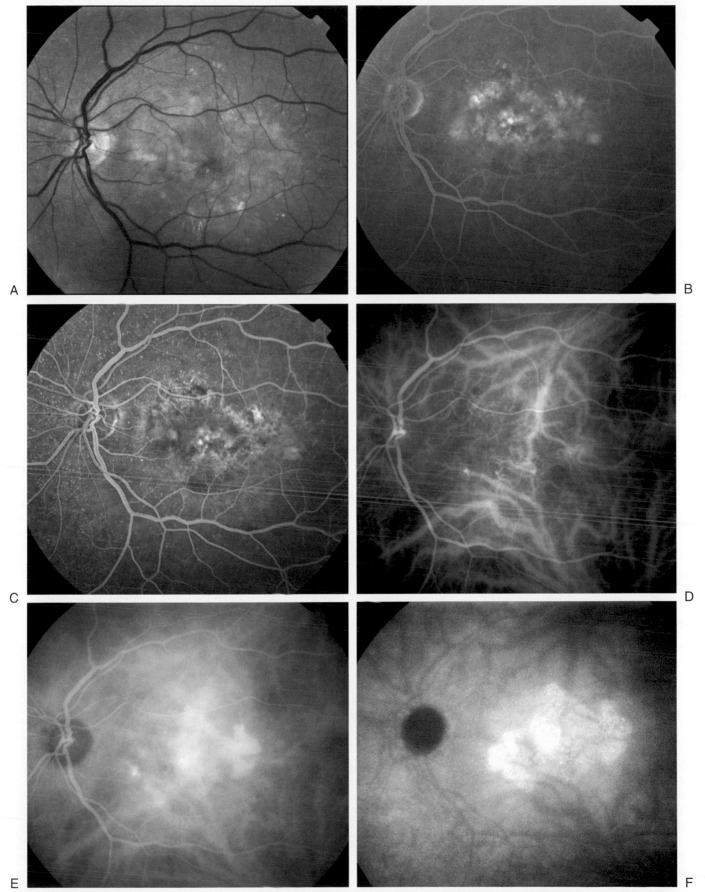

Figure 2–8 *A:* Red-free photograph of a patient with AMD. *B,* and *C:* Early-phase (*B*) and late-phase (*C*) fluorescein angiograms demonstrate occult choroidal neovascularization without serous PED. *D, E,* and *F:* ICG angiograms show early vascular hyperfluorescence (*D*) and staining of the abnormal vessels during the mid (*E*) and late (*F*) phases of the study.

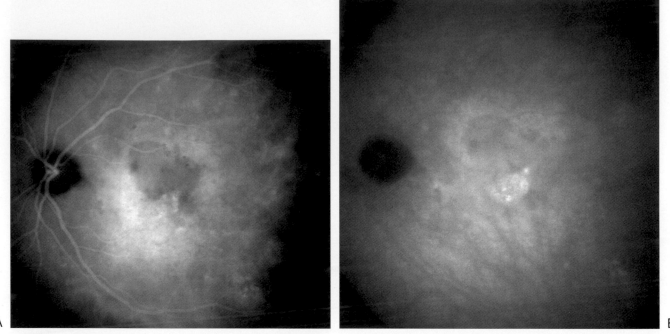

Figure 2–9 *A:* Early-phase ICG angiogram reveals hypofluorescence of serous PED in a patient with AMD. *B:* Late-phase ICG angiogram shows staining of the abnormal vessels and hypofluorescent serous PED.

They appear to leak slowly as the surrounding hypofluorescent area becomes increasingly hyperfluorescent. In the later phase of the angiogram there is uniform disappearance of dye ("washout") from the bulging polypoidal lesions. The late characteristic ICG staining of occult CNV is not seen in the PCV vascular abnormality. Although the first reports of PCV were in middle-aged black women, it is now recognized that PCV may be a variant of CNV seen in white patients with AMD. PCV may be localized in the macular area without any peripapillary component (**Figure 2–16**), and it may be formed by a network of small branching vessels ending in polypoidal dilation that is difficult to image without ICG angiography.

Retinal angiomatous proliferation. RAP is a distinct subgroup of neovascular AMD.[37] Angiomatous proliferation within the retina is the first manifestation of the neovascularized process. Dilated retinal vessels, pre-, intra-, and subretinal hemorrhages, and exudates evolve surrounding the angiomatous proliferation as the process extends into the deep retina and subretinal space. One or more dilated compensatory retinal vessels perfuse and drain the neovascularization, sometimes forming a retinal-retinal anastomosis. FA in these patients usually reveals indistinct staining simulating occult CNV. ICG angiography is useful for making an accurate diagnosis in most cases. It reveals a focal area of intense hyperfluorescence corresponding to the neovascularization (hot spot) (**Figure 2–17**) and some late extension of the leakage within the retina from the intraretinal neovascularization (IRN). As the IRN progresses toward the subretinal space, the CNV becomes part of the neovascular complex. At this stage

there is often clinical and angiographic evidence of a V-PED. ICG angiography is better for imaging the presence of a V-PED because the serous component of the PED remains dark during the study and the vascular component appears as a hot spot (**Figure 2–18**). At this stage, ICG angiography may sometimes be able to image a direct communication between the retinal and the choroidal component of the neovascularization to form a retinal-choroidal anastomosis (RCA) (**Figure 2–19**).

2.5.2 INTERPRETATION OF ICG ANGIOGRAPHY FINDINGS IN CENTRAL SEROUS CHORIORETINOPATHY

The application of ICG angiography to the study of central serous chorioretinopathy (CSC) has expanded our knowledge of the disease.[1,7,36,38] The common findings in patients with CSC are multifocal areas of hyperfluorescence in the early and mid phases of the study, which tend to fade in the late phases (**Figure 2–20**). Typically, these areas of hyperfluorescence are found not only in corresponding areas of leakage as seen on FA but also with areas of the fundus that appear normal on both FA and clinical examination. One may also find hyperfluorescent spots on ICG angiography in otherwise normal-appearing fellow eyes. The areas of early hyperfluorescence are believed to represent diffuse choroidal hyperpermeability. The multifocal hyperpermeable areas noted on wide-angle ICG angiography are presumed to be "occult" PEDs that extend far beyond the posterior pole.[32] Both the multifocal hyperfluorescent spots seen throughout the fundus and

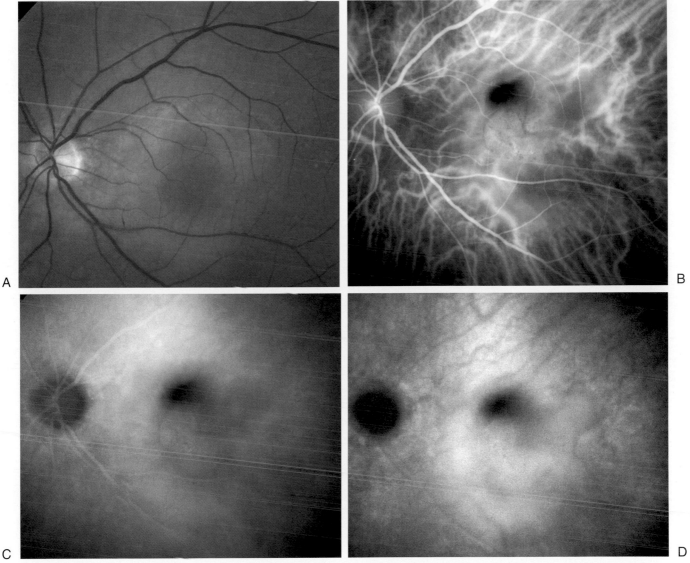

Figure 2–10 *A:* Red-free photograph of a patient with AMD shows a PED. *B, C,* and *D:* All phases of the ICG study reveal a well-defined vascularized PED. A small choroidal nevus superior of the fovea blocks the fluorescence throughout the study.

the presumed occult PEDs that are visible only on ICG angiography emphasize the fact that this disease may be more diffuse and widespread than previously believed.

It is important to remember the difference in appearance on ICG angiography of a serous PED in AMD and a serous PED in CSC. In fact, in CSC there is increased permeability of the choriocapillaris that causes leakage of the ICG molecules under the PED. As a result, a serous PED in CSC appears bright (hyperfluorescent) with ICG angiography (**Figure 2–21**).

2.5.3 INTERPRETATION OF ICG ANGIOGRAPHY FINDINGS IN INTRAOCULAR TUMORS

Guyer and associates[12] used ICG angiography to study 40 patients with intraocular tumors and found that

certain tumors have characteristic ICG videoangiographic patterns. Pigmented choroidal melanomas block ICG fluorescence because the near-infrared light is absorbed by melanin. The choroidal and tumor vasculature cannot be visualized through dense tumor pigmentation. ICG angiography can distinguish pigmented choroidal melanomas from nonpigmented tumors, such as hemangiomas and osteomas. In our experience, ICG videoangiography cannot distinguish melanomas from other pigmented lesions such as nevi or metastatic cutaneous melanoma.

Marked progressive hyperfluorescence is observed during ICG angiography of choroidal hemangiomas because of the vascularity of the lesion.[29] A speckled pattern with stellate borders is observed. In early stages of a ICG study, a network of small-caliber vessels is seen. These vessels completely obscure the choroidal pattern.

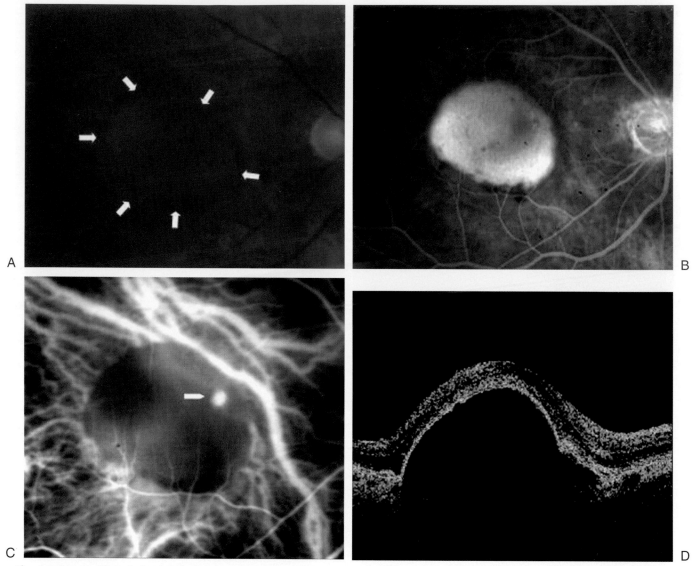

Figure 2–11 *A:* Clinical photograph showing a large PED (*white arrows*) in a patient with focal occult CNV. *B:* Late-phase fluorescein angiogram illustrating late staining of the PED. *C:* Mid-phase ICG angiogram showing a focal area of abnormal hyperfluorescence (hot spot). *D:* The OCT scan confirms a large PED.

The technique is also useful in evaluating vascular lesions with overlying hemorrhage. ICG angiography, unlike FA, may allow visualization of the tumor through an overlying hemorrhage.

Choroidal metastatic lesions show different patterns on ICG videoangiography depending on vascularity, pigmentation, and the primary location of the lesion.[12] In the early study phase, choroidal metastasis shows diffuse, homogenous hypofluorescence. The normal perfusing choroidal pattern can often be visualized underneath.

The early ICG phase in choroidal osteomas reveals characteristic small vessels that often leak too quickly to be detected by FA.[29] Variable hypofluorescence is observed in the bony areas. These lesions may show mid to late ICG hyperfluorescence.

2.5.4 INTERPRETATION OF ICG ANGIOGRAPHY FINDINGS IN CHORIORETINAL INFLAMMATORY DISEASES

Serpiginous choroidopathy is a rare, progressive condition that appears to affect primarily the inner choroidal and RPE layers with secondary retinal involvement, beginning at the optic nerve and advancing centrifugally. ICG videoangiography typically shows two patterns according to the stage of the disease. In the acute phase, ICG angiography is characterized by generalized hypofluorescence through all phases of the study (**Figure 2–22**). In the subacute stage of the disease, mid- and large-sized choroidal vessels are visualized within the lesions. Persistent delay or nonperfusion of the choriocapillaris and smaller choroidal vessels is noted, giving the area a generalized hypofluorescent

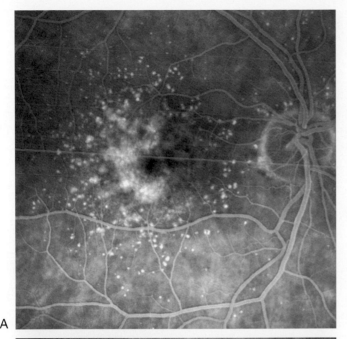

A

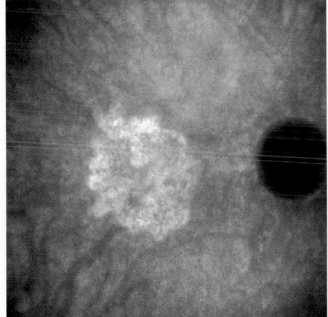

B

Figure 2–12 *A:* FA reveals occult choroidal neovascularization. *B:* Late-phase ICG angiogram shows a well-defined plaque.

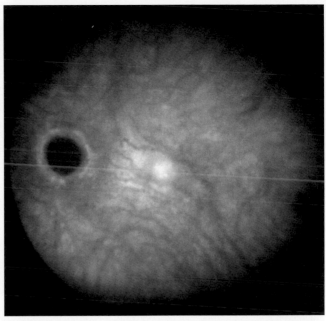

Figure 2–13 Late-phase ICG angiogram reveals an ill-defined plaque with indistinct margins.

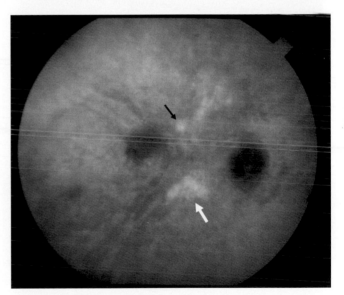

Figure 2–14 Late-phase ICG angiogram shows a plaque (*white arrow*) with a remote hot spot (*black arrow*).

appearance but with less distinct margins and a more heterogeneous appearance. This pattern is more typically seen after resolution of acute inflammatory changes and associated edema. In the late phase of the study, lesions present with sharp, well-demarcated borders. This is due to a combination of choroidal perfusion abnormalities as demonstrated on SLO and blockage by inflammatory exudative material or edema of the RPE and outer retina. In the healed stages, deeper choroidal vessels become better visualized because of

the associated development of RPE and choriocapillaris atrophy.[11]

Acute multifocal placoid pigment epitheliopathy (AMPPE) is a syndrome of young adults characterized by the development of multifocal, yellow-white, flat, placoid lesions of the RPE in the posterior pole and midperipheral fundus.[18] The lesions are hypofluorescent by ICG angiography in both early and late phases of the study (**Figure 2–23**). The hypofluorescence may be due to a partial choroidal vascular occlusion caused by

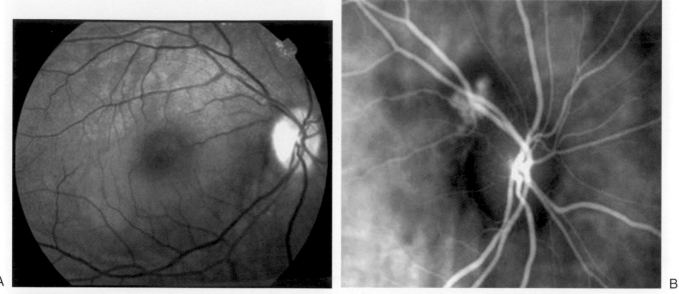

Figure 2–15 *A:* Red-free photograph of a 62-year-old woman illustrating a neurosensory retinal detachment in the central macula. *B:* ICG angiogram reveals the presence of a polypoidal choroidal vascular abnormality in the superior temporal juxtapapillary region.

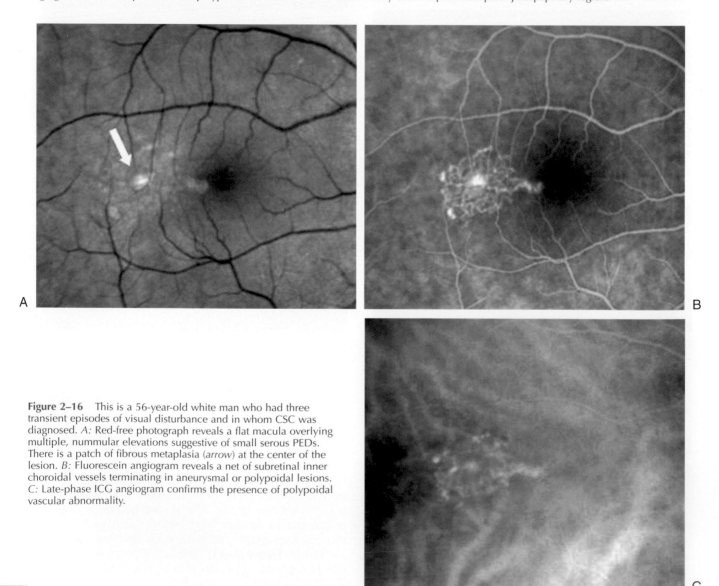

Figure 2–16 This is a 56-year-old white man who had three transient episodes of visual disturbance and in whom CSC was diagnosed. *A:* Red-free photograph reveals a flat macula overlying multiple, nummular elevations suggestive of small serous PEDs. There is a patch of fibrous metaplasia (*arrow*) at the center of the lesion. *B:* Fluorescein angiogram reveals a net of subretinal inner choroidal vessels terminating in aneurysmal or polypoidal lesions. *C:* Late-phase ICG angiogram confirms the presence of polypoidal vascular abnormality.

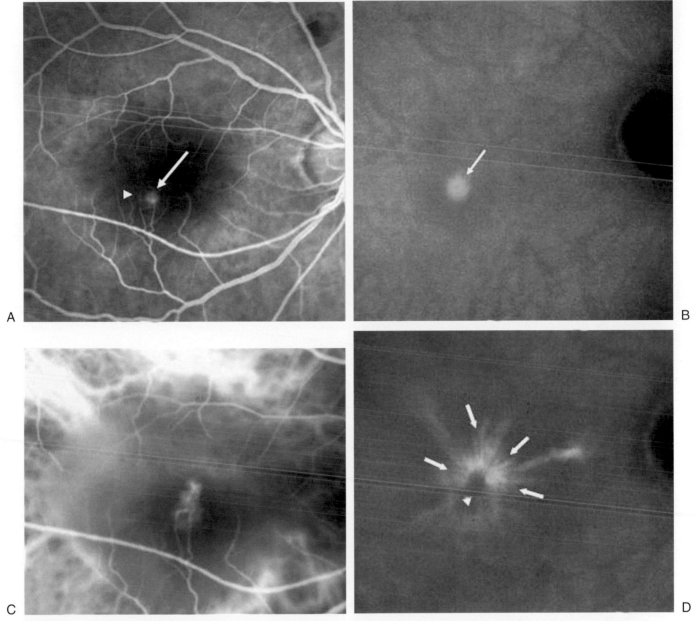

Figure 2–17 *A:* Fluorescein angiogram of a 73-year-old patient reveals RAP stage I (*arrow*). Note the telangiectasia surrounding this area (*arrowhead*). *B:* ICG angiogram showing a focal area of intense hyperfluorescence (*arrow*) or so-called "hot spot." *C:* The ICG angiogram 1 year later illustrates a retinal-retinal anastomosis and subretinal neovascularization. *D:* The late-phase ICG angiogram shows intraretinal leakage (*arrows*) surrounding the fading angiomatous proliferation (*arrowhead*).

occlusive vasculitis. ICG angiography study of healed lesions also demonstrates early hypofluorescence and more clearly delineates late choroidal hypofluorescence.

Multiple evanescent white dot syndrome (MEWDS) typically presents with unilateral acute loss of vision in healthy young women. It is a clinical condition of unknown cause, but it is thought to affect primarily the RPE-photoreceptor complex.[19] With ICG angiography, a pattern of hypofluorescent spots throughout the posterior pole and peripheral retina is seen. These hypofluorescent spots appear approximately 10 minutes

after dye injection in the mid phase of the study and persist throughout the remainder of the study. These spots appear larger than the white dots seen clinically, varying in diameter from less than 50 to about 500 microns. Many more lesions can easily be identified with ICG angiography than with fundus examination or FA. A ring of hypofluorescence surrounding the optic disc is seen in some patients (**Figure 2–24**). In these patients a blind spot enlargement on visual field examination is always present. During the convalescent phase, the return of visual function and normalization of the

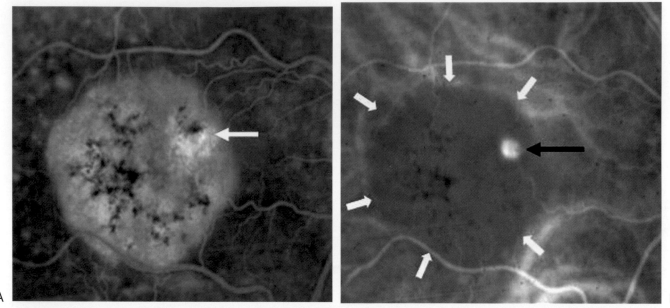

Figure 2–18 *A:* The fluorescein angiogram of a patient with stage II RAP reveals late staining of a PED. There is an increase in the intensity of fluorescence in the area of the RAP lesion (*arrow*). *B:* The ICG angiogram shows hypofluorescence in the area of the PED (*white arrows*) and a "hot spot" corresponding to the RAP (*black arrow*).

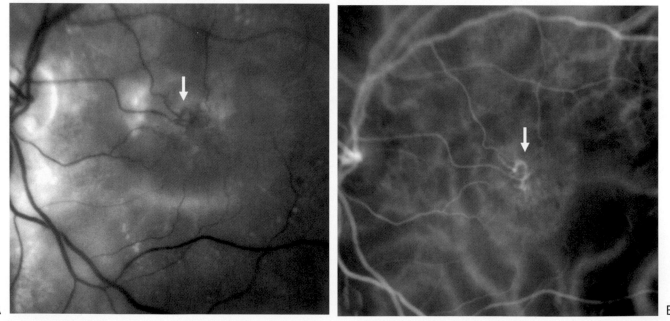

Figure 2–19 *A:* Red-free photograph of a patient with RAP demonstrates a RCA (*arrow*). *B:* Early ICG angiogram confirms the retinal choroidal anastomosis (*arrow*).

clinical examination findings do not correlate completely with resolution of the hypofluorescent spots seen on ICG angiography.

Birdshot retinochoroidopathy is an uncommon, but potentially serious, inflammatory disorder that involves both the choroid and retina. No relation to any systemic disease has been observed, whereas a strong association with the HLA-A29 class I antigen suggests a genetic predisposition. ICG angiography reveals multiple hypofluorescent lesions resembling "holes" in the fluorescence of the choriocapillaris (**Figure 2–25**). These lesions correspond to the clinical creamy lesions. The distribution of the patches follows the larger choroidal vessels. Howe and colleagues[17] found that ICG angiography detects birdshot lesions more rapidly than FA and may be of benefit in assessing disease activity.

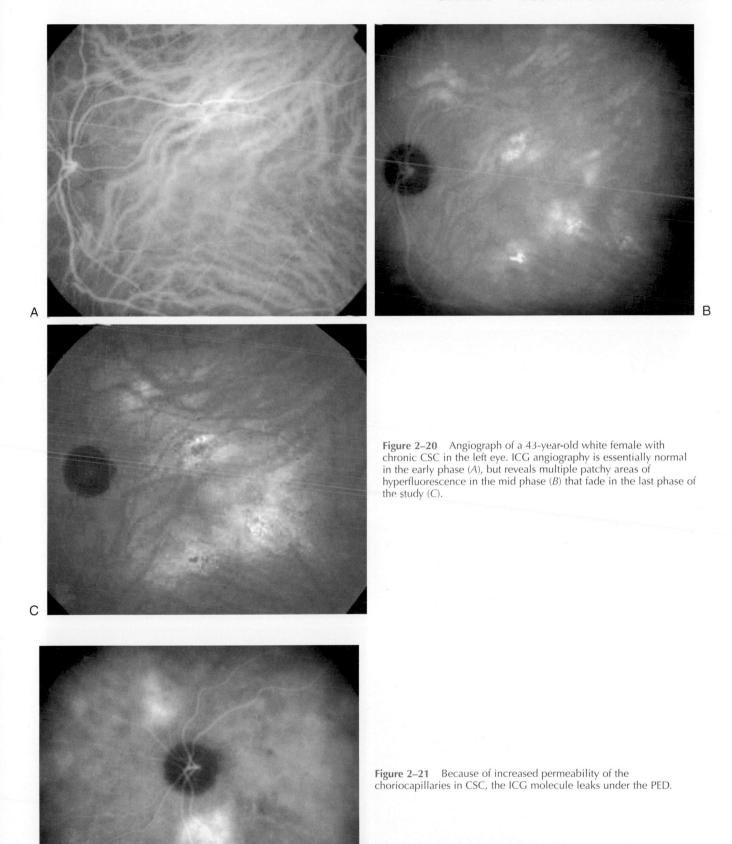

Figure 2–20 Angiograph of a 43-year-old white female with chronic CSC in the left eye. ICG angiography is essentially normal in the early phase (A), but reveals multiple patchy areas of hyperfluorescence in the mid phase (B) that fade in the last phase of the study (C).

Figure 2–21 Because of increased permeability of the choriocapillaries in CSC, the ICG molecule leaks under the PED.

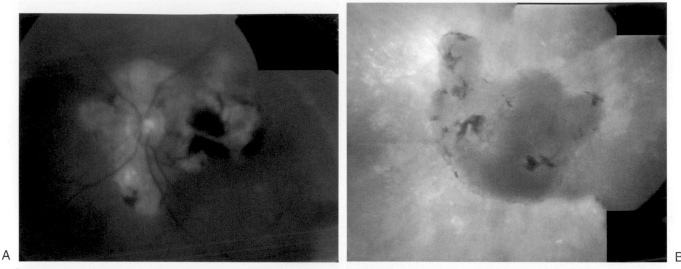

Figure 2–22 *A:* Composite color photograph of a patient with serpiginous choroidopathy. *B:* The composite of the ICG angiogram reveals a large area of hypofluorescence typical for the acute phase of the disease. The dark pigmented areas represent healed regions.

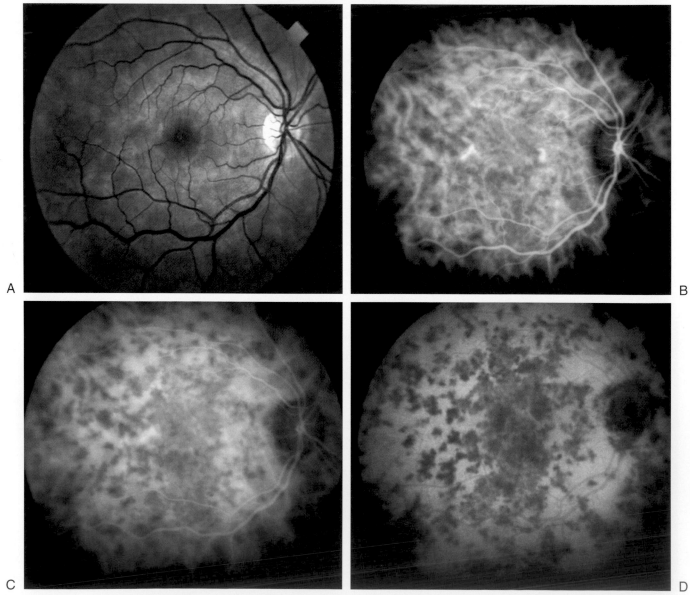

Figure 2–23 *A:* Red-free photograph of a patient with AMPPE shows multiple white flat placoid lesions. The lesions are hypofluorescent hy ICG angiography in early (*B*), mid (*C*), and late (*D*) phases of the study.

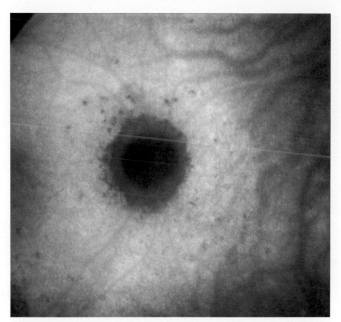

Figure 2-24 In this patient with MEWDS, the late-phase ICG angiogram reveals a hypofluorescent ring surrounding the optic disc.

Multifocal choroiditis (MFC) is an idiopathic choroidal inflammatory disorder with varied presentation and clinical course. Clinical features include "punched out" chorioretinal spots, peripapillary atrophy, peripheral chorioretinal curvilinear lesions, and neovascularized macular degeneration or disciform scar. MFC lesions block fluorescence on ICG videoangiography (**Figure 2-26**). Hyperfluorescent foci that do not correlate with lesions seen clinically or by FA can also be observed. These hyperfluorescent areas may represent subclinical foci of choroiditis.

2.6 Clinical Applications

2.6.1 CLINICAL APPLICATION OF ICG ANGIOGRAPHY TO THE STUDY OF AMD

Bischoff and Flower[2] studied 100 ICG angiograms of patients with AMD. They found "delayed and/or irregular choroidal filling" in some patients. The significance of this finding is unclear, however, because these authors did not include an age-matched control group. Tortuous choroidal vessels and marked dilation of macular choroidal arteries, often with loop formation, were also observed.

Hayashi and DeLaey[15] found that ICG videoangiography was useful in the detection of CNV. ICG angiography was able to confirm the FA appearance of CNV in patients with well-defined CNV. It revealed a well-defined neovascularization in 27 eyes with occult CNV by FA. In a subgroup of patients with poorly defined occult CNV, t ICG angiography, but not FA, showed a well-defined CNV in 9 of 12 (75%) eyes. ICG videoangiography of the other three eyes revealed suspicious areas of neovascularization. Hayashi and DeLaey[15] were also the first to show that leakage of ICG with CNV was slow compared with the rapid leakage seen with sodium fluorescein. Destro and Puliafito[6] reported that ICG videoangiography was particularly useful in studying occult CNV with overlying hemorrhage and recurrent CNV. Yannuzzi and associates[38] have shown that ICG angiography is extremely useful in converting occult CNV into a well-defined pattern of CNV. In their study, 39% of 129 patients with occult CNV were converted to a well-defined CNV based on the information added by ICG angiography. These authors reported that ICG angiography was especially useful in identifying occult

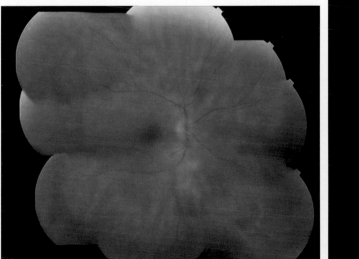

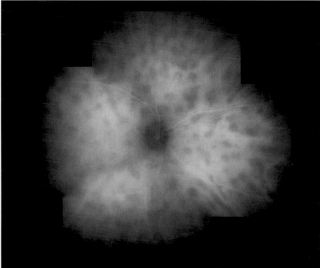

A   B

Figure 2-25 A 46-year-old white female with newly diagnosed birdshot retinochoroidopathy. *A:* Clinical photograph composite reveals multiple creamy round lesions. *B:* Mid-phase ICG angiography illustrates multiple hypofluorescent lesions resembling "holes" in the fluorescence of the choriocapillaris.

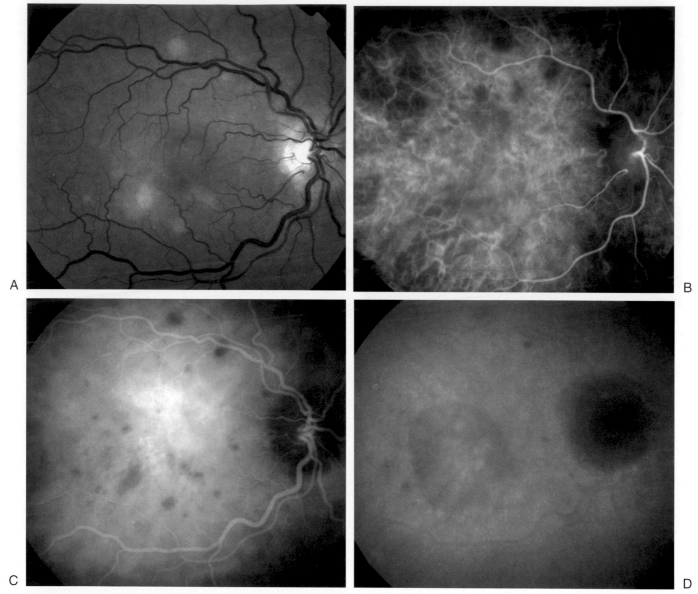

Figure 2–26 *A:* Red-free photograph of a patient with MFC demonstrates white chorioretinal lesions at the posterior pole. *B, C,* and *D:* The chorioretinal lesions block the fluorescence of all phases of the ICG angiography study. Note the hypofluorescence surrounding the optic disc caused by peripapillary atrophy (*D*).

CNV in patients with serous PED or with recurrent CNV. Chang and co-authors[3] demonstrated that in patients with newly diagnosed unilateral occult CNV due to AMD the fellow eye tended to develop the same morphologic type of CNV.

These studies demonstrate that ICG angiography is an important adjunctive study to FA in the detection of CNV. Although FA may image well-defined CNV better than ICG angiography in some cases, ICG videoangiography can enable treatment of about 30% of occult CNV lesions by the detection of well-defined CNV eligible for ICG-guided laser treatment.[13] Thus, the best imaging strategy to detect the CNV is to perform both FA and ICG angiography.

ICG Angiography–Guided Laser Treatment of CNV in AMD

Patients potentially eligible for laser photocoagulation therapy guided by ICG angiography are those with clinical and FA evidence of occult CNV (**Figure 2–27**). Of the two types of occult CNV that can be identified by ICG angiography study, hot spots and plaques, we recommend direct laser photocoagulation of only the hot spots.

Two subtypes of hot spots are RCA and polypoidal-type CNV. When RCA is present, the success of laser photocoagulation is negatively influenced by the presence of an associated serous PED.

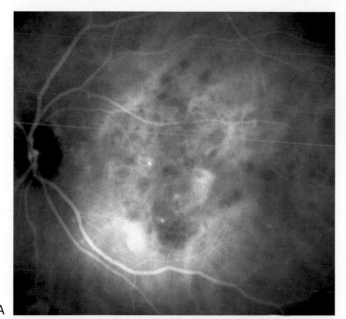

A

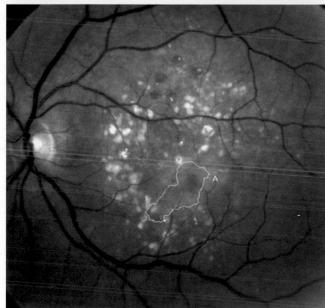

B

Figure 2–27 *A:* Mid-frame ICG angiograph showing hyperfluorescence in the macula corresponding to the area of activity within CNV. *B:* Corresponding ICG angiography tracing of active CNV applied to a red-free photograph that can be displayed during laser treatment for easy reference.

Slakter and associates[31] performed ICG angiography–guided laser photocoagulation in 79 eyes with occult CNV. Occult CNV was successfully eliminated in a majority of the eyes. Visual acuity was stabilized or improved in 29 (66%) of 44 eyes with occult CNV associated with neurosensory retinal elevations and in 15 (43%) of 35 eyes with occult CNV associated with PED. This study demonstrated that in some cases ICG angiography imaging can successfully guide laser photocoagulation of occult CNV.

In a recent report by Kuhn and co-workers,[21] RCAs were identified in 93% of patients with CNV associated with a serous PED. They reported a poor success rate with laser treatment.

From the work of Freund and associates,[9] it is known that only approximately 13% of patients with CNV due to AMD have a classic or well-defined extrafoveal CNV by FA that is eligible for laser treatment. With a recurrence rate of approximately 50% after FA-guided laser photocoagulation for classic CNV, only approximately 6.5% of patients will benefit from treatment. The remaining 87% of patients have occult CNV by fluorescein imaging. About 30% of these eyes have a focal spot that is potentially treatable by ICG angiography. Therefore about one-fourth of all eyes with exudative maculopathy may be treated by the ICG angiography–guided laser photocoagulation. With a success rate of 35%, this means that an additional 9% of patients can be successfully treated using the ICG angiography–guided laser photocoagulation.

Staurenghi and associates[34] considered a series of 15 patients with subfoveal CNV in whom feeder vessels (FVs) could be clearly detected by means of dynamic ICG angiography but not necessarily by FA (**Figure 2–28**). FVs were treated using an argon green laser. CNV was obliterated after the first treatment in only one patient; five patients needed more than one treatment, and obliteration failed in nine patients (40% success rate). The width and the number of the FVs affected the rate of success. The success rate in the second series of 16 patients was higher (75%). The authors concluded that dynamic ICG angiography may detect smaller FVs. It allows control of the laser effect and initiation of immediate retreatment for incomplete FV closure.

Polypoidal Choroidal Vasculopathy

In a series of 374 consecutive eyes diagnosed with occult CNV, 14 eyes (4%) were diagnosed with PCV by means of ICG angiography.[22] Pauleikhoff and colleagues[25] diagnosed PCV in 13.9% of 101 consecutive patients with clinical signs of PCV and drusen (**Figure 2–29**). Yannuzzi and associates[40] diagnosed PCV in 13 (7.8%) of 167 consecutive patients with presumed neovascularized AMD. ICG angiography has led to the early discovery of polyps in the peripapillary, the macular, and the extramacular areas (**Figure 2–30**).

Retinal Angiomatous Proliferation

In 1995, Kuhn and co-workers[21] identified RCA as a potential manifestation of this form of neovascular AMD. They specifically related the development of RCA to an associated vascularized PED. Utilizing ICG angiography for enhanced imaging of the choroid, this group found evidence of RCA in 50 of 186 (28%) patients with AMD and an associated vascularized PED. Fernandes and co-workers[7] reported in a series of 190 patients with neovascular AMD that in 34 eyes (16%), the neovascularization was related to RAP lesions as identified on ICG angiography. ICG angiography is helpful in

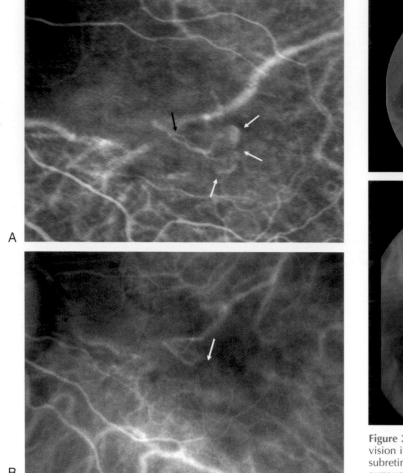

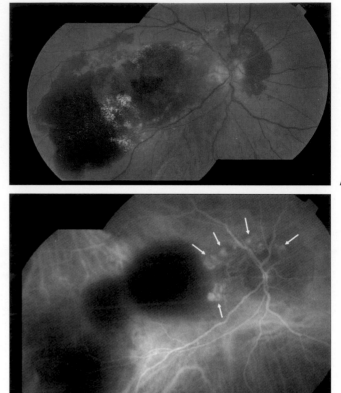

Figure 2–28 *A:* High-speed angiography of a patient with CNV (*white arrows*) demonstrates clearly the perfusing and draining feeder vessels (*black arrow*). *B:* After focal thermal laser treatment of the FVs, the ICG angiogram reveals closure of these vessels (*arrow*).

Figure 2–29 A 66-year-old white male with sudden deterioration of vision in his right eye. *A:* Color photograph composite shows large subretinal and intraretinal hemorrhages at the posterior pole and surrounding the optic nerve. There are areas with dense lipid exudation. *B:* Mid-phase ICG angiogram illustrates a large hypofluorescent area. In the peripapillary area, there is a net of subretinal inner choroidal vessels that terminate in polypoidal lesions (*white arrows*).

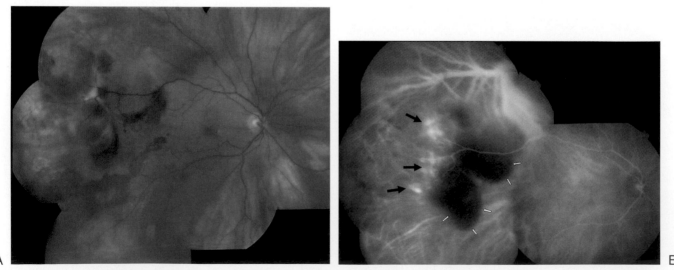

Figure 2–30 *A:* Color photograph composite of the fundus of a patient with PCV demonstrates hemorrhagic PED in the temporal periphery and subretinal hemorrhages. Note the subretinal fluid exudation involving the macula. *B:* ICG angiography composite of the right fundus reveals a cluster of actively leaking polypoidal vessels in the retinal periphery (*black arrows*). Note the two hemorrhagic PEDs blocking the background fluorescence (*white arrows*).

making an accurate diagnosis when IRN has progressed beneath the neurosensory retina (**Figure 2–31**).

2.6.2 CLINICAL APPLICATION OF ICG ANGIOGRAPHY TO THE STUDY OF CSC

Yannuzzi and co-workers[36] reported a rapid reduction in subretinal fluid in patients with chronic CSC when treated with ICG angiography–guided photodynamic therapy.

Some patients with CSC may have associated clinical and fluorescein angiographic manifestations, which are indistinguishable from PCV. In such cases, ICG angiography is helpful for confirming the accurate diagnosis. Katsimpris and co-workers[20] demonstrated that ICG hyperfluorescence appears in CSC-affected eyes and in fellow eyes in areas that demonstrate no clinical or fluorescein angiographic signs of active disease. They suggested that the persistence of abnormal ICG findings in eyes with inactive disease is related to chronic and not recurrent disease (**Figure 2–32**).

2.6.3 CLINICAL APPLICATION OF ICG ANGIOGRAPHY TO THE STUDY OF OCULAR TUMORS

Sallet and associates[27] demonstrated that ICG angiography can yield additional information that is useful in differentiating among choroidal tumors.

In pigmented choroidal tumors, the hypofluorescence caused by blockage from the tumor pigment may appear to be larger with ICG videoangiography than suspected clinically. When a pigmented choroidal melanoma thickens or otherwise develops prominent intrinsic vasculature, ICG angiography shows an increase in fluorescence in the late phase.[29]

ICG angiography can usually distinguish between metastatic choroidal lesions and choroidal hemangiomas. However, Bacin and co-authors[1] reported a patient in whom an extensively vascularized metastatic lesion was interpreted as a choroidal hemangioma by ICG videoangiography. This report emphasized that ICG angiographic findings must be evaluated along with the results of clinical examination, ultrasound examination, and FA before arriving at a diagnosis.

2.6.4 CLINICAL APPLICATION OF ICG ANGIOGRAPHY TO THE STUDY OF INTRAOCULAR INFLAMMATORY DISEASE

Giovannini and co-workers[11] reported the presence of occult satellite choroidal lesions found on ICG angiography with no clinical or fluorescein angiographic evidence in 17 patients with serpiginous choroiditis. The ICG pattern shows hypofluorescent areas up to the late phase of angiography that is characteristic for choriocapillaris nonperfusion. It is useful to distinguish this disorder from other choroidal vascular inflammatory diseases, such as ocular sarcoidosis, ocular tuberculosis, and birdshot choroidopathy, in which diffuse choroidal hyperfluorescence in the late ICG phase is caused by involvement of large choroidal vessels.

The location of lesions in MEWDS with ICG angiography has been compared with the presence of scotomas and enlargement of the blind spot in visual fields.[19] The perimetric findings correspond with hypofluorescent spots observed around the optic disc and at the macula in the late phase of ICG angiography. Resolution of the enlarged blind spot and return of vision does not completely correlate with the disappearance of the hypofluorescent areas on ICG angiography. These findings suggest that MEWDS may result in persistent abnormalities in choroidal circulation even after clinical symptoms disappear. Hypofluorescent spots were also present in periphlebitic areas (**Figure 2–33**).

Slakter and co-workers[30] reported on ICG angiography findings in a series of 14 patients with MFC. Fourteen (50%) of the 28 eyes were found to have large hypofluorescent spots in the posterior pole that did not correspond to clinically or fluorescein angiographically detectable lesions (**Figure 2–34**). In seven eyes exhibiting enlargement of the blind spot on visual field testing, ICG angiography showed confluent hypofluorescence surrounding the optic nerve. The ICG angiogram was useful in evaluating the natural course in two patients with MFC, as well as evaluating the response to oral prednisone treatment in four others. ICG angiography in these patients showed changes correlating with the clinical course. After administration of oral prednisone, the patients were noted to have decreased symptoms and less vitreitis on clinical examination. ICG

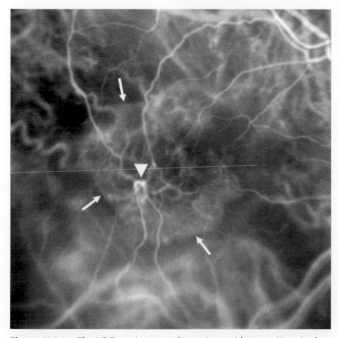

Figure 2–31 The ICG angiogram of a patient with stage III retinal angiomatous proliferation shows intraretinal and subretinal neovascularization (*arrowhead*) overlying a large area of choroidal neovascularization (*arrows*) with multiple RCAs.

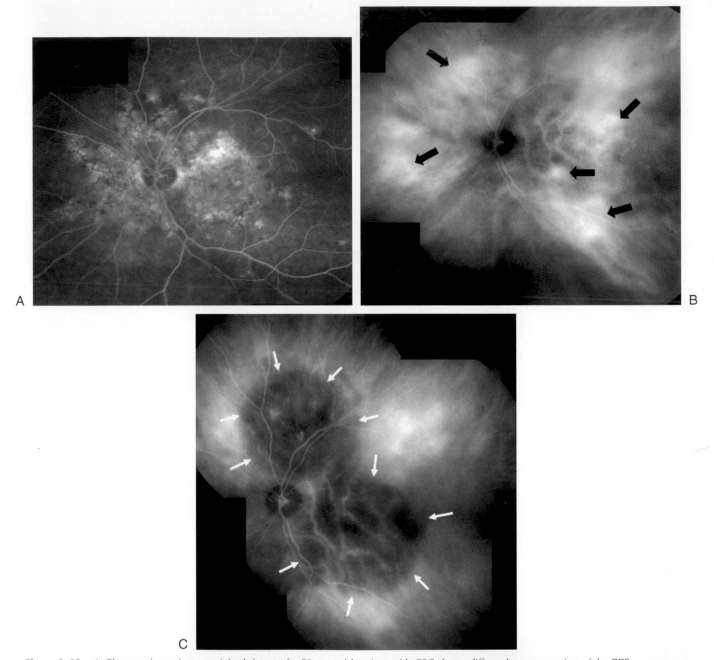

Figure 2–32 *A:* Fluorescein angiogram of the left eye of a 53-year-old patient with CSC shows diffuse decompensation of the RPE. *B:* The mid-phase ICG angiogram reveals multifocal areas of hyperfluorescence (*black arrows*) that do not always correspond with the leaking points seen on FA. *C:* ICG angiography 3 weeks after photodynamic therapy (*white arrows*). Leaking choroidal areas show resolution of the inner choroidal staining.

angiography showed a reduction in the size and number of the hypofluorescent spots in three patients with complete resolution of these angiographic lesions in the fourth patient. ICG angiography was also helpful in differentiating MFC from presumed ocular histoplasmosis syndrome, which has a similar clinical appearance. Patients with MFC clearly have hypofluorescent spots in the posterior pole during periods of relative activity, whereas patients with presumed ocular histoplasmosis syndrome may exhibit focal areas of hyperfluorescence.

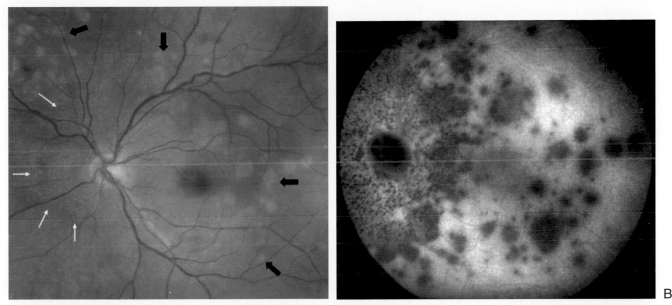

Figure 2–33 A 29-year-old woman with unilateral visual disturbance caused by MEWDS. *A:* The clinical photograph shows multiple round, white to yellow-white spots (*black arrows*) distributed over the posterior fundus. In the peripapillary region, there are multiple small yellow dots (*white arrows*). *B:* The mid-phase ICG angiogram reveals multiple large and small hypofluorescent spots in the posterior pole. Note the ring of hypofluorescence surrounding the optic disc.

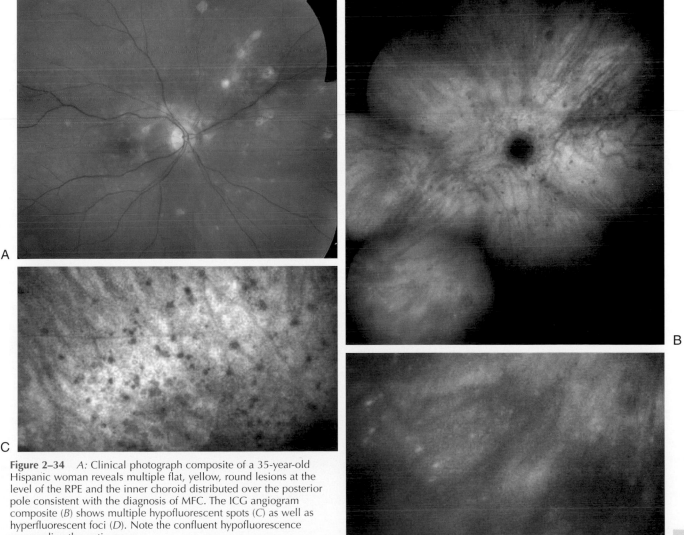

Figure 2–34 *A:* Clinical photograph composite of a 35-year-old Hispanic woman reveals multiple flat, yellow, round lesions at the level of the RPE and the inner choroid distributed over the posterior pole consistent with the diagnosis of MFC. The ICG angiogram composite (*B*) shows multiple hypofluorescent spots (*C*) as well as hyperfluorescent foci (*D*). Note the confluent hypofluorescence surrounding the optic nerve.

REFERENCES

1. Bacin F, Buffet JM, Mutel N. Angiographie par absorption, en infrarouge, au vert d'inocyanine, aspects chez le sujet normal et dans les tumeurs choridenned. Bull Soc Ophthalmol Fr. 1981;81:315.

2. Bischoff PR, Flower RW. Ten years experience with choroidal angiography using indocyanine green dye: a new routine examination or an epilogue? Doc Ophthalmol. 1985;60:235–291.

3. Chang B, Yannuzzi LA, Ladas ID, et al. Choroidal neovascularization in second eyes of patients with unilateral exudative age-related macular degeneration. Ophthalmology. 1995;102:1380–1386.

4. Cherrick GR, Stein SW, Leevy CM, et al. Indocyanine green: observations on its physical properties, plasma decay, and hepatic extraction. J Clin Invest. 1960;39:592–596.

5. David NJ. Infrared absorption fundus angiography. In Proceedings of International Symposium on Fluorescein Angiography, Albi, France, 1969. Basel, Switzerland: S Karger, 1971.

6. Destro M, Puliafito CA. Indocyanine green videoangiography of choroidal neovascularization. Ophthalmology. 1988;96:846–853.

7. Fernandes LHS, Freund BK, Yannuzzi LA, et al. The nature of focal areas of hyperfluorescence or hot spots imaged with indocyanine green angiography. Retina. 2002;22:557–568.

8. Flower RW, Hochheimer BF. Clinical infrared absorption angiography of the choroid. Am J Ophthalmol. 1972;73:458–459.

9. Freund KB, Yannuzzi LA, Sorenson JA, et al. Age-related macular degeneration and choroidal neovascularization. Am J Ophthalmol. 1993;115:786–791.

10. Geeraets WJ, Berry ER. Ocular spectral characteristics as related to hazards from lasers and other light sources. Am J Ophthalmol. 1968;66:15–20.

11. Giovannini A, Ripa E, Scassellati-Sforzolini B, et al. Indocyanine green angiography in serpiginous choroidopathy. Eur J Ophthalmol. 1996;6:299–306.

12. Guyer DR, Yannuzzi LA, Krupsky S, et al. Digital indocyanine green angiography of intraocular tumors. Semin Ophthalmol. 1993;8:224–229.

13. Guyer DR, Yannuzzi LA, Ladas I, et al. Indocyanine green guided laser photocoagulation of focal spots at the edge of plaques of choroidal neovascularization: a pilot study. Arch Ophthalmol. 1996;114:693–697.

14. Guyer DR, Yannuzzi LA, Slakter JS, et al. Classification of choroidal neovascularization by digital indocyanine green videoangiography. Ophthalmology. 1996;103:2054–2060.

15. Hayashi K, DeLaey JJ. Indocyanine green angiography of neovascular membranes. Ophthalmologica. 1985;190:30–39.

16. Hochheimer BF. Angiography of the retina with indocyanine green. Arch Ophthalmol. 1971;86:564–565.

17. Howe LJ, Stanford MR, Graham EM, et al. Choroidal abnormalities in birdshot chorioretinopathy: an indocyanine green angiography study. Eye. 1997;11:554–559.

18. Howe LJ, Woon H, Graham EM, et al. Choroidal hypoperfusion in acute multifocal posterior placoid pigment epitheliopathy: an indocyanine green angiography study. Ophthalmology. 1995;102:790–798.

19. Ie D, Glaser BM, Murphy RP, et al. Indocyanine green angiography in multiple evanescent white-dot syndrome. Am J Ophthalmol. 1994;117:7–12.

20. Katsimpris J, Donati G, Kapetanios A, et al. The value of indocyanine green angiography in detection of central serous chorioretinopathy. Klin Monatsbl Augenheilkd. 2001;218:335–337.

21. Kuhn D, Meunier I, Soubrane G, Coca G. Imaging of chorioretinal anastomoses in vascularized retinal pigment epithelium detachments. Arch Ophthalmol. 1995;113:1392–1396.

22. Lafaut BA, Leyes AM, Snyers B, et al. Polypoidal choroidal vasculopathy in Caucasians. Graefes Arch Clin Exp Ophthalmol. 2000;238:752–759.

23. Macular Photocoagulation Study Group. Occult choroidal neovascularization. Influence on visual outcome in patients with age-related macular degeneration. Arch Ophthalmol. 1996;114:400–412.

24. Patz A, Flower RW, Klein ML, Orth DH, Fleishman JA, MacLeod D. Clinical applications of indocyanine green angiography. Doc Ophthalmol Proc Ser. 1976;9:245–251.

25. Pauleikhoff D, Loffert D, Spital G, et al: Pigment epithelial detachment in the elderly. Clinical differentiation, natural course and pathogenetic implications. Graefes Arch Clin Exp Ophthalmol. 240:533–538, 2002.

26. Probst P, Paumgartner G, Caucig H, Froehlich H, Grabner G. Studies on clearance and placental transfer of indocyanine green during labor. Clin Chim Acta. 1970;29:157–160.

27. Sallet S, Amoakn WM, Lafaut BA, et al. Indocyanine green angiography of choroidal tumors. Graefes Arch Clin Exp Ophthalmol. 1995;223:677–689.

28. Scheider A, Schroedel C. High resolution indocyanine green angiography with scanning laser ophthalmoscope. Am J Ophthalmol. 1989;108:458–459.

29. Shields CL, Shields JA, De Potter P. Patterns of indocyanine green videoangiography of choroidal tumors. Br J Ophthalmol. 1995;79:237–245.

30. Slakter JS, Giovannini A, Yannuzzi LA, et al. Indocyanine green angiography of multifocal choroiditis. Ophthalmology. 1997;104:1813–1819.

31. Slakter JS, Yannuzzi, LA, Sorenson, JA, et al. A pilot study of indocyanine green videoangiography-guided laser photocoagulation of occult choroidal neovascularization in age-related macular degeneration. Arch Ophthalmol. 1994;112:465–472.

32. Spaide RF, Orlock DA, Herrmann-Delamazure B, et al. Wide-angle indocyanine green angiography. Retina. 1998;18:44–49.

33. Spaide RF, Orlock DA, Yannuzzi LA, et al. Digital subtraction indocyanine green angiography of occult choroidal neovascularization. Ophthalmology. 1998;105:680–688.

34. Staurenghi G, Orzalesi N, La Capria A, Aschero M. Laser treatment of feeder vessels in subfoveal choroidal neovascular membranes: a revisitation using dynamic indocyanine green angiography. Ophthalmology. 1998;105:2297–2305.

35. Webb RH, Hughes GW, Delori FC. Confocal scanning laser ophthalmoscope. Appl Opt. 1987;26:1492–1499.

36. Yannuzzi LA, Freund KB, Goldbaum M, et al. Polypoidal choroidal vasculopathy masquerading as central serous chorioretinopathy. Ophthalmology. 2000;107:767–777.

37. Yannuzzi LA, Negrao S, Iida T, et al. Retinal angiomatous proliferation in age-related macular degeneration. Retina. 2001;21:416–34

38. Yannuzzi LA, Slakter JS, Sorenson JS, Guyer DR, Orlock DA. Digital indocyanine green videoangiography and choroidal neovascularization. Retina. 1992;12:191–223.

39. Yannuzzi LA, Sorenson JS, Spaide RF, et al. Idiopathic polypoidal choroidal vasculopathy. Retina. 1990;10:1–8.

40. Yannuzzi LA, Wong DW, Sforzolini SB, et al. Polypoidal choroidal vasculopathy and neovascularized age-related macular degeneration. Arch Ophthalmol. 1999;17:1503–1510.

Chapter 3

Optical Coherence Tomography

DAVID HUANG, MD, PhD • OU TAN, PhD • JAMES G. FUJIMOTO, PhD • WOLFGANG DREXLER, PhD • JOHANNES F. DE BOER, PhD • MACIEJ WOJTKOWSKI, PhD • ANDRZEJ KOWALCZYK, PhD

3.1 Physical Principles

Optical coherence tomography (OCT) is based on the imaging of reflected light. However, unlike a simple camera image that only has transverse dimensions (left/right and up/down), it also resolves depth. The depth resolution of OCT is extremely fine, typically on the order of 0.01 mm or 0.4 thousandth of an inch. This provides cross-sectional views (tomography) of internal tissue structures similar to those of tissue sections under a microscope, but unlike histologic analysis, OCT does not disturb the tissue. Thus, OCT has been described as a method for noninvasive tissue "biopsy." This section explains the technical details of how OCT accomplishes this magic.

3.1.1 REFLECTOMETRY

In OCT, a beam of light (typically 800 to 1400 nm wavelength in the near infrared) is scanned across the tissue sample. The OCT system then collects the reflected light and measures its time-of-flight delay. Light reflected from deeper layers has a longer propagation delay than that reflected from more superficial layers (**Figure 3–1**). The amplitude of reflected light can be plotted against delay (**Figure 3–2**) to demonstrate tissue reflectivity at successively deeper levels of tissue penetration along the axis of beam propagation. This is called an axial scan (A-scan). As the OCT probe beam is scanned across a sample, many A-scans are acquired to form an image (**Figure 3–3**). A color or gray scale is used to represent the signal amplitude.

Ultrasound imaging and radio detection and ranging (RADAR) are also reflectometry-based imaging methods. Because OCT uses light, several advantages are gained. The wavelength of light (~0.001 mm) is shorter than that of ultrasound (~0.1 mm) and radio waves (>10 mm). Therefore, the spatial resolution of OCT is much higher. And unlike ultrasound imaging, OCT does not require probe-tissue contact or an immersion fluid because light passes through the air-tissue interface easily.

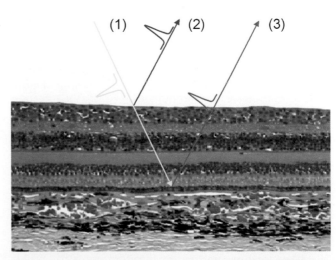

Figure 3–1 The OCT beam is scanned across the retina *(1)*. The delay of a superficial reflection *(2)* is shorter than that of a deeper reflection *(3)*.

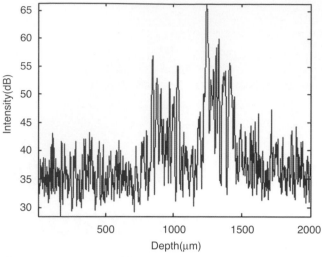

Figure 3–2 An A-scan of the retina. The amplitude of reflection on a decibel scale is plotted against depth.

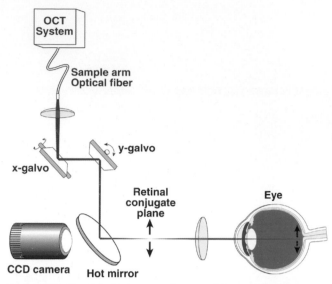

Figure 3–4 Simplified schematic diagram of the transverse scanning mechanism of a retinal OCT system.

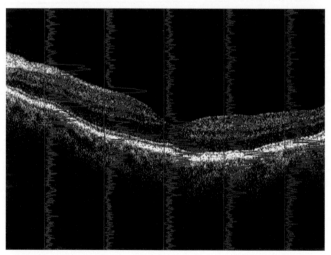

Figure 3–3 An OCT cross-sectional image (gray-scale image) is built up from many A-scans (*red plot lines*).

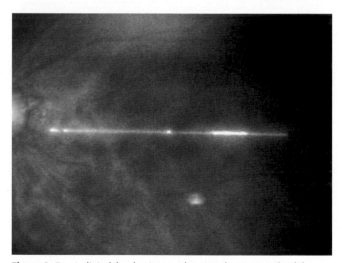

Figure 3–5 A digital fundus image showing the scan path of the OCT beam used to acquire the OCT image shown in **Figure 3–3**.

A retinal OCT system uses a transverse scanning system to steer the OCT beam across the fundus (**Figure 3–4**). The transverse scanning setup of the OCT system is essentially a confocal scanning laser ophthalmoscope (cSLO) in which the tip of the sample arm fiber serves as the confocal aperture. The OCT beam coming out of the fiber tip is focused on a retinal conjugate plane. The beam is steered by a pair of galvanometer-driven mirrors in two dimensions. An objective lens and the eye's own focusing system relay the beam from the conjugate plane to the retina. The OCT beam is focused on the retina and reflections are collected along the same beam path in the reverse direction back to sample arm fiber. The fiber is connected to an interferometer to resolve the delay (depth) of reflections (see next section). The depth-resolving capability of the retinal OCT system distinguishes it from an ordinary cSLO. A digital camera is also often included to capture the en face fundus image (**Figure 3–5**) so the OCT beam path can be visualized and aligned.

3.1.2 LOW-COHERENCE INTERFEROMETRY

Because light travels very rapidly (3×10^8 m/sec), it is not possible to directly measure the time-of-flight delay on a small spatial scale. The micron-scale resolution of OCT is achieved by comparing the delays of sample reflections with the known delay of a reference reflection in an interferometer. The classic OCT system (**Figure 3–6**) uses a "low-coherence" fiberoptic Michelson interferometer.[18] Interferometry measures the effect of combining two light waves. Low coherence means that the system uses a wide range of wavelengths. We will explain the concepts of interferometry and coherence separately.

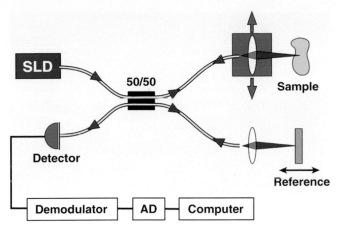

Figure 3–6   Schematic diagram of the classic OCT system.

The interferometer (**Figure 3–6**) has source, sample, reference, and detector arms all centered on a 50/50 fiber coupler. Output of the superluminescent diode (SLD) light source is launched into the source arm fiber and split by the coupler into the sample and reference arms. Sample and reference reflections are recombined at the coupler and produce interference. This interferometric signal is converted from light to electrical current by a photodetector, processed electronically, and transferred to computer memory.

To understand how the Michelson interferometer works, let us start with the simple case (**Figure 3–7**) in which the sample arm reflection comes from a simple mirror surface and the light source emits only one wavelength. Think of the sample and reference reflections as two waves of light. The coupler partially transfers these waves to the detector arm, where they combine and produce an interference signal. Interference can be thought of as the addition of the amplitude of two waves. When the two waves are in phase (lined up peak to peak), they interfere constructively, forming a peak in the interference waveform. When the two waves are exactly out of phase (lined up peak to trough), they interfere destructively, forming a trough in the interference waveform. As the reference mirror is moved, the phase of the reference wave changes, producing a sinusoidal interference signal. As the reference mirror moves through one-half cycle of the source wavelength, the round trip delay of the reference wave varies by one

wavelength and the interference signal goes through one cycle of sinusoidal oscillation.

To resolve the delay of sample reflections, the OCT system uses a light source that has a wide range of wavelengths (low coherence). When the interference signals are added together over the range of wavelengths, the interferometric oscillation fades as the delay mismatch between the reference and sample reflections increases (**Figure 3–8**). To understand why this occurs, look carefully at the phase relationship between the wavelength components shown schematically in the *left panel* of **Figure 3–8**. When the delay mismatch is near zero (center of waveforms), the interference signals from all wavelength components have the same phase (peaks and troughs lined up) or are "coherent." This adds up to large interferometric modulation (see large peaks and troughs in the center of the right-side waveform). When the mismatch is large (away from the center of the waveforms), the interference waveforms vary widely in phase over the wavelength range (peaks and troughs not lined up) and add up to near a flat line. The summed interference signal (**Figure 3–8**, *right panel*) forms a wave pulse. In an OCT system, the pulse is demodulated electronically to extract the pulse envelope (shape of the pulse without the sinusoidal oscillation). The width of the pulse envelope is the coherence length, which determines the axial resolution of the OCT system. The coherence length is inversely proportional with the wavelength range or *bandwidth*.

When the OCT system is used to image an actual tissue sample, there are many reflections at different depths. As the reference mirror is scanned, each sample reflection gives rise to a signal pulse when the reference delay matches it. The plot of the demodulated interferometric signal is the A-scan (**Figure 3–2**) waveform, which represents amplitude of reflection versus depth.

All clinical OCT systems use SLD light sources. SLDs are similar to the diode lasers inside the common compact disc (CD) player, but are made to emit over a wider range of wavelengths. SLDs are used because they are economical, compact, and long-lasting, and they emit high-quality beams that couple efficiently with an

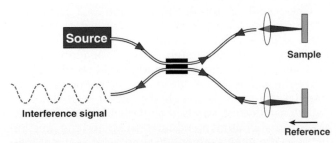

Figure 3–7   In a single-wavelength Michelson interferometer, varying the reference delay produces a sinusoidal oscillation of optical power in the detector arm.

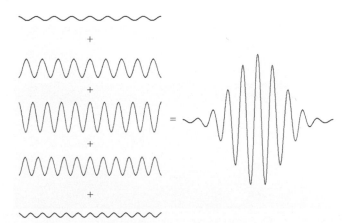

Figure 3–8   Combining interference signals from a range of wavelengths (*left*) produces a pulse (*right*). The width of this pulse determines the axial resolution of the OCT system.

optical fiber. The resolution of clinical OCT is basically limited by the state of SLD technology. Early retinal OCT systems typically used SLDs emitting around an 820-nm center wavelength over a bandwidth of 20 nm full-width at half-maximum (FWHM).[13,30] This limits the axial resolution to roughly 15 microns FWHM in air and 11 microns in tissue. The axial resolution may be further degraded by the mismatch of chromatic aberration between the sample and reference arms and other limitations of the optical and electrical components.

3.2 Technology Development

OCT was first developed by David Huang and colleagues in James Fujimoto's laboratory at the Massachusetts Institute of Technology (MIT) in 1991.[18] A retinal scanner that was fast enough for clinical use was first developed by Swanson and associates at MIT.[30] OCT was first commercially introduced as a retinal scanner in the mid-1990s and has now become a widespread tool for ophthalmologists. Advanced OCT technologies developed in several laboratories have resulted in improved resolution, speed, and capabilities to measure flow and birefringence. These new OCT technologies will greatly enhance both research applications and clinical practice in the coming years.

3.2.1 COMMERCIAL OCT RETINAL SCANNERS

The OCT technology[13,18,30] developed at MIT was licensed by Humphrey Instruments, Inc., and developed into a clinical retinal scanner (OCT1 or System 2000). A more compact and ergonomic system was later marketed under the name OCT2 or System 2010. Both systems had 12- to 16-micron FWHM axial resolution in tissue. The data acquisition rate was 100 A-scans/sec. The transverse resolution was 20 microns, as determined by the beam size and focusing property of the eye. Images were limited to 100 A-scans and appeared grainy (**Figure 3–9**).

Humphrey Instruments was subsequently acquired by Carl Zeiss Meditec, Inc. Zeiss recently introduced the

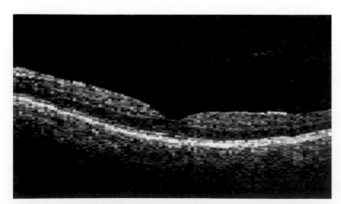

Figure 3–9 OCT cross section of the macula produced by the Humphrey OCT1 system. The image is 6 mm wide (transverse) × 1.46 mm high (axial) and the corresponding pixel counts are 100 × 512.

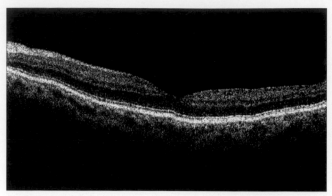

Figure 3–10 OCT cross section of the macula produced by the Zeiss Stratus system. The image is 6 mm wide (transverse) × 2 mm high (axial) and the corresponding pixel counts are 512 × 1024.

OCT3 (Stratus System). The Stratus system has a higher axial resolution of 9 to 10 microns FWHM in tissue. The axial sampling interval was halved to 2 microns. More importantly, the system has a much higher acquisition rate of 400 A-scans/sec by the use of high-speed, grating-based, reference delay scanning.[27] Thus, although the transverse resolution (focused spot size) is unchanged, the transverse sampling density can be greatly improved. The number of A-scans per image is adjustable and ranges from 128 to 768. The increased axial and transverse pixel counts produced dramatically improved image quality (**Figure 3–10**).

3.2.2 ULTRAHIGH-RESOLUTION OCT

Although the Stratus system produces beautifully detailed OCT images of the retina, it is possible to obtain three times better performance with ultrahigh-resolution technology. The examples in this section will demonstrate the importance of higher resolution.

The axial resolution of an OCT system can approach the source wavelength if one uses a very broad-band light source such as the femtosecond titanium:sapphire laser. An axial resolution down to 1 micron has been demonstrated.[2] Imaging of the human retina in vivo is limited to 3 microns axial resolution by the chromatic aberration of the ocular media. Drexler and Fujimoto were the first to demonstrate clinical retinal imaging at this level of resolution,[9] which they called *ultrahigh-resolution* OCT because it approached the fundamental physical limits of OCT imaging.

One benefit of ultrahigh-resolution OCT is the improved delineation of retinal layers. Correlation between these scans and histologic analysis helps us interpret OCT images more accurately.[10] The ultrahigh-resolution OCT image of the macula (**Figure 3–11**) clearly defines all of the major retinal layers and even shows further internal structures. In the photoreceptor layer, there are two thin reflective bands that probably correspond to the external limiting membrane (ELM) and the junction between the inner segment (IS) and outer segment (OS) of the photoreceptors.[10] However, this interpretation leads to a relatively thin OS layer on OCT compared with

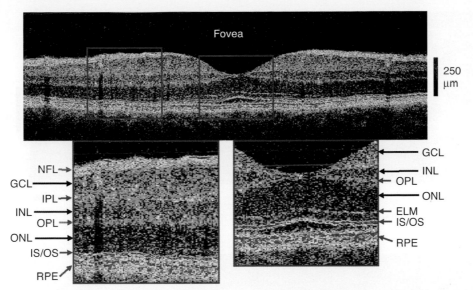

Figure 3–11 Ultrahigh-resolution OCT cross section of normal human macula showing the nerve fiber layer (NFL), ganglion cell layer (GCL), inner plexiform layer (IPL), inner nuclear layer (INL), outer nuclear layer (ONL), external limiting membrane (ELM), inner/outer segments (IS/OS) of photoreceptors, and retinal pigment epithelium (RPE). (Courtesy J. G. Fujimoto.)

histologic analysis. An alternative interpretation may be that the inner band represents the IS/OS junction and the outer band represents a layer in the OS.

Ultrahigh-resolution OCT improves the localization of retinal pathologic changes and provides a more detailed assessment of fine anatomic changes. In a case of central serous retinopathy (CSR) shown in **Figure 3–12**, the photoreceptor layer is visibly thickened and more reflective (except where the retina is oblique to the OCT beam) in the area of retinal detachment. The preservation of the photoreceptor structure is consistent with the clinical observation that vision often fully recovers after the resolution of the retinal detachment in CSR.

Figure 3–13 shows a full-thickness macular hole. Ultrahigh-resolution OCT localizes the cystic changes to the inner and outer nuclear layers. The internal structure of the photoreceptor layer appears intact despite being lifted off the retinal pigment epithelium (RPE). This may indicate a potential for recovery if the hole can be surgically closed.

Figure 3–14 shows a case of age-related macular degeneration (AMD) with choroidal neovascularization (CNV). Both RPE and retinal detachments are present, and the planes of separation are consistent with the identification of outer retinal layers shown in **Figure 3–11**.

Figure 3–15 shows a case of adult-onset foveomacular vitelliform dystrophy. Ultrahigh-resolution OCT shows foveal changes that include thickening of the RPE-Bruch's membrane-choriocapillaris complex and disruption of the photoreceptor IS/OS structures.

These examples demonstrate some of the benefits of ultrahigh resolution in the visualization of the internal structure of the retina. In diseases such as CNV, CSR, and macular hole, this may help us plan treatment and predict prognosis. In inherited retinal diseases such as adult-onset foveomacular vitelliform dystrophy and retinoschisis, ultrahigh resolution may allow us to further localize the affected retinal layers and improve phenotypic characterization.

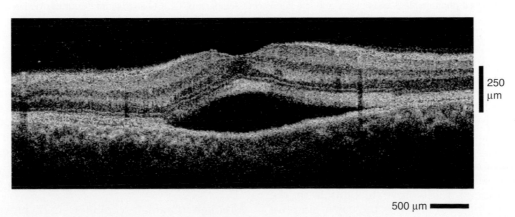

Figure 3–12 Ultrahigh-resolution OCT section of CSR with serous retinal detachment. (Courtesy J. G. Fujimoto.)

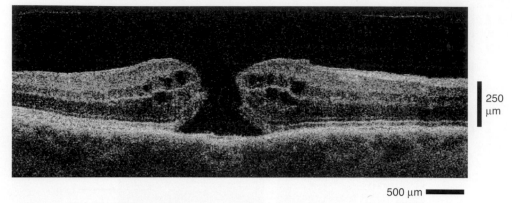

250 μm

500 μm

Figure 3–13   Ultrahigh-resolution OCT section of a stage IV macular hole. (Courtesy J. G. Fujimoto.)

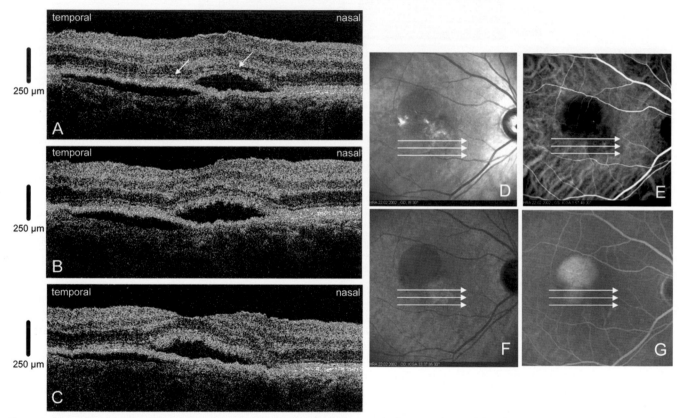

Figure 3–14   AMD with CNV. *A–C:* Ultrahigh-resolution OCT sections showing both RPE and retinal detachment. Lines of scan shown to the bottom in *D–G*. *D:* Infrared photograph. *E* and *F:* Early and late fluorescein angiograms. *G:* ICG angiogram. (Courtesy W. Drexler.)

The femtosecond lasers used in ultrahigh-resolution OCT are still too expensive, bulky, and unreliable to be used in commercial clinical OCT systems. However, the bandwidth of SLD light sources is incrementally improving, and we can anticipate that commercial OCT systems will gradually approach ultrahigh resolution in the coming years.

So far we have been discussing ultrahigh resolution only along the axial dimension. New technology has also been developed to improve resolution in the transverse dimensions. For instance, the use of adaptive optics to compensate for ocular aberrations can greatly improve the focusing of the OCT beam, which determines the transverse resolution. Recently the improvement of transverse resolution to 5 microns (from 20) and signal-to-noise ratio (SNR) by 9 dB have been demonstrated.[17] Adaptive-optic OCT images can show very fine details such as small capillaries. The clinical implications of this new technology are still being tested.

3.2.3 FOURIER-DOMAIN (ULTRAHIGH-SPEED) OCT

Although ultrahigh-resolution OCT provides us with stunningly detailed images, ultrahigh-speed OCT with

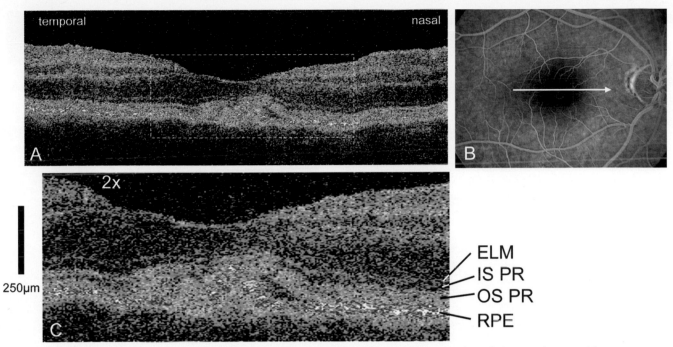

Figure 3–15   Adult-onset foveomacular vitelliform dystrophy. *A:* Ultrahigh-resolution OCT section through the macula. *B:* Red-free photograph. *C:* Magnified OCT section of the foveal region. (Courtesy W. Drexler.)

the Fourier-domain (FD) technology (also called *spectral domain* or SD) may bring even greater practical improvement in clinical utility and ease of use. Laboratory results have shown that FD-OCT can achieve nearly 100-fold speed improvement over conventional time-domain (TD) OCT.

In FD-OCT (**Figure 3–16**), the detector arm of the Michelson interferometer uses a spectrometer instead of a single detector. The spectrometer measures spectral modulations produced by interference between the sample and reference reflections. A Fourier transform

of this spectrum produces a waveform that represents the amplitude of sample reflections as a function of depth. Although the information provided by a single spectrometer measurement is equivalent to an A-scan in TD-OCT, it has two important advantages. First, no physical scanning of the reference mirror is required; thus, FD-OCT can be much faster than TD-OCT. And second, the simultaneous detection of reflections from a broad range of depths is much more efficient than TD-OCT, in which signals from various depths are scanned sequentially. This allows a gain in either the image

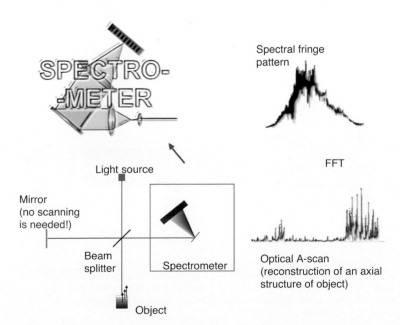

Figure 3–16   Schematic representation of FD-OCT. *Lower left:* A spectrometer is placed in the detector arm of the interferometer. *Upper left:* In the spectrometer, a grating disperses light into a spectrum on the detector array. *Upper right:* The detected spectrum contains an interferometric fringe pattern. *Lower right:* Fast Fourier transform (FFT) of the spectral fringe pattern yields the A-scan. (Courtesy M. Wojtkowski.)

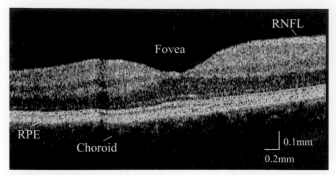

Figure 3–17 FD-OCT of the human macula in vivo with 1125 A-scans acquired in 0.072 second. (Courtesy M. Wojtkowski.)

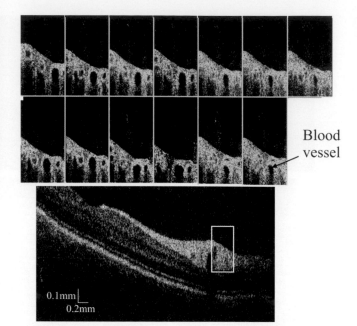

Figure 3–18 FD-OCT of the human retina. Large blood vessels are seen near the optic nerve head (*inset lower panel*). Successive images acquired at 9 frames/sec (*upper panels*) with a magnified view of the blood vessels (*arrow*) show pulsation during the cardiac cycle. (Courtesy M. Wojtkowski.)

acquisition rate or the SNR by a factor proportional to the number of detector elements in the spectrometer (typically 1024 or 2048). Thus, FD-OCT not only dramatically improves imaging speed but also produces more detailed and brighter images.

Very high-speed FD-OCT was first accomplished by Maciej Wojtkowski and co-workers in Andrzej Kowalczyk's laboratory at Nicholas Copernicus University in Poland[32–34] and then by Nassif and associates in Johannes de Boer's laboratory at Harvard University.[25,26] They have demonstrated an improvement in image acquisition rate (A-scans per second) of nearly 100-fold while simultaneously improving the SNR.

FD-OCT of the macula (**Figure 3–17**) shows greater detail (1125 A-scans versus 512 A-scans) than a similar Stratus TD-OCT system image (see **Figure 3–10**). Because the image acquisition time is much shorter (0.072 versus 1.23 seconds), the FD-OCT image (**Figure 3-17**) does not have the problem of motion artifact, which manifests itself as an undulation of the RPE layer in the slower TD-OCT image. The lack of motion artifacts can be a significant advantage in the interpretation of images in which the surface contours of the RPE and other layers may carry diagnostic information such as the thickness and location of a choroidal neovascular membrane. FD-OCT is also fast enough for sequential image frames to track the pulsation of blood vessels

during the cardiac cycle (**Figure 3–18**). The fastest result so far acquired by Nassif and co-workers[26] (**Figure 3–19**) is 1000 A-scans in 0.034 second (29,000 A-scans/sec).

Ultrahigh-speed OCT may also have great importance in diseases such as glaucoma for which precise measurement of the nerve fiber layer (NFL) and other structures over time is critical. A major limitation on biometric accuracy is that the position of the measurement may not be properly centered on the optic disc, and sequential measurements may not be made at the same point. This complicates the use and interpretation of OCT data. With the speed of FD-OCT, a wide area of the retina (i.e., macula or optic nerve head [ONH]) can be scanned within a fraction of a second. A fundus image can be generated directly from the OCT data and

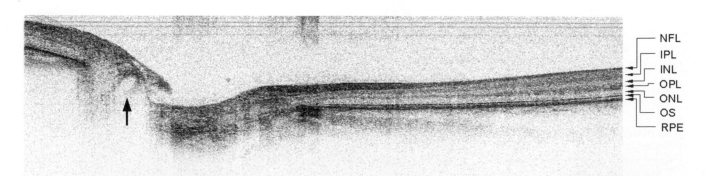

Figure 3–19 FD-OCT of the optic nerve head region with 1000 A-scans acquired in 0.034 second in a human eye in vivo. Note the high detail and lack of motion artifact. The *arrow* points to a blood vessel in the ONH. The gray scale is reversed (black = high reflectivity). From Nassif N, Cense B, Park BH, et al. In-vivo human retinal imaging by ultrahigh-speed spectral domain optical coherence tomography. Opt Lett. 2004;29:480–482, with permission from the Optical Society of America. (Courtesy J. F. de Boer.)

centration on fundus features can be done very precisely in postprocessing. This should improve the accuracy and reliability of any application that requires tracking of anatomic measurements or mapping of retinal features (i.e., retinal thickness in macular edema).

The components of FD-OCT technology, such as the detector array and high-speed digital signal processing, are now mature. There is no cost-prohibitive barrier for commercialization of FD-OCT. It can be anticipated that FD-OCT will be the basis of the next generation of clinical retinal OCT systems.

3.2.4 DOPPLER OCT FOR BLOOD FLOW IMAGING

Measurement of blood flow based on the Doppler principle can be achieved with both TD-OCT[36–39] and FD-OCT.[19,20,31] In Doppler imaging, the flow velocity produces a frequency shift in the reflected light. Flow toward the incident beam increases the reflected optical frequency (blue shift) whereas flow away from the beam decreases the optical frequency (red shift). The Doppler shift is measured in each pixel of the OCT image (**Figures 3–20** and **3–21**). In **Figure 3–20,** the structural and flow information is presented in separate images of reflectivity and Doppler shift. The high frame rate of FD-OCT allows dynamic tracking of blood flow with excellent time resolution (**Figure 3–22**).

The clinical significance of Doppler OCT merits further investigation. Measuring the blood flow of the retina, choroid, and ONH contributes to our understanding of the pathophysiology of diabetic retinopathy, glaucoma, and AMD. It may also be useful for the management of these diseases once we know how to interpret the data clinically. Doppler OCT offers better spatial resolution than Doppler ultrasound and Doppler scanning laser ophthalmoscopy. Unlike fluorescein

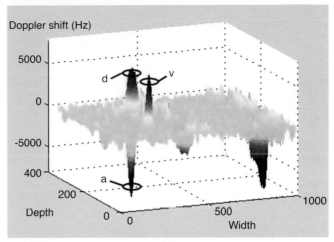

Figure 3–21 Plot of chorioretinal blood flow corresponding to the image in Figure 3–20. Image width and depth are mapped onto the horizontal plane and the Doppler shift is shown on the vertical axis. From White BR, Pierce MC, Nassif N, et al. In vivo dynamic human retinal blood flow imaging using ultra-high-speed spectral domain optical Doppler tomography. Opt Express. 2003;11:3490–3497, with permission from the Optical Society of America. (Courtesy J. F. de Boer.)

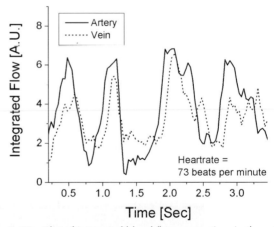

Figure 3–22 Plot of integrated blood flow versus time in the retinal artery and vein pair in Figure 3–20. A total of 95 frames were acquired at 29 frames/sec over 3.28 seconds. From White BR, Pierce MC, Nassif N, et al. In vivo dynamic human retinal blood flow imaging using ultra-high-speed spectral domain optical Doppler tomography. Opt Express. 2003;11:3490–3497, with permission from the Optical Society of America. (Courtesy J. F. de Boer.)

and indocyanine green angiography, Doppler OCT does not require injection of a contrast agent and is more quantitative.

3.2.5 OTHER OCT TECHNOLOGIES

Polarization-sensitive OCT systems have been developed to measure tissue birefringence.[8,12] Birefringence contains information on the status of the retinal nerve fiber layer (RNFL) in addition to its thickness.[4,5] This may be useful in the diagnosis of glaucoma and other optic nerve diseases.

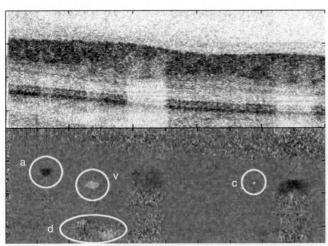

Figure 3–20 Doppler FD-OCT of human retina and choroid showing structure (reflectivity image, *upper panel*) and flow (Doppler shift image, *lower panel*). a, artery, v, vein, c, capillary, d, choroidal vessel. From White BR, Pierce MC, Nassif N, et al. In vivo dynamic human retinal blood flow imaging using ultra-high-speed spectral domain optical Doppler tomography. Opt Express. 2003;11:3490–3497, with permission from the Optical Society of America. (Courtesy J. F. de Boer.)

OCT can also detect spectral shifts due to absorption in the imaged tissue.[24] This spectroscopic measurement is made even simpler with the new FD-OCT technology[21] and could enable imaging of oxyhemoglobin and deoxyhemoglobin concentrations and measurement of oxygenation. Injection of a dye that absorbs the OCT beam and alters its spectrum might also be useful for contrast enhancement with spectroscopic OCT.

3.3 Image Interpretation

Because the Zeiss Stratus OCT system is the current clinical standard, the examples in this section are obtained using the Stratus system from human subjects in vivo.

3.3.1 RETINAL LAYERS

The major layers of the retina can be resolved in Stratus OCT system images (**Figure 3–23**), although the contrast of some boundaries is less distinct than in ultrahigh-resolution OCT images. The reflectivities of the layers vary in predictable manners. The NFL is typically the brightest retinal layer because the fibers are uniformly perpendicular to the OCT beam. The nasal macula (*left side* of **Figure 3–23**) is closer to the ONH and has a thicker NFL. The plexiform layers are of intermediate reflectivity because they contain fibers of varied orientation. The nuclear layers have low reflectivity. The photoreceptor layer has two bright and two dark bands (**Figure 3–23**). The two bright bands are probably the ELM and the IS/OS junctions. The ELM is not always resolvable with the Stratus system. The RPE is highly reflective because of its high concentration of melanin granules. The choroidal structures are very faint owing to blocking by the RPE through both scattering and absorption. Dark holes corresponding to large choroidal vessels can sometimes be discerned under the RPE.

3.3.2 COLOR VERSUS GRAY-SCALE DISPLAYS

OCT images are presented using either a gray-scale (**Figure 3–24**) or a color-scale (**Figure 3–25**) representation of reflected signal strength. The standard gray scale runs continuously from high signal (white) to no signal (black). The standard color scale uses a modified continuous rainbow spectrum in which signal level from high to low is represented by white-red-orange-yellow-green-blue-black. A low signal below or near the noise level is typically blacked out.

The gray scale is better for impartial delineation of retinal layers. Identification of a retinal layer with a color (i.e., "the NFL is the red layer on top") is tempting on a color image, but may be misleading. The color scale is arbitrary, and the color transition boundary may shift because of extrinsic factors (focusing and polarization matching) that affect the signal strength. On the other hand, the color scale maintains high display brightness over most of the signal scale and is better for visualizing faint structures. For example, a thin epiretinal membrane is much easier to visualize on a color scale (**Figure 3-25**) than on a gray scale (**Figure 3–24**). Most clinicians seem to favor the color scale because it is more attractive, and images are easier to read. Many engineers and scientists tend to favor the gray scale as a more accurate representation.

3.3.3 MACULAR THICKNESS PROFILE AND MAP

OCT cross-sectional images provide a wealth of biometric data such as the thickness of the retina and its

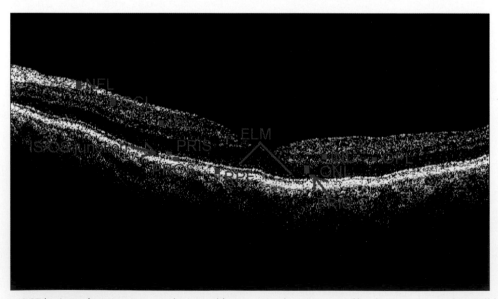

Figure 3–23 Stratus OCT horizontal section (6 mm) of a normal human macula. NFL, nerve fiber layer; GCL, ganglion cell layer; IPL, inner plexiform layer; INL, inner nuclear layer; OPL, outer plexiform layer; ONL, outer nuclear layer; ELM, external limiting membrane; PR, photoreceptor; IS, inner segment; OS, outer segment; RPE, retinal pigment epithelium.

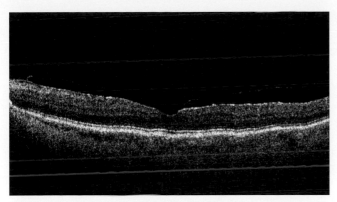

Figure 3–24   Gray-scale OCT horizontal section (6 mm) of a macula with epiretinal membrane.

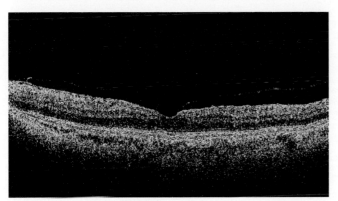

Figure 3–25   Color-scale OCT horizontal section (6 mm) of a macula with epiretinal membrane. The OCT data are the same as in Figure 3–24.

component layers. Although it is possible to measure this manually by positioning cursors on the computer screen, fully automatic measurement by an image-processing algorithm is much faster and more practical.

With the Stratus system, it is possible to map the retinal thickness over the entire macular area relatively quickly using the "fast macular thickness map" scan pattern. The scan consists of 6-mm radial lines along six meridians, forming a clockhour spoke pattern. Each radial line consists of 128 A-scans and the entire pattern of 768 A-scans is completed in less than 2 seconds. The retinal thickness profile is computed from each cross-sectional image. On the retinal thickness profile display (**Figure 3–26**), a selected OCT cross-sectional image is displayed with superimposed outlines of the inner and outer retinal boundaries as determined by the image-processing software. The user should inspect the boundary outline to confirm that the computer has made a correct boundary determination on all six cross sections. The Stratus system also provides a fundus image from a digital camera with a superimposed computer-generated scan pattern outline. The user should inspect this to confirm that the scan pattern is centered on the macula. Interpolation of the thickness profiles from the six cross sections produces a color-scale retinal thickness map of the macula (**Figure 3–27**). On the normal map, one should be able to recognize a well-centered foveal depression in the central 1-mm-diameter circular area, and a relatively thicker nasal area formed by the maculopapular and arcuate nerve fiber bundles.

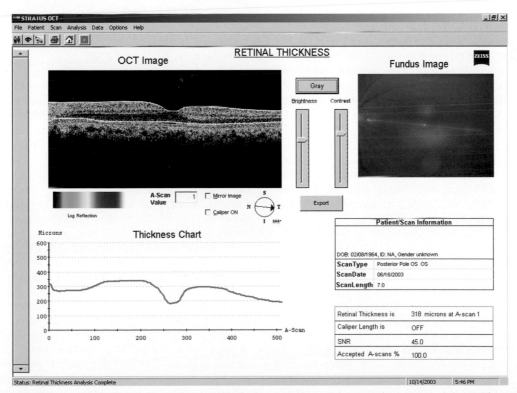

Figure 3–26   Retinal thickness profile display from a fast macular thickness map scan of a normal eye. *Upper left:* OCT horizontal cross section with retinal boundaries outlined in *white*. *Lower left:* Retinal thickness plot. *Upper right:* Fundus image showing the scan pattern.

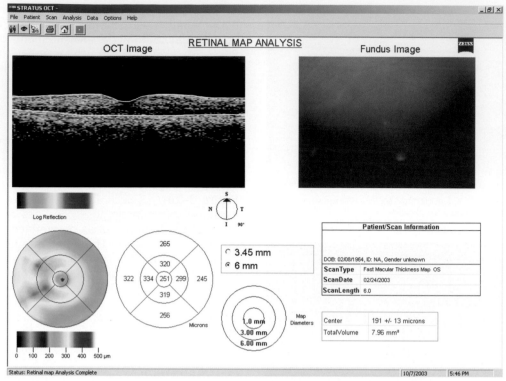

Figure 3–27 Fast macular thickness map of a normal eye. *Upper left:* Vertical OCT cross section with retinal boundaries outlined in *white.* *Lower left:* Color-scale OCT thickness map and sector thickness averages. *Upper right:* Fundus image showing the scan pattern.

The Zeiss OCT software measures the retinal thickness from the inner surface of the NFL to the outer retinal signal complex. Because of the faintness of the ELM signal, the outer surface picked up by the segmentation algorithm is usually what we now believe to be the IS/OS junction (compare **Figures 3–23** and **3–26**). The software does not attempt to search further outward to the RPE border. Therefore, the "retinal thickness" measurement does not include the thickness of the photoreceptor outer segment. This is a developmental holdover from OCT1 images, in which the lower resolution blended the IS/OS junction signal with the RPE signal and the signal complex. Even with the Stratus system, the IS/OS junction and the RPE cannot always be distinguished, especially with attenuated signal levels and in pathologic conditions (i.e., in macular edema). In practice, this minor drawback does not usually affect clinical diagnosis.

3.4 Clinical Applications

OCT has become an indispensable tool to the retina specialist for the diagnosis of macular diseases. Glaucoma is another application for which the precise measurements made possible by OCT are used to diagnose and track the disease. Examples of applications of OCT in major diseases are shown here. More detailed descriptions and correlation with other imaging modalities are shown in later chapters on specific diseases.

3.4.1 MACULAR DISEASES

OCT imaging of macular diseases was first demonstrated by Michael Hee and others at MIT in collaboration with Carmen Puliafito's clinical research group.[11,14–16] The most important applications are macular edema, macular hole, CNV, and CSR.

In cystoid macular edema, the OCT cross-sectional image shows intraretinal cysts in the central macula and loss of the foveal depression on the inner retinal contour (**Figures 3–28** to **3–30**). The retinal thickness map shows increased thickness in the central macula (**Figures 3–28** and **3–29**). The fast macular thickness map pattern provides a better global view of the areas of edema (**Figures 3–28** and **3–29**). However, a more detailed cross-sectional scan (512 A-scan) is useful for confirming the cystoid nature of edema (**Figure 3–30**) and determining whether vitreous traction is a causative mechanism.

In diabetic macular edema (DME), the OCT cross-sectional image shows intraretinal and subretinal fluid accumulation (**Figures 3–31** and **3–32**). The retinal thickness map shows thickening in a distribution that usually matches areas of leakage on a fluorescein angiogram. The area of edema may be localized (**Figure 3–31**) or diffuse. Our example of DME is clinically significant because it involves the central 1-mm-diameter area of the macula. The fast macular thickness map pattern provides a better global view of the area of edema (**Figure 3–31**). However, a more detailed cross-sectional scan (512 A-scan) is useful for confirming whether

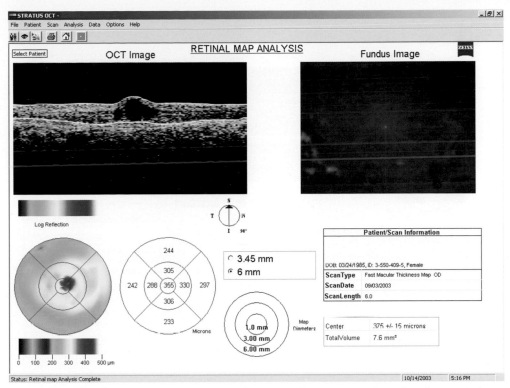

Figure 3–28 Fast macular thickness map scan of mild cystoid macular edema. The OCT image shows foveal intraretinal cysts and the map shows foveal thickening.

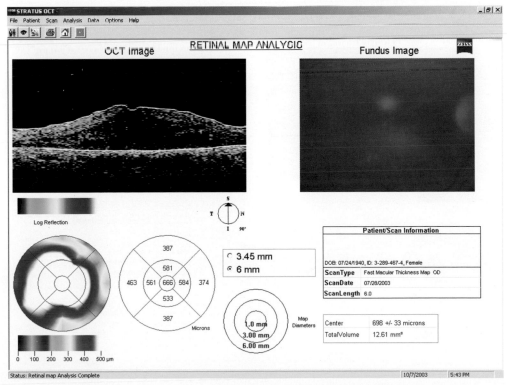

Figure 3–29 Fast macular thickness map scan of severe cystoid macular edema. The OCT image shows intraretinal fluid, and the map shows retinal thickening over a large area.

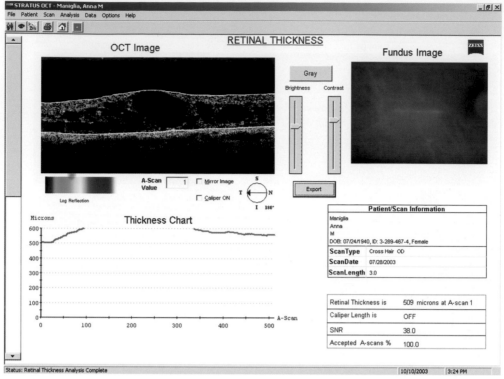

Figure 3–30   Horizontal line scan (3 mm) of severe cystoid macular edema. The detailed image (512 A-scans) shows complex cystic structures.

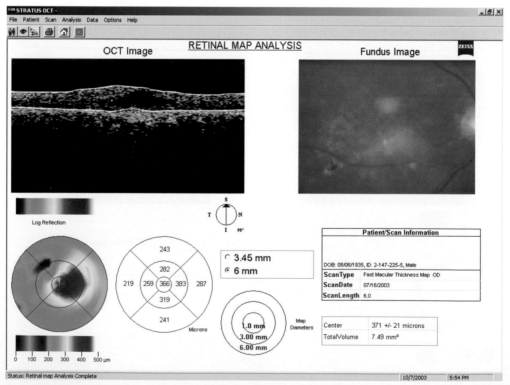

Figure 3–31   Fast macular thickness map scan of localized diabetic macular edema. The cross-sectional image shows retinal thickening and intraretinal fluid. The retinal thickness map shows a region of thickening.

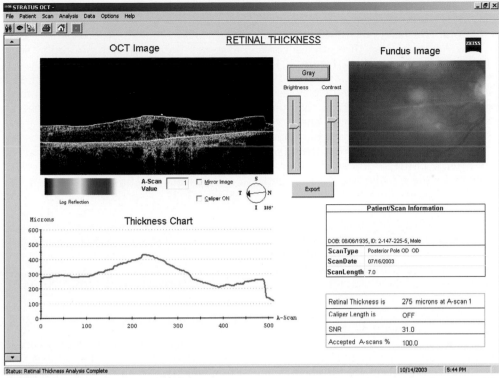

Figure 3–32 Horizontal scan (7 mm) of diabetic macular edema. The OCT image shows a complex pattern of intraretinal fluid space. There is no subretinal fluid nor tractional vitreous membrane in this case.

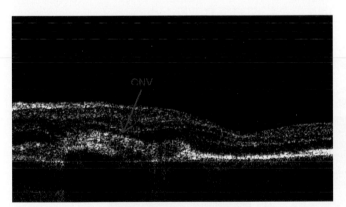

Figure 3–33 OCT line scan image showing a choroidal neovascular membrane located above the RPE.

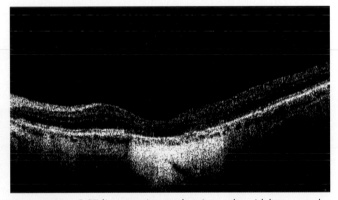

Figure 3–34 OCT line scan image showing a choroidal neovascular membrane located below the RPE. The photoreceptor IS/OS junctional signal is absent above the choroidal neovascular membrane but visible elsewhere.

the fluid accumulation is intraretinal (**Figure 3–32**) or subretinal and whether a vitreous traction is a causative mechanism.

OCT is useful in exudative AMD. In some (but not all) high-quality OCT images, one can visualize whether the choroidal neovascular membrane is above (**Figure 3–33**) or below the RPE (**Figure 3–34**). This information may be useful in the planning of submacular surgery and other therapies. OCT mapping of macular edema and subretinal fluid is also useful in assessing the effectiveness of photodynamic therapy and tracking subsequent reactivation of the choroidal neovascular membrane (CNV).

OCT is also useful for the staging of macular holes (**Figure 3–13**) and the planning of surgical repair.

In CSR, OCT is useful for visualizing retinal detachment (**Figure 3–12**) and RPE detachment.

3.4.2 GLAUCOMA AND OPTIC NERVE DISEASES

The high axial resolution of OCT is ideal for the detection and tracking of glaucomatous damage to the RNFL, ONH, and macula.

The RNFL is the easiest to measure because of its high reflectivity on OCT images. This application was pioneered by Joel Schuman and co-workers in 1995.[28,29]

On the Stratus OCT system, the RNFL is measured by scanning the retina around the optic disc in a 3.4-mm-diameter circular pattern. The "fast RNFL thickness" scan pattern performs 256 A-scan circles three times consecutively. The "RNFL thickness analysis" (**Figure 3–35**) display is used to analyze each circular scan. The cylindrical cross section is unfolded for display as a rectangular image (**Figure 3–35,** *upper left*). A computer algorithm automatically identifies the inner and outer borders of the RNFL and outlines them on the image with thin white lines. The user should inspect the image to confirm that the RNFL borders are drawn correctly. The RNFL thickness from the circular scan is averaged in clockhour sectors, quadrants, and the overall circle. These parameters are again averaged over the three repeat circular scans in the fast RNFL thickness pattern. Because the Stratus system provides normative standards based on measurements from a population of normal eyes, RNFL thickness parameters from an individual can then be compared with the database for percentile classification as either normal (>5%), borderline (1% to 5%), or abnormal (<1%). This is shown in the RNFL thickness average analysis display (**Figure 3–36**). The display shows both right and left eyes side by side to facilitate the identification of any asymmetry. RNFL analysis by OCT has high sensitivity and specificity for glaucoma. The area under the receiver operating curve for Stratus OCT system RNFL parameters in the most recent studies is better than 0.9.[3,23,35] In addition to glaucoma, OCT measurement of the RNFL has also been used in studying traumatic,[22] toxic,[40] and inherited[1] optic neuropathies.

Increased ONH cupping (or rim thinning) is the hallmark of glaucoma and the basis of anatomic diagnosis by human observers. The Stratus OCT system assesses the ONH with six radial scans. A computer algorithm identifies the edges of the optic disc on the RPE plane. The neural rim is identified as tissue above a reference plane that is a fixed distance above the RPE (**Figure 3–37**). Interpolation from the six radials scans provides a map of the rim and cup areas. The rim width and area and the cup/disk area ratios are found to have sensitivity and specificity for diagnosis of glaucoma that are comparable to the RNFL parameters.[23,35]

The average retinal thickness in the macular area (**Figure 3–27**) also provides information on glaucoma, probably based on thinning of the ganglion cell layer. However, clinical data so far suggest that it is not as sensitive and specific as RNFL and ONH parameters.

3.5 Strengths and Limitations

3.5.1 RESOLUTION

High spatial resolution is the primary strength of OCT. The axial resolution of the Stratus OCT system (9 to 10 microns) is at least 10 times better than that of any other noninvasive imaging modality such as ultrasound, x-ray computed tomography (CT), magnetic resonance imaging (MRI), and scanning laser ophthalmoscopy/tomography (SLO/SLT). With further improvement toward ultrahigh resolution (~3 micron axial resolution) and

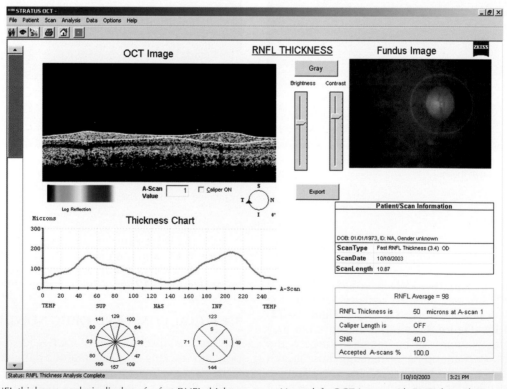

Figure 3–35 RNFL thickness analysis display of a fast RNFL thickness scan. *Upper left:* OCT image with RNFL boundaries outlined in *white*. *Middle left:* RNFL thickness plot. *Lower left:* RNFL thickness averages by clockhours and quadrants. *Upper right:* Fundus image showing scan circle around the optic disc.

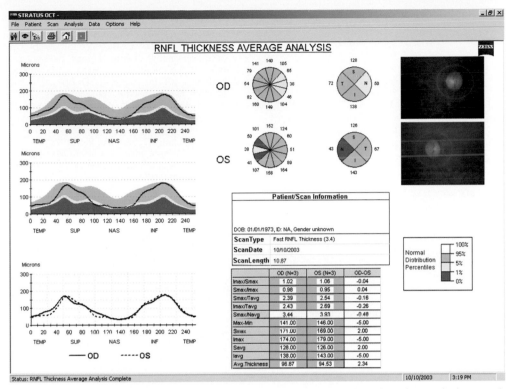

Figure 3–36 RNFL thickness average analysis display of a fast RNFL thickness scan. *Upper left:* Plots of RNFL thickness with reference ranges (*green* = normal, *yellow* = borderline, and *red* = abnormal). *Lower left:* OD/OS RNFL thickness plot to detect asymmetry. *Upper center:* OD/OS color-coded classification of RNFL thickness by clockhours and quadrants.

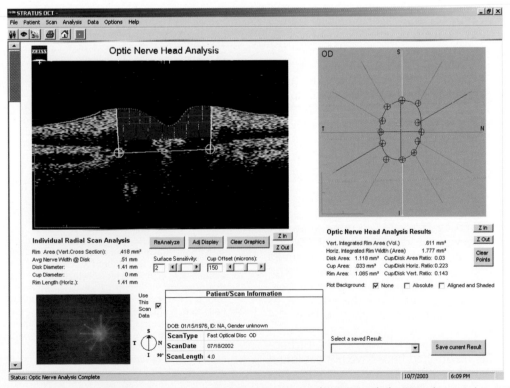

Figure 3–37 ONH display of a fast optic disc scan. *Upper left:* OCT section across the ONH with the RPE edges (*circles*), surface contour, and neural retinal rim (*red hash*) automatically outlined by a computer algorithm. *Lower left:* Fundus image showing six radial scans across the ONH. *Upper right:* Composite drawing of disc (*red*) and cup (*green*) boundaries based on the radial scans (*blue/yellow*).

adaptive optics (5 micron transverse resolution), OCT will further surpass other imaging methods.

3.5.2 PENETRATION

The penetration of OCT is primarily limited by tissue scattering. In highly pigmented tissue such as the RPE, absorption is also significant. In posterior segment imaging, the RPE blocks most of the choroidal signal. Scattering by choroidal blood further decreases the signal from the outer choroid. Therefore, conventional TD-OCT provides limited information on choroidal anatomy except in rare cases of CNV. The increased SNR of FD-OCT may allow better imaging of the choroids because of its deeper penetration. Generally speaking, the reach of OCT is similar to that of SLO/SLT and not as good as that of ultrasound, MRI, and CT.

3.5.3 SPEED

Speed is an important limitation for current retinal OCT systems. When one looks at a Stratus OCT cross section carefully, there is usually some noticeable motion effect in the contour of the RPE. Further inspection of the fundus image may show that the scan is not perfectly centered on the intended landmark such as the optic disc. Most of the motion problem is actually hidden because transverse motion error during the scan does not show up on the single frame of a captured fundus image. Motion and position error are usually not critical for the diagnosis of macular diseases. However, in applications such as glaucoma in which accurate and repeatable measurement of the RNFL and other anatomic parameters is important, motion is a significant issue.

The motion and centration problem should be ameliorated by the introduction of ultrahigh-speed FD-OCT technology into clinical practice. FD-OCT has been demonstrated at 29,000 A-scans/sec or nearly 100 times faster than the Stratus system. With the assumption of 256 to 1024 lines per frame, this translates into 30 to 100 frames/sec, which means that most images should contain no significant biologic motion artifact.

3.5.4 SUMMARY

The spatial resolution of OCT is far better than that of other noninvasive imaging modalities. Speed is currently a major limiting factor for accurate anatomic measurements. However, the development of FD-OCT technology provides an effective solution to the speed problem. Other limitations, such as the limited penetration of OCT into the choroids, are harder to overcome. Furthermore, OCT cannot measure fluorescence or any other inelastic scattering process that destroys the coherence of light.

Because OCT is relatively new, many of the technologic developments mentioned here have not yet found their way into clinical practice. To the researcher, this represents an exciting challenge. The clinician can anticipate that the breadth of applications and ease of use of OCT will continually improve for many years to come.

REFERENCES

1. Barboni P, Savini G, Valentino ML, et al. Retinal nerve fiber layer evaluation by optical coherence tomography in Leber's hereditary optic neuropathy. Ophthalmology. 2005;112:120–126.
2. Boppart SA, Bouma BE, Pitris C, Southern JF, Brezinski ME, Fujimoto JG. In vivo cellular optical coherence tomography imaging. Nat Med. 1998;4:861–865.
3. Budenz DL, Michael A, Chang RT, McSoley J, Katz J. Sensitivity and specificity of the StratusOCT for perimetric glaucoma. Ophthalmology. 2005;112:3–9.
4. Cense B, Chen TC, Park BH, Pierce MC, de Boer JF. In vivo depth-resolved birefringence measurements of the human retinal nerve fiber layer by polarization-sensitive optical coherence tomography. Opt. Lett. 2002;27:1610–1612.
5. Cense B, Chen TC, Park BH, Pierce MC, de Boer JF. Thickness and birefringence of healthy retinal nerve fiber tissue measured with polarization sensitive optical coherence tomography. Invest Ophthalmol Vis Sci. 2004;45:2606–2612.
6. Choma MA, Sarunic MV, Yang CH, Izatt JA. Sensitivity advantage of swept source and Fourier domain optical coherence tomography. Opt Express. 2003;11:2183–2189.
7. de Boer JF, Cense B, Park BH, Pierce MC, Tearney GJ, Bouma BE. Improved signal-to-noise ratio in spectral-domain compared with time-domain optical coherence tomography. Opt Lett. 2003;28:2067–2069.
8. de Boer JF, Milner TE, Nelson JS. Determination of the depth-resolved Stokes parameters of light backscattered from turbid media by use of polarization-sensitive optical coherence tomography. Opt Lett. 1999;24:300–302.
9. Drexler W, Morgner U, Ghanta RK, Kärtner FX, Schuman JS, Fujimoto JG. Ultrahigh-resolution ophthalmic optical coherence tomography. Nat Med. 2001;7:502–507.
10. Gloesmann M, Hermann B, Schubert C, Sattmann H, Ahnelt PK, Drexler W. Histologic correlation of pig retina radial stratification with ultrahigh-resolution optical coherence tomography. Invest Ophthalmol Vis Sci. 2003;44:1696–1703.
11. Hee MR, Baumal CR, Puliafito CA, et al. Optical coherence tomography of age-related macular degeneration and choroidal neovascularization. Ophthalmology. 1996;103:1260–1270.
12. Hee MR, Huang D, Swanson EA, Fujimoto JG. Polarization-sensitive low-coherence reflectometer for birefringence character-ization and ranging. J Opt Soc Am B Opt Phys. 1992;9:903–908.
13. Hee MR, Izatt JA, Swanson EA, et al. Optical coherence tomography of the human retina. Arch Ophthalmol. 1995;113:325–332.
14. Hee MR, Puliafito CA, Wong C, et al. Optical coherence tomography of central serous chorioretinopathy. Am J Ophthalmol. 1995;120:65–74.
15. Hee MR, Puliafito CA, Wong C, et al. Optical coherence tomography of macular holes. Ophthalmology. 1995;102:748–756.
16. Hee MR, Puliafito CA, Wong C, et al. Quantitative assessment of macular edema with optical coherence tomography. Arch Ophthalmol. 1995;113:1019–1029.
17. Hermann B, Fernandez EJ, Unterhuber A, et al. Adaptive-optics ultrahigh-resolution optical coherence tomography. Opt Lett. 2004;29:2142–2144.
18. Huang D, Swanson EA, Lin CP, et al. Optical coherence tomography. Science. 1991;254:1178–1181.
19. Leitgeb RA, Schmetterer L, Drexler W, Fercher AF, Zawadzki RJ, Bajraszewski T. Real-time assessment of retinal blood flow with ultrafast acquisition by color Doppler Fourier domain optical coherence tomography. Opt Express. 2003;11:3116–3121.
20. Leitgeb RA, Schmetterer L, Hitzenberger CK, et al. Real-time measurement of in vitro flow by Fourier-domain color Doppler optical coherence tomography. Opt Lett. 2004;29:171–173.
21. Leitgeb R, Wojtkowski M, Kowalczyk A, Hitzenberger CK, Sticker M, Fercher AF. Spectral measurement of absorption by spectroscopic frequency-domain optical coherence tomography. Opt Lett. 2000;25:820–822.
22. Medeiros FA, Moura FC, Vessani RM, Susanna R Jr. Axonal loss after traumatic optic neuropathy documented by optical coherence tomography. Am J Ophthalmol. 2003;135:406–408.
23. Medeiros FA, Zangwill LM, Bowd C, Vessani RM, Susanna R Jr, Weinreb RN. Evaluation of retinal nerve fiber layer, optic nerve head, and macular thickness measurements for glaucoma

detection using optical coherence tomography. Am J Ophthalmol. 2005;139:44–55.

24. Morgner U, Drexler W, Kartner FX, et al. Spectroscopic optical coherence tomography. Opt Lett. 2000;25:111–113.

25. Nassif N, Cense B, Park BH, et al. In vivo high-resolution video-rate spectral-domain optical coherence tomography of the human retina and optic nerve. Optics Express.2004;12:367–376.

26. Nassif N, Cense B, Park BH, et al. In-vivo human retinal imaging by ultrahigh-speed spectral domain optical coherence tomography. Opt Lett. 2004;29:480–482.

27. Rollins AM, Kulkarni MD, Yazdanfar S, Ung-arunyawee R, Izatt JA. In vivo video rate optical coherence tomography. Opt Express. 1998;3:219–229.

28. Schuman JS, Hee MR, Puliafito CA, et al. Quantification of nerve fiber layer thickness in normal and glaucomatous eyes using optical coherence tomography. Arch Ophthalmol. 1995; 113:586–596.

29. Schuman JS, Pedut-Kloizman T, Hertzmark E, et al. Reproducibility of nerve fiber layer thickness measurements using optical coherence tomography [see comments]. Ophthalmology. 1996; 103:1889–1898.

30. Swanson EA, Izatt JA, Hee MR, et al. In vivo retinal imaging by optical coherence tomography. Opt Lett. 1993;18:1864–1866.

31. White BR, Pierce MC, Nassif N, et al. In vivo dynamic human retinal blood flow imaging using ultra-high-speed spectral domain optical Doppler tomography. Opt Express. 2003;11:3490–3497.

32. Wojtkowski M, Bajraszewski T, Targowski P, Kowalczyk A. Real-time in vivo imaging by high-speed spectral optical coherence tomography. Opt Lett. 2003;28:1745–1747.

33. Wojtkowski M, Kowalczyk A, Leitgeb R, Fercher AF. Full range complex spectral optical coherence tomography technique in eye imaging. Opt Lett. 2002;27:1415–1417.

34. Wojtkowski M, Leitgeb R, Kowalczyk A, Bajraszewski T, Fercher AF. In vivo human retinal imaging by Fourier domain optical coherence tomography. J Biomed Opt. 2002;7.457–463.

35. Wollstein G, Ishikawa H, Wang J, Beaton SA, Schuman JS. Comparison of three optical coherence tomography scanning areas for detection of glaucomatous damage. Am J Ophthalmol. 2005;139:39–43.

36. Yazdanfar S, Rollins AM, Izatt JA. Imaging and velocimetry of the human retinal circulation with color Doppler optical coherence tomography. Opt Lett. 2000;25:1448–1450.

37. Yazdanfar S, Rollins AM, Izatt JA. Noninvasive imaging and velocimetry of human retinal blood flow using color Doppler optical coherence tomography. Invest Ophthalmol Vis Sci. 2000;41:S548–S548.

38. Zhao YH, Chen ZP, Saxer C, et al. Doppler standard deviation imaging for clinical monitoring of in vivo human skin blood flow. Opt Lett. 2000;25:1358–1360.

39. Zhao YH, Chen ZP, Saxer C, Xiang SH, de Boer JF, Nelson JS. Phase-resolved optical coherence tomography and optical Doppler tomography for imaging blood flow in human skin with fast scanning speed and high velocity sensitivity. Opt Lett. 2000;25:114–116.

40. Zoumalan CI, Agarwal M, Sadun AA. Optical coherence tomography can measure axonal loss in patients with ethambutol-induced optic neuropathy. Graefes Arch Clin Exp Ophthalmol. Nov 23, 2004 [Epub ahead of print].

Chapter 4

Optical Coherence Tomographic Ophthalmoscopy

RICHARD B. ROSEN, MD, FACS • ADRIAN PODOLEANU, PhD •
SHANE DUNNE, PhD • PATRICIA M. T. GARCIA, MD

4.1 Introduction

Retinal imaging moved beyond the confines of classical optics in the early 1980s with the introduction of the scanning laser ophthalmoscope (SLO) by Webb, Pomeranzeff, and colleagues at the Schepens Eye Research Institute.[6,29] High-resolution, nonmydriatic images composed of sequential streams of reflected points revealed the fundus surface in exquisite detail, often despite cataracts or other media opacities. The discrete method of illumination and image assembly also offered the capability of introducing complex stimuli for perimetry and acuity testing. However, this technique is still subject to the optical limitations of the eye, fixing its maximum resolution at about 300 microns—greater than the maximum thickness of the retina.

Optical coherence tomography (OCT) was developed almost a decade later, through the efforts of Fujimoto, Huang, Puliafito, and associates at the Massachusetts Institute of Technology.[10,26] For the first time, clinicians could study cross-sectional images of the macula, optic nerve, and anterior segment with near-histologic resolution in the living eye. By using the technique of low-coherence interferometry, resolutions in the 10- to 15-micron range could be achieved, dependent solely on the bandwidth of the light source.[7,32] This technology has been commercialized by Carl Zeiss, Inc. As exciting as these new images appeared, it soon became apparent that precise correlation with standard fundus views was very difficult to achieve.

An innovative fusion of SLO and OCT technologies, which we now call OCT *ophthalmoscopy*, was achieved by Podoleanu, Jackson, and associates at the University of Kent at Canterbury (UKC) in 1995.[15–17,23,28] Combining the transverse or C-scan acquisition approach of SLO with the optical processing methods of OCT, the UKC device generates simultaneous pairs of images that document both surface anatomy and subsurface detail. Use of a single illuminating source to produce both images ensures point-to-point correspondence, permitting accurate overlays and accurate location of B-scan OCT slices with respect to the SLO image. This technology is presently under commercial development by Ophthalmic Technologies, Inc. (OTI) (Toronto, ON, Canada). Its unique features and clinical images are the subject of this chapter.

4.2 Technical Principles

The fundamental principles of OCT are presented in detail elsewhere in this book. This chapter focuses on the distinctive aspects of the OCT ophthalmoscopy approach.

4.2.1 CONCEPT

Figure 4–1A–C illustrates the basic concept of OCT ophthalmoscopy. Subsurface structure, obtained by OCT, is related (ideally in three dimensions) to surface landmarks on an accompanying SLO image.

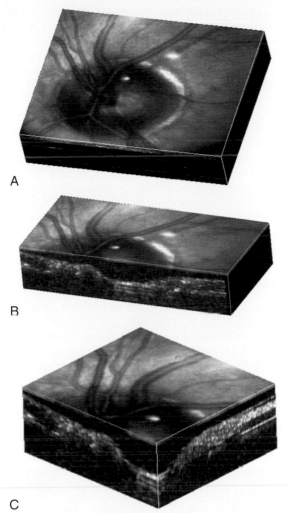

A

B

C

Figure 4–1 Concept of OCT ophthalmoscopy: a block of tissue is imaged with OCT for subsurface structure, and a simultaneously acquired SLO image provides an accurate positional reference (*A*). Cutting into the block reveals OCT cross sections (*B* and *C*). True three-dimensional OCT ophthalmoscopy as shown here is not always practical in the clinic, but the principle of SLO-based landmarking can be usefully applied to individual B-scan and C-scan OCT images as well.

4.2.2 SCANNING ABC'S

Refer to **Figure 4–2.** In OCT, as in ultrasound, an A-*scan* is a one-dimensional scan along the depth axis (usually close to the optical axis of the eye). In ultrasound, A-scan data are sometimes presented individually as graphs of signal strength versus depth, but in OCT (as in ultrasound) A-scans are usually captured in groups and assembled to form B-scans. A B-*scan* is a cross-sectional image in which signal strength is translated to brightness. In OCT, a B-scan is also called a *longitudinal* image.[8]

A C-*scan*, also called a *transversal* or *en face* image, is a cross-sectional image acquired on a plane at a fixed distance (depth) from the scanning apparatus. C-scans are not yet widely used in ophthalmology, but they are not entirely unknown. Their orientation is similar to that

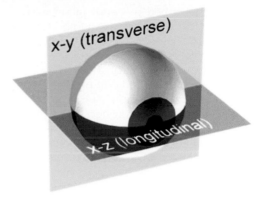

Figure 4–2 A-, B-, and C-scan orientations defined relative to the eye. An *A-scan* is a one-dimensional scan along the depth axis. A *B-scan* is any two-dimensional cross section in which one axis is the depth axis. A *C-scan* is a two-dimensional cross section in which all points have the same depth. Three-dimensional scans can be assembled as stacks of parallel B- or C-scans.

of the coronal scans used in radiology. Three-dimensional (3D) ultrasound systems can reconstruct C-scans from a captured set of B-scan images, and scanning confocal devices such as the Heidelberg HRT and HRA also produce C-scans.

The C-scan orientation is particularly interesting, because the arrangement of detail in the image corresponds to that seen in fundus photographs.

4.2.3 SCANNING STRATEGIES: SCAN ACQUISITION SEQUENCE

B- and C-scan images consist of a matrix of pixels. Conventional OCT systems, such as the Stratus OCT machine made by Carl Zeiss Meditec, Inc. (Dublin, CA), use a fast-moving reference mirror (*z*-dimension) within the interferometry optics and a slower-moving scanning mirror for transverse (*xy*-dimensions) scanning: as a result they capture B-scans one pixel-*column* at a time, as a sequence of A-scans. This *z*-priority scanning sequence is similar to the way ultrasound B-scans are assembled—as a series of A-scan lines captured rapidly as the transducer sweeps laterally across the target at a much slower rate.

The principle used in ultrasound imaging, in which time-of-flight events are registered, is difficult to extend to optical waves owing to the much greater speed of light. To obtain images based on the time of flight of light for micron-scale tissue structures would require electronic devices to respond to femtosecond temporal events. No such devices exist. Therefore, researchers have found a way around this limitation of OCT with the use of interferometry to allow low-speed electronics to track matching of temporal events happening on a femtosecond scale.[10]

In OCT (except for spectrometric OCT), all dimensions are scanned mechanically, and so the question of which dimension is scanned most rapidly and which less rapidly is one of engineering. The research group at UKC, whose work is described in detail in the next section, designed their OCT apparatus using a fast-moving transverse (*xy*-dimensions) scanning mirror and a much slower interferometry reference mirror (*z*-dimension). In this *xy*-priority scanning sequence, the B-scan and C-scan images are assembled one pixel-*row* at a time.[9]

The order of scan acquisition is unimportant in theory but very important in practice when the target is a living eye. During the time period required to assemble a single image, the eye will exhibit saccadic, micro-saccadic, and drift motions laterally, and there will also be motion along the Z or depth axis owing to head motion and pulsatile blood flow in the retina.[3] The *z*-priority scanning used in the Zeiss OCT system and the *xy*-priority scanning strategy used in the UKC design have different strengths and weaknesses, of which diagnosticians should be keenly aware.[25]

In *z*-priority scanning, the target area is repeatedly probed with fast A-scans. This allows for accurate detection of Z-axis motions, which manifest as imperfect alignment of adjacent pixel columns. By using suitable image-processing techniques, this effect can be compensated for entirely automatically; this is a major strength of *z*-priority scanning. It is not possible, however, to detect or compensate for lateral eye motion during the scan. This effectively means there is no

guarantee that the B-scan image actually contains backscattering events all from the same vertical position if the lateral movement was horizontal or all from the same horizontal position if the lateral movement was vertical and implies that any lateral measurements are suspect.

In *xy*-priority scanning, the target is repeatedly imaged in lateral stripes at different depths. This ensures that lateral measurements are accurate (because each line scan is fast enough to freeze even rapid eye movements) but provides no assurance that the pixels in each en face scan originate from the same target or that the image has not been compromised by Z-axis motion of the eye. By using information in the same OCT image, movements along the fast scanning direction (*x* or *y*) can be corrected by information acquired from the SLO image. This is illustrated in **Figures 4–3** and **4–4**.

Three-Dimensional Scanning

Modern digital imaging systems make it practical to consider scanning in three dimensions rather than just two. A 3D OCT scan, for example, could be built up from a series of closely spaced, parallel B- or C-scans. Scanning in three dimensions takes much longer than scanning in only two dimensions, because many more data points (voxels) are required. When the living eye is scanned, the question of which dimension is scanned least frequently becomes important, because the eye

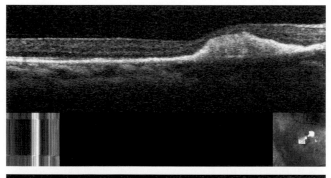
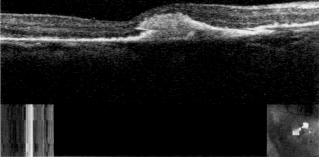

Figure 4–3 Detecting lateral motion in B-scans. Each pair of images features an OCT B-scan image *above* and the corresponding vertical stripes (*lower left*) and image obtained on the SLO channel (*lower right*). The stripes on the *top* show a highly regular structure, indicating little or no lateral motion of the eye during scan. We can thus confidently assume that the corresponding B-scan OCT image (*above*) represents a true planar cross section of the fundus. The stripes on the image *below* show variation from top to bottom, indicating that the scanned area of the fundus has changed between the beginning and the end of the scan, i.e., the eye has moved. The corresponding OCT image (*bottom right*) should be considered suspect.

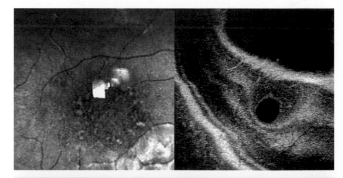
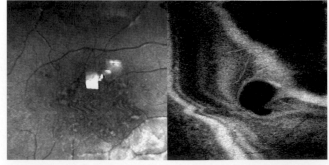

Figure 4–4 Detecting saccadic motions in C-scans. These two SLO/OCT image pairs were captured in the course of a 3D scan sequence. The SLO image on the *top left* shows a clean view of the fundus. The SLO image on the *bottom left* shows a characteristic "tearing" appearance, because the eye moved rapidly about two-thirds of the way through the scan from top to bottom of the frame. Interestingly, in this case the eye also moved back to approximately its original position immediately after the brief saccade.

is likely to move as the scan progresses. Hence, with current scanning technology, 3D OCT is not yet practical for all patients in the clinic.

In Praise of the C-Scan

C-scan OCT images are an unfamiliar format, but as has been the case with all other diagnostic imaging modalities in the past, experience brings understanding. The most compelling aspect of C-scan OCT images is that the layout is comparable to that of well-understood fundus photographs; every C-scan OCT image comes with a companion SLO fundus image that makes this layout obvious. In fact, there is a precise point-to-point correspondence between the paired images. To exploit the utility of this association, software has been developed that allows marking or encircling specific features on either image that then appear on its matching image. In addition, an adjustable transparency feature on the SLO image invites a view of the underlying C-scan OCT slice through the window of the SLO surface features. This display permits the observer to easily understand the relationship between surface landmarks and subsurface anatomy (**Figure 4–5A–D**).

C-scan OCT images can, however, be difficult to interpret in isolation, because what is imaged is a slab of tissue less than 15 microns thick. There is a tendency for individual slices to appear patchy because of the way the scanning plane intersects with curved layers of the retina. Tilting of the macular plane due to normal saccadic shifts even under the influence of controlled fixation often splays overlying retinal layers from their vertical orientation to reveal multiple depth structures within a single slice. Interpretation therefore depends upon understanding of this unique orientation and recognition of these movement-induced artifacts. Simulation of C-scanning has been attempted in cutting of histopathologic specimens and computer animation

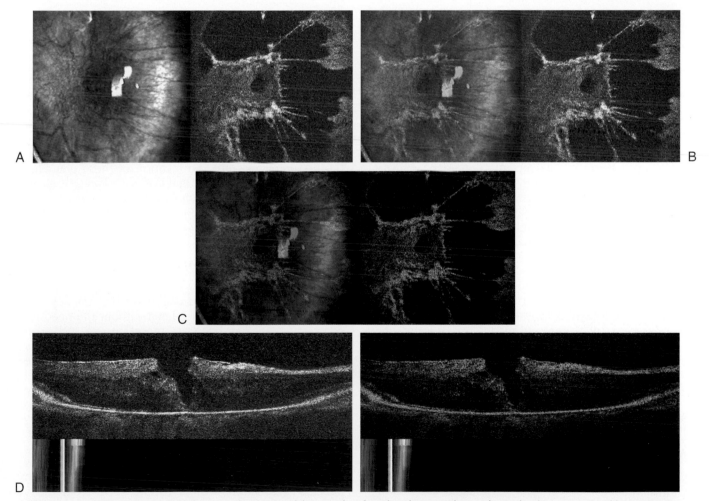

Figure 4–5 *A:* The image on the *left* is a confocal view of the retinal surface that shows evidence of vascular distortion caused by contraction of the surface membrane. On the *right* the C-scan OCT image reveals the ridges of the membrane surface. *B:* With the overlay feature of the software, the pair of images reveal the contours of the membrane in relation to vessels that may be valuable in planning the surgical approach. *C:* The overlay effect is enhanced by the use of pseudo-color. *D:* B-scan OCT slices emphasize the constriction of the foveal cone and the tractional flattening of the inner retinal surface induced by the membrane, creating the illusion of a full-thickness macular hole on clinical examination.

models developed to further familiarize and orient clinicians to the images.

Three additional techniques have been explored to enhance the readability of the C-scans: (1) combining multiple adjacent OCT images to increase the effective slab thickness; (2) 3D reconstruction; and (3) successive and repetitive switching of the system from B-scan to C-scan and vice versa. The first technique approximates the lower axial resolution of the SLO, masking much of the granular detail revealed by the OCT processing. The second technique is more versatile, preserves the OCT features, and is used in the clinical prototypes built by UKC and OTI. Its full implementation is currently still limited to the most cooperative subjects, but the stacks of images collected reveal most of the essential aspects of the 3D form while still maintaining the resolution of the original scans. The third technique is the method of choice when the patient is noncooperative or lacks fixation. 3D stacking of C-scans is not feasible, however, because switching the system between orthogonal acquisition directions leads to filling gaps in the 3D profile the user tries to generate in her or his own mind.

4.3 Clinical Examples

This section presents a series of recent cases from the New York Eye and Ear Infirmary, concentrating on OCT ophthalmoscopy results obtained using a prototype of the OTI/UKC imaging system.

Most of the image examples in this chapter are presented in gray scale rather than the false-color representation popularized by Zeiss. The superiority of gray-scale representation was recently argued by Ishikawa and colleagues.[11] The combination of a semitransparent gray-scale SLO with a false-color C-scan OCT image provides a powerful superimposition of surface and depth. However, the color thresholding, although pleasing in appearance, often masks considerable fine anatomic detail, negating some of the benefits of the technology.

A key aspect of C-scan imaging to consider in evaluating clinical studies is the ability and necessity of reviewing the full sequence of slices and not merely an isolated scan as with conventional B-scan OCT imaging. The assembly of features from different depths when examined alongside associated B-scans presents a comprehensive picture of the internal anatomy of the subject (**Figure 4–6A–D**).

4.3.1 DISTURBANCES AT THE VITREORETINAL INTERFACE

Macular Pucker

OCT has been especially helpful in conditions requiring surgical management. C-scan OCT imaging extends this utility by providing the surgeon with a perspective seen under the surgical microscope. This case of macular pucker due to an epiretinal membrane demonstrates the effect. The first pair of images (see **Figure 4–6A**) of

this example show the confocal view on the *left* with the corresponding C-scan OCT image on the *right*. The C-scan image shows a characteristic stellate pattern of epiretinal membrane proliferation, which is difficult to appreciate in the confocal fundus image despite the notable vascular pattern distortion.

Macular Hole

Confirmation of macular hole development and staging was one of the earliest recognized advantages observed after the introduction of B-scan OCT imaging. Early clinical diagnosis was able to move from the subjective visual symptoms, using the Watzke sign, to objective findings in the cross-sectional images. C-scan OCT images expand upon this facility, presenting the orthogonal component of the anatomy, which demonstrates the encircling garland of cystic formations that develop surrounding the central dehiscence. The appearance is flower-like, changing with almost kaleidoscopic fluidity as the sequence of images of increasing depth in **Figure 4–7A–E** demonstrate.

4.3.2 DISTURBANCES OF THE INNER RETINA

Diabetic Maculopathy

The microvascular events that cause diabetic maculopathy produce an array of space-occupying lesions, ranging from remodeled vascular structures with proteinaceous fluid accumulations and hemorrhages to fibrous membranes that distort the normal anatomy through cicatricial contraction. B-scan OCT images gave the first glimpses into the location of these elements within the depths of the retinal layers. C-scan OCT slices further expand on these visual descriptions by providing the contextual surroundings of specific structures (**Figure 4–8A–C**)

Cystoid Macular Edema (Aphakic, Pseudophakic, or Uveitic)

The ability to confirm and document the diagnosis of suspected cystoid macular edema without the need for contrast agents has been an important use of B-scan OCT imaging since its introduction. The availability of the en face perspective adds to the sensitivity of the technique because it often only involves a segment of the perifoveal capillary circle early in the course of the disease and may be missed by single B-scan OCT cuts. In addition, several varieties of the condition display anatomic changes without involving fluorescein leakage, such as retinitis pigmentosa, nicotinic acid maculopathy, and hereditary juvenile X-linked retinoschisis, that show up on OCT. The multilobulated nature of the lesion appears as a section through a sponge or piece of Swiss cheese. With resolution of the acquired forms of the condition after anti-inflammatory treatment, OCT nicely demonstrates the collapse of cysts and restoration of the normal anatomy (**Figure 4–9A–C**).

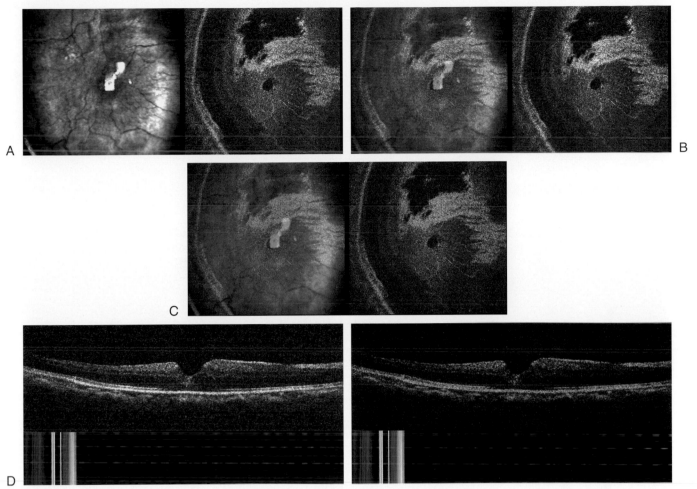

Figure 4–6 *A:* After pars plana vitrectomy and membrane peeling, macular vessels and contour relax to a more normal configuration (*left*). The C-scan OCT image (*right*) reveals some residual sweep of distortion superiorly in the macular periphery. *B:* The overlay mode localizes the persistent edema in relation to the surface features highlighted in the confocal image. *C:* The pseudo-color version of the overlay helps differentiate the surface features from those of the inner retina. *D:* Corresponding B-scan OCT slices display the restoration of fovea curvature in cross section.

Hereditary Cystoid Macular Edema—Juvenile X-Linked Retinoschisis

Changes in this condition can be seen on OCT imaging (**Figure 4–10A** and **B**).

4.3.3 DISTURBANCES OF THE OUTER RETINA

Central Serous Retinopathy

The neurosensory retinal detachments and retinal pigment epithelium (RPE) detachments that are the anatomic lesions of this disorder have characteristic appearances and are particularly well suited for diagnosis and monitoring with OCT imaging. The points of leakage found with fluorescein angiography are often flat and may not be readily detected with this technology; however, these lesions are rarely treated. Clinical improvement in acute conditions generally parallels restoration of macular anatomy, which is revealed by OCT (**Figure 4–11A–L**).

RPE Detachment

Elevation of the RPE shows up as a bright "ring of light" on C-scan OCT images because the RPE region is the most highly reflective component of the retinal image. Viewed in cross-section using B-scan OCT, the bright line actually appears to be composed of three layers that are thought to include the external limiting membrane, a region of outer retina-RPE interdigitation, and the actual RPE layer itself. The enclosed region in the lesion is usually dark if it is serous in composition but may appear brighter if the elevation is due to hemorrhage as is often the case with polypoidal choroidal vasculopathy (**Figure 4–12 A** and **B**).

Myopic Staphyloma

Myopic distension of the globe and the accompanying retinal degeneration is a challenging disorder that heretofore has defied adequate explanation or been treated satisfactorily. Appreciation of the geometry of

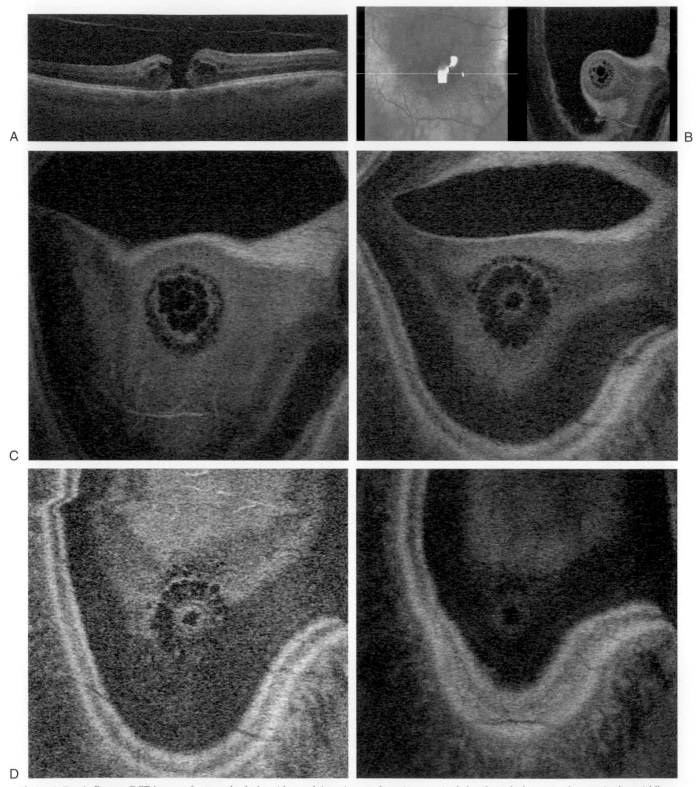

Figure 4–7 *A:* B-scan OCT image of a macular hole with overlying vitreous face. Inner retinal details include cystic changes in the middle layers and elevated edematous edges of the hole. *B:* Confocal image of the hole (with reflex artifact) (*left*) shows radial distortion of the retina converging on the hole. The C-scan OCT image (*right*) cuts through cysts surrounding the hole. *C–E:* C-scan OCT slices at progressively deeper levels reveal the complex cystic changes in the perifoveal macula, which appear like the variety of petal configurations of chrysanthemum flowers. As the hyperreflective base of the hole is reached, details of surrounding choroidal vessels are seen.

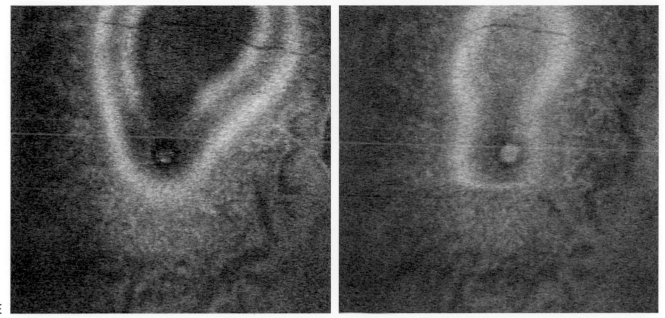

E

Figure 4–7—cont'd

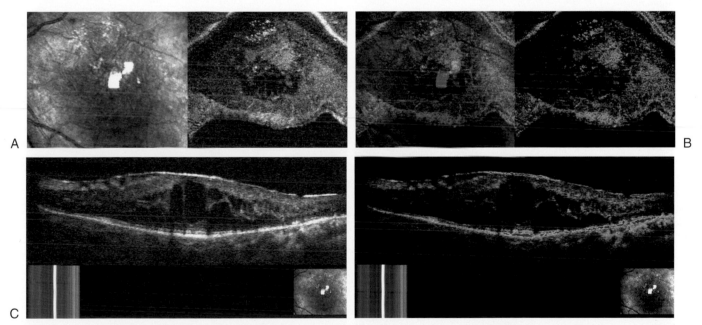

A

B

C

Figure 4–8 *A:* Confocal image (*left*) shows scattered hemorrhages, edema residues, and loss of foveal reflex. C-scan OCT image (*right*) reveals the multilobulated cystic configuration of the edematous macula. *B:* Color overlay images of the cystic changes. *C:* B-scan OCT image and color overlay of the same region reveal the location of the cysts within the middle retinal layers.

these changes is often additionally hampered by the extreme optics of the crystalline lens in affected eyes, which add distortion and further challenge the examiner's understanding of the particular anatomy. The coronal slicing strategy of C-scan OCT overcomes some of the apparent flattening of conventional ophthalmoscopy and outlines the area of protrusion of the posterior pole. When viewed in the overlay mode, the can be distention related to specific fundus features (**Figure 4–13A–C**).

4.3.4 DISTURBANCES OF THE RETINA-CHOROID INTERFACE

Drusen

These warty excrescences on Bruch's membrane exemplify the notion of the mysterious within the commonplace. Their appearance often signifies an underlying disturbance in physiology that threatens the onset of degenerative change, but the time course is quite

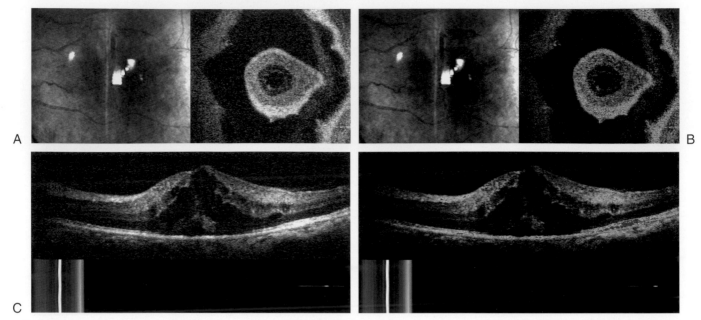

Figure 4–9 *A:* Confocal imaging (*left*) of the macula demonstrates minimal changes. C-scan OCT image (*right*) reveals a garland of perifoveal cysts similar to that seen with diabetic maculopathy or macular holes. *B:* Color overlay highlights the extent of swelling in relation to the surface features of the confocal image. *C:* B-scan OCT image and color overlay show the full extent of cystic degeneration of the middle layers of the retina.

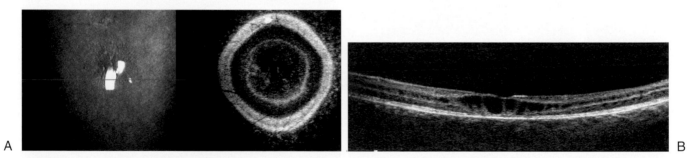

Figure 4–10 *A:* Confocal image of juvenile X-linked retinoschisis (*left*) demonstrates the classic spoke wheel appearance of the macula. C-scan OCT image (*right*) reveals fine cystic changes. *B:* B-scan OCT image shows the relative flatness of the retina compared with the appearance of acquired cystoid macular edema.

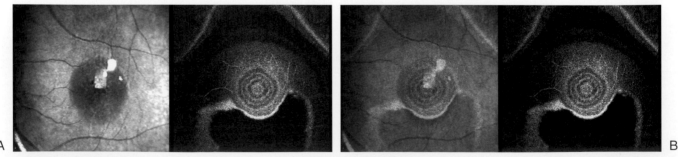

Figure 4–11 *A:* Confocal image (*left*) suggests central macular elevation due to loss of normal foveal sheen. C-scan OCT image (*right*) demonstrates a characteristic "bulls-eye" pattern produced by planar slicing through the dome-shaped elevation of the neurosensory retina. The concentric pattern of alternating light and dark rings appears to parallel the alternating layers of the retina seen histologically or with B-scan OCT. *B:* Overlay image pairs demonstrate how the concentric pattern follows the elevation contour.

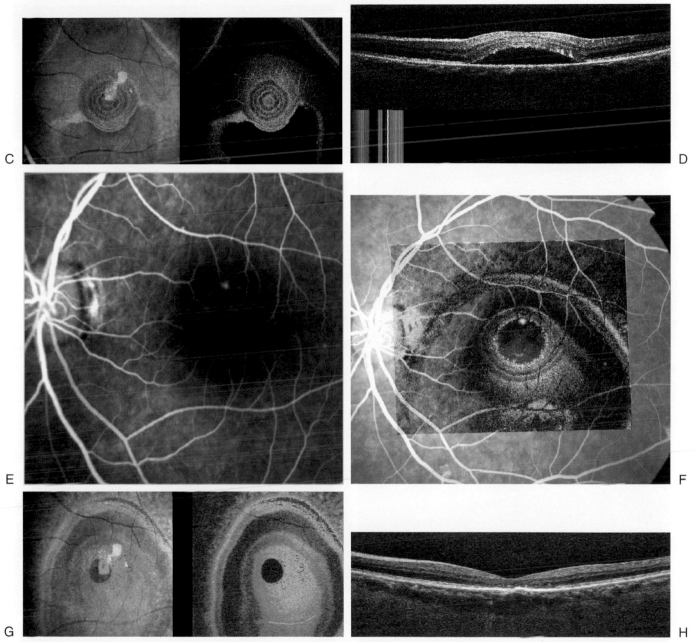

Figure 4–11—cont'd *C:* Overlay image pairs demonstrate how the concentric pattern follows the elevation contour. *D:* B-scan OCT image highlights the subretinal blister of fluid responsible for the convex geometry of retinal displacement. The tightness of the rings in the C-scan image appears to directly relate to the small radius of curvature of the blister. *E* Fluorescein angiogram reveals a focal spot of hyperfluorescence in the macula. *F:* C-scan OCT overlay localizes the spot at the upper edge of the blister. *G:* After laser treatment to the hyperfluorescent spot, the blister resolved with restoration of foveal depression. *H:* B-scan OCT image shows restoration the macular contour in cross section.

Continued

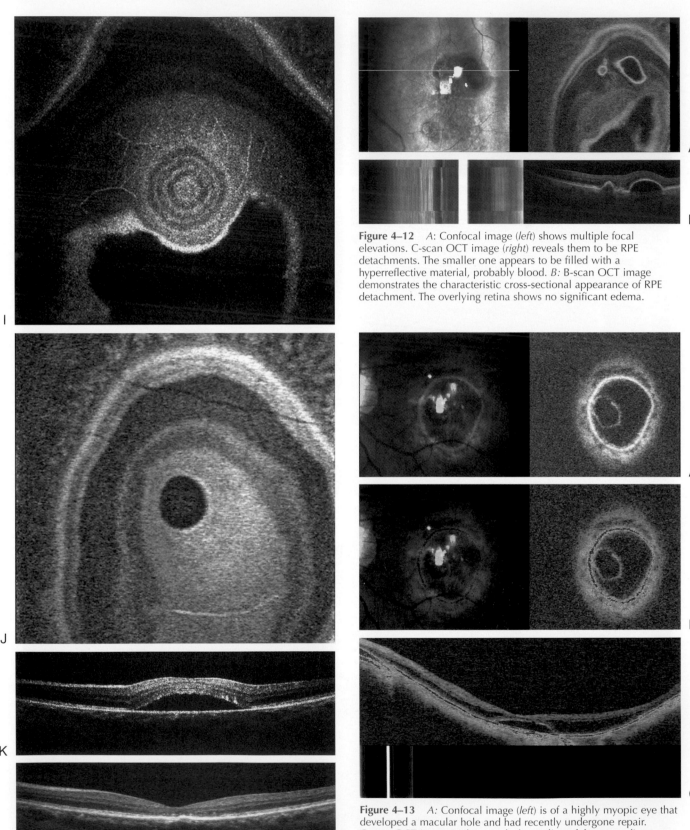

Figure 4–12 *A:* Confocal image (*left*) shows multiple focal elevations. C-scan OCT image (*right*) reveals them to be RPE detachments. The smaller one appears to be filled with a hyperreflective material, probably blood. *B:* B-scan OCT image demonstrates the characteristic cross-sectional appearance of RPE detachment. The overlying retina shows no significant edema.

Figure 4–11—cont'd *I–L:* Side-by-side comparison of macular anatomy before and after treatment.

Figure 4–13 *A:* Confocal image (*left*) is of a highly myopic eye that developed a macular hole and had recently undergone repair. C-scan OCT image (*right*) reveals the outline of the protruding cone. The choroidal features are seen outside the bright RPE region, and a small inner circle corresponds to an area of persistent serous detachment beneath the closed hole. *B:* Color overlay versions of the same image pair localize the edge of the staphyloma and the serous bleb against the surface fundus features. *C:* Corresponding B-scan OCT image shows the complex anatomy in cross section.

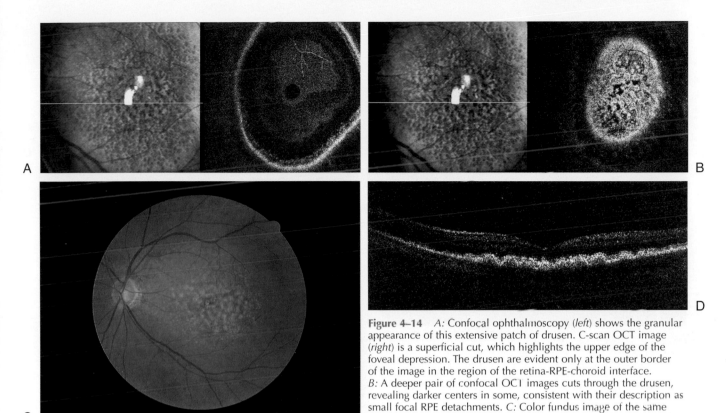

Figure 4–14 *A:* Confocal ophthalmoscopy (*left*) shows the granular appearance of this extensive patch of drusen. C-scan OCT image (*right*) is a superficial cut, which highlights the upper edge of the foveal depression. The drusen are evident only at the outer border of the image in the region of the retina-RPE-choroid interface. *B:* A deeper pair of confocal OCT images cuts through the drusen, revealing darker centers in some, consistent with their description as small focal RPE detachments. *C:* Color fundus image of the same eye. *D:* B-scan OCT cross section shows the normal contour of the inner retina overlying the granular RPE region.

variable. The near-infrared wavelengths used by the OCT ophthalmoscope penetrate to a level beneath the retina that highlight these disturbances (**Figure 4–14A–D**).

Choroidal Neovascular Membranes

Neovascular membranes that develop from choroidal vessels and extend into the sub-RPE and subretinal spaces create complex lesions featuring areas of hemorrhage, serous detachment, cystoid edema, and fibrosis. Attempts to characterize these lesions using fluorescein angiography have been somewhat disappointing and misleading, producing descriptive terms that acknowledge their own limitations, e.g., occult, Although B-scan OCT can help dissect the various layers and components, understanding of the convoluted layout of these components requires the broad picture of the standard ophthalmoscopic perspective **Figure 4–15A–C**).

Idiopathic Polypoidal Choroidal Vasculopathy

Polypoidal choroidal vasculopathy often presents with hemorrhagic events and is reported more commonly in pigmented populations that typically do not develop choroidal neovascular membranes.[31] Characteristic lesions include poorly defined collections of hemorrhagic RPE detachments, dilated choroidal vessels, and subretinal hemorrhage that lack any neovascular focus.

C-scan OCT is able to capture the complexity of these fundi and complement the selective cross-sectional imaging of B-scan OCT (**Figure 4–16A–C**).

Integration of Confocal Indocyanine Green Angiography and OCT Imaging

The simultaneous dual-imaging design of the OCT ophthalmoscope opens the possibility of incorporating angiographic studies in the confocal channel. The similarity of operating spectra between OCT and indocyanine green imaging allowed development of a system that could utilize the same illumination source for the two functions, maintaining the precise correspondence between paired images. Because the OCT B- and C-scans are also precisely related, it becomes feasible to use fluorescent phenomena in the confocal channel to guide acquisition of B-scan cross sections (**Figure 4–17A–H**).

4.4 Next Steps

OCT ophthalmoscopy is a exciting new fusion of clinical imaging technologies at an early stage of what promises to be a multidimensional, multimodal vehicle for retinal exploration. Expansion of the initial efforts discussed in this chapter will feature integration—a variety of tools aimed to develop "functional OCT." Refinement of

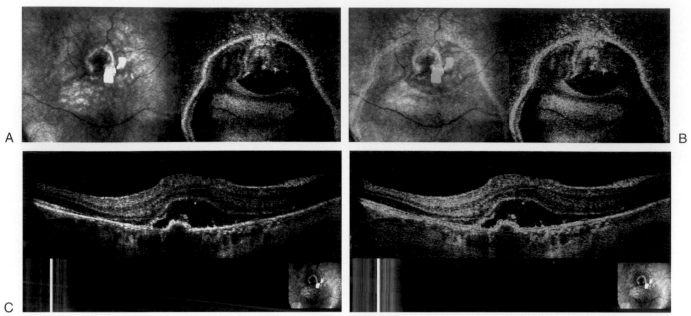

Figure 4–15   *A:* Confocal image (*left*) of a macula with a subfoveal choroidal neovascular membrane (CNVM) complex surrounded by drusen. C-scan OCT image (*right*) shows a slight downward tilt with a splaying of the layers. The CNVM is seen extending through the RPE zone with a dark circular space that can be partially seen below surrounding the vascular mass. *B:* Color overlay versions of the same image pair reveal how the serous elevation relates to the surface features of the fundus. *C:* B-scan OCT image pair provide the cross-sectional perspective of the same slices, showing the thickening of the overlying retina and the pocket of serous fluid overlying the membrane.

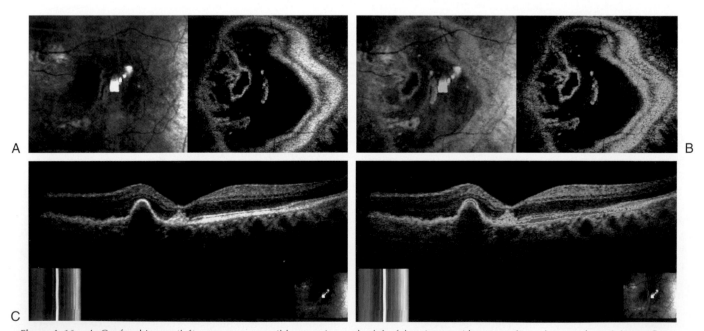

Figure 4–16   *A:* Confocal image (*left*) suggests some mild convexity on the *left* of the picture with surrounding edema and precipitates. C-scan OCT (*right*) reveals a heterogeneous collection of RPE detachments. *B:* Color overlay versions of the same image pair. The overlay on the *left* shows the outline of the normally hidden underlying lesions against the surface features of the macula. *C:* B-scan OCT images reveal the RPE detachment, dilated choroidal vessels, thickened RPE region, and edema precipitates on the RPE.

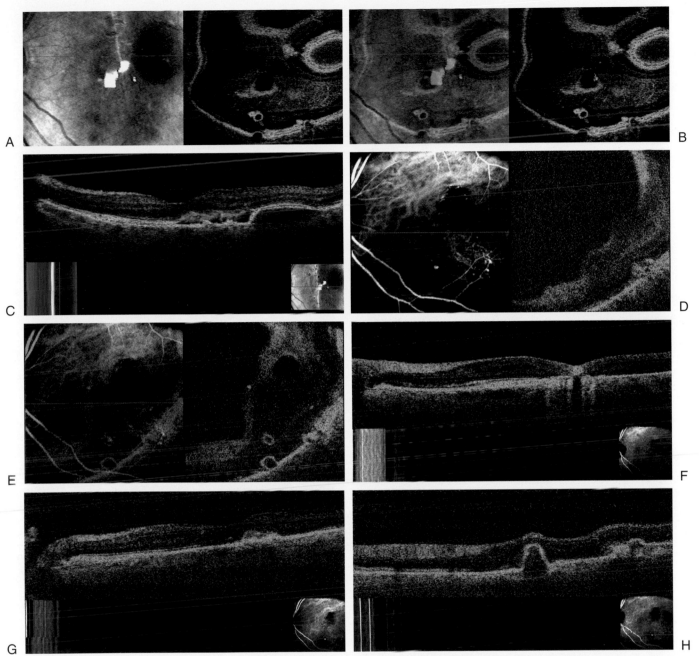

Figure 4–17 *A:* Confocal image (*left*) shows a large, dark, round lesion along with several smaller lesions. C-scan OCT image (*right*) highlights the multiple RPE detachments, including the one in the *upper right,* which appears hemorrhagic, and a central black circle that represents the foveal depression. *B:* Color overlay images outline the RPE detachments against the surface features shown in the confocal picture. *C:* B-scan OCT image shows the subretinal complex in cross section pretreatment. *D:* Simultaneous confocal ICG angiogram (*left*) with paired C-scan OCT image (*right*) after focal laser treatment to the source of the hemorrhagic RPE detachment. The ICG angiogram shows a variety of hyperfluorescent lesions. The OCT image shows invasion through the RPE into the subretinal space. *E:* Color overlay image (*left*) with matching C-scan OCT image (*right*) showing area of vascular leakage within one of several RPE detachments. *F:* B-scan OCT image through an area of macula treated with a laser showing a focal scar. *G:* B-scan OCT image through the central macula showing the foveal depression with a temporal area of RPE thickening. *H:* B-scan OCT image through the lower area of the macula in a region of multiple RPE detachments.

hardware and software will allow more rapid acquisition to enable fully automated 3D imaging, higher resolution, topographic mapping, Doppler blood flow, and spectral analysis.[1,2,4,5,13,14,18–20,30] As OCT ophthalmoscopy evolves and becomes available to more investigators and clinicians, the tremendous expansion of experience and observations can be expected to foster better appreciation of the information contained within its images.[12]

REFERENCES

1. Bouma BE, Tearney GJ, Bilinsky IP, et al. Self-phase-modulated Kerr-lens mode-locked Cr:forsterite laser source for optical coherence tomography. Opt Lett. 1996;21:1839–1841.

2. Bouma B, Tearney GJ, Boppart SA, et al. High-resolution optical coherence tomographic imaging using a mode-locked Ti:Al$_2$O$_3$ laser source. Opt Lett. 1995;29:1486–1488.

3. Carpenter RHS. Movements of the Eyes. 2nd ed. London, England: Pion, 1988.

4. Drexler W, Morgner U, Kärtner FX, et al. In vivo ultrahigh-resolution optical coherence tomography. Optics Lett. 1999;24:1221–1223.

5. Drexler W, Morgner U, Ghanta RK, et al. Ultrahigh-resolution ophthalmic optical coherence tomography. Nat Med. 2001; 7:502–507.

6. Elsner AE, Burns SA, Weiter JJ, et al. Infrared imaging of subretinal structures in the human ocular fundus. Vision Res. 1996; 36:191–205.

7. Gilgen HH, Novak RP, Salathe RP, et al. Submillimeter optical reflectometry. J Lightwave Technol 1989;7:1225–1233.

8. Hecht E, Zajac A. Optics. 4th ed. Reading, Mass: Addison-Wesley, 2001.

9. Henney K, ed. Radio Engineering Handbook. 5th ed. New York, NY: McGraw-Hill Book Co, 1959.

10. Huang D, Swanson EA, Lin CP, et al. Optical coherence tomography. Science. 1991;254:1178–1181.

11. Ishikawa H, Gurses-Ozden R, Hoh ST, et al. Grayscale and proportion-corrected optical coherence tomography images. Ophthalmic Surg Lasers. 2000;31:223–228.

12. Podoleanu AG, Charalambous I, Plesea, L,Dogariu A, Rosen RB. Correction of distortions in OCT imaging of the eye. Phys Med Biol. 2004;49:1277–1294.

13. Podoleanu AG, Dobre GM, Cucu RG, et al. Sequential OCT and confocal imaging. Opt Lett. 1995;29:364–366.

14. Podoleanu AG, Dobre GM, Cucu RG, et al. Combined multiplanar optical coherence tomography and confocal scanning ophthalmoscopy. J Biomed Opt. 2004;9:86–93.

15. Podoleanu AG, Dobre GM, Jackson DA. En-face coherence imaging using galvanometer scanner modulation. Opt Lett. 1998;23:147–149.

16. Podoleanu AG, Dobre GM, Webb DJ, et al. Coherence imaging by use of a Newton rings sampling function. Opt Lett. 1996; 121:1789–1791.

17. Podoleanu AG, Dobre GM, Webb DJ, et al. Fiberised set-up for retinal imaging of the living eye using low coherence interferometry. In: IEE Colloquium on Biomedical Applications of Photonics, London, 1997. IEE Seminar Digest Ref No. 1997/124. London, England: Institution of Electrical Engineers, 1997.

18. Podoleanu AG, Dobre GM, Webb DJ, et al. Simultaneous enface imaging of two layers in the human retina by low coherence reflectometry. Opt Lett. 1997;22:1039–1041.

19. Podoleanu AG, Rogers JA, Dobre GM, et al. Multi-planar OCT/confocal ophthalmoscope in the clinic. In: Ophthalmic Research, Supplement. Basel, Switzerland: S Karger; 2002:112.

20. Podoleanu AG, Rogers JA, Jackson DA. Dynamic focus applied for correct determination of flow speed of a biological liquid using OCT. In: Kim BY, Hotate, K, eds. OFS-13, International Conference on Optical Fiber Sensors, Kyongju, Korea, 12–16 April, 1999. Proceedings of SPIE. Vol. 3746. Bellingham, WA: SPIE, 1999:288–291.

21. Podoleanu AG, Rogers JA, Jackson DA, et al. Three-dimensional OCT images from retina and skin. Opt Express. 2000;7:202–298.

22. Podoleanu AG, Rogers JA, Jackson DA. OCT En-face images from the retina with adjustable depth resolution in real time. IEEE J Selected Top Quantum Electron 1999;5:1176–1184.

23. Podoleanu AG, Rogers JA, Webb DJ, et al. Compatibility of transversal OCT imaging with confocal imaging of the retina in vivo. In: SPIE Conference on Coherence Domain Optical Methods in Biomedical Science and Clinical Applications III, San Jose, Calif, 27–29 January 1999. Proceedings of SPIE. Vol. 3598. Bellingham, Wash: SPIE; 1999:61–67.

24. Podoleanu AG, Rogers JA, Webb DJ, et al. Criteria in the simultaneous presentation of the images provided by a stand alone OCT/SLO system. In: EUROPTO Conference on Lasers in Ophthalmology, Stockholm, Sweden, 11–12 September 1998. Proceedings of SPIE. Vol 3564. Bellingham, Wash: SPIE; 1998:163–168.

25. Podoleanu AG, Seeger M, Dobre GM, et al. Transversal and longitudinal images from the retina of the living eye using low coherence reflectometry. J Biomed Opt. 1998;3:12–20.

26. Puliafito CA, Hee MR, Schuman JS, et al. Optical coherence tomography of ocular diseases. Thorofare, NJ: SLACK; 1996.

27. Saleh BEA, Teich MC. Fundamentals of photonics. New York, NY: John Wiley & Sons, 1991.

28. Seeger M, Podoleanu AG, Jackson DA. Preliminary results of retinal tissue imaging using coherence radar technique. In: Applied Optics Division Conference, Reading (UK), 16–19 September 1996. Bristol, England: IOP Publishing, 1996.

29. Webb RH, Hughes GW, Pomeranzeff O. Flying spot TV ophthalmoscope. Appl Opt. 1980;19:2991–2997.

30. Wojtkowski M, Leitgeb R, Kowalczyk A, et al. In vivo human retinal imaging by Fourier domain optical coherence tomography. J Biomed Opt 2002;7:457–463.

31. Yanuzzi LA, Flower RW, Slatker JS, eds. Indocyanine Green Angiography. St Louis, Mo, Mosby; 1997.

32. Youngquist RC, Carr S, Davies DEN. Optical coherence-domain reflectometry: a new optical evaluation technique. Opt Lett. 1987;12:158–160.

Chapter 5

Ultrasound

FIONA J. EHLIES, BSC (HONS), RDMS •
DIANE CHIALANT, RN, RDMS, ROUB •
CATHY W. DiBERNARDO, RN, RDMS, ROUB

5.1 Physical Principles

Ophthalmic ultrasound echography uses high-frequency sound waves (ultrasound) to obtain images of intra ocular pathologic changes. A piezoelectric crystal, contained within a hand-held probe, emits ultrasonic waves that then penetrate the ocular structures. As the sound wave encounters the various ocular structures, some of the energy is reflected back to the transducer. The reflected sound waves (echoes) are converted to electrical signals by the transducer and processed for display on the monitor or screen. This conversion is referred to as the *piezoelectric effect*. Depending on the acoustic impedance of the adjacent media, the amount of the energy being reflected back to the probe will vary. This variation in reflected energy produces the image on the oscilloscope screen. The gain or sensitivity setting changes the intensity of the echoes, but not the energy from the transducer. To obtain accurate diagnostic information, the clinician must understand that the velocity or speed of sound depends on the media through which it is passing. In ophthalmic ultrasound for diagnostic purposes the average tissue velocity used is 1550 m/sec. Distance measurements are obtained by multiplying the velocity times the time it takes for the sound wave to travel to a reflective interface and return to the probe. The distance in millimeters is automatically displayed on the screen when measurement cursors are placed. The frequency of the ultrasound wave generated by the probe is measured in megahertz (MHz): 10 MHz indicates that the ultrasound oscillates at a rate of 10 million cycles/sec. It is useful to remember that the higher the frequency, the shorter the wavelength and the better the resolution. However, higher-frequency ultrasound is more quickly absorbed by tissue and has reduced penetration. Typically, the frequencies used in ophthalmic ultrasound imaging are higher than those used in other organ systems because of the relatively small size of the eye and its superficial location. The frequency of the sound wave depends on the probe being used.

A one-dimensional ultrasound scan is called an A-*scan* because the amplitude of echoes is plotted as vertical height against distance along the axis of ultrasound propagation (see **Figure 5–3A**). A two-dimensional ultrasound scan is called a B-*scan*, for which the amplitude of echoes is represented by brightness on a gray-scale image (see **Figure 5–3B**). The image is typically fan shaped because the ultrasound beam is scanned by changing the direction of propagation but not the position of the transducer.

A standardized A-scan probe has a non-focused 8-MHz transducer that emits a parallel sound beam. The design of the amplifier in this equipment makes it more sensitive to variations in tissue. Standardized echography refers to an examination using a specifically designed A-scan probe and a specific decibel setting or tissue sensitivity, combined with B-scan evaluation for the detection and differentiation of intraocular pathologic lesions. The specialized A-scan probe used for axial biometry measurements has a focused sound beam and a 10-MHz transducer that gives a one-dimensional image and cannot be used to differentiate one tissue from another.

There are four types of B-scan probes. The most commonly used probe has a frequency of 10 MHz (**Figure 5–1**) and is used to examine the posterior segment. There are two probes with higher frequencies (20 MHz): one is designed specifically for evaluation of the anterior segment, lens, and ciliary body and a newer one is designed for evaluation of the posterior segment (**Figure 5–2**). Ultrasound biomicroscopy, using 50 to 100 MHz, is also available for evaluation of the anterior segment.

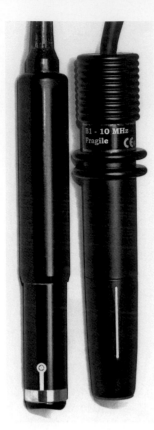

Figure 5–1 Examples of 10-MHz B-scan probes.

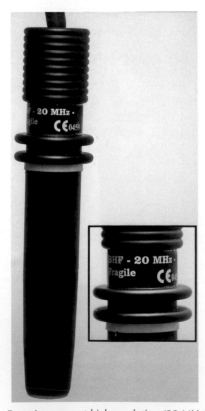

Figure 5–2 Posterior segment high-resolution (20-MHz) B-scan probe.

5.2 Technology Development

Ultrasound has been used in ophthalmology for more than 40 years. In 1956 Mundt and Hughes were the first to use an A-scan technique for tumor detection. Shortly thereafter, in 1958, Baum and Greenwood developed an immersion B-scan to document intraocular pathologic lesions. Bronson and Turner developed the first commercially available contact B-scan machine in 1972, and from this early technology rapid improvements were made in the equipment, as ultrasound examinations became easier for the patients to tolerate and for the sonographers and technicians to perform and interpret. Basically, all ultrasound machines have a probe, pulse emitter, receiver, amplifier, signal processor, and display screen. Ossoinig believed that to allow for reproducible comparisons and differentiation of intraocular pathologic conditions among different echographers, a standardization of instrumentation and techniques was needed. His work in the 1960s and 1970s led to the development of the standardized A-scan. The practice of standardized echography produces reproducible differentiation of intraocular tissues.

5.3 Image Interpretation

5.3.1 STANDARDIZED A- AND B-SCANS

With the patient reclined, the basic examination of the posterior segment is performed in a systematic fashion using specific examination techniques to ensure that all areas of the eye are screened. Both the standardized A-scan and the B-scan may be used. The A-scan is composed of a series of one-dimensional vertical deflections from a baseline, and the B-scan is a series of multiple bright dots. The denser the echo source on the A-scan becomes, the higher the spike produced. Similarly, the denser the echo on the B-scan becomes, the brighter the dot. Generally pathologic lesions are seen as a combination of a point-like, membrane-like, band-like, or mass-like source. The histologic structure of the pathologic lesion is reflected in the standardized A-scan. A normal A-scan (**Figure 5–3A**) has a flat baseline, and a normal B-scan (**Figure 5–3B**) shows a black or echolucent vitreous cavity. It is essential that the echographer be able to build a three-dimensional picture from the two-dimensional B-scan topographic images obtained. This information is combined with the standardized A-scan vertical echo patterns and properties observed during the dynamic examination to interpret the diagnostic findings.

5.3.2 OPACITIES AND MEMBRANES

Opacities and membranes within the vitreous show up echographically as bright echoes on the B-scan or as vertical deviations from the baseline on the A-scan. Various forms of vitreous opacities can be detected with

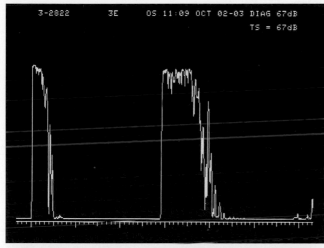

A

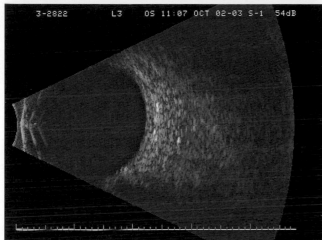

B

Figure 5–3   Normal echograms. *A:* A-scan. *B:* B-scan.

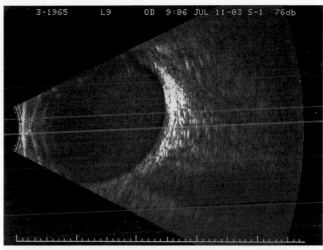

Figure 5–4   Diffuse hemorrhage filling the vitreous cavity.

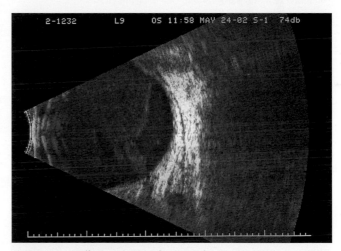

Figure 5–5   Diffuse vitreitis with a partial posterior vitreous detachment, adherent to the peripapillary fundus, and subhyaloid opacities.

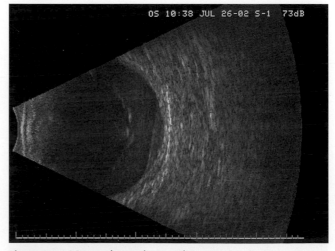

Figure 5–6   Vitreous hemorrhage with a posterior vitreous detachment and diffuse subhyaloid hemorrhage, some of which is layered on the posterior fundus.

ultrasound, but they may have a similar appearance, echographically; e.g., vitreous hemorrhage (**Figure 5–4**) and vitritis (**Figure 5–5**) can only be differentiated with the aid of clinical history.

Vitreous hemorrhage or opacities that are layered on the posterior fundus have a distinctive appearance (**Figure 5–6**) on the B-scan. The surface of the layered opacities may appear flat, and the opacities may slowly slide over the fundus as the patient moves his or her eyes or turns his or her head.

Asteroid hyalosis, due to calcium soaps within the vitreous, produces a unique image (**Figure 5–7**) on the B-scan with highly reflective echoes floating within the vitreous. These echo sources exhibit a swirling motion with eye movement that makes them distinctive.

Elevated membranes within the globe can be differentiated by their echographic characteristics (brightness and thickness on the B-scan, spike thickness and height on the A-scan, and their mobility on both A- and B-scans), which can vary a great deal. Vitreous membranes are generally highly mobile, and they usually appear thin on both A- and B-scans (**Figure 5–8A** and **B**).

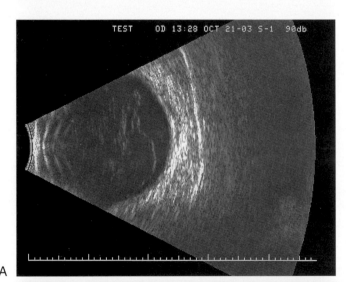

Figure 5–7 Asteroid hyalosis showing many bright echoes contained within a posterior vitreous detachment.

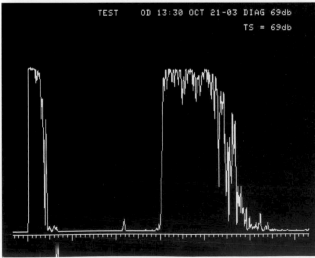

Figure 5–8 *A:* B-scan of vitreous opacities and thin posterior vitreous detachment. *B:* A-scan of posterior hyaloid, showing only a very low reflective posterior hyaloid spike in the mid-vitreous.

5.3.3 RETINA

Sometimes a vitreous membrane may have an acoustic appearance similar to that of an extensive retinal detachment on the B-scan (**Figure 5–9A** and **B**), and in these instances standardized echography is crucial for differentiating one from the other. By evaluating the mobility on both B- and A-scans and the spike height on the A-scan the two membranes can usually be differentiated. Retinal detachments are usually less mobile and have a more dense, folded appearance on the B-scan (**Figure 5–10A**) and almost always exhibit a 100% spike on the A-scan (**Figure 5–10B**).

Retinoschisis can usually be identified by the smooth, dome-shaped appearance on the B-scan (**Figure 5–11A**) and a 100%, very thin, slightly mobile spike on the A-scan (**Figure 5–11B**). Evaluation of the other eye for the presence of a similar membrane in the same location can also be useful in making this diagnosis.

5.3.4 CHOROID

Choroidal detachments (**Figure 5–12A**) are always thicker on the B-scan and do not insert into the optic disc. On A-scan evaluation, a maximally high (100%), double-peaked spike will be produced (**Figure 5–12B**).

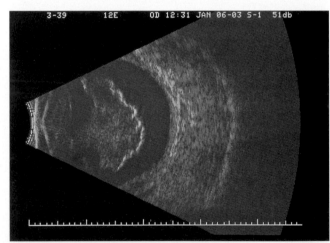

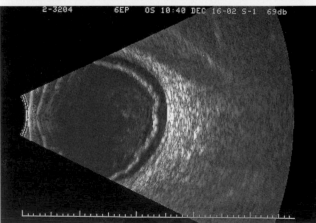

Figure 5–9 *A:* Vitreous hemorrhage with a posterior vitreous detachment. *B:* Vitreous hemorrhage with a retinal detachment and subretinal hemorrhage.

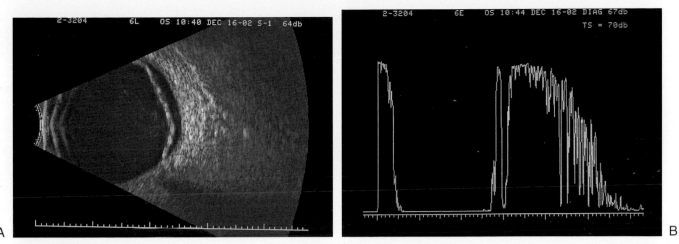

Figure 5–10 Retinal detachment. *A:* B-scan showing folded membrane inserting into the disc. *B:* A-scan showing 100% high retinal spike.

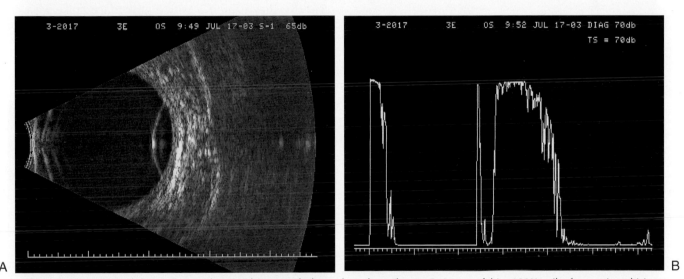

Figure 5–11 Retinoschisis. *A:* B-scan showing thin, smooth dome-shaped membrane. *B:* A-scan of thin, 100% spike from retinoschisis.

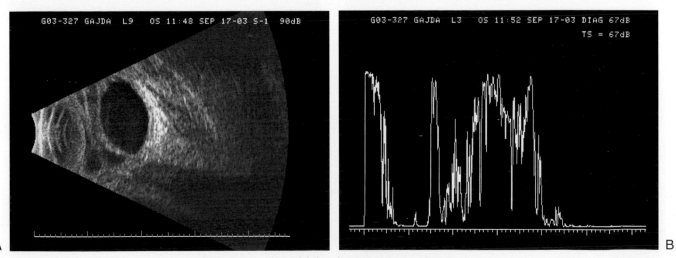

Figure 5–12 Choroidal detachment. *A:* B-scan. *B:* A-scan.

5.3.5 INTRAOCULAR TUMORS

A large amount of information can be obtained about the acoustic features of intraocular tumors by using the techniques of standardized echography, thus aiding in their differentiation and management. Assessing the shape, internal structure and reflectivity, degree of sound attenuation, and presence or absence of internal vascularity can yield a diagnosis of the type of tumor that is present. Standardized echography can also be useful in tracking the size and internal characteristics of a lesion for changes, either during serial observation or after treatment.

Some intraocular tumors have very distinctive echographic characteristics. Choroidal melanomas typically exhibit regular internal structure, low to medium reflectivity, and strong sound attenuation (**Figure 5–13**), and vascularity can usually be detected. They may present in one of several shapes, the most common being a dome shape (**Figure 5–14**). A collar-button shape may be seen (**Figure 5–15A** and **B**) when a tumor has broken through Bruch's membrane. Ultrasound is also helpful in diagnosing extrascleral extension of melanoma into the orbit (**Figure 5–16**).

Several predominantly dome-shaped lesions, which are regularly structured but usually highly reflective and nonvascular, are nevi (**Figure 5–17A** and **B**), choroidal hemangioma (**Figure 5–18A** and **B**), and melanocytoma (**Figure 5–19**).

Other intraocular lesions that can be differentiated using standardized echography include metastatic tumors, which typically have a somewhat lobulated shape (**Figure 5–20A** and **B**), and disciform lesions, which tend to be irregularly shaped (**Figure 5–21**) and structured, and nonvascular.

Osteomas exhibit very distinctive echographic features that include an extremely high reflective, plaque-like image on the B-scan (**Figure 5–22A**), with marked shadowing of the orbital tissue. On the A-scan (**Figure 5–22B**), they exhibit a very high surface spike with an absence of echoes posterior to the lesion. This absence of echoes represents shadowing because all of the sound is being absorbed by the calcified tumor.

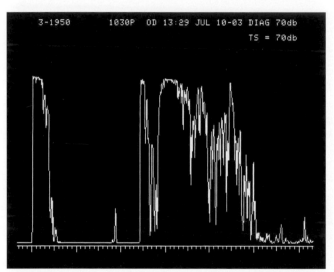

Figure 5–13 A-scan of melanoma with mainly low to medium internal reflectivity.

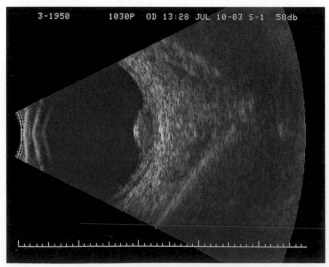

Figure 5–14 Dome-shaped melanoma.

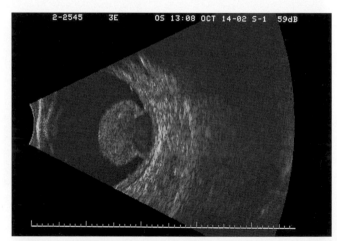

A

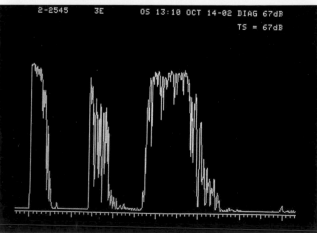

B

Figure 5–15 *A:* B-scan of collar-button–shaped melanoma. *B:* A-scan showing mainly medium internal reflectivity of the button of the lesion and very low reflectivity of the base.

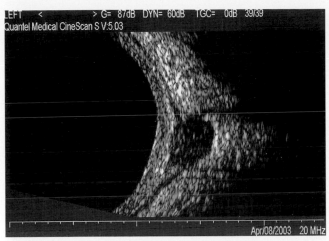

Figure 5–16 High-resolution B-scan of extrascleral extension of a melanoma after radiation plaque therapy.

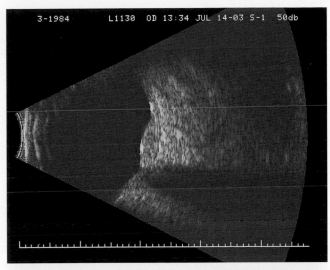

A

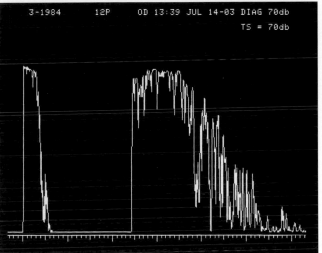

B

Figure 5–18 *A:* B-scan of a dome-shaped choroidal hemangioma. *B:* A-scan showing regular internal structure and high internal reflectivity.

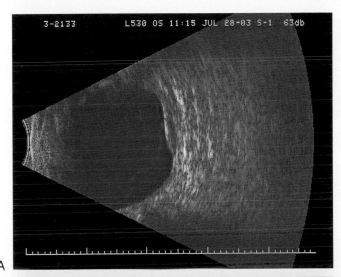

A

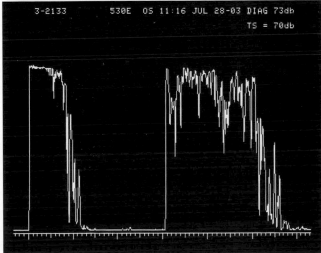

B

Figure 5–17 *A:* B-scan of a dome-shaped nevus. *B:* A-scan showing regular internal structure and medium to high internal reflectivity.

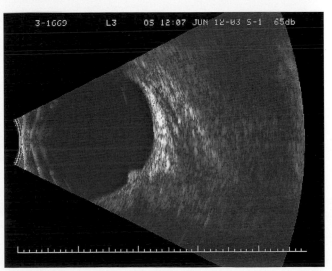

Figure 5–19 B-scan of a small dome-shaped melanocytoma at the optic nerve head.

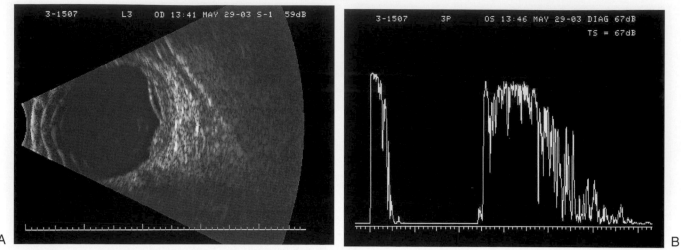

Figure 5–20 *A:* B-scan of a lobulated metastatic lesion with a shallow overlying retinal detachment. *B:* A-scan showing a slightly irregular structure.

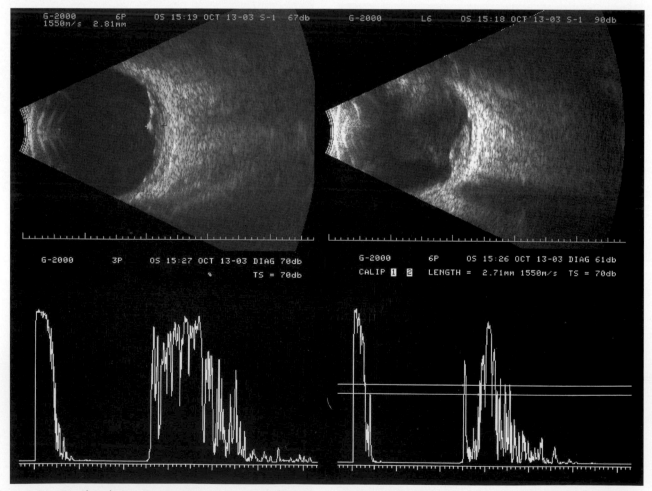

Figure 5–21 Disciform lesion. *Top:* Transverse B-scan on (*left*) and longitudinal on (*right*). *Bottom:* A-scan at tissue sensitivity (*left*) and at measuring sensitivity (*right*).

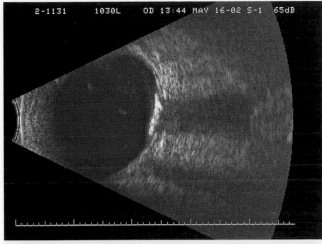

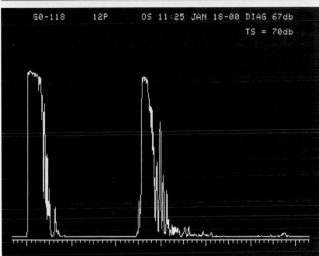

Figure 5–22 *A:* Calcified osteoma with marked shadowing. *B:* A-scan of a highly reflective surface spike and nearly total absorption of posterior echoes.

Figure 5–23 Retinoblastoma with vitreous seeding and shadowing from marked calcification.

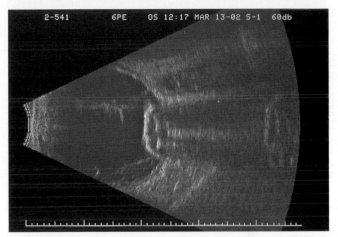

Figure 5–24 Dislocated, calcified lens lying on the fundus and causing shadowing of the orbital tissues.

Retinoblastomas (**Figure 5–23**) can vary in shape but generally exhibit high internal reflectivity. Marked orbital shadowing is usually present due to the high calcium content.

5.4 Clinical Applications

Ultrasound has numerous uses in ophthalmology. It can be used to evaluate the posterior segment of the eye when the ophthalmoscopic view is hindered due to the presence of opaque media, including corneal opacification, cataracts, and vitreous hemorrhage or opacities from inflammation or infection. In these cases the sonographer can evaluate the posterior segment for the presence or absence of any atypical pathologic change such as a mass lesion or retinal detachment. This evaluation can be particularly valuable before surgery to help avoid surprises (**Figure 5–24**).

When hemorrhage is very dense, ultrasound can often reveal and localize a retinal tear (**Figure 5–25A** and **B**).

When elevated membranes are present, a skilled echographer can often differentiate one membrane from another. Ultrasound is very helpful in diagnosing and documenting total retinal detachments (**Figure 5–26**) as well as the extent of a retinal detachment and whether or not the detachment has a tractional component (**Figure 5–27A** and **B**). It can also be useful in assessing the elevation and extent of choroidal detachments and whether or not they are "kissing" (**Figure 5–28**). When retinal or choroidal detachments are present, ultrasound can be used to determine whether there is serous or hemorrhagic fluid in the underlying space (**Figure 5–29A** and **B**).

Tumor differentiation and measurement are important aspects of echography. This test is also helpful to the clinician in the observation of lesions or to evaluate changes in their dimensions and characteristics after treatment.

Another valuable use for ultrasound in ophthalmology is in the localization of intraocular foreign bodies (**Figure 5–30**). Certain objects, such as glass and metal,

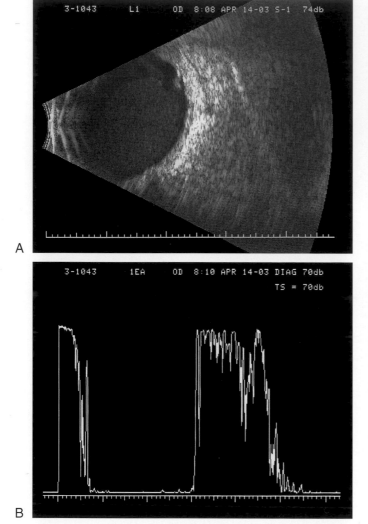

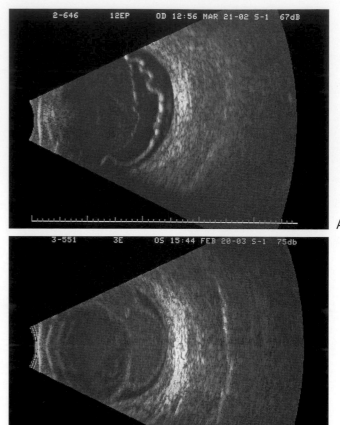

Figure 5–27 *A:* Exudative retinal detachment. *B:* Posterior hyaloid is adherent to the retina, causing a traction retinal detachment.

Figure 5–25 *A:* Posterior hyaloid adherent to a small, peripheral retinal tear. *B:* A-scan showing a highly reflective spike from retinal tear.

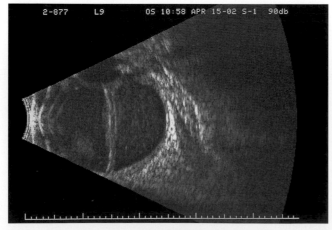

Figure 5–26 Total, closed funnel-shaped retinal detachment, adherent to the posterior lens surface, with subretinal opacities.

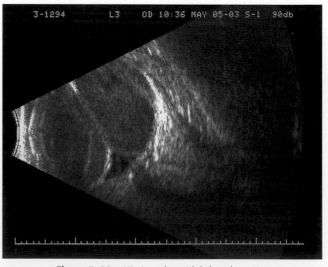

Figure 5–28 Kissing choroidal detachments.

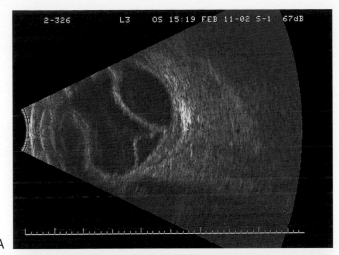

A

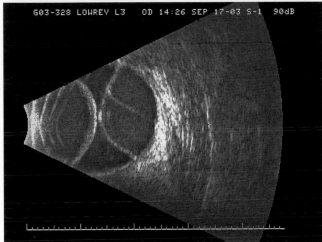

B

Figure 5–29 *A:* Serous choroidal detachments with posterior retinal detachment. *B:* Hemorrhagic, nearly kissing choroidal detachments. Note the vortex vein extending from the choroid to the sclera.

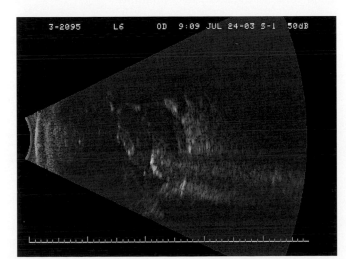

Figure 5–30 Intraocular foreign body (BB gun injury) presents as a very bright echo (with marked reverberations) among the lower reflective echoes of the hemorrhage.

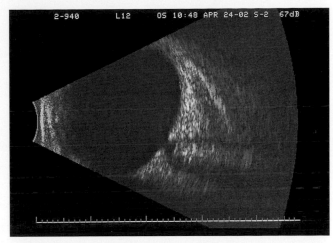

Figure 5–31 Longitudinal B-scan showing a large optic nerve cup.

reflect sound waves strongly and produce distinctive echoes on the oscilloscope. Other foreign bodies, such as vegetation, produce weaker echoes but can also sometimes be identified. Ultrasound is often used as the primary imaging method to rule out or confirm the presence of an intraocular foreign body, or it can be used in conjunction with computed tomography scans or other forms of imaging to accurately localize the position of a foreign body.

For the glaucoma patient with opaque media, the extent of optic nerve cupping can be evaluated with ultrasound (**Figure 5–31**).

5.5 Strengths and Limitations

5.5.1 STRENGTHS

The relative low cost of echography equipment, compared with that for other imaging modalities, provides the opportunity for an increased number of facilities to purchase their own equipment. Thus, the examination can be requested and performed in a timely fashion. The size of the machine allows evaluations to be carried out in fairly small patient examination areas, and the portability of the equipment allows the technician to work at a bedside or in an operating room, when necessary.

The examination procedure is noninvasive and harmless because ultrasound is not associated with ionizing radiation or a high magnetic field. The energy emitted is slowly absorbed and converted to heat while it passes through different media; however, the low amount of heat generated has not been shown to have any harmful effects on tissues.

5.5.2 LIMITATIONS

There are some instances in which echographic evaluation is limited or images cannot be obtained. If the eye is filled with silicone oil (after surgery to repair a retinal detachment), the view of the posterior segment is poor

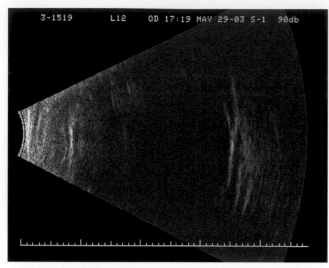

Figure 5–32 Silicone oil–filled eye.

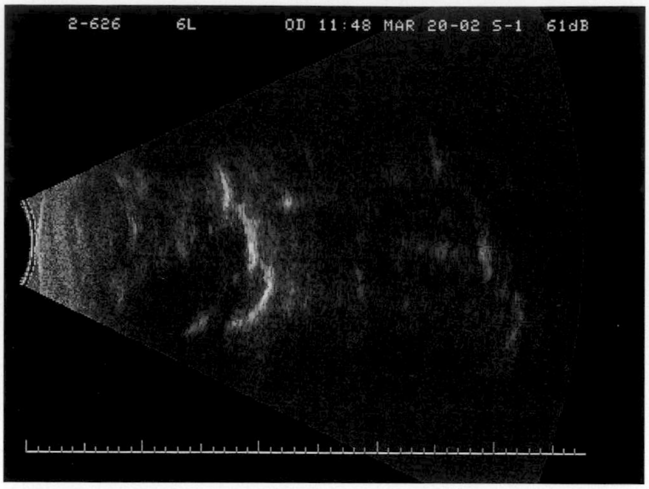

Figure 5–33 Phthisical eye with calcification of globe wall and shadowing of the orbital tissues.

owing to the slow speed of the sound through the silicone, which returns a distorted picture (**Figure 5–32**).

Air and gas bubbles placed in the vitreous during retinal surgery can also limit the view with ultrasound. To get useful information in these cases it may be necessary to have the patient remain in an upright position or turn the head from side to side to move the gas bubble away from the sound beam.

In traumatized eyes, in which small bubbles of air have entered the globe, care must be taken to differentiate gas bubbles from true intraocular foreign bodies. One way to do this is to reexamine the patient after a few days; generally, small air bubbles reabsorb and are no longer present.

Sound waves do not travel through bone or calcium, so areas of plaque-like calcification, as in prephthisical or phthisical eyes (**Figure 5–33**), cause shadowing that block the tissue behind from view. The presence of calcification within a retinoblastoma (especially if it is marked) can be a problem because the shadowing limits the echographer's ability to rule out extraocular extension and, in some cases, does not allow evaluation of the retrobulbar optic nerves.

Because ultrasound does not cross the air-tissue interface well, the probe, coupling gel, or immersion fluid must contact the tissue. An anesthetic eyedrop may be used. In general, the procedure is well tolerated.

To perform a diagnostic echography examination, specific instrumentation must be used. A contact B-scan probe as well as a standardized A-scan probe must be available. The standardized A-scan probe, which uses a specific decibel setting referred to as *tissue sensitivity*, is used for diagnostic evaluations. This probe can be used for biometry as well. The reverse is not true, however, as a biometry probe cannot be used for diagnostic examinations.

Because the ultrasound examination is dynamic and directed by the ultrasonographer, the examiner's training and experience are of utmost importance. Use of the techniques of standardized echography enables a thorough examination to be performed. Clinical experience and exposure to a large variety of ophthalmic conditions are also essential to the ultrasonographer's ability to provide valuable information for the referring physician. Experienced, trained professionals are of great value to the medical community.

SUGGESTED READINGS

Atta HR. Ophthalmic Ultrasound: A Practical Guide. New York, NY: Churchill Livingstone; 1996.

Byrne SF, Green RL. Ultrasound of the Eye and Orbit. 2nd ed. St Louis, Mo: Mosby; 2002.

DiBernardo C, Schachat A, Fekrat S. Ophthalmic Ultrasound: A Diagnostic Atlas. New York, NY: Thieme; 1998.

Kendall CJ. Ophthalmic Echography. Thorofare, NJ: Slack; 1990.

Chapter 6

Scanning Laser Tomography

ADAEL S. SOARES, MD • RAYMOND P. LeBLANC, MD, FRCSC

6.1 Physical Principles

Scanning laser tomography (SLT) was introduced in ophthalmology more than a decade ago. Although it has been used to evaluate retinal disorders,[2,15] its main use is to perform three-dimensional evaluation of the optic nerve head (ONH). At present, two commercial instruments are available: the Heidelberg retina tomograph and the Heidelberg retina tomograph II (HRT and HRT II, respectively; Heidelberg Engineering GmbH, Heidelberg, Germany).

SLT devices consist of a camera head mounted on a slit-lamp–type stand, a control panel for operation, and a computer for the display, acquisition, processing, and storage of data (**Figure 6-1**). The camera head holds the confocal scanning illumination and imaging systems. The scanning laser tomograph is illuminated by a near-infrared diode laser (675 nm in the HRT and HRT II). Light reflected from the fundus is collected and filtered by a confocal pinhole that is conjugate to the retinal focal plane (**Figure 6-2**). The pinhole ensures that only light reflected from a narrow spot at the focal plane of the laser is recorded by the detector, whereas reflections from other locations and planes are highly suppressed. By varying the depth of the laser focus, cross-sectional images at different positions on the axial plane of the structure (z-axis) can be acquired (**Figure 6-3**). The number of confocal images along the z-axis, the image resolution, and the total image acquisition time vary according to the device used (see Section 6.2).

After acquisition, the confocal images are aligned for horizontal, vertical, and rotational shifts that may result from small eye movements. The sum of reflectivity measurements along the z-axis for each aligned pixel is used to generate a *reflectivity* image, whereas the location along the z-axis where the maximum reflectivity is registered is assumed to be the height of the location and is used to generate a *topographic* image. Because the average of three 3D data sets has been associated with higher reproducibility,[19] the final product is composed of a mean topographic image and a mean reflectivity image (**Figure 6-4**).

6.2 Technology Development

Heidelberg Engineering has produced two generations of scanning laser tomographs. The HRT II is a more compact device than the HRT and has different features such as automatic setting of scan depth and fine focus; a series of three complete examinations are performed

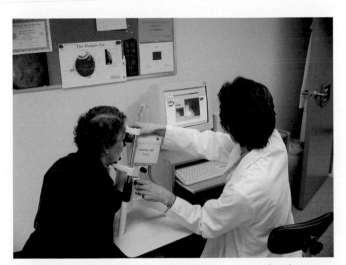

Figure 6–1 Heidelberg retina tomograph II: a camera head mounted on a slit-lamp–type stand and a computer for the display, acquisition, processing, and storage of data.

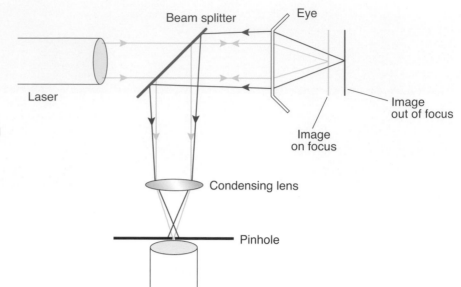

Figure 6–2   Schematic diagram of a confocal system. The pinhole is conjugate to the focal plane of the laser and prevents reflections outside the focal plane from reaching the detector.

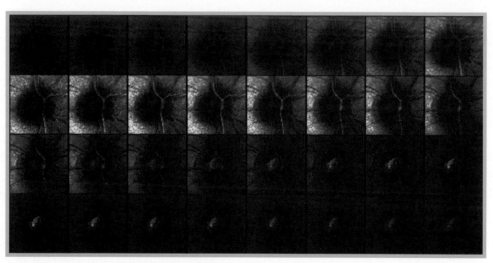

Figure 6–3   Thirty-two color–coded confocal image sections (HRT). The *top left* shows the first and most anterior image, whereas the *bottom right* shows the last image at the level of the retrolaminar optic nerve.

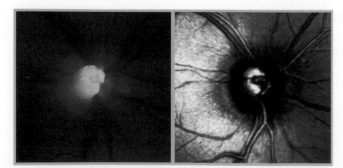

Figure 6–4   After processing of the confocal images, a mean topographic image (*left*) and a mean reflectivity image (*right*) are obtained.

automatically, which decreases examination time with measurements that are less influenced by the operator experience. **Table 6–1** shows a comparison of the specifications of the two SLT devices.

6.3 Image Interpretation

SLT is most often used clinically to objectively evaluate and monitor the surface contour of the ONH in glaucoma. **Figure 6–5** shows a HRT II scan of a glaucomatous eye. By using each topographic image generated and without interaction of the operator, the average height of a reference ring is calculated.[5] The width of this reference

TABLE 6–1
Specifications of SLT Devices

	HRT	HRT II
Digital image size (pixels)	256 × 256	84 × 384
Number of images	32	16–64
Laser source	Diode 675 nm	Diode 675 nm
Acquisition time (3D image)	1.4 sec	1.0 sec
Field of view	10° × 10°, 15° × 15° or 20° × 20°	15° × 15°
Optical resolution		
Transverse	10 μm	300 μm
Longitudinal	10 μm	300 μm

ring is 8 pixels, and the outside diameter is 240 pixels. The position of the reference ring (average height of all reference ring pixels) is normalized to zero, and all parameter values are evaluated in their position relative to it. The operator then defines the disc border by drawing a "contour line" along Elschnig's scleral ring. The software then computes a reference plane 50 μm below the mean height of the contour line (i.e., nerve fiber layer) between 350 and 356 degrees in the inferior temporal quadrant (clockwise direction with 0 degrees being at the 9 o'clock position in the right eye and counterclockwise direction with 0 degrees at the 3 o'clock position in the left eye). This location represents the position of the papillomacular bundle, which was thought to be the last location affected in glaucoma and

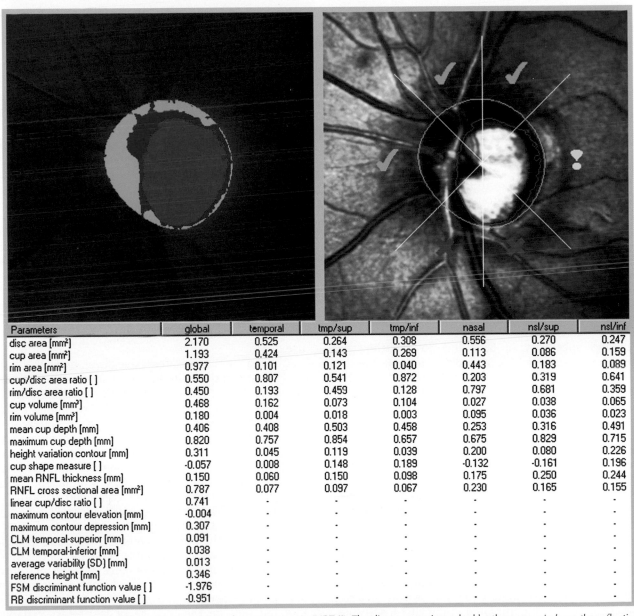

Parameters	global	temporal	tmp/sup	tmp/inf	nasal	nsl/sup	nsl/inf
disc area [mm²]	2.170	0.525	0.264	0.308	0.556	0.270	0.247
cup area [mm²]	1.193	0.424	0.143	0.269	0.113	0.086	0.159
rim area [mm²]	0.977	0.101	0.121	0.040	0.443	0.183	0.089
cup/disc area ratio [ ]	0.550	0.807	0.541	0.872	0.203	0.319	0.641
rim/disc area ratio [ ]	0.450	0.193	0.459	0.128	0.797	0.681	0.359
cup volume [mm³]	0.468	0.162	0.073	0.104	0.027	0.038	0.065
rim volume [mm³]	0.180	0.004	0.018	0.003	0.095	0.036	0.023
mean cup depth [mm]	0.406	0.408	0.503	0.458	0.253	0.316	0.491
maximum cup depth [mm]	0.820	0.757	0.854	0.657	0.675	0.829	0.715
height variation contour [mm]	0.311	0.045	0.119	0.039	0.200	0.080	0.226
cup shape measure [ ]	-0.057	0.008	0.148	0.189	-0.132	-0.161	0.196
mean RNFL thickness [mm]	0.150	0.060	0.150	0.098	0.175	0.250	0.244
RNFL cross sectional area [mm²]	0.787	0.077	0.097	0.067	0.230	0.165	0.155
linear cup/disc ratio [ ]	0.741	·	·	·	·	·	·
maximum contour elevation [mm]	-0.004	·	·	·	·	·	·
maximum contour depression [mm]	0.307	·	·	·	·	·	·
CLM temporal-superior [mm]	0.091	·	·	·	·	·	·
CLM temporal-inferior [mm]	0.038	·	·	·	·	·	·
average variability (SD) [mm]	0.013	·	·	·	·	·	·
reference height [mm]	0.346	·	·	·	·	·	·
FSM discriminant function value [ ]	-1.976	·	·	·	·	·	·
RB discriminant function value [ ]	-0.951	·	·	·	·	·	·

Figure 6–5 Stereometric analysis of the ONH in a glaucomatous eye (HRT II). The disc contour is marked by the *green circle* on the reflectivity image (*top right*). On the topographic image (*top left*), the disc is color coded in *red* (cup), *green*, and *blue* (neuroretinal rim). The stereometric parameters are provided for six sectors (*bottom*). RNFL, retinal nerve fiber layer; SD, standard deviation; RB, retinoblastoma.

therefore the most steady position for the reference plane. However, this hypothesis has been contested in recent studies using newer technologies.[11] After reference plane determination, various stereometric ONH parameters are estimated (**Figure 6–5**). These include the neuroretinal rim area (the area enclosed by the contour line and located above the reference plane), the disc cup area (the area enclosed by the contour line and below the reference plane), and a cup-shaped measure (the value describing the steepness of the optic disc cupping).

The contour line, once determined, is exported to subsequent images to maintain a constant size and location.

6.4 Clinical Applications

6.4.1 GLAUCOMA DETECTION

The possibility of objective and quantitative optic disc measurements with accuracy to differentiate glaucomatous optic neuropathy from normal optic nerves would be of great value in the field of glaucoma because of the huge variation of optic disc characteristics in the normal population, which often overlap with those of patients with glaucoma[12] and also because optic disc damage in glaucoma often precedes visual field loss.[18] Several studies have reported good correlations between HRT stereometric parameters and visual field indices on automated perimetry. However, although the correlations were statistically significant, the degree of correlation was not adequate to allow diagnosis of glaucoma using any of these parameters alone.[14] Other researchers have evaluated the sensitivity and specificity of separating normal patients from patients with glaucoma with the use of linear discriminant functions, which are statistical formulas that combine various stereometric parameters. Using this approach, Mikelberg and colleagues[16] reported a sensitivity and specificity of 83% and 86%, Bathija and associates[2] reported 78% and 88%, and Mardin and co-workers[14] reported 83.6% and 95%, respectively. It is important to note that these levels of sensitivity and specificity usually are higher when they are applied to the study population from which they were derived. Subsequent studies have shown that the performance of these formulas in other study populations was far from ideal.[10]

Wollstein and colleagues,[20] using the 99% prediction interval from the linear regression between optic disc area and the log of the neuroretinal rim area, also reported high specificity (96.3%) and sensitivity (84.3%) values to separate normal patients from patients with early glaucoma in their study population. However, cross-validation in a different population showed lower diagnosis precision.[10] The regression analysis performed by Wollstein and colleagues (also known as *Moorfields regression analysis*) is incorporated in the HRT II software . On the printout provided (**Figure 6–6**), if the measured rim area is 95% confidence interval (CI) of the database,

the respective disc sector is classified as normal (symbolized by a *green check mark*). If, on the other hand, the value measured is between the 95% and 99.9% CI, the sector is classified as borderline (symbolized by a *yellow exclamation point*). If the measured value is below the 99.9% CI, the sector is classified as outside normal limits (symbolized by a *red cross*).

The detection of localized retinal nerve fiber layer defects[4] in patients with glaucoma is also possible using SLT, which can be very helpful in diagnostic decision making, particularly for inexperienced observers. **Figure 6–7** shows the HRT scan in a patient with a history of glaucoma who was referred because of suspicious optic discs. The visual field shows a questionable superior arcuate defect but is nominally "within normal limits" by the Glaucoma Hemifield Test (GHT). The HRT scan clearly shows a nerve fiber bundle defect and neuroretinal rim defect identified by the Moorfields regression classification.

6.4.2 MONITORING PROGRESSION OF GLAUCOMA

The detection of ONH changes in patients with ocular hypertension and glaucoma is essential to the care of such patients. Stereoscopic disc photography is currently the standard method of monitoring optic disc changes. However, less than optimal agreement has been reported in subjective assessment of optic disc photographs performed by different observers and even among glaucoma subspecialists.[17] Other significant drawbacks are the facts that optic disc photographs are not always readily available for immediate clinical use and that their subjective evaluation is time consuming. The prospect of supplementing the clinician's judgment with objective data is very attractive.

Quantitative measurements performed with SLT have been shown to have high levels of reliability and reproducibility. Thus, recognition of the progression of glaucomatous damage is the most important potential use of SLT.

Chauhan and associates[6] have developed a technique to evaluate optic disc changes using SLT—the *change probability map* (CPM) analysis. In this method, three 3D image series are acquired at each examination (from which the software computes the mean topography). Before baseline and follow-up images are compared, the topographic images are aligned to correct for shift, rotation, and magnification differences among images. In each image, clusters of 4 × 4 adjacent height measurements (or pixels) are combined to form the so-called *superpixels*. Thus, for each superpixel we have 48 (4 × 4 × 3) baseline height measurements and 48 follow-up height measurements. The use of such superpixels allows more reliable estimates of test-retest variability. An analysis of variance is then performed to evaluate changes in these height measurements among the baseline and follow-up images. Changes that fall outside the 95% CI of test-retest variability on the follow-up image are considered significant. The resulting CPM is color coded. Regions that are more

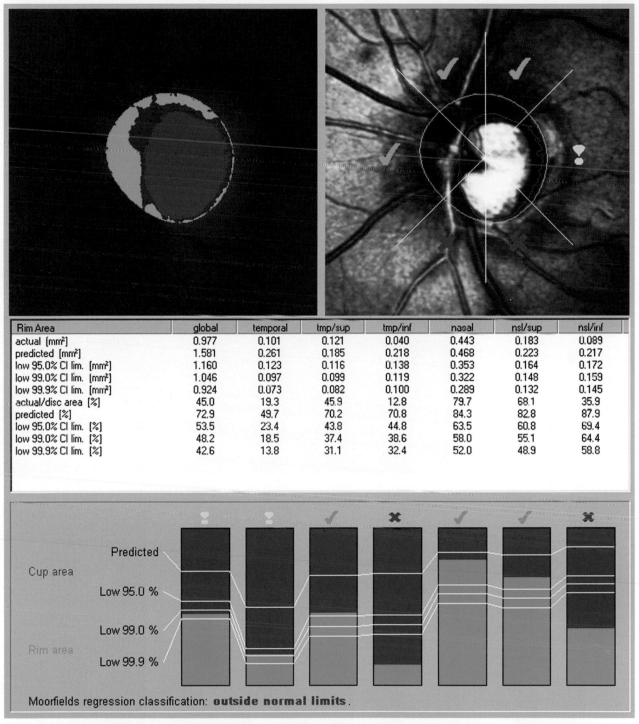

Rim Area	global	temporal	tmp/sup	tmp/inf	nasal	nsl/sup	nsl/inf
actual [mm²]	0.977	0.101	0.121	0.040	0.443	0.183	0.089
predicted [mm²]	1.581	0.261	0.185	0.218	0.468	0.223	0.217
low 95.0% CI lim. [mm²]	1.160	0.123	0.116	0.138	0.353	0.164	0.172
low 99.0% CI lim. [mm²]	1.046	0.097	0.099	0.119	0.322	0.148	0.159
low 99.9% CI lim. [mm²]	0.924	0.073	0.082	0.100	0.289	0.132	0.145
actual/disc area [%]	45.0	19.3	45.9	12.8	79.7	68.1	35.9
predicted [%]	72.9	49.7	70.2	70.8	84.3	82.8	87.9
low 95.0% CI lim. [%]	53.5	23.4	43.8	44.8	63.5	60.8	69.4
low 99.0% CI lim. [%]	48.2	18.5	37.4	38.6	58.0	55.1	64.4
low 99.9% CI lim. [%]	42.6	13.8	31.1	32.4	52.0	48.9	58.8

Moorfields regression classification: **outside normal limits**.

Figure 6–6   Moorfields regression analysis on the same glaucomatous ONH as in **Figure 6–5.** The measured rim areas in six sectors are compared with predicted values and classified as normal, borderline, or outside normal limit.

depressed in the follow-up examination appear in *red*, whereas regions that are more elevated in the follow-up examinations appear in *green* (**Figure 6–8**). The significant changes must occur in the same location on two or three consecutive examinations (clinician's option) to be shown on the reflectivity image. An important advantage of this method is that no contour line is required. On a subsequent study in a cohort of patients

with open-angle glaucoma, Chauhan and co-workers[8] showed that CPM analysis detects significantly more progression than automated perimetry (**Figure 6–9**).

Another approach to assess disc progression is analysis of changes in the stereometric parameters over time. Using this approach, Kamal and co-workers[13] showed that SLT detected optic disc changes before confirmed visual field changes in a group of patients

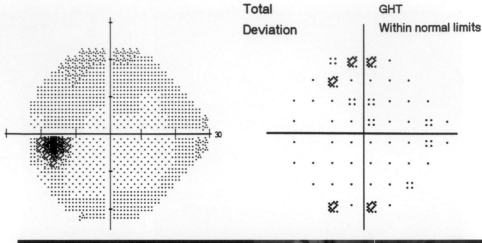

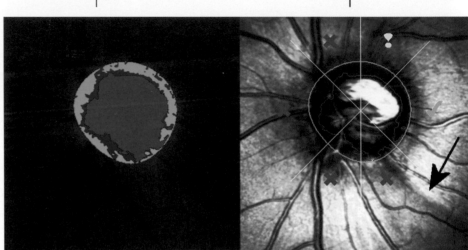

Figure 6–7 The HRT image shows a neuroretinal rim defect (Moorfields regression value outside normal limits) and nerve fiber layer defect (*black arrow*) in a patient with suspected glaucoma with a visual field "within normal limits" by the Glaucoma Hemifield Test.

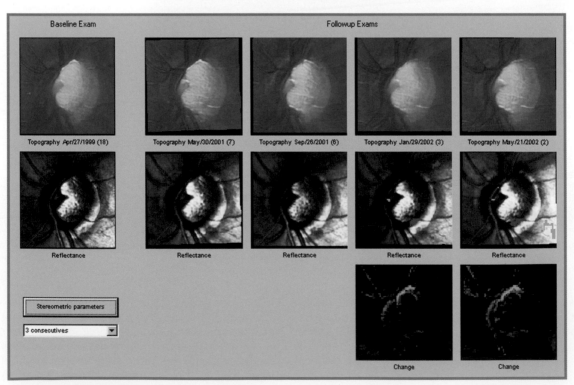

Figure 6–8 CPM. *Red* superpixels superimposed on the reflectivity images indicate *significant* depression and *green* superpixels indicate *significant* elevation.

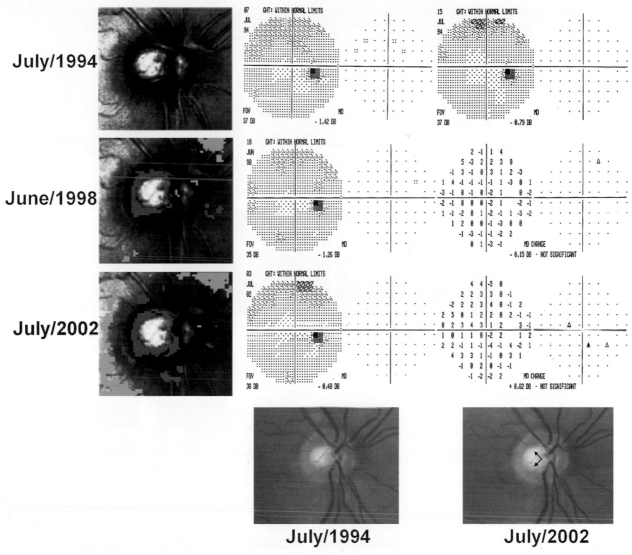

Figure 6–9 CPM showing concentric progression (*red* superpixels) of neuroretinal rim loss confirmed on optic disc photographs (*arrows*) in the right eye of a patient with ocular hypertension. The visual field remained normal.

with ocular hypertension that developed into early glaucoma. With this approach, however, the contour line is required. **Figure 6–10** shows a patient with glaucoma progression as shown by the stereometric parameters of SLT.

6.4.3 RETINAL DISORDERS

A less common use of SLT is the evaluation of retinal diseases, mainly macular disorders.[1,3]

6.5 Strengths and Limitations

6.5.1 STRENGTHS

Strengths of SLT include the following:

- Quick and easy image acquisition with the possibility of immediate data evaluation

- Quantitative analysis for diagnosis and progression
- Good-quality images without pupil dilation
- Reproducibility

6.5.2 LIMITATIONS

Limitations of SLT include the following:

- The stereometric ONH analysis depends on an operator-defined disc contour and an arbitrarily defined reference plane. Subtle differences in the drawing of the disc contour can lead to significant difference in the analysis of the rim status (**Figure 6–11**). The standard reference plane assumes that the papillomacular bundle thickness is 50 μm, not considering the interindividual variation in retinal nerve fiber layer thickness. Moreover, Chen and colleagues[9] have shown that the papillomacular bundle may vary between eyes of patients with asymmetrical glaucoma, underestimating the

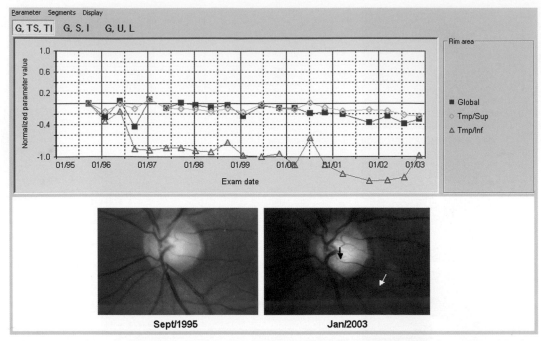

Figure 6–10 Stereometric analysis of a glaucomatous ONH shows progressive rim loss on the temporal inferior sector (*blue line*) confirmed by disc photography (*black arrow*). A retinal nerve fiber layer defect is also observed (*white arrow*).

Figure 6–11 Different contour lines on the same optic disc. Subtle differences between the contour lines lead to significant differences in the stereometric parameters and on the Moorfields regression analysis classification.

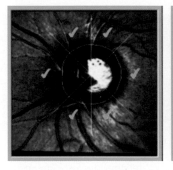 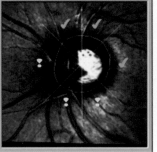 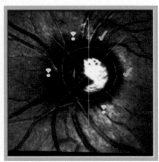

glaucoma damage in advanced cases. Another aspect relates to temporally tilted discs, for which the nasal neuroretinal rim is incorrectly overestimated by this conventional standard reference plane. Because myopia is a risk factor for glaucoma, tilted discs are often encountered in this disease. If the neuroretinal rim is overestimated in such a situation, the ability of HRT in detect glaucoma may also be reduced.

- Cost
- Variability increases with age[7] and media opacities,[21] which can increase test-retest variability and consequently impair detection of change.

REFERENCES

1. Akiba J, Yanagiya N, Konno S, Hikichi T, Yoshida A. Three-dimensional characteristics of macular pseudoholes using confocal laser tomography. Ophthalmic Surg Lasers. 1999;30:513–517.
2. Bartsch DU, Intaglietta M, Bille JF, Dreher AW, Gharib M, Freeman WR. Confocal laser tomographic analysis of the retina in eyes with macular hole formation and other focal macular diseases. Am J Ophthalmol. 1989;108:277–287.
3. Bathija R, Zangwill L, Berry CC, Sample PA, Weinreb RN. Detection of early glaucomatous structural damage with confocal scanning laser tomography. J Glaucoma. 1998;7:121–127.
4. Burk RO, Tuulonen A, Airaksinen PJ. Laser scanning tomography of localised nerve fibre layer defects. Br J Ophthalmol. 1998;82:1112–1117.
5. Burk RO, Vihanninjoki K, Bartke T, et al. Development of the standard reference plane for the Heidelberg retina tomograph. Graefes Arch Clin Exp Ophthalmol. 2000;238:375–384.
6. Chauhan BC, Blanchard JW, Hamilton DC, LeBlanc RP. Technique for detecting serial topographic changes in the optic disc and peripapillary retina using scanning laser tomography. Invest Ophthalmol Vis Sci. 2000;41:775–782.
7. Chauhan BC, LeBlanc RP, McCormick TA, Rogers JB. Test-retest variability of topographic measurements with confocal scanning laser tomography in patients with glaucoma and control subjects. Am J Ophthalmol. 1994;118:9–15.
8. Chauhan BC, McCormick TA, Nicolela MT, LeBlanc RP. Optic disc and visual field changes in a prospective longitudinal study of patients with glaucoma: Comparison of scanning laser tomography with conventional perimetry and optic disc photography. Arch Ophthalmol. 2001;119:1492–1499.
9. Chen E, Gedda U, Landau I. Thinning of the papillomacular bundle in the glaucomatous eye and its influence on the reference plane of the Heidelberg retinal tomography. J Glaucoma. 2001;10:386–389.

10. Ford BA, Artes PH, McCormick TA, Nicolela MT, LeBlanc RP, Chauhan BC. Comparison of data analysis tools for detection of glaucoma with the Heidelberg retina tomograph. Ophthalmology. 2003;110:1145–1150.

11. Greenfield DS, Bagga H, Knighton RW. Macular thickness changes in glaucomatous optic neuropathy detected using optical coherence tomography. Arch Ophthalmol. 2003;121:41–46.

12. Jonas JB, Gusek GC, Naumann GO. Optic disc, cup and neuro-retinal rim size, configuration and correlations in normal eyes. Invest Ophthalmol Vis Sci. 1988;29:1151–1158.

13. Kamal DS, Viswanathan AC, Garway-Heath DF, Hitchings RA, Poinoosawmy D, Bunce C. Detection of optic disc change with the Heidelberg retina tomograph before confirmed visual field change in ocular hypertensives converting to early glaucoma. Br J Ophthalmol. 1999;83:290–294.

14. Mardin CY, Horn FK, Jonas JB, Budde WM. Preperimetric glaucoma diagnosis by confocal scanning laser tomography of the optic disc. Br J Ophthalmol. 1999;83:299–304.

15. Menezes AV, Giunta M, Chisholm L, Harvey PT, Tuli R, Devenyi RG. Reproducibility of topographic measurements of the macula with a scanning laser ophthalmoscope. Ophthalmology. 1995; 102:230–235.

16. Mikelberg FS, Parfitt CM, Swindale NV, et al. Ability of the Heidelberg retina tomograph to detect early glaucomatous field loss. J Glaucoma. 1995;4:242–247.

17. Nicolela MT, Drance SM, Broadway DC, Chauhan BC, McCormick TA, LeBlanc RP. Agreement among clinicians in the recognition of patterns of optic disk damage in glaucoma. Am J Ophthalmol. 2001;132:836–844.

18. Quigley HA, Addicks EM, Green WR. Optic nerve damage in human glaucoma. III. Quantitative correlation of nerve fiber loss and visual field defect in glaucoma, ischemic optic neuropathy, papilledema and toxic neuropathy. Arch Ophthalmol. 1989; 107:453–464.

19. Weinreb RN, Lusky M, Bartsch DU, Morsman D. Effect of repetitive imaging on topographic measurements of the optic nerve head. Arch Ophthalmol. 1993;111:636–638.

20. Wollstein G, Garway-Heath DF, Hitchings RA. Identification of early glaucoma cases with the scanning laser ophthalmoscope. Ophthalmology. 1998;105:1557–1563.

21. Zangwill L, Irak I, Berry CC, Garden V, de Souza Lima M, Weinreb RN. Effect of cataract and pupil size on image quality with confocal scanning laser ophthalmoscopy. Arch Ophthalmol. 1997;115:983–990.

Chapter 7

Scanning Laser Polarimetry

HARMOHINA BAGGA, MD • DAVID S. GREENFIELD, MD

7.1 Physical Principles

7.1.1 SCANNING LASER POLARIMETRY

Scanning laser polarimetry (SLP) uses a confocal scanning laser ophthalmoscope with an integrated polarimeter to quantitatively evaluate the retardation of the retinal nerve fiber layer (RNFL) by measuring the change in polarization of incident light as it doubly passes through the birefringent RNFL (**Figure 7–1**). The parallel arrangement of the microtubules within the retinal ganglion cell axons causes the RNFL to behave like a form birefringent medium. As a result, the slow axis of birefringence is aligned with the orientation of the RNFL bundles and its retardation is proportional to its thickness.[12,39] In normal eyes, the superior and inferior peripapillary regions exhibit much higher

retardance compared with the nasal and temporal regions, thereby corresponding to the normal anatomic distribution pattern of RNFL. **Figure 7–2** illustrates the retardation map of a normal eye. Note the high retardation superiorly and inferiorly displayed in *red* and *yellow* and the relatively low retardation nasally and temporally displayed in *blue* and *green*.

7.1.2 CALCULATION AND COMPENSATION OF CORNEAL BIREFRINGENCE ARTIFACT

Because all birefringent structures cause a change in the polarization of an illuminating beam, the total retardance consists of contributions from the anterior segment (cornea and lens) and the RNFL. The accuracy of RNFL measurements with SLP depends on the ability to extract the RNFL retardance from the measured total

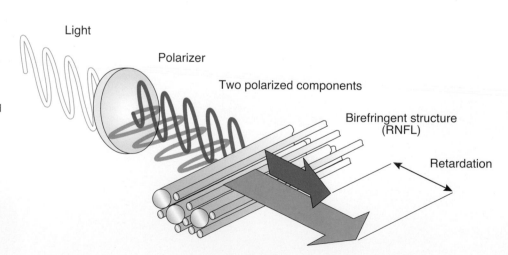

Figure 7–1 Retardation of polarized light after passing through a birefringent medium. (Courtesy of Laser Diagnostic Technology, San Diego, CA.)

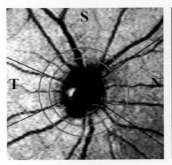
Fundus image

Retardation map

Figure 7–2 Fundus image (*left*) and retardance image (*right*) of a normal eye. Note the high retardation superiorly and inferiorly displayed in *red* and *yellow*.

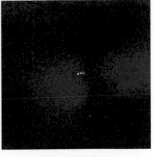
Before compensation

After complete compensation

Figure 7–3 A well-defined bow-tie pattern (*left*) with uncompensated corneal birefringence and a uniform pattern of retardation (*right*), indicating complete compensation of corneal birefringence. (From Bagga H, Greenfield DS, Knighton RW. Scanning laser polarimetry with variable corneal compensation: Identification and correction for corneal birefringence in eyes with macular disease. Invest Ophthalmol Vis Sci. 2003;44:1969–1976.)

retardance. To neutralize the confounding influence of corneal birefringence on RNFL thickness, the latest commercial polarimeter has an integrated variable corneal compensator, which determines and neutralizes the eye-specific corneal polarization axis (CPA) and magnitude (CPM) using the concept of the macula as an intraocular polarimeter.[13,15,25,37,38,43] Henle's layer of the macula is radially birefringent owing to the uniform arrangement of the photoreceptor axons.[5,11,23] Macular polarimetry images obtained without compensating for the corneal birefringence demonstrate a distinct "bow-tie" or "double-humped" pattern. Based on the assumption that the corneal birefringence interacts with an intact Henle's layer to produce the bow-tie patterns, the macular bow-tie patterns are used to determine corneal birefringence. The bright arms of the bow-tie are formed where the slow axis of the cornea is parallel with the slow axis of Henle's layer, resulting in summation of retardation. The dark arms are formed where the slow axis of the cornea is perpendicular to the slow axis of Henle's layer and retardation cancels. Thus, the slow axis of the anterior segment birefringence can be read out directly from the orientation of the bright arms of the bow-tie. The shape of the retardation profile on a circle around the macula reflects the combined magnitude of the anterior segment birefringence and that of the Henle's layer from which it is possible to extract the magnitude of the anterior segment birefringence.[43] **Figure 7–3** illustrates a well-defined bow-tie pattern (*left*

panel). After compensation of the corneal birefringence axis and retardance, a uniform pattern of retardation can be observed (*right panel*), suggesting complete neutralization of the influence of corneal birefringence.

The adequacy of corneal compensation can be assessed by inspection of the macular retardation image. A fully compensated macular image shows a uniform pattern of retardation with a magnitude of <28 nm. A persistent macular bow-tie after "compensation" is suggestive of residual corneal birefringence.

Macular pathologic lesions may disrupt the integrity of Henle's layer and produce indeterminate bow-tie patterns, resulting in failure of the bow-tie algorithm for corneal compensation.[2] **Figure 7–4** illustrates an indeterminate bow-tie in an eye with dry age-related macular degeneration. Note the persistence of the bow-tie after neutralization of the corneal birefringence axis and retardance.

Alternative strategies for corneal compensation in eyes with maculopathy have been described.[2,24] A "screen method" has been reported for successful neutralization of anterior segment birefringence in eyes with maculopathy based on the assumption that the fundus acts as a polarization-preserving reflector, i.e., the polarization state of the deflected beam results from

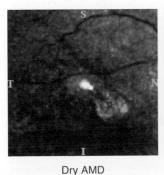
Dry AMD

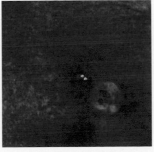
Before compensation

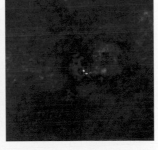
Residual birefringence after compensation

Figure 7–4 An indeterminate bow-tie (*center*) in an eye with dry age-related macular degeneration. Note the persistence of the bow-tie after compensation, indicating incomplete neutralization of the corneal birefringence. (From Bagga H, Greenfield DS, Knighton RW. Scanning laser polarimetry with variable corneal compensation: identification and correction for corneal birefringence in eyes with macular disease. Invest Ophthalmol Vis Sci. 2003;44:1969–1976.)

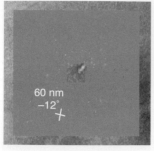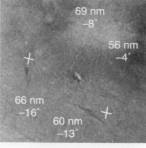

Figure 7–5 An eye with an epiretinal membrane showing a 213 × 213 pixel area (*uniform gray square*) averaged for determination of corneal birefringence using the screen method. The magnitude and orientation of birefringence was similar over the entire image (*right*). (From Bagga H, Greenfield DS, Knighton RW. Scanning laser polarimetry with variable corneal compensation: identification and correction for corneal birefringence in eyes with macular disease. Invest Ophthalmol Vis Sci. 2003;44:1969–1976.)

the cumulative effect of all the birefringent structures through which it is passed. In the screen method anterior segment birefringence information is extracted from both within and outside the potential zone of macular artifacts to provide a more robust measure of the anterior segment birefringence in such eyes. **Figure 7–5** illustrates the concept underlying the screen method in which an average is obtained over a large area in each birefringence image to determine the retardation (*left panel*). The central region containing the bright optical artifact and saturated pixels in the image were excluded. The *right panel* displays single-pass retardance (nanometers) at selected pixels (*crosses*) on an enhanced retardation image. Cross orientation shows the slow and fast axes of the retardation, which is high and similarly oriented over the entire image. This strategy is successful in normal eyes and eyes with maculopathy.

7.2 Technology Development

Recent advances in SLP have provided a means to obtain accurate, objective, quantitative, and reproducible structural measurements of RNFL thickness. Since its introduction more than a decade ago, SLP has undergone several hardware and software changes.

7.2.1 NERVE FIBER ANALYZER

The first generation device (NFA I) became commercially available in 1992 and was equipped with a single detector, which was later replaced by a double detector (NFA II). The detector incorporated a fixed retarder to adjust for corneal retardation, and the assumption was that all individuals have a slow axis of corneal birefringence 15 degrees nasally downward and a corneal birefringence magnitude of 60 nm. The measured total retardation was assumed to be the retardance of the RNFL.

High levels of reproducibility have been reported using the NFA,[35,36,39,41] and retardation measurements have been demonstrated to be strongly correlated with

visual function.[21,35,39] Chi and colleagues[6] reported mean coefficients of variability of 3.59% and 5.65% for normal eyes and eyes with glaucoma, respectively. Hoh and colleagues[22] described excellent intraoperator reproducibility and found that variability between operators can be minimized by using a single measurement ellipse acquired from the original baseline image.

7.2.2 GDx NERVE FIBER ANALYZER

The GDx nerve fiber analyzer became commercially available in 1996. It included a normative database consisting of 400 eyes matched for age and race, and a blood vessel removal algorithm to augment reproducibility. High reproducibility has been reported in phakic and pseudophakic eyes of normal and glaucomatous subjects.[9,32]

As with previous devices, the GDx nerve fiber analyzer incorporated a fixed corneal compensator to neutralize corneal birefringence. Several studies have demonstrated that the magnitude and axis of corneal polarization are variable and are strongly correlated with RNFL thickness assessments obtained with SLP.[16,25,38] This produced incomplete neutralization of corneal birefringence and erroneous RNFL thickness assessment in eyes that deviate from the fixed compensator settings. **Figure 7–6** demonstrates the influence of residual corneal birefringence on RNFL thickness measurements. Note that the greater the deviation of corneal birefringence measurements from the fixed compensator settings becomes, the stronger the apparent RNFL retardation.

Moreover, uncorrected corneal birefringence falsely broadened the distribution of normative RNFL thickness data and significantly reduced the sensitivity and specificity of this technology. Correction for CPA significantly reduced the distribution of normative RNFL data by up to 35%[19] and increased the discriminating power of this technology for glaucoma detection.[18] Correction for both CPA and CPM has been reported to further increase the diagnostic accuracy of this technology.[8,38]

7.2.3 GDx-VARIABLE CORNEAL COMPENSATION

The GDx with variable corneal compensation (VCC) utilizes macular birefringence patterns to determine eye-specific corneal birefringence. The screen method[1] is commercially available for corneal birefringence neutralization in eyes with macular pathologic lesions. A new normative database consisting of 540 eyes corrected for CPA and CPM is incorporated. Retardation parameters are color-coded to indicate statistical deviation from the normative database. Two-dimensional RNFL probability maps that indicate the statistical likelihood of glaucomatous damage are available.

Compared with fixed corneal compensation (FCC), VCC provides increased correlation with visual function,[8] greater discriminating power for glaucoma detection,[38] and greater correlation with RNFL assessments obtained with optical coherence tomography (OCT).[1] **Figure 7–7** illustrates OCT and SLP images of the peripapillary

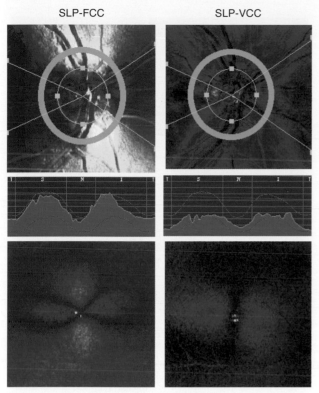

SLP-FCC   SLP-VCC

Figure 7–6 Peripapillary RNFL (*top*) and macular image (*bottom*) using FCC and VCC in a normal eye (CPA 44 degrees nasally downward, CPM 53 nm). The bright macular bow-tie pattern using FCC indicates a high degree of uncompensated corneal birefringence. After VCC note the absence of a macular bow-tie pattern indicative of complete neutralization of corneal birefringence. (From Bagga H, Greenfield DS, Feuer W, Knighton RW. Scanning laser polarimetry with variable corneal compensation and optical coherence tomography in normal and glaucomatous eyes. Am J Ophthalmol. 2003;135:521–529.)

RNFL using FCC and VCC in a glaucomatous eye with thinning of the inferior neuroretinal rim and a corresponding superior arcuate field defect (corneal polarization axis 35 degrees nasally downward, corneal polarization magnitude 18 nm). The SLP FCC image demonstrates poor correlation with the visual field defect as a result of uncompensated corneal birefringence. After VCC, note the absence of inferior retardation and marked reduction in the inferior RNFL thickness plot consistent with the OCT-derived RNFL thickness values (mean superior RNFL thickness 112 μm; mean inferior RNFL thickness 42 μm).

7.3 Image Interpretation

The GDx-VCC uses a fixed scan circle of 3.2 mm diameter centered on the optic disc. A high-quality scan is sharply focused and is well centered around the optic nerve with minimal eye movement and even illumination. An image with abnormal definition of the edges of blood vessels or with black borders indicates eye movement and is unacceptable. The most recent software version automatically generates a quality score of 1 through 10 based on various criteria including fixation, refraction, and ocular alignment. An acceptable quality score has been suggested to be 8 or greater.

A normal RNFL thickness map is characterized by bright yellows and reds (thicker) in the superior and inferior sectors and greens and blues (thinner) in the nasal and temporal sectors. The TSNIT (temporal, superior, nasal, inferior, temporal) graph should display the RNFL thickness values along the calculation circle for a given normal value within the shaded area

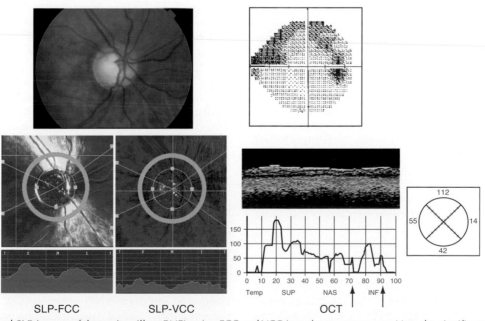

SLP-FCC   SLP-VCC   OCT

Figure 7–7 OCT and SLP images of the peripapillary RNFL using FCC and VCC in a glaucomatous eye. Note the significant improvement in the correlation of VCC with visual field (VF) and OCT compared with FCC. (From Bagga H, Greenfield DS, Feuer W, Knighton RW. Scanning laser polarimetry with variable corneal compensation and optical coherence tomography in normal and glaucomatous eyes. Am J Ophthalmol. 2003;135:521–529.)

indicating the normal range. Retardation parameters generated automatically by the software include the TSNIT average, superior average, inferior average, TSNIT standard deviation, intereye symmetry, and nerve fiber ndex (NFI). These are color-coded to indicate statistical deviation from the normative database.

A consensus on the definition of an abnormal scan has not been established. A GDx-VCC scan may be considered abnormal if the TSNIT average, superior average, inferior average, TSNIT standard deviation, intereye symmetry, or NFI is abnormal at the $p < 1\%$ level. A GDx-VCC scan may be considered borderline if the TSNIT average, superior average, inferior average, TSNIT standard deviation, intereye symmetry, or NFI is outside normal at the $p < 5\%$ level. It has been suggested that the cutoff value for NFI is >47 at the $p < 1\%$ level and >30 at the $p < 5\%$ level (personal communication, Michael J. Sinai, PhD, Director of Clinical Research, Laser Diagnostic Technologies, Inc.).

There is no commonly accepted criterion for judging progression either on the RNFL thickness map or the retardation parameters. The Serial Analysis report displays a selection of up to four scans of the same eye displayed chronologically to help track RNFL changes over time. This report presents an RNFL thickness map, deviation from a normal map, deviation from a reference map, TSNIT parameters, and NFI for each eye. In addition, a combination TSNIT graph provides an overlay showing the TSNIT values for each eye as a different colored line. The examination at the top of the report is considered the baseline measurement for the selected serial analysis. The Deviation from Reference map highlights changes in the RNFL thickness since the first visit for a given eye. Points or areas highlighted in color indicate possible clinically significant changes. The color legend defines change in 20-micron increments.

7.4 Clinical Applications

7.4.1 DIAGNOSIS OF GLAUCOMA

Numerous studies have reported high discriminating power for separating normal eyes from eyes with glaucoma,[7,26,40] and good agreement with other structural technologies.[1,15,21,33,42] Recently, a Fourier-based linear discriminant function has been reported to have sensitivity of 84% for a specificity set at 92% compared with the GDx software-provided parameters with sensitivities ranging from 24% to 69%.[28] **Figure 7–8** illustrates a patient with juvenile open-angle glaucoma with an inferior RNFL defect and a small wedge-shaped superior RNFL defect (*white arrows*) with a corresponding superonasal visual field defect. The GDx-VCC peripapillary RNFL retardation map shows markedly reduced retardation, and the RNFL thickness plot demonstrates reduction of both the superotemporal and inferotemporal nerve fiber layer consistent with the visual field defect.

Differences in RNFL have been reported between normal eyes and eyes with ocular hypertension.[4,34]

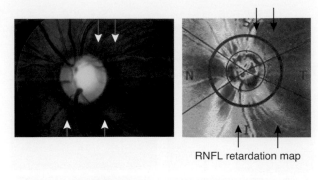

RNFL retardation map

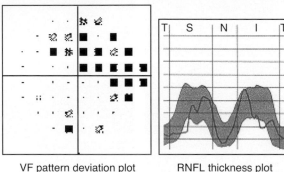

VF pattern deviation plot   RNFL thickness plot

Figure 7–8 A left eye with juvenile open-angle glaucoma and an RNFL defect (inferior > superior) with a corresponding superonasal field defect. GDx-VCC illustrates diminished retardation and RNFL loss consistent with the visual field (VF) defect.

Others have reported that no structural differences exist in eyes with ocular hypertension with normal short-wavelength perimetry.[30] Early structural abnormalities may be more likely to be identified in high-risk ocular hypertensive eyes such as eyes in patients with large cup-to-disc ratios, eyes in older patients, eyes with increased intraocular pressure, and eyes with reduced central corneal thickness.[14] Considerable RNFL atrophy may precede functional loss as detected using standard automated perimetry. **Figure 7–9** demonstrates preperimetric glaucoma in an eye with pigment dispersion, elevated intraocular pressure, marked glaucomatous optic nerve damage, and normal automated perimetry. **Figure 7–10** demonstrates an eye with hemifield visual loss due to primary open-angle glaucoma with marked RNFL atrophy in both retinal hemifields detected using SLP and OCT.

7.4.2 DETECTION OF PROGRESSION

Several reports have demonstrated that SLP can detect progressive RNFL atrophy. Colen and associates[10] and Medeiros and co-workers[27] reported progressive RNFL loss in eyes with anterior ischemic optic neuropathy. Meier and colleagues[29] demonstrated similar findings after ocular trauma. Poinoosawmy and associates[31] compared median RNFL thicknesses in 75 eyes of patients with normal pressure glaucoma over 2 years with those in eyes of 35 normal control subjects and found a significant difference in the decrease in RNFL thickness (8% versus 2.4%, respectively). In contrast,

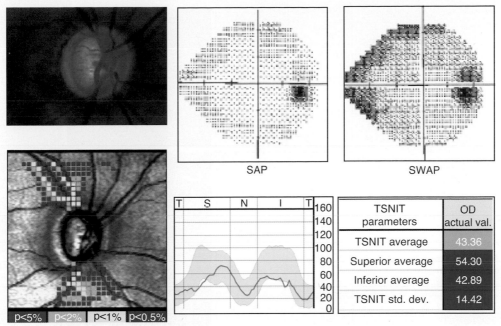

Figure 7-9 A right eye with pigmentary glaucoma with advanced glaucomatous optic nerve damage but with normal standard automated perimetry and superonasal field defect on short wavelength automated perimetry. GDx-VCC demonstrates marked reduction of retardation and RNFL loss consistent with the appearance of the optic nerve head.

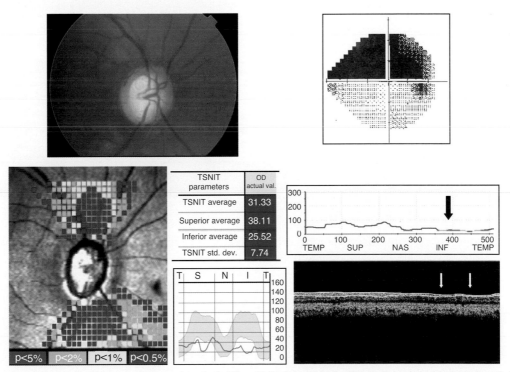

Figure 7–10 A right eye with hemifield visual loss and marked diffuse RNFL loss on both GDx-VCC and OCT in both hemifields.

Boehm and colleagues[3] did not find a significant change in SLP parameters among 10 glaucomatous eyes with reproducible visual field progression in patients who were followed for an average of 31 months after optic disc hemorrhage. Fifty-nine percent of the eyes developed reproducible visual field progression, but only 29%

of eyes had reproducible progression on SLP. Furthermore, in 10 eyes (59%) with suspected progression on SLP, progression was not confirmed on subsequent testing. **Figure 7–11** illustrates a left eye with primary open-angle glaucoma with established progression on visual fields over a 5-year period. Note the inferior

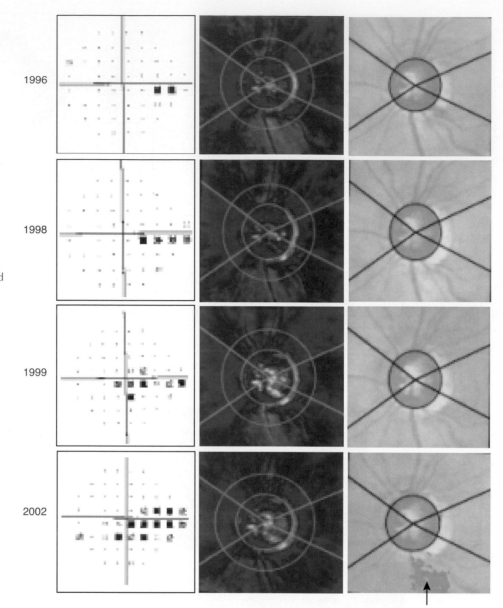

Figure 7–11 A left eye with primary open-angle glaucoma with established progression on visual fields over a 5-year period. Note the inferior area (*arrow*) of progressively diminished retardation corresponding to the development of a new superior field defect.

area (*arrow*) of progressively diminished retardation corresponding to the development of a new superior field defect.

7.5 Strengths and Limitations

7.5.1 STRENGTHS

SLP is a sophisticated technology that has evolved considerably over the last decade and provides highly reproducible, objective measurements of the peripapillary RNFL in eyes with glaucomatous and nonglaucomatous optic neuropathy. SLP imaging offers certain specific advantages: it is easy to perform, does not require pupillary dilatation, is highly reproducible, does not use a reference plane, does not require correction for ocular magnification, and incorporates an age-matched normative database of 540 eyes. In

contrast to earlier versions of this technology, the GDx-VCC has largely eliminated the problems associated with uncompensated corneal birefringence. Finally, a 2D probability map is a sensitive way to identify early RNFL abnormalities and generates statistical values to illustrate the likelihood of deviation from normal.

7.5.2 LIMITATIONS

Incorporation of a variable corneal compensator has considerably reduced the frequency of anterior segment-induced artifacts. However, anterior and posterior segment pathologic lesions may produce spurious RNFL measurements,[20] and caution should be used when one interprets images in eyes with ocular surface disease, previous keratorefractive surgery, advanced media opacification, and extensive peripapillary atrophy. Examination of eyes with macular pathologic lesions requires caution to ensure the adequacy of corneal compensation. Finally, although there is good 1-year stability for CPA measurements,[17] long-term stability and the effect of intraocular and refractive surgery upon such measurements remain unknown.

New strategies for detection of progressive structural change need to be validated against accepted measures of structural (stereoscopic disc photography) and functional (psychophysical) change. Statistical units of change probability are absent at this time and are essential to differentiate true biologic change from variability (e.g. microsaccades during fixation, vessel pulsations, instrument, or operator-induced variability). As with other imaging technologies, prospective studies are necessary to validate change analysis strategies.

7.6 Conclusions

Studies have shown that glaucomatous injury to the RNFL can precede functional loss by as long as 5 years. Thus, accurate and objective methods of detecting disc and RNFL abnormalities and their progression are essential to facilitate the diagnosis and monitoring of glaucomatous optic neuropathy. SLP provides rapid, accurate, highly reproducible, and objective measurements of RNFL thickness. Very good correlation exists between structural damage to the RNFL as assessed by SLP and visual field loss, and SLP is a highly sensitive tool for detection of early glaucomatous RNFL injury. As with perimetry, it is not recommended that isolated clinical decisions be based solely upon SLP imaging results, and confirmatory testing is essential. Clinical correlation should be determined, and treatment recommendations should be individualized.

ACKNOWLEDGMENTS

This work was supported in part by the New York Community Trust, New York, NY; a grant from Mr. Barney Donnelley, Palm Beach, FL; and National Institutes of Health Grant R01-EY08684, Bethesda, MD.

The authors have no financial interest in any device or technique described in this paper.

REFERENCES

1. Bagga H, Greenfield DS, Feuer W, Knighton RW. Scanning laser polarimetry with variable corneal compensation and optical coherence tomography in normal and glaucomatous eyes. Am J Ophthalmol. 2003;135:521–529.
2. Bagga H, Greenfield, DS, Knighton RW. Scanning laser polarimetry with variable corneal compensation: Identification and correction for corneal birefringence in eyes with macular pathology. Invest Vis Sci Ophthalmol. 2003;44:1969–1976.
3. Boehm MD, Nedrud C, Greenfield DX, Chen PP. Scanning laser polarimetry and detection of progression after optic disc hemorrhage in patients with glaucoma. Arch Ophthalmol. 2003;121:189–194.
4. Bozkurt B, Irkec M, Karaagaoglu E, Orhan M. Scanning laser polarimetric analysis of retinal nerve fiber layer thickness in Turkish patients with glaucoma and ocular hypertension. Eur J Ophthalmol. 2002;12:406–412.
5. Brink HB, Van Blokland GJ. Birefringence of the human foveal area assessed in vivo with Mueller-matrix ellipsometry. J Opt Soc Am. 1988;5:49–57.
6. Chi QM, Tomita G, et al. Evaluation of the effect of aging on the retinal nerve fiber layer thickness using scanning laser polarimetry. J Glaucoma. 1995;4:406–413.
7. Choplin NT, Lundy DC, Dreher AW. Differentiating patients with glaucoma from glaucoma suspects and normal subjects by nerve fiber layer assessment with scanning laser polarimetry. Ophthalmology. 1998;105:2068–2076.
8. Choplin NT, Zhou Q, Knighton RW. Effect of individualized compensation for anterior segment birefringence on retinal nerve fiber layer assessments as determined by scanning laser polarimetry. Ophthalmology. 2003;110:719–725.
9. Colen TP, Tjon-Fo-Sang MJH, Mulder PG, Lemij HG. Reproducibility of measurements with the nerve fiber analyzer (NFA/GDx). J Glaucoma. 2000;9:363–370.
10. Colen TP, Van Everdingen JAM, Lemij HG. Axonal loss in a patient with anterior ischemic optic neuropathy as measured with scanning laser polarimetry. Am J Ophthalmol. 2000;130: 847–850.
11. Delori FC, Webb RH, et al. Macular birefringence. Invest Ophthalmol Vis Sci. 1979;53(19 Suppl).
12. Dreher AW, Reiter K, et al. Spatially resolved birefringence of the retinal nerve fiber layer assessed with a retinal ellipsometer. Appl Opt. 1992;31:3730–3749.
13. Garway-Heath DF, Greaney MJ, Caprioli J. Correction for the erroneous compensation of anterior segment birefringence with the scanning laser polarimeter for glaucoma diagnosis. Invest Ophthalmol Vis Sci. 2002;43:1465–1474.
14. Gordon MO, Beiser JA, Brandt JD, et al. The Ocular Hypertension Treatment Study: Baseline factors that predict the onset of primary open-angle glaucoma. Arch Ophthalmol. 2002;120:714–720.
15. Greaney MJ, Hoffman DC, Garway-Heath DF, Nakla M, Coleman AL, Caprioli J. Comparison of optic nerve imaging methods to distinguish normal eyes from those with glaucoma. Invest Vis Sci Ophthalmol. 2002;43:140–145.
16. Greenfield DS, Knighton RW, Huang XR. Effect of corneal polarization axis on assessment of retinal nerve fiber layer thickness by scanning laser polarimetry. Am J Ophthalmol. 2000;129:715–722.
17. Greenfield DS, Knighton RW. Stability of corneal polarization axis measurements for scanning laser polarimetry. Ophthalmology. 2001;108:1065–1069.
18. Greenfield DS, Knighton RW, Feuer WJ, Schiffman JC, Zangwell L, Weinreb RN. Correction for corneal polarization axis improves the discriminating power of scanning laser polarimetry. Am J Ophthalmol. 2002;134:27–33.
19. Greenfield DS, Knighton RW, Feuer WJ, Schiffman JC. Normative retardation data corrected for corneal polarization axis using scanning laser polarimetry. Ophthalmic Surg Lasers Imaging. 2003;34:165–171.
20. Hoh ST, Greenfield DS, Liebmann JM, et al. Factors affecting image acquisition during scanning laser polarimetry. Ophthalmic Surg Lasers. 1998;29:545–551.
21. Hoh ST, Greenfield DS, Mistlberger A, Lievmann JM, Iskikawa H, Ritch R. Optical coherence tomography and scanning laser polarimetry in normal, ocular hypertensive, and glaucomatous eyes. Am J Ophthalmol. 2000;129:129–135.
22. Hoh ST, Ishikawa H, Greenfield DS, Liebmann JM, Chew SJ, Ritch R. Peripapillary nerve fiber layer thickness measurement reproducibility using scanning laser polarimetry. J Glaucoma. 1998;7:12–15.
23. Hunter DG, Patel SN, et al. Automated detection of foveal fixation by use of retinal birefringence scanning. Appl Opt. 1999; 39:1273–1279.
24. Knighton RW, Huang XR. Analytical methods for scanning laser polarimetry. Opt Express. 2002;10:1179–1189.
25. Knighton RW, Huang XR, Greenfield DS. Analytical model of scanning laser polarimetry for retinal nerve fiber layer assessment. Invest Ophthalmol Vis Sci. 2002;43:383–392.
26. Lee VW, Mok KH. Retinal nerve fiber layer measurement by nerve fiber analyzer in normal subjects and patients with glaucoma. Ophthalmology. 1999;106:1006–1008.
27. Medeiros FA, Susanna R. Retinal nerve fiber layer loss after traumatic optic neuropathy detected by scanning laser polarimetry. Arch Ophthalmol. 2001;119:920–921.
28. Medeiros FA, Zangwill LM, Bowd C, Bernd AS, Weinreb RN. Fourier

analysis of scanning laser polarimetry measurements with variable corneal compensation in glaucoma. Invest Ophthalmol Vis Sci. 2003;44: 2606–2612.

29. Meier FM, Bernasconi P, Sturmer J, Caubergh MJ, Landau K. Axonal loss from acute optic neuropathy documented by scanning laser polarimetry. Br J Ophthalmol. 2002;86:285–287.

30. Mistlberger A, Liebmann JM, Greenfield DS, et al. Assessment of optic disc anatomy and nerve fiber layer thickness in ocular hypertensive subjects with normal short-wavelength automated perimetry. Ophthalmology. 2002;109:1362–1266.

31. Poinoosawmy D, Tan JCH, Bunce C, Membrey LW, Hitchings RA. Longitudinal nerve fibre layer thickness change in normal-pressure glaucoma. Graefes Arch Clin Exp Ophthalmol. 2002;238:965–969.

32. Rhee DJ, Greenfield DS, Chen PP, Schiffman J. Reproducibility of retinal nerve fiber layer thickness measurements using scanning laser polarimetry in pseudophakic eyes. Ophthalmic Surg Lasers. 2002;33:117–122.

33. Sanchez-Galeana C, Bowd C, Blumenthal EZ, Gokhale PA, Zangwell LM, Weinreb RN. Using optical imaging summary data to detect glaucoma. Ophthalmology. 2001;108:1812–1818.

34. Tjon-Fo-Sang MJ, de Vries J, Lemiz HG. Measurement by nerve fiber analyzer of retinal nerve fiber layer thickness in normal subjects and patients with ocular hypertension. Am J Ophthalmol. 1996;122:220–227.

35. Tjon-Fo-Sang MJ, Lemij HG. The sensitivity and specificity of nerve fiber layer measurements in glaucoma as determined with scanning laser polarimetry. Am J Ophthalmol. 1997;123:62–69.

36. Tjon-Fo-Sang MJH, van Strik R, de Vries J, Lemij HG. Improved reproducibility of measurements with the nerve fiber analyzer. J Glaucoma. 1997;6:203–211.

37. Weinreb RN, Bowd C, Greenfield DS, Zangwell LM. Measurement of the magnitude and axis of corneal polarization with scanning laser polarimetry. Arch Ophthalmol. 2002;120:901–906.

38. Weinreb RN, Bowd C, Zangwell LM. Glaucoma detection using scanning laser polarimetry with variable corneal polarization compensation. Arch Ophthalmol. 2003;120: 218–224.

39. Weinreb RN, Shakiba S, Sample PA, et al. Scanning laser polarimetry to measure the nerve fiber layer of normal and glaucomatous eyes. Am J Ophthalmol. 1995;119:627–636.

40. Weinreb RN, Zangwill L, Berry CC, Bathija R, Sample PA. Detection of glaucoma with scanning laser polarimetry. Arch Ophthalmol. 1998;116:1583–1589.

41. Zangwill L, Berry CA, et al. Reproducibility of retardation measurements with the Nerve Fiber Analyzer II. J Glaucoma. 1997;6:384–389.

42. Zangwill LM, Bowd C, Berry CC, et al. Discriminating between normal and glaucomatous eyes using the Heidelberg retina tomograph, GDx nerve fiber analyzer, and optical coherence tomograph. Arch Ophthalmol. 2001;119:985–993.

43. Zhou Q, Weinreb RN. Individualized compensation of anterior segment birefringence during scanning laser polarimetry. Invest Ophthalmol Vis Sci. 2002;43:2221–2228.

Chapter 8

Retinal Thickness Analyzer

SANJAY ASRANI, MD • RAN ZEIMER, PhD

8.1 Physical Principles

The retinal thickness analyzer (RTA) is an automated, computerized slit-lamp biomicroscopic system. It uses a green (543 nm) He-Ne laser in the form of a slit beam. It allows acquisition of optical cross sections of the retina and the disc. In the macula, the optical cross sections provide visualization of pathologic changes and are analyzed to generate two- and three-dimensional quantitative maps of the retinal thickness. At the disc, the RTA delineates the surface of the nerve fibers and yields a topographic map of the disc.

8.2 Description

The RTA was invented by Ran Zeimer and his colleagues[20,21] and was developed into a commercial clinical instrument (**Figure 8–1**) by Talia Technology (Neve Ilan, Israel). **Figure 8–2** schematically illustrates the principle of optical sectioning with the RTA. Sixteen optical cross sections, 200 μm apart, are acquired in 330 msec, fast enough to avoid eye movement. To perform a scan (**Figure 8–3**), the operator centers and focuses the pupil viewed on a monitor. The 16 optical cross sections yield a scan over a 3 mm × 3 mm area (**Figure 8–4a**) and a record of the location on the fundus. The posterior pole (6 mm × 6 mm) is covered by five scans (**Figure 8–4b**).

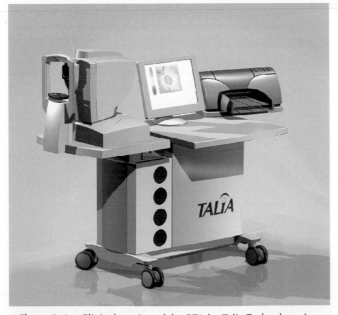

Figure 8–1   Clinical version of the RTA by Talia Technology, Inc.

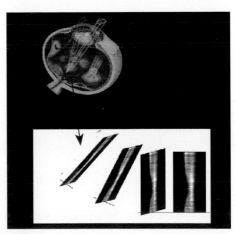

Figure 8–2   Principle of the RTA. *Top:* A thin slit from a green laser is projected obliquely onto the retina and imaged at a known angular separation. *Bottom:* The retinal thickness is derived from the separation between the vitreoretinal interface and the retinal pigment epithelium on the cross-sectional image.

Figure 8–3 Alignment of the RTA before scanning. *Top right:* The scan area is marked by a *yellow square* on the fundus image. *Top center:* Pupil image and buttons for centration and focusing. *Bottom right:* the slit image is focused by buttons on the left or automatically. *Center left:* Control buttons for fixation target/scan location.

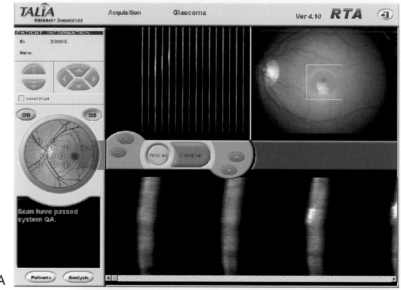

Figure 8–4 *A:* Results of a single 270 msec RTA scan. *Top right:* 3 mm × 3 mm scan area documented on the fundus. *Top center:* 16 linear optical cross sections, 200 μm apart. *Bottom right:* scans viewed at higher magnification. The inner (*left*) and outer (*right*) retinal boundaries are visualized. The dark anteroposterior streaks are due to shadows cast by retinal vessels. *B:* The five macular areas scanned by the RTA are shown by *yellow squares* superimposed on a fundus image. *Top right:* 3 mm × 3 mm scan area documented on the fundus. *Top center:* 16 linear optical cross sections, 200 μm apart.

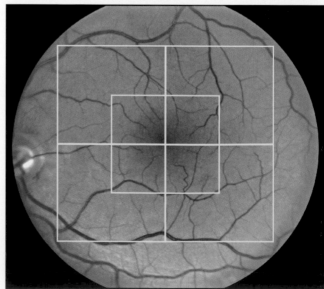

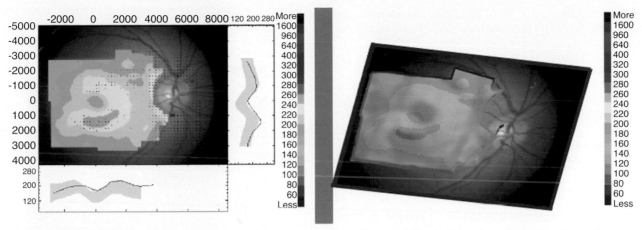

Figure 8–5 Typical normal retinal thickness map. *Left:* Two-dimensional map of retinal thickness with color code on the adjacent bar. *Right:* Three-dimensional topographical elevation map of the same. The deleted points (large deviations due to major blood vessels or exudates or hemorrhages) are displayed on the map as *black dots* indicating lack of reliable data.

An automatic algorithm analyzes the optical cross sections and generates a two- or three-dimensional map of the retinal thickness (**Figure 8–5**). An automated algorithm detects deviations from fixation and rasters the individual maps into a composite map. The operator-free algorithm performs quality tests and deletes points that deviate from their neighbors by a preset value. These large deviations are typically due to major blood vessels or large pathologic lesions (exudates or hemorrhages) that cast a shadow on the retinal pigment epithelium.

8.3 Performance and Interpretation

8.3.1 SHAPE OF THE RETINAL THICKNESS MAP

The composite shown in **Figure 8–5** illustrates the retinal thickness map of the normal macula.[3] The central crater corresponds to the foveal depression. A thick doughnut-shaped region surrounds the fovea and extends toward the disc, creating a typical "C" shape. The doughnut is due to the thick layer of ganglion cells around the fovea that is distorted into a C shape by the nerve fibers running their course toward the optic nerve head.

8.3.2 REPRODUCIBILITY

The RTA has been designed to minimize many of the factors that could adversely affect reproducibility. The short acquisition time minimizes artifacts generated by eye movements, the operator-free algorithm avoids the variability that may be induced by an operator (e.g., marking the disc margin), and the registration of the scans with the fundus landmarks corrects for deviations in fixation.

The reproducibility of the RTA map was assessed in normal subjects by a number of investigators. Regions 1 disc diameter in size were reported to have, on average, a reproducibility of 13 μm for scans in the same day and

14 μm for scans performed in different sessions.[4,7,8,11,14] Similar values were obtained in glaucomatous eyes. In edematous eyes, the variability was reported to be higher (27 μm)[11] (of little clinical impact because macular edema is accompanied by large retinal thickness changes that can reach 10 times this value). Assuming correct operation of the instrument, the main factor limiting the reproducibility is, as for most other ophthalmic imaging methods, the quality of the image, which depends mainly on the degree of ocular media opacity.

8.3.3 CHANGE SENSITIVITY

When investigators compare the mean values of a study cohort at two time points, the sensitivity to change is determined by the variation of the mean (the standard error of the mean [SEM]) and depends on the cohort size. Such studies are valuable to assess overall change, but they do not help the clinician faced with an individual patient. In this case, the clinician needs to know the sensitivity, referred to here as the *change sensitivity*, which is determined by the intervisit reproducibility to detect a change in a given individual. Change sensitivity is the change needed to determine, with 97.5% confidence, that there is an increase (or a decrease) and that it is equal to twice the reproducibility between visits. For the RTA, the change sensitivity for an area 1 disc in diameter is 26 μm for nonedematous eyes and most likely twice this value in the presence of edema.

8.3.4 RETINAL THICKNESS IN NORMAL SUBJECTS

Different investigators have found similar values for the mean macular thickness (230 μm) over a 6 × 6 mm area centered over the fovea. The values reported for the fovea (150 to 180 μm) differed more, probably because of differences in the size of the area being averaged. The values reported for the standard deviation of macular and foveal thicknesses in a normal population are quite consistently around ±15 μm.[3,4,11] This consistency is encouraging because it indicates that the anatomy of the healthy retina is well defined and constant among subjects.

For the retinal thickness of an individual to be considered (with 97.5% confidence) to be greater than (or less than) the normal range, it needs to deviate by twice the standard deviation of normal values. Accordingly, the RTA has a diagnostic sensitivity of 30 μm.

8.4 Clinical Applications

8.4.1 RTA IN GLAUCOMA

Glaucoma has traditionally been diagnosed by observing the optic nerve head (ONH) and visual field (VF). Unfortunately, the structure of the ONH varies dramatically among normal individuals, thereby inherently lowering the diagnostic sensitivity that can be achieved by many modern objective techniques of optic disc imaging and hindering the task of separating glaucomatous eyes from normal eyes. VF testing is a subjective psychophysical test that has poor reproducibility. We have proposed that the retinal thickness at the macula could play an important role in the evaluation of glaucoma.[19] The ganglion cell layer in the macula is up to six layers thick and, along with the retinal nerve fiber layer, constitutes 30% to 40% of macular retinal thickness. The ganglion cell layer is thicker in the macula (**Figure 8–6**) and accounts for half of the ganglion cells in the eye. Most importantly, anatomic studies have shown that the number of ganglion cells varies less at the macula. finally, because 70% of ganglion cells need to be lost for the development of a 3-dB VF loss close to fixation (versus only 10% at 24 degrees from fixation),[5] there is a potential for considerable loss of retinal thickness in the macula before perimetry findings become apparent.

Figures 8–7 and **8–8** show two instances in which the RTA detected glaucomatous changes before a definitive VF defect occurred. In **Figure 8–7**, a patient with a family history of glaucoma shows normal VFs with a large cup-to-disc ratio in the right eye. The RTA shows both global and focal thinning in the macula. In **Figure 8–8,** the RTA shows trench-like thinning in the inferior macula that corresponds to an inferior disc hemorrhage in the absence of a definite superior VF defect.

The RTA may also be helpful when the diagnosis of glaucoma is uncertain. In **Figure 8–9**, the RTA demonstrates superior macular thinning that is consistent with the presence of an inferior scotoma, despite the normal appearance of the ONH. In **Figure 8–10**, the RTA confirms that a large ONH cupping is physiologic rather than glaucomatous.

We also show examples in which the RTA results agree with both the appearance of the ONH and the VF (**Figures 8–11** and **8–12**).

The examples shown illustrate the utility of RTA macular thickness mapping in glaucoma diagnosis. The objective assessment of loss of ganglion cells and nerve fibers provides the clinician with a useful complement

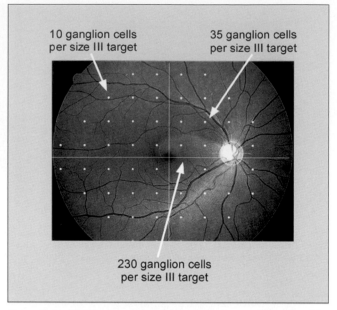

Figure 8–6 Distribution of ganglion cells in the macular region. The density of ganglion cells varies significantly among the visual field test points. (Courtesy of Ted Garway-Heath, Glaucoma Research Unit, Moorfields Eye Hospital, UK.)

to optic nerve evaluation and perimetry. However, only long-term prospective studies (now under way) will reveal the diagnostic and prognostic power of macular retinal thickness mapping.

8.4.2 RETINAL THICKNESS MAPPING IN DIABETIC MACULAR EDEMA

The comparison of retinal thickness measurements and stereophotographs read by the Wisconsin Reading Center suggested that stereophotography does not identify locations with mild or localized thickening.[17]

Cross-sectional studies have shown good correlation between foveal thickness and visual acuity ($r \cong 0.7$)[11,16,18] but they cannot reveal the true relationship, because vision changes could have been affected by past events or could lag behind thickness changes. Only a longitudinal study could elucidate this relationship.

The finding that in some patients with clinically significant macular edema the fovea can be three times thicker than normal implies that thickening can be accompanied by large tissue distortions that are likely to cause irreversible damage to the structure and function of the retina. The fact that no association was found between retinal thickening and the presence of hard exudates, soft exudates, hemorrhages, or microaneurysms[9,17] is clinically important because it provides evidence for the recommendation to detect macular edema only on the basis of thickening.

Pilot studies have demonstrated that drugs can reduce macular edema and that changes in thickening can occur in a short period.[12,13] Objective mapping of the retinal thickness has begun to elucidate the relationship between focal laser treatment and reduction of

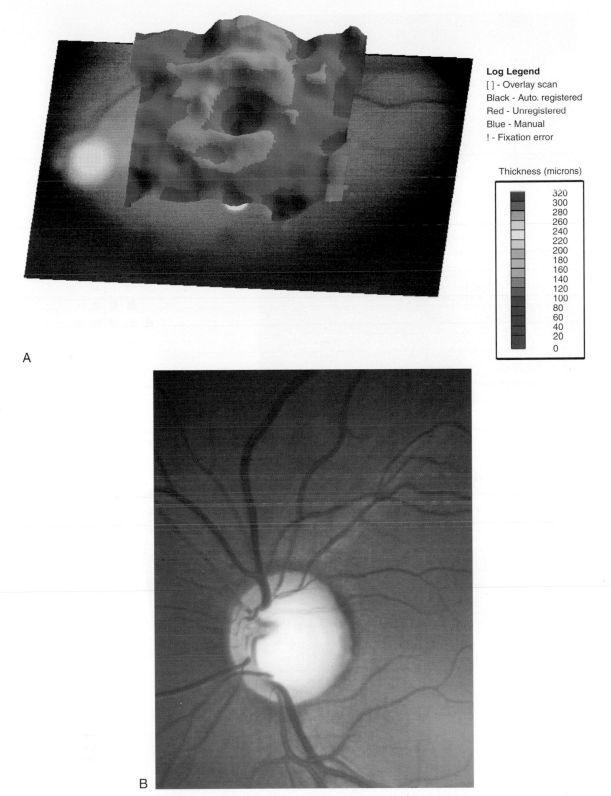

Log Legend
[ ] - Overlay scan
Black - Auto. registered
Red - Unregistered
Blue - Manual
! - Fixation error

Thickness (microns)

320
300
280
260
240
220
200
180
160
140
120
100
80
60
40
20
0

A

B

Figure 8–7   RTA thinning without visual field changes in a glaucoma suspect. The RTA macular thickness map (*A*) shows considerable generalized depression along with localized loss inferiorly in the ganglion cell rim. There is an enlarged cup (B) but a normal VF.

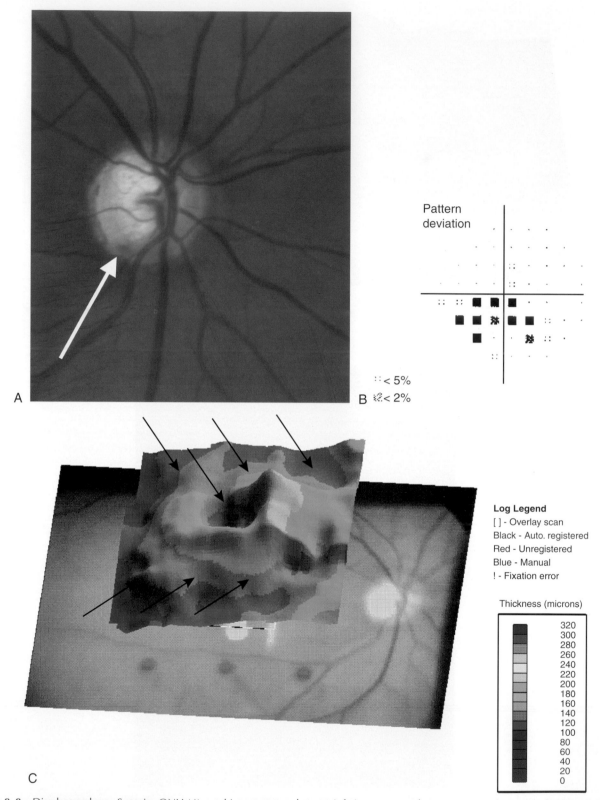

Pattern deviation

:: < 5%

< 2%

Log Legend
[ ] - Overlay scan
Black - Auto. registered
Red - Unregistered
Blue - Manual
! - Fixation error

Thickness (microns)

	320
	300
	280
	260
	240
	220
	200
	180
	160
	140
	120
	100
	80
	60
	40
	20
	0

Figure 8–8   Disc hemorrhage. Superior ONH (*A*) notching corresponds to an inferior paracentral scotoma (*B*) and superior thinning on the RTA (*C*). A disc hemorrhage inferiorly (*A*) is associated with retinal thinning (*C*) but not with a VF defect (*B*). (From Asrani S, Challa P, Herndon L, Lee P, Stinnett S, Allingham R. Correlation between retinal thickness analysis, optic nerve and visual fields in glaucoma patients and suspects. J Glaucoma. 2003;12:119–128.)

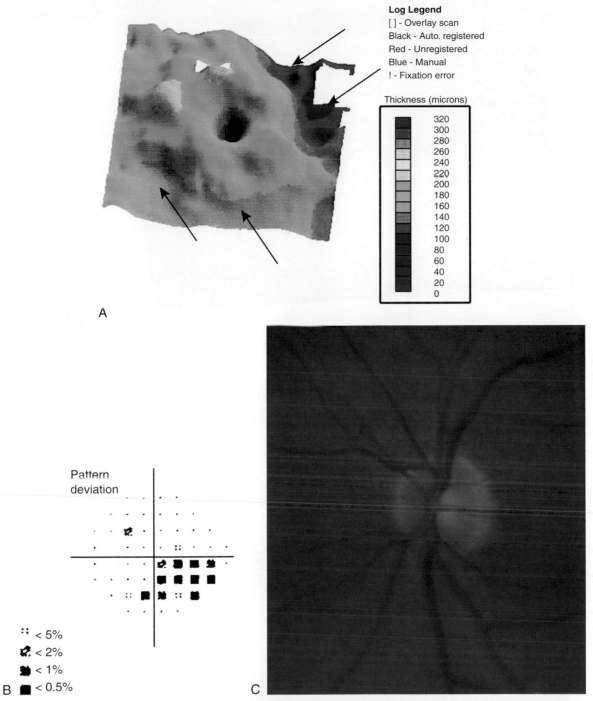

Log Legend
[ ] - Overlay scan
Black - Auto. registered
Red - Unregistered
Blue - Manual
! - Fixation error

Thickness (microns)

	320
	300
	280
	260
	240
	220
	200
	180
	160
	140
	120
	100
	80
	60
	40
	20
	0

A

Pattern
deviation

:: < 5%
✿ < 2%
✹ < 1%
■ < 0.5%

B

C

Figure 8–9 Glaucomatous eye *(left)* with inferior scotoma and normal ONH appearance. The RTA *(A)* shows localized superior thinning corresponding to the inferior scotoma *(B)*. Also note the early groove-like thinning inferiorly in the RTA. The ONH *(C)* appears normal.

117

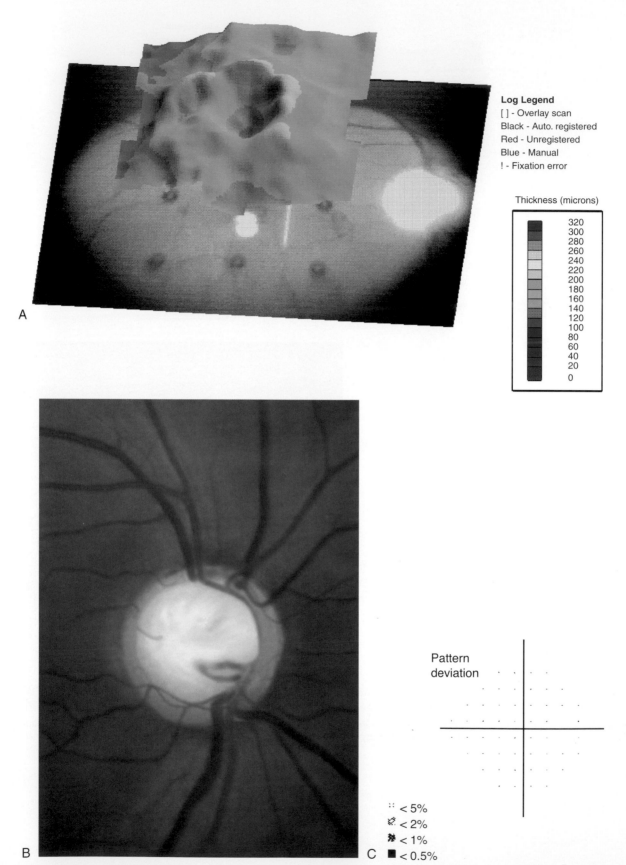

Log Legend
[ ] - Overlay scan
Black - Auto. registered
Red - Unregistered
Blue - Manual
! - Fixation error

Thickness (microns)

	320
	300
	280
	260
	240
	220
	200
	180
	160
	140
	120
	100
	80
	60
	40
	20
	0

Pattern
deviation

∷ < 5%
< 2%
< 1%
■ < 0.5%

Figure 8–10   Large physiologic ONH cupping (right eye). The RTA (*A*) shows normal macular thickness in this eye with a deep and large cup in a large ONH (*B*). *C:* The VF was normal.

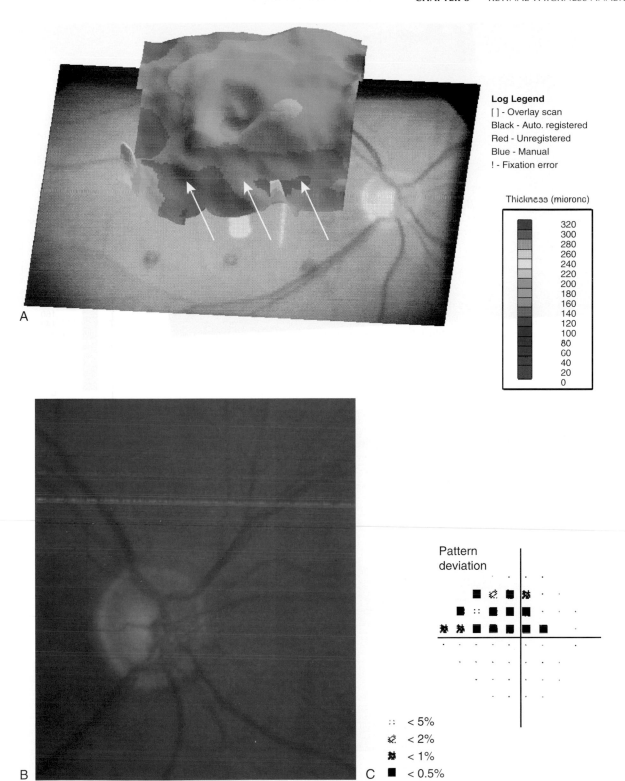

Log Legend
[ ] - Overlay scan
Black - Auto. registered
Red - Unregistered
Blue - Manual
! - Fixation error

Thickness (microns)

	320
	300
	280
	260
	240
	220
	200
	180
	160
	140
	120
	100
	80
	60
	40
	20
	0

Pattern
deviation

::   < 5%

✳   < 2%

✷   < 1%

■   < 0.5%

Figure 8–11   Glaucomatous eye. The RTA macular thickness map (*A*) demonstrates a deep inferior trench-like thinning (*arrows*) extending toward the optic nerve. It matches an inferior notch in the ONH (*B*) and a dense superior paracentral scotoma on the VF (*C*).

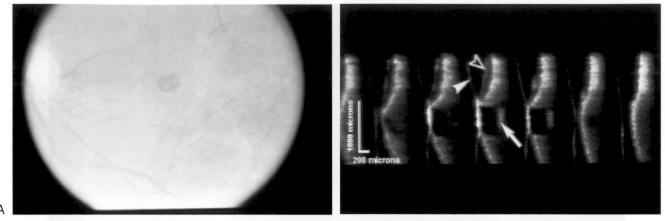

Figure 8–15 Pseudo-macular hole. Fundus photograph (*A*) and RTA sections (*B*) showing a pseudo-macular hole with an epiretinal membrane (*empty arrowhead*) and an attached posterior hyaloid at edges of foveal cyst (*solid arrowhead*). (From Asrani S, Zeimer R, Goldberg M, Zou S. Serial optical sectioning of macular holes at different stages of development. Ophthalmology. 1998;105:66–77.)

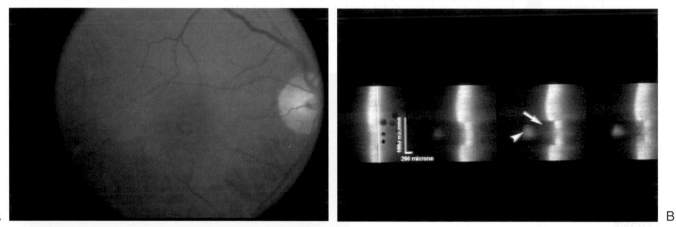

Figure 8–16 Macular hole (stage 3). Fundus photograph (*A*) and RTA sections (*B*) demonstrate a macular hole with an operculum (*arrow*). (From Asrani S, Zeimer R, Goldberg M, Zou S. Serial optical cross sectioning of macular holes at different stages of development. Ophthalmology. 1998;105:66–77.)

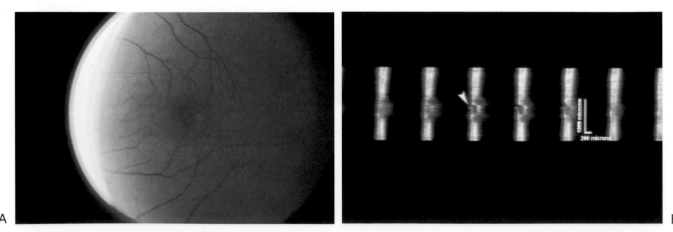

Figure 8–17 Macular hole (stage 2). Fundus photograph (*A*) and RTA sections (*B*) show an eccentric break (*arrowhead*) in a foveal cyst. (From Asrani S, Zeimer R, Goldberg M, Zou S. Serial optical cross sectioning of macular holes at different stages of development. Ophthalmology. 1998;105:66–77.)

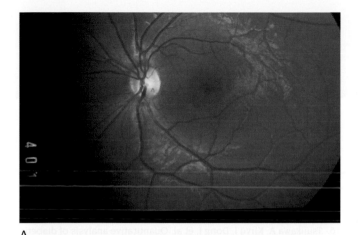

A

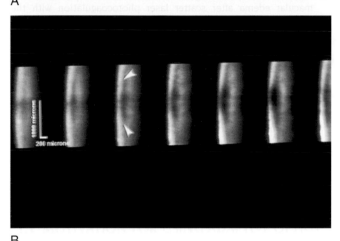

B

Figure 8–18   Juvenile X-linked retinoschisis. Fundus photograph (A) and RTA sections (B) show separation of retinal layers at the fovea (space between the nerve fiber and ganglion cell layer and the rest of the retina). (From Tanna A, Asrani S, Zou S, Zeimer R, Goldberg M. Foveal optical sectioning with the retinal thickness analyzer in patients with juvenile X-linked retinoschisis. Arch Ophthalmol. 1998;116:1036–1041.)

8.5 Strengths and Limitations

The necessity for a 5-mm dilation of the pupil may be inconvenient in some cases but is typically not restrictive in the ophthalmic environment because patients' eyes are often dilated for other clinical reasons. The quality of RTA scans can be affected by dislocated intraocular lenses, irregular and decentered pupils, and marked astigmatism. But the main limitation of the RTA, as for most optical methods, is the need for clear media. It is not possible to obtain high-quality RTA images in persons with corneal pathologic lesions (except for mild to moderate symptoms of dry eye), visually significant cataracts, or vitreous opacity.

It is important to realize that, ultimately, the interpretation of images obtained with various imaging techniques necessitates clinical judgment. It is not only needed to identify images that are less reliable because of poor quality but also to identify confounding

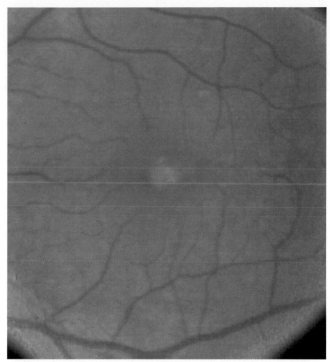

A

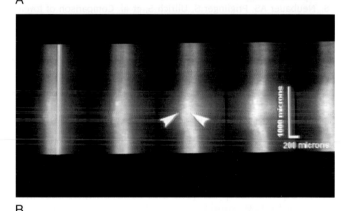

B

Figure 8–19   Adult Vitelliform Dystrophy. Fundus photograph (A) with hypo pigmented foveal lesion and RTA sections (B) show elevation of the retina (arrowheads point to elevation of both surfaces of the retina). (From Asrani S, Zeimer R, Goldberg MF, Zou S: Application of rapid scanning retinal thickness analysis in retinal pathologies. Ophthalmology 104:1145–51, 1997.)

pathologic changes that can yield artifactual results. For example, preretinal membranes or strong reflections can yield falsely thick values, a macular hole may confound the analysis algorithm, and a number of retinopathies other than glaucoma and diabetic macular edema could affect retinal thickness (e.g., diabetic or hypertensive retinopathy, cystoid macular edema, age-related macular degeneration, retinal-vascular occlusion, or uveitis).

ACKNOWLEDGMENT

Under a licensing agreement with Talia Technology, Ltd., Dr. Zeimer is entitled to a share of royalty received

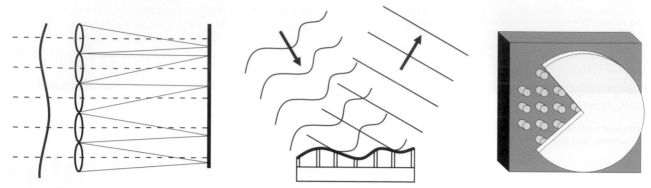

Figure 9–1 Basic components of an AO system. The wavefront sensor (*left*) measures the wavefront aberration, which is then corrected by a DM that is shaped by a series of electromechanical pistons glued to its back surface.

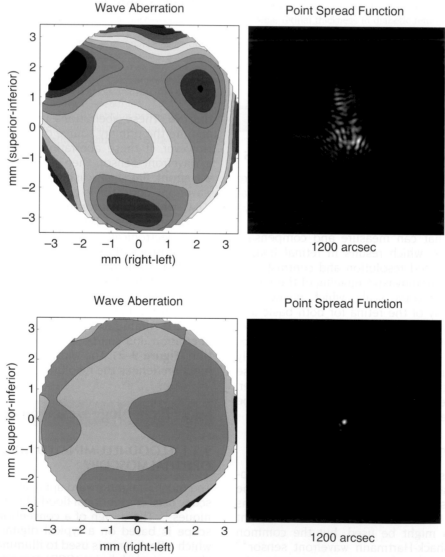

Figure 9–2 Before AO (*top*), the wavefront is distorted, which gives rise to a broad point spread function. After AO (*bottom*), the wavefront is nearly flat, and the corresponding point spread function is very small.

integrates a wavefront sensor and a wavefront corrector into the path. The layout of the conventional AO ophthalmoscope is shown in **Figure 9–3.**

The wavefront sensor uses a superluminescent diode to illuminate a small spot on the retina at the location of the desired image. Light scattered by the retina emerges from the eye and bounces off the DM, which is originally in a flat state. The wavefront sensor measures the aberrations and sends the signal to the mirror to compensate. In each subsequent cycle, the wavefront sensor measures the eye-plus-DM combination, and continues to correct in a closed loop until the wave aberration reduces to near diffraction-limited levels. Once the wave aberration is sufficiently low, the camera automatically takes a picture. The illumination for the picture is from a separate incoherent light source. The flash from the imaging source is brief enough (about 4 msec) to freeze the motion of the retina, which is constantly moving, even while fixating. If the source is broadband, then interference filters can be used in the path to control the wavelength. The light source uniformly illuminates a patch on the retina, generally less than 1 mm across. **Figure 9–4** shows the benefit of using AO on images of the photoreceptor mosaic in a living

eye. All three images are of the same retinal area located 1 degree from the central fovea. Images were taken with 550-nm light (25-nm bandwidth) through a 6-mm pupil. The *leftmost* image shows a single snapshot taken after defocus and astigmatism have been corrected. The *middle* image is a snapshot after additional aberrations have been corrected with AO. The *rightmost* image shows the benefits in image quality obtained by registering and averaging multiple frames.

9.2.2 ADAPTIVE OPTICS SCANNING LASER OPHTHALMOSCOPY

More recently, AO has been applied to the scanning laser ophthalmoscope (SLO).[9] Scanning laser ophthalmoscopy differs from conventional imaging in that the SLO captures an image over time by detecting the scattered light from a focused point as it scans across the retina in a raster pattern. This imaging modality offers several noted advantages over conventional ophthalmoscopes. First, one can use more sensitive detectors, such as photomultiplier tubes or avalanche photodiodes, to detect the light rather than using an inherently noisier and less sensitive CCD camera. More importantly, SLOs

Figure 9–3 Schematic diagram of the Rochester flood-illuminated AO ophthalmoscope.

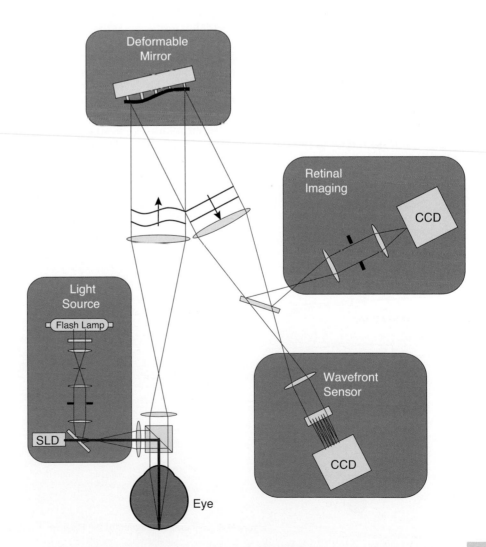

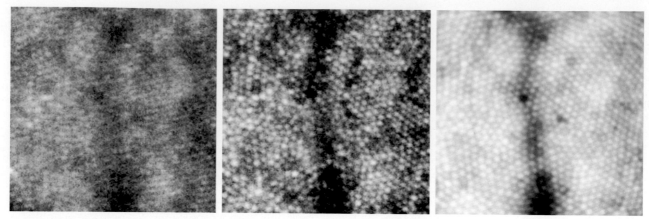

Figure 9–4   Retinal images from a live human subject before (*left*) and after (*center*) AO compensation, and after further enhancement (*right*) by registering and averaging multiple frames.

are relatively insensitive to image degradation owing to scatter in the optics, and SLOs have the ability to do optical sectioning in the retina. The latter two advantages are facilitated by passing the scattered light through a small aperture conjugate to the retina, called the confocal pinhole, before detection. A schematic diagram of the adaptive optics scanning laser ophthalmoscope (AOSLO) is shown in **Figure 9–5**. The AOSLO uses a laser. The laser light is scanned on the retina with the scanning mirrors. Light that scatters back from the retina is split into a light detection path, for forming the image, and into the wavefront sensing path, for measuring the wave aberration of the eye. The wavefront sensor combines with the DM to measure and compensate the wavefront.

The AOSLO is similar to a conventional ophthalmoscope in that both rely on the optical system of the eye as the objective lens for imaging. Hence, an SLO shows

the same image quality losses due to aberrations. It follows that the AO technique can offer the same benefits to this imaging technique. There are several differences in the AO system of the AOSLO compared with a flood-illuminated system. First, the AOSLO wavefront sensor uses the same light source for imaging as it uses for wavefront sensing. A consequence of using the same light source is that the AOSLO wavefront sensor measures aberrations from the entire raster-scanned area of the retina. In conventional imaging systems this is not possible because the large field of illumination on the retina makes wavefront sensing impossible. However, in the AOSLO it is possible because the light from the raster is "descanned" on its return path in the SLO and appears to originate from a single point, even though it does not. The second difference is that the wave aberrations are corrected on the way into the eye (to get a small focused spot on

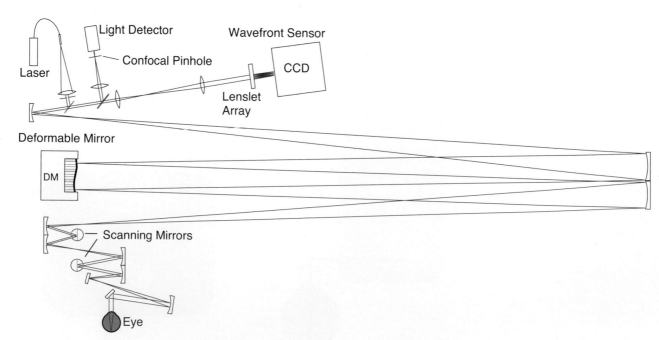

Figure 9–5   Schematic diagram of the Houston AOSLO.

the retina) and on the way out of the eye (to get a small focused spot at the confocal pinhole), the result being that the potential lateral resolution is moderately higher than that with conventional imaging systems.[12] There are several advantages of using the SLO as the imaging method. The first is that the high detection and scanning speed are conducive to taking retinal images at video rates, making it possible to see dynamic changes in the retina, such as blood flow. The AOSLO in Houston generates 512 × 480 pixel images at 30 frames/sec. Another advantage of using the AOSLO is its ability to image optical sections of the retina. This is shown in **Figure 9–6,** which presents images of three layers from a single location on the retina. The retinal location and image size are indicated in the conventional fundus photograph. The *right* image shows the nerve fiber layer,

which overlies some of the vessels, and then a deeper layer, which reveals more blood vessels, but otherwise shows little detail because of the transparent retina. The *left* image shows the photoreceptor layer, which lies about 300 μm deeper than the nerve fibers. The high contrast of each layer is achieved by blocking the light from out-of-focus layers with the confocal pinhole.

9.3 Imaging Results and Applications

9.3.1 BASIC SCIENCE APPLICATIONS

Some of the most dominant features in microscopic images of living human eyes are the cone photoreceptors. They appear bright because light is guided through

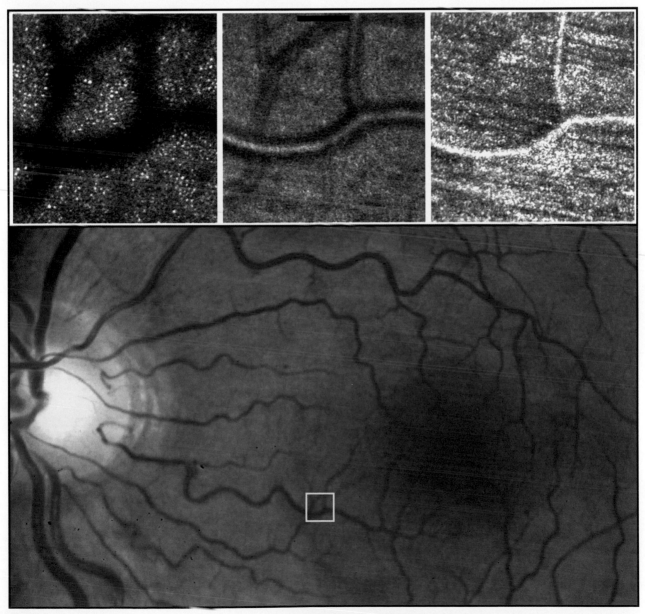

Figure 9–6 The retinal location indicated by the *yellow box* on the fundus photograph (*top*) is imaged by the AOSLO at the level of the photoreceptors (*left*), mid-retina (*center*), and nerve fiber layer (*right*). Scale bar = 100 μm.

them, reflects from their base at the retinal pigment epithelium, which is the location of the strongest retinal reflections, and reemerges from the inner segments of the fibers again. The cones are very effective waveguides, with very high contrast, and preferentially direct the reflected light toward the pupil. Most effort to date has been concentrated on measuring the cone photoreceptors and their properties. **Figure 9–7,** from the Rochester AO ophthalmoscope, is a composite image showing the entire central 3.25 degrees (0.975 mm) of the retina of a human fovea. Cone photoreceptors appear with high contrast, even at the foveal center, where they are about 2.5 μm in diameter.

The Three Cone Classes in the Human Eye

The ability to image cone photoreceptors with AO provided the first opportunity to measure their properties directly.[10] **Figure 9–8** shows the first ever maps of the arrangement of the three cone classes in the human eye. The images use a color scale so that blue (S), green (M), and red (L) cones are shown in their respective colors. Images were taken at either 1 or 1.25 degrees from the

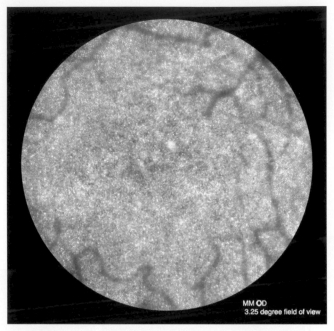

Figure 9–7 Living human fovea imaged with the Rochester AO ophthalmoscope, showing bright spots corresponding to cones.

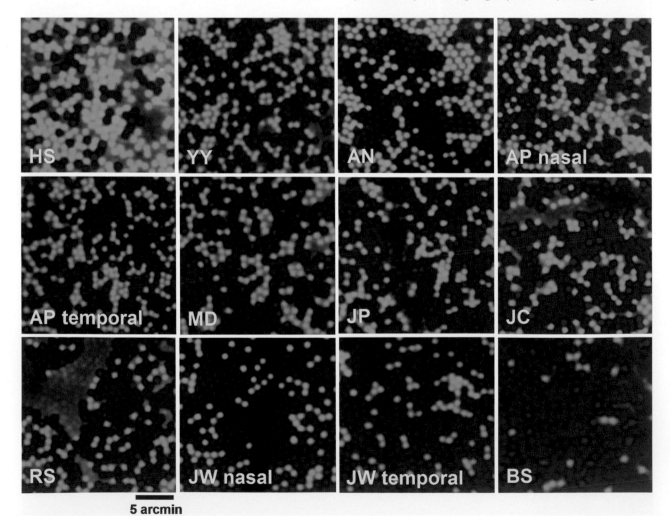

Figure 9–8 The cone mosaics in 12 locations from 10 normal subjects imaged with adaptive optics and retinal densitometry. The false-color scale represent S, M, and L cones in *blue, green,* and *red,* respectively.

foveal center. The study revealed some interesting facts about the retina. The first was that the proportions of cones vary remarkably between individuals. The L-to-M cone ratios are (from left to right and top to bottom) 0.37, 1.11, 1.14, 1.24, 1.77, 1.88, 2.32, 2.35, 2.46, 3.67, 3.90, and 16.54. Despite the large range of L-to-M ratios, every one of the subjects demonstrated normal color vision by all conventional tests.[2] The arrangement of cones, which was never known until imaged with AO, was essentially random in the locations where we imaged.

Cones as Waveguides

The waveguiding, or optical fiber, property of cones has several advantages, including the rejection of stray light in the retina and maximizing efficiency in light collection. AO imaging has revealed that the cone photoreceptors demonstrate a remarkable precision in the alignment of their optical axes. **Figure 9–9** shows an image of the cone photoreceptors superimposed with small arrows that indicate the pointing direction of each of the cones. The length of the arrows indicates the amount of deviation in pointing direction that each cone has with respect to the ensemble of cones. Although this image may suggest that the cones are disarrayed, projecting each cone axis into the pupil plane shows that the cones are remarkably well-tuned, all pointing into an area in the pupil that is less than 0.15 mm across.[11]

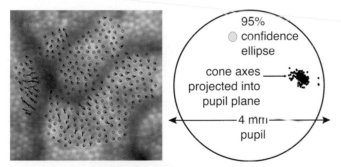

Figure 9–9 Angular tuning of cone photoreceptors. The photoreceptor image on the *left* is superimposed with lines that indicate the pointing direction and the amount of deviation of each cone. The deviation is very small in a healthy eye.

9.3.2 CLINICAL APPLICATIONS

The basic science benefits of microscopic retinal imaging are clear, but they may eventually be surpassed by the clinical benefit of this technology. Noninvasive images of the fundus with high contrast and showing microscopic details offer potential for all clinical applications, from early detection of disease to studying the mechanisms of the disease to monitoring and studying the efficacy of treatments for the disease.

Blood Flow

High-contrast and high-resolution imaging makes it possible to visualize the flow of single white blood cells through the retinal capillaries. This has been used to measure the velocity of white blood cells in the smallest capillaries near the fovea. The movement of the white blood cells is best seen in video frames, which can be downloaded from http://www.uh.edu/research/aroorda/aoslo/htm.

Hard Exudates

Imaging of an eye from a type 1 diabetic patient showed detailed features of a hard exudate that was located about 700 μm from the foveal center. **Figure 9–10** shows how the microscopic features of the hard exudate changed over time.

Microaneurysms

Imaging in the same type 1 diabetic patient of the retina just nasal to the fovea showed images of photoreceptors and shadows of many microaneurysms (**Figure 9–11**). Many of the microaneurysms were not detectable in a subsequent conventional fluorescein angiogram. When serial AOSLO images are viewed in a real-time movie, one can see blood flow in the vessels with the microaneurysms.

Solar Retinopathy

Figure 9–12 shows an image near the fovea in one patient who had a dark patch where photoreceptors were expected. Through-focus imaging revealed that the

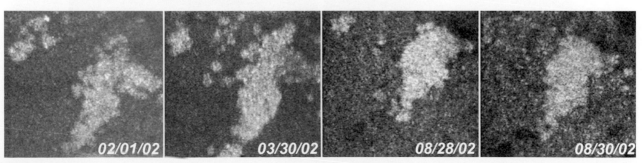

Figure 9–10 Evolution of a hard exudate in type 1 diabetic retina imaged with the AOSLO. The hard exudate appears bright and sits anterior to the photoreceptors.

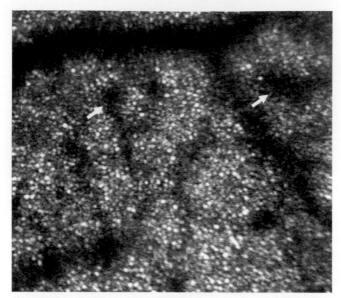

Figure 9–11 Microaneurysms in a type 1 diabetic retina. The AOSLO is focused on the cones in the photoreceptor layer. The shadows are from the capillaries that contain numerous microaneurysms (*yellow arrows*).

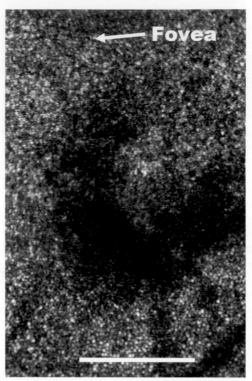

Figure 9–12 The solar retinopathy appears as a region of missing cones, close to the foveal center, which is indicated by the *yellow arrow*. The size of the burn is consistent with the image of the sun (0.5 degrees or 150 microns). Scale bar = 150 microns.

feature was in the plane of the photoreceptors and was not a shadow from overlying tissue. The image quality was excellent, as demonstrated by the visibility of photoreceptors surrounding the burned area. The features were not visible in a conventional fundus photograph but were only visible by indirect ophthalmoscopy. The patient had done previous research as a solar astronomer and reported that he had looked directly at the sun during a solar eclipse about 5 years earlier.

New Cause for Color Blindness

New genotypes for retinal disease are being found,[8] but the physical manifestation of the diseases are often more difficult to assess. Most of what we do know about

retinal diseases has come from studying donor tissue, which obviates the possibility of studying visual function in the same subjects. Microscopic AO retinal images can reveal phenotypes of retinal disease to better understand the mechanisms for the disorder. For example, **Figure 9–13** shows retinal images from individuals with two different forms of red-green color blindness. Color blindness occurs when one of the cone classes is functionally absent. A lack of long, middle, or short

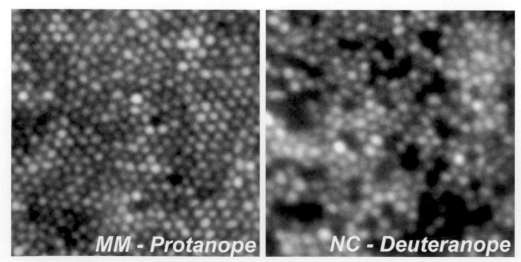

Figure 9–13 The images are from two patients who are color-blind. *Left:* Complete mosaic, devoid of L cones. *Right:* Sparse mosaic in which the gaps are presumably the intended locations of the absent M-cone class.

wavelength cone function is referred to as *protanopia*, *deuteranopia*, or *tritanopia*, respectively. The *left* image is from a protanope who has a well-known genotype for the disorder. It appears as an absence of the gene to produce the L-cone pigment. His retina shows a full complement of cones, but none of the cones are of the L-type. In other words, the L cones have all been replaced by those with M-cone pigment. The *right* image shows a deuteranope who does not show a classic genotype for the disorder. In his case, the genes that produce the L- and M-cone pigment are present, but for some reason the M-pigment gene does not produce a functional photopigment (hence his gross phenotype of deuteranopia). The retinal image from this subject is very different; it shows a subset of "missing" or non-reflecting cones. We hypothesize that this is where the M cones would have resided in that retina, but because of the lack of functioning photopigment, those cones have been physically lost. This loss indicates that the defect in his M-pigment gene manifests itself at a rather late stage in retinal development and is one example for which precise classification of the phenotypes can help us understand the etiology of a retinal disease. Applications for this capability are broad ranging and include the study of many of the cone dystrophies, such as retinitis pigmentosa, for which tremendous phenotypic and genotypic variability is seen.

9.4 Future Developments

AO technology may be used for applications other than imaging. An AO system can be adapted to deliver light to the retina with precision. In the AOSLO, for example, a spot of light is already delivered to the retina with microscopic precision. For microretinal stimulation, it is simply a matter of modulating the scanning laser beam. For therapeutic applications, it is a matter of coupling a second, more powerful, laser into the path, while the laser is scanning over the region of interest.

There are only a few working AO ophthalmoscopes in the world at this time, and they are relatively large and expensive. However, new technology that will make these instruments more compact and inexpensive, as well as more effective for imaging the human eye, is on the horizon. The main size and cost limitations of the current instruments are related to the DMs, which will soon be replaced by small microelectrical mechanical systems (MEMS) mirrors.[1] MEMS mirrors are small, they can be mass produced, and several groups are developing MEMS devices that are specifically suited for vision applications.

9.5 Conclusion

AO ophthalmoscopes offer unprecedented microscopic lateral resolution in images of the living human eye. This chapter shows results from two instruments. The range of results and applications will, no doubt, continue to expand as this technology becomes more widely available.

REFERENCES

1. Doble N, Yoon G, Bierden P, Chen L, Olivier S, Williams DR. Use of a microelectromechanical mirror for adaptive optics in the human eye. Opt Lett. 2002;27:1537–1539.
2. Hofer H. Implications of the Trichromatic Mosaic for Color Vision. Rochester, NY: University of Rochester; 2003.
3. Hofer H, Chen L, Yoon G, Singer B, Yamauchi Y, Williams DR. Improvement in retinal image quality with dynamic correction of the eye's aberrations. Opt Express. 2001;8:631–643.
4. Liang J, Grimm B, Goelz S, Bille JF. Objective measurement of wave aberrations of the human eye with use of a Hartmann-Shack wave-front sensor. J Opt Soc Am A. 1994;11:1949–1957.
5. Liang J, Williams DR. Aberrations and retinal image quality of the normal human eye. J Opt Soc Am A. 1997;14:2873–2883.
6. Liang J, Williams DR, Miller D. Supernormal vision and high-resolution retinal imaging through adaptive optics. J Opt Soc Am A. 1997;14:2884–2892.
7. Porter J, Guirao A, Cox IG, Williams DR. Monochromatic aberrations of the human eye in a large population. J Opt Soc Am A. 2001;18:1793–1803.
8. Rattner A, Sun H, Nathans J. Molecular genetics of human retinal disease. Annu Rev Genet. 1999;33:89–131.
9. Roorda A, Romero-Borja F, Donnelly WJ, Queener H, Hebert TJ, Campbell MCW. Adaptive optics scanning laser ophthalmoscopy. Opt Express. 2002;10:405–412.
10. Roorda A, Williams DR. The arrangement of the three cone classes in the living human eye. Nature. 1999;397:520–522.
11. Roorda A, Williams DR Optical fiber properties of individual human cones. J Vision. 2002;2:404–412.
12. Wilson T, Sheppard CJR. Theory and Practice of Scanning Optical Microscopy. London, England: Academic Press; 1984.

Chapter 10

Imaging of Ocular Blood Flow

BRENT A. SIESKY, PhD • ALON HARRIS, MS, PhD • LARRY KAGEMANN, MS, BME

10.1 Physical Principles

10.1.1 BLOOD FLOW TO THE EYE

Imaging ocular blood flow (OBF) requires analysis of the complex vascular anatomy of the eye. The eye has two separate and distinct circulatory systems, the retinal and the uveal.[2] The retinal vascular system nourishes the inner retina, whereas the uveal system supplies the choroid, ciliary body, and iris. The choroidal circulation nourishes the outer retina. Both the uveal and the retinal circulations are supplied by the ophthalmic artery (OA) via retrobulbar vessels.[29] The posterior ciliary arteries (PCAs) and the central retinal artery (CRA) are branches of the OA. One to five PCAs branch off from the OA, dividing into approximately 10 to 20 short PCAs that perfuse the posterior choroid and anterior optic nerve.[2] In addition, two long PCAs track anteriorly along the outside of the globe before penetrating the sclera along with one or more anterior ciliary arteries (ACAs) to supply the iris, ciliary body, and the anterior region of the choroid.[2,29]

The complex interaction of ocular vessels and tissues and their regulatory abilities require careful individual interpretation. Currently, no single imaging device is capable of accurately and completely assessing OBF. Several technologies do exist, however, that allow imaging of select vasculature within and behind the eye. If these are used together in a "multitissue analysis" approach, meaningful information about an individual's OBF may be obtained and discussed.

10.2 Technology Development

10.2.1 COLOR DOPPLER IMAGING

Color Doppler imaging (CDI) is an ultrasound technique combining B-scan gray-scale imaging and blood velocity measurements based on Doppler shifted frequencies and pulsed Doppler.[26] **Figure 10–1** shows a CDI probe about to be applied to the outside of a patient's closed eyelid for CDI analysis. During CDI examination of the eye, the operator identifies the desired vessel and places

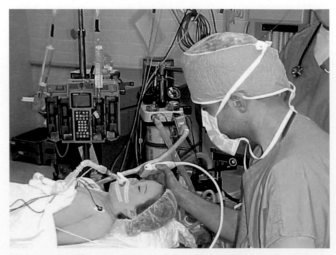

Figure 10–1 The CDI probe from the CDI cart about to be applied to the outside of a patient's closed eyelid during an examination.

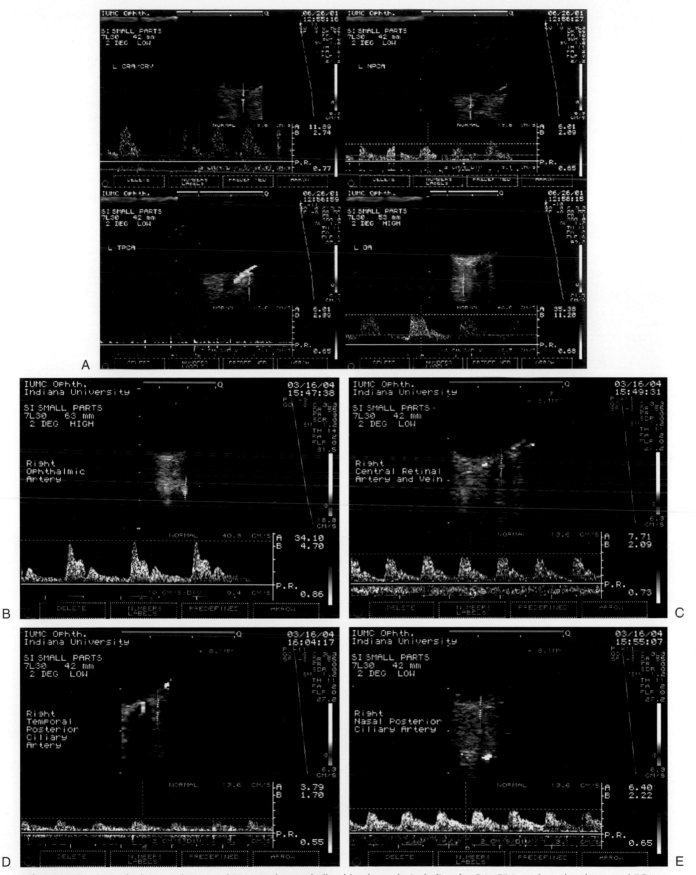

Figure 10–2 CDI calculations of PSVs and EDVs in the retrobulbar blood vessels, including the OA, CRA, and nasal and temporal PCAs.

a sampling window for pulsed-Doppler measurements on the vessel to obtain flow velocity, which is graphed over time.

CDI can be used to calculate peak systolic velocities (PSVs) and end-diastolic velocities (EDVs) in the retrobulbar blood vessels, including the OA, CRA, and nasal and temporal PCAs, which are located immediately posterior to the globe. **Figure 10–2** shows the retrobulbar vessels and measured sampling area on a CDI color printout. The peak and trough of the wave are identified by the operator, and the computer calculates the PSV and EDV, respectively, as seen in **Figure 10–3.**

Pourcelot's resistive index is then calculated, which represents downstream vascular resistance, where higher values indicate higher distal vascular resistance.[25]

CDI is noninvasive, allowing hemodynamic data to be obtained in eyes with poor optical media and without regard to pupil size.[18] Furthermore, validity and reproducibility of Doppler ultrasound measures of flow velocity have both been thoroughly studied.[10] The greatest limitation impeding the clinical use of CDI is its cost. Additionally, obtaining reproducible data requires an experienced CDI technician.

10.2.2 CANON LASER BLOOD FLOWMETER

The Canon laser blood flowmeter (CLBF) is a recently developed device used to simultaneously quantify the velocity of blood within large retinal vessels and their diameter. Similar to a fundus camera, the CLBF provides an image from which a large retinal artery or vein can be tracked and measured to provide an immediate measurement of retinal blood flow in units of microliters per minute.[9,35]

Doppler shifts are analyzed with the CLBF to determine maximum blood velocity using an assumed relationship between the maximum Doppler shift and the true average blood velocity. In a turbulent flow system, the average velocity is equal to the maximum velocity, whereas in a laminar flow system, the average velocity is equal to half the maximum velocity. The average velocity is estimated with a value between 0.5 to 1 time the maximum velocity. The CLBF compensates for the axial length of the eye (found by A-mode ultrasound) and the ocular refractive error to accurately calculate vessel diameter. **Figure 10–4** shows the CLBF computer screen during a CLBF analysis.

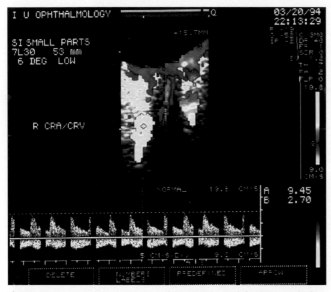

Figure 10–3 A CDI computer analysis printout of the CRA with the PSV and EDV calculated.

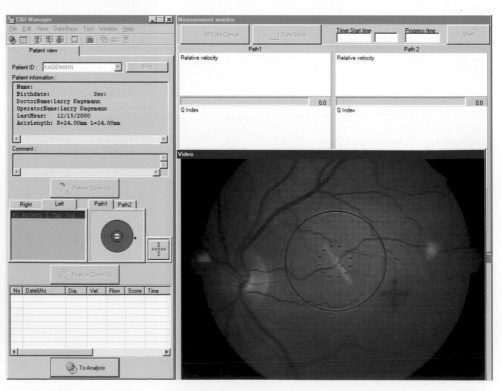

Figure 10–4 CLBF computer screen as seen during a patient's OBF examination.

Use of the CLBF is limited by its calculated flow assumptions, cataracts, vitreous opacities, small pupils, and eye movements.[18] Several validation and technology comparison studies have been performed on the CLBF, including one that showed a significant correlation of CLBF flow measurements in retinal arteries and flow velocity measured in the CRA by CDI.[22]

10.2.3 HEIDELBERG LASER DOPPLER FLOWMETRY

The confocal scanning laser Doppler flowmeter, also known as the r Heidelberg retina flowmeter (HRF), combines a laser Doppler flowmeter with a confocal scanning laser tomograph.[23] **Figure 10–5** shows the HRF head mount used during a patient's examination.

The HRF images a 2560×640 μm^2 area of the retina or optic nerve head at a resolution of approximately 10 μm/pixel. Every line is scanned 128 times with a 790-nm laser, at a sampling rate of 4000 Hz, resulting in a total scan time of 2.048 seconds. After the scan is completed, the HRF computer performs a fast Fourier transform to extract the Doppler shift spectrum from each measured pixel of reflected light. Each frequency location on the *x*-axis of the spectrum represents a blood velocity, and the height of the spectrum at that point represents the number of blood cells required to produce that intensity. Integrating the spectrum yields total blood flow.

To compensate for noise within the flow measurement, the HRF mathematically removes noise from the raw measurement of Doppler shifts. Noise is presumed to be a function of image brightness:

$$Noise = f(brightness)$$

For the final flow measurement presented by the HRF, noise is subtracted from the raw Doppler analysis:

$$HRF_{final} = HRF_{raw} - Noise$$

which can be rewritten as:

$$HRF_{final} = HRF_{raw} - f(brightness)$$

Higher levels of overall image brightness result in the subtraction of a larger correction factor. Because noise is subtracted to produce the final HRF flow measurement, a higher noise term relates to a lower final HRF flow measurement. This can be seen in **Figure 10–6**, in which a series of HRF images has been obtained at five different levels of brightness. Notice the progression from dark to light in the reflectance image. On the right, are the resulting HRF flow maps. In these maps, brighter pixels represent higher flow. Notice the measurements in the center of the optic disc. In the darkest of the images, the flow measurements in the vessels are very bright, suggesting very high measurements. This is an artifact due to the extremely low brightness level. To a lesser extent, the progression from higher to lower flow levels can be observed on the left side of the flow maps within the capillary beds of the peripapillary retina. In this area of the flow map, each image contains progressively lower flow levels. In the same area of the reflectance image, it is obvious that the brightness level within the same area is becoming progressively greater.

Advantages of HRF include the facts that it is simple to use and, in most cases, does not require pupillary dilation. HRF is also very sensitive and able to detect small changes in blood flow in the same eye over time. However, the flow measurements are displayed in arbitrary units. The HRF provides the mean and standard deviation of flow in an image. However, if all HRF flow measurements from a single image are displayed on a histogram, it can be seen that HRF data are not normally distributed, making data interpretation more difficult.

The HRF obtains digital samples of light intensity at a rate of 4000 samples/sec. This limits the detectable level of Doppler shifts to 2000 Hz. Doppler shifts at high frequencies would be mistaken as lower-frequency shifts. With application of the Doppler equation, the maximum detectable velocity by HRF is 0.78 mm/sec. Because of this limit, use of the HRF is limited to quantification

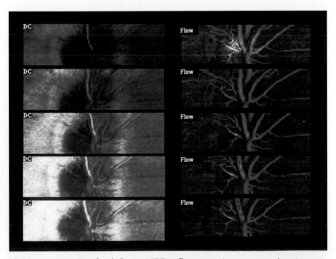

Figure 10–6 On the *left* are HRF reflectance images ranging (*top* to *bottom*) from low to high signal levels. On the *right* are the resulting HRF flow maps in which brighter pixels represent higher flow. Notice areas of artifactually high flow in the *top right* flow map obtained with low reflectance signal (*top left*).

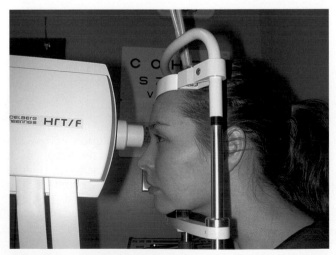

Figure 10–5 The HRF head mount keeps the patient's eye in position during a HRF OBF examination.

of blood moving slowly through the capillaries. Flow readings for large vessels will be erroneously low because of the sample rate limitation.

10.2.4 SCANNING LASER OPHTHALMOSCOPE ANGIOGRAPHY

Fluorescein angiography (FA) and indocyanine green (ICG) angiography performed with a scanning laser ophthalmoscope (SLO) can be used to quantitate blood flow. Two commercial SLO systems are currently available: the analog Rodenstock SLO (**Figure 10–7**), which records data on an S-VHS video recorder or in a digital format and the more recently developed Heidelberg retina angiography (HRA) system, which records data digitally onto a computer. The SLO uses a laser beam that scans across the retina and collects reflected light through a confocal aperture. The confocal aperture blocks light reflected and scattered from sources outside of the focal plane, thus reducing the effects of lens and corneal opacities. The detector measures the intensity of the reflected light in real time, creating a video signal.[23] The SLO provides valuable data concerning the passage of blood through the retinal or choroidal vasculature by recording an injected dye at a speed of 30 frames/sec with the Rodenstock SLO and 20 frames/sec with the HRA system.[7] For both the SLO and HRA, a 488 nm argon blue laser with a 530 nm barrier filter is provided for FA, and a 790 nm infrared diode laser with an 830 nm barrier filter is installed for ICG angiography.[15]

In SLO angiography fluorescein dye may be used to evaluate the retinal vasculature to yield hemodynamic measurements such as arteriovenous passage (AVP) time and mean dye velocity (MDV). AVP time can be estimated by noting the time between the arrival of dye at the measuring point on the designated artery and that on a corresponding vein (**Figure 10–8**).[32] MDV can be calculated by placing a second measuring window at a known distance downstream on the artery from the first arterial measuring window (**Figure 10–9**).[7,34]

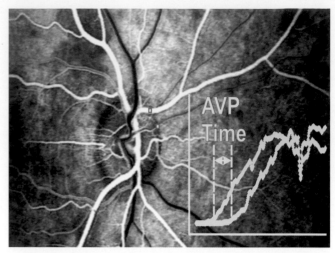

Figure 10–8 AVP time can be estimated by noting the time between the arrival of dye at the measuring point on the designated artery with that on a corresponding vein.

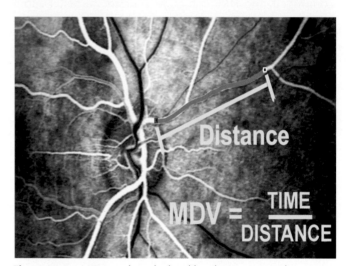

Figure 10–9 MDV can be calculated by placing a second measuring window at a known distance downstream on the artery from the first arterial measuring window.

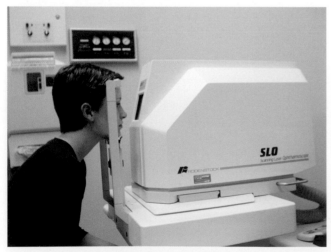

Figure 10–7 A patient sits in front of the SLO for examination of the retinal and choroidal blood flow. Both ICG and fluorescein dye will be used during the angiography examination.

Because the choroid supplies the bulk of OBF, a method for the evaluation of this ocular tissue is important. ICG angiography uses near-infrared light, which penetrates the pigmented layers of the retina much more efficiently than the shorter wavelength light used in FA.[11] In an analysis method developed by the Indiana University Glaucoma Research and Diagnostic Center, the entire 40-degree ICG angiogram is divided into a number of small regions, and dye dilution curves are created for each region. Six locations on the image, each a 6-degree square, are identified for analysis (**Figure 10–10**). The average brightness of the area contained in each box is computed for each frame of the angiogram. Area dye-dilution analysis identifies three parameters from the dye-dilution curves: 10% filling time, the slope of the curve, and maximum brightness. The 10% filling time is the amount of time required to reach brightness 10% above baseline. This parameter describes the

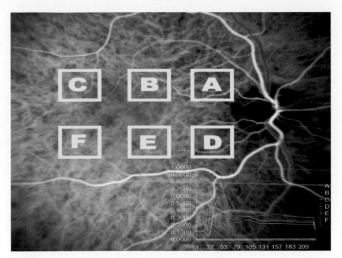

Figure 10–10 ICG angiography analysis of the choroid with six digital analysis windows identified for statistical analysis of blood flow.

rapidity of dye movement from the time of injection to the earliest choroidal filling. Slope of the filling curve is calculated by first noting the difference between the intensity at 40% filling and that at 60% filling and then dividing the difference by the number of frames during that time, where each frame represents a known time interval. This parameter represents the overall speed of blood flow as it enters the choroid.[15]

The resolution of the images obtained during FA and ICG angiography provide great details of an individual's OBF. However, the assessment of OBF requires knowledge of both blood velocity and vessel diameter; therefore, studies in which the vessel diameter is not measured must be interpreted with caution. Additionally, use of MCT or AVP times assumes that an area supplied by one specific artery is completely drained by the corresponding vein, which may not hold true in all cases. The invasive nature of dye injections during imaging remains highly undesirable.

10.2.5 PULSATILE OCULAR BLOOD FLOW MEASUREMENT

Pulsatile ocular blood flow (POBF) devices consist of a modified pneumotonometer interfaced with a microcomputer that records the ocular pulse.[30] POBF monitors the rhythmic change in intraocular pressure (IOP) during the cardiac cycle, which fluctuates up to 2 mm Hg in a sinusoidal fashion. The pneumotonometer sends an analog signal to the computer, where it is digitized and recorded. The amplitude of the IOP pulse wave is used to calculate the change in ocular volume using the relationship described by Silver et al.[30]

Despite their attractiveness, use of POBF systems has been impeded by their limitations. POBF flow measurements are not obtained through direct measurement of ocular blood flow but rather are derived mathematically by estimating ocular pulse volume changes on the basis of a preset relationship between ocular volume and IOP.

This relationship incorporates a model of the cardiac cycle and a standard value for scleral rigidity. POBF measurements are therefore affected by individual differences in scleral rigidity, ocular volume, heart rate, systemic blood pressure, and IOP.

10.3 Clinical Applications

10.3.1 GLAUCOMATOUS OPTIC NEUROPATHY

Elevated IOP is the most important risk factor for the development and progression of glaucoma. However, in some patients glaucoma continues to progress despite therapeutic reduction of the IOP. This has led investigators to study other risk factors, such as OBF and/or other hemodynamic factors that could possibly be responsible for the progression of the disease.

Many published studies suggest that low OBF may be present in many glaucoma patients, and reduced blood flow in the retina, choroid, and optic nerve head has also been demonstrated. For instance, CDI has revealed lower PSVs and EDVs in the ophthalmic and posterior ciliary arteries of glaucoma patients.[28] Reduced velocities on central retinal arteries of high-tension glaucoma patients have been documented.[20] Harris et al.[19] found that CDI of ophthalmic arteries of normal-tension glaucoma patients showed significantly lower EDV and higher resistance indices than those in healthy control subjects. Glaucoma patients have also been shown to have significantly reduced POBF than healthy subjects.[12,18] Many other publications on OBF and glaucoma showing an array of findings are available. The magnitude of OBF defects in glaucoma has yet to be fully defined.

10.3.2 DIABETIC RETINOPATHY

Diabetic retinopathy (DR) is a leading cause of blindness in the United States. Pathologic vascular changes in diabetes may precede detectable vision loss; therefore, it is necessary to evaluate further the vascular changes and their implication on the progression of the disease. The development of retinal ischemia often begins early in the course of DR. Before the development of neovascularization in DR, abnormalities in retinal circulatory regulation occur. Decreases in retinal blood flow and retinal artery velocities have been measured in very early nonproliferative DR, and increases in retinal blood flow were observed in patients with advanced nonproliferative and proliferative DR compared with nondiabetic patients. The increase in retinal blood flow is accompanied by vasodilatation of the retinal vessels, especially the primary retinal veins.[8]

A CDI study revealed decreased mean PSV in the CRA in subjects with nonproliferative DR compared with that in diabetic subjects in a preretinopathy control group.[28] Similarly, the presence of proliferative retinopathy has been found to correlate strongly with reduced flow velocities in the retrobulbar vessels, most markedly in the CRA.[24] Pigment epitheliopathy can be diagnosed when there is minimal DR or macular edema, yet diffuse fluorescent leakage occurs across the macular retinal pigment epithelium.[33] Similarly, both intrachoroidal neovascularization and choriocapillaris degeneration are observed more frequently in diabetic patients than in healthy individuals.[4,13] Some studies show a strong correlation between elevation in blood flow and degree of retinopathy in advanced stages of nonproliferative retinopathy.[8] These increases may be associated with the growth of new retinal vessels with advanced disease.

10.3.3 AGE-RELATED MACULAR DEGENERATION

The pathogenesis of age-related macular degeneration (AMD), the leading cause of irreversible visual loss in the United States, remains elusive. Several theories have been proposed; these include primary retinal pigment epithelium senescence,[3,36] genetic defects such as mutations of the ABCR gene (which encodes a retinal rod photoreceptor protein),[1] and primary ocular perfusion abnormalities. The exact nature of the relationship between OBF and AMD is currently unknown; however, several prior studies demonstrated ocular perfusion abnormalities in AMD.

10.4 Summary

Many varied and unique methods for assessing OBF in the living human eye have been developed. It is important to note that each technique evaluates a portion of the ocular circulation in a distinct way, using various signal sources, which causes difficulty when one is comparing results among different methods and imaging devices. Each ocular vascular bed supplies an important portion of the total ocular blood flow. With careful interpretation of each technology's limitations, new information on the interplay between OBF and disease continues to emerge.

REFERENCES

1. Allikmets R, Shroyer N, Singh N, et al. Mutation of the Stargardt disease gene (ABCR) in age-related macular degeneration. Science. 1997;277:1805–1807.
2. Alm A: Ocular circulation. In: Adler's Physiology of the Eye. 6th ed. Hart WM, editor. St Louis, Mo: Mosby, 1992:198–227.
3. Eagle RJ. Mechanisms of maculopathy. Ophthalmology. 1984; 91:613–625.
4. Cao J, McLeod S, Mergus CA, Lutty GA. Choriocapillaris degeneration and related pathologic changes in human diabetic eyes. Arch Ophthalmol. 1998;116:589–597.
5. Chauhan BC. The relationship between intraocular pressure and visual field progression in glaucoma. In: Drance SM, ed. Update to Glaucoma, Blood Flow and Drug Treatment. Amsterdam, Netherlands: Kugler, 1995:1–6.
6. Cherrrick GR, Stein SW, Levy CM. Indocyanine green: Observations on its physical properties, plasma decay, and hepatic extraction. J Clin Invest. 1960;39:592.
7. Ciulla TA, Regillo CD, Harris A. Retina and Optic Nerve Imaging. Philadelphia, PA: Lippincott Williams & Wilkins, 2003.
8. Clermont AC, Aiello LP, Mori F, Aiello LM, Bursell SE. Vascular endothelial growth factor and severity of nonproliferative diabetic retinopathy mediate retinal haemodynamics in vivo: A potential role for vascular endothelial growth factor in the progression of nonproliferative diabetic retinopathy. Am J Ophthalmol. 1998; 124:433–446
9. Feke GT, Delori F, Webb R. U.S. Patent 5, 633, 695, 1997.
10. Flaharty PM, Priest DL, Eaton AM, et al. Reproducibility of orbital hemodynamic parameters as measured by color Doppler imaging in normal volunteers [abstract]. Invest Ophthalmol Vis Sci. 1994; 35(suppl):1630.
11. Flower RW, Hochheimer BF. Clinical infrared absorption angiography of the choroids. Am J Ophthalmol. 1972;73:458–459.
12. Fontana L, Poinoosawmy D, Bunce CV, O'Brien C, Hitching RA. Pulsatile ocular blood flow investigation in asymmetric normal tension glaucoma and normal subjects. Br J Ophthalmol. 1998;82:731–736.
13. Fukushima I, McLeod DS, Lutty GA. Intrachoroidal microvascular abnormality: a previously unrecognized form of choroidal neovascularization. Am J Ophthalmol. 1997;124:473–487.
14. Goebel W, Lieb WE, Ho A, Sergott RC, Farhoumand R, Grehn F. Colour Doppler imaging: A new technique to assess orbital blood flow in patients with diabetic retinopathy. Invest Ophthalmol Vis Sci. 1995;36:864–870.
15. Garzozi HJ, Shohom N, Chung HS, Kagemann L, Harris A. Ocular blood flow measurements and their importance in glaucoma and age-related macular degeneration. Israeli Med Assoc J. 2001; 3(1–6):443–448.
16. Grunwald J, Hariprasad S, DuPont J, et al. Foveolar choroidal blood flow in age-related macular degeneration. Invest Ophthalmol Vis Sci. 1998;39:385–390.
17. Guven D, Ozdemir H, Hasanreisoglu B. Haemodynamic alterations in diabetic retinopathy. Ophthalmology. 1996;103:1245–1249.
18. Harris A, Jonescu-Cuypers CP, Kagemann L, Ciulla TA, Krieglstein GK. Atlas of Ocular Blood Flow—Vascular Anatomy, Pathophysiology, and Metabolism. Philadelphia: Butterworth Heinemann, 2003:19–70.
19. Harris A, Sergott RC, Spaeth GL, Katz JL, Shoemaker JA, Martin BJ. Color Doppler analysis of ocular vessel blood velocity in normal tension glaucoma. Am J Ophthalmol. 1994;118:642–649.
20. Konigsreuther KA, Michelson G. Retinal hemodynamics in glaucoma [abstract]. Invest Ophthalmol Vis Sci. 1994;35(suppl):1842.
21. Langham ME, Farrel R, Krakau T, Silver D. Ocular pulsatile blood flow, hypotensive drugs and differential light sensitivity in glaucoma. In: Krieglstein GK, ed. Glaucoma Update IV. Berlin, Germany: Springer-Verlag, 2000:162–172.
22. Kagemann L, Harris A, Jonescu-Cuypers C, et al. Comparison of ocular hemodynamics measured by a new retinal blood flowmeter and color Doppler imaging. Ophthalmic Surg Lasers Imaging. 2003;34:342–347.
23. Michelson G, Langhans MJ, Groh MJ. Clinical investigation of the combination of scanning laser ophthalmoscope and laser Doppler flowmeter. Ger J Ophthalmol. 1995;4:342–349.
24. Dimitrova G, Kato S, Yamashita H, Tamaki Y, Nagahara M, Fukushima H, Kitano S, Relation between retrobulbar circulation and progression of diabetic retinopathy. Br J Ophthalmol. 2003;87:622–625.
25. Pourcelot L. Indications de l'ultrasonographie Doppler dans l'etude des vaisseaux peripheriques. Rev Prat. 1975,25:4671–4680.
26. Powis RL. Color flow imaging: Understanding its science and technology. J Diag Med Ultrasound. 1988;4:236–245.
27. Rossetti L, Marchetti I, Orzalesi N, Scorpiglione N, Torri V, Liberati A. Randomized clinical trials on medical treatment of glaucoma. Are they appropriate to guide clinical practice? Arch Ophthalmol. 1993;111:96–103.
28. Sergott RC, Aburn NS, Trible JR, Costa VP, Lieb WE Jr, Flaharty PM. Color Doppler Imaging: Methodology and preliminary results in glaucoma [Published erratum appears in Surv Ophthalmol. 1994;39: 165]. Surv Ophthalmol. 38(suppl):S65–S70.
29. Sigelman J, Ozanics V. Retina and ocular anatomy. In: Jacobiec FA, ed. Embryology and Teratology. Hoboken, NJ: Wiley, 1982:441:506.
30. Silver DM, Farrell RA, Langham ME, O'Brien V, Schilder P. Estimation of pulsatile ocular blood flow from intraocular pressure. Acta Ophthalmol. 1989;191(suppl):25–29.
31. Takamine Y. Disorders of choroidal circulation in diabetic maculopathy [article in Japanese]. Nippon Ganka Gakkai Zasshi. 1998;102:487–494.

32. Tomic L, Maepea O, Sperber GO, Alm A. Comparison of retinal transit times and retinal blood flow: a study in monkeys. Invest Ophthalmol Vis Sci. 2001;42:752–755.

33. Weinberger D, Fink-Cohen S, Gaton DD, Priel E, Yassur Y. Non-retinovascular leakage in diabetic maculopathy. Br J Ophthalmol. 1995;79:728–731.

34. Wolf S, Toonen H, Koyama T, Meyeer-Ebrecht D, Reim M. Scanning laser ophthalmoscopy for the quantification of retinal blood-flow parameter: a new imaging technique. In: Row B, ed. Scanning Laser Ophthalmoscopy and Tomography. Munich, Germany: Quintessenz, 1990.

35. Yosida A, Feke GT, Mori F, et al. Reproducibility and clinical application of a newly developed stabilized retinal laser Doppler instrument. Am J Ophthalmol. 2003;135:356–361.

36. Young R. Pathophysiology of age-related macular degeneration. Surv Ophthalmol. 1987;31:291–306.

Section II

Macular Diseases

Chapter 11

Non-Neovascular Age-Related Macular Degeneration

RAFAEL L. UFRET-VINCENTY, MD • LEONID E. LERNER, MD, PhD • PETER K. KAISER, MD

11.1 Introduction and Epidemiology

Age-related macular degeneration (AMD) is the leading cause of irreversible blindness and low vision among people older than 60 years of age. It leads to significant emotional distress, a need for help with key daily activities, and profoundly reduced quality of life. An estimated 30% of the population older than 75 years of age has some degree of macular degeneration. It accounts for about 54% of all cases of blindness (visual acuity <20/200) in white Americans. AMD is classified into a "dry" or non-neovascular or nonexudative form (90% of cases) and a "wet" or neovascular form (see Chapter 12 on neovascular AMD). About 11.7% of patients with AMD end up having advanced disease (7.1% neovascular AMD and 4.6% central geographic atrophy [GA]). Presentations of dry AMD include drusen and a wide range of abnormalities of the retinal pigment epithelium (RPE), going from focal areas of hypopigmentation and hyperpigmentation, to the more advanced GA.

Several potential risk factors for AMD have been identified including advanced age, family history of AMD, cigarette smoking, exposure to blue light, and cardiovascular factors such as systemic hypertension and obesity. Although the impact of most of these factors on AMD is still controversial, patients should be made aware of the possible association, particularly of modifiable risk factors such as smoking, obesity, hypertension, and blue light exposure.

11.2 Clinical Signs and Symptoms

Most patients with non-neovascular AMD are asymptomatic and maintain excellent visual acuity. Some patients with confluent, central drusen may complain of a decreased ability to read, particularly in dimmed illumination, and mild metamorphopsia. Significant loss of contrast sensitivity is common, but it is rarely tested. Noncentral areas of GA can lead to paracentral scotomas that can have a great impact on visual functioning despite excellent central acuity.

The earliest sign of AMD is the development of *druse* (plural *drusen*), which means nodule or crystal within a stone in German. Drusen (**Figures 11–1** to **11–3**) tend to be bilateral and may be present in the macula and/or in an extramacular location. Drusen can be classified by size: small (<63 microns in diameter), intermediate (63 to 124 microns), and large (≥125 microns, which is the average diameter of a retinal venule at the edge of the optic disc). Other important characteristics of drusen that should be noted are whether they are confluent or calcified. The borders of small drusen are almost always distinct and well defined, contributing to the designation of *hard drusen*. Small, hard drusen are not sufficient to diagnose AMD. Their mere presence is not associated with an increased risk of the development of the neovascular form of AMD. In fact, at least one small druse can almost always be found in the macula of individuals older than 40 years of age. However, eyes

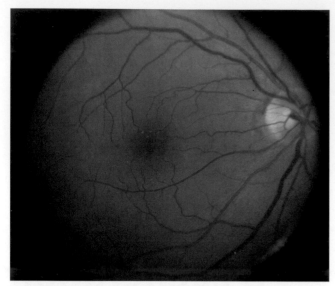

Figure 11–1 Several small hard drusen are seen in this eye. All are less than 63 microns in diameter (one half of the diameter of a retinal vein at the edge of the optic nerve head) and are thus classified as small. These findings would place the patient in category 2 of the AREDS classification. If there were fewer than five small drusen, the patient would fall in category 1. With even one drusen larger than 63 microns the patient would fall in category 2. Using the AREDS grading system this eye would have 0 points because there are no large drusen or extensive intermediate drusen and no significant pigmentary changes.

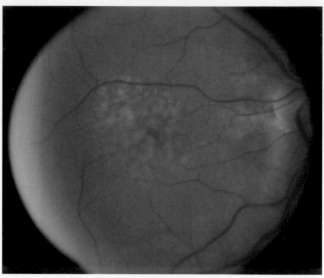

Figure 11–3 Extensive large soft drusen, many of which are confluent. Because there is no neovascular component, no central geographic atrophy in either eye, and the vision is better than 20/32 in both eyes, this patient still has category 3 AMD by the AREDS classification. It would be assigned only 1 point in the AREDS grading system given the absence of significant pigmentary abnormalities.

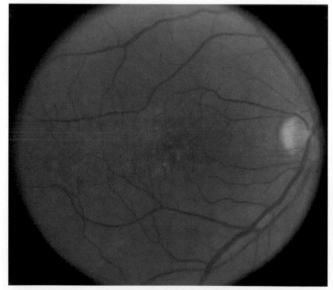

Figure 11–2 Many small and intermediate drusen with at least one large druse and significant pigmentary abnormalities. This patient would be classified as category 3 of the AREDS classification because of the large soft druse inferior to the fovea. This would also be the classification if the patient did not have any large drusen but had extensive intermediate drusen. Using the Ferris et al. grading system this eye would be assigned 2 points given the large druse (1 point) and the pigmentary changes (1 point). This is the maximum number of points that can be assigned to an eye in this grading system. For complete grading, the other eye needs to be examined.

with numerous small, hard drusen are at increased risk of developing soft or larger drusen over time.

Large, soft drusen (**Figure 11–3**) are the defining feature of dry AMD. The incidence and prevalence of soft drusen have been shown to be age related. Their presence is associated with an increased risk for the development of RPE abnormalities, GA, and choroidal neovascularization. Large drusen can become confluent, which may make it impossible to distinguish them from localized serous detachments of the RPE. Larger and more numerous drusen seem to be associated with an increased risk of visual loss from AMD.

Early in their development, drusen may be imperceptible ophthalmoscopically because of their small size and relatively normal overlying RPE. Often, however, they can be detected in retroillumination with the slit lamp or with fluorescein angiography. As the deposit enlarges and the overlying RPE thins, drusen assume a yellow or gray color and are more easily detected. In general, the distribution of drusen is similar in both eyes. In some patients, drusen may be present nasal to the optic disc or along the major vascular arcades. When many widely scattered drusen with a halo of pigment are seen in the midperipheral fundus, they are referred to as senile reticular degeneration of the pigment epithelium. Drusen change in size, shape, distribution, color, and consistency with the passing years. Although they tend to increase in number and size, drusen may also fade from view and decrease in number (**Figures 11–4** and

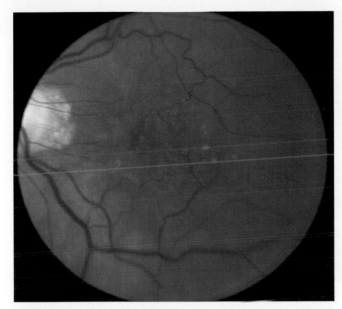

Figure 11–4 A few large and intermediate drusen are seen. Prominent pigmentary changes are observed. There is also an epiretinal membrane.

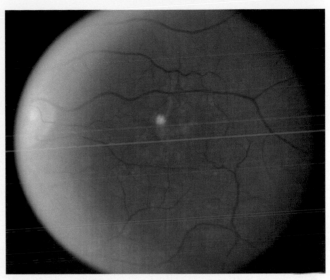

Figure 11–6 Prominent pigmentary changes and a large druse are present in this patient.

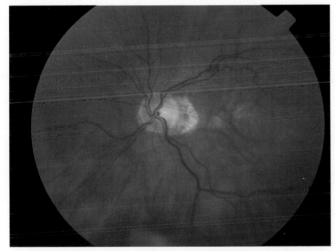

Figure 11–5 Ten years later, the same eye in **Figure 11–4** has developed a large area of GA. Most of the drusen have faded or disappeared.

11–5). In some cases, areas of GA of the pigment epithelium may remain after disappearance of drusen (**Figures 11–4 to 11–7**).

Other signs of non-neovascular AMD include RPE alterations (**Figures 11–2 and 11–4 to 11–8**), hypopigmentation, hyperpigmentation, or mottling, and GA. GA is observed clinically as a well-demarcated round or oval area(s) of RPE depigmentation and atrophy in which choroidal vessels are seen more clearly.

11.3 Classification Schemes for Age-Related Macular Degeneration

The Age-Related Eye Disease Study (AREDS) demonstrated that using high doses of certain vitamins and minerals (15 mg of β-carotene, 500 mg of vitamin C, 400 IU of vitamin E, 80 mg of zinc oxide, and 2 mg of cupric oxide) leads to a 25% to 30% reduction in the risk of development of advanced AMD in a subgroup of patients with AMD. This formulation of antioxidants and minerals specifically benefited patients whose AMD characteristics placed them in categories 3 or 4 of the AREDS classification:

Category 1. Essentially no age-related macular abnormalities, with a total drusen area less than five small drusen and visual acuity of 20/32 or better in both eyes

Category 2. Mild or borderline age-related macular degeneration features with extensive small drusen or at least one intermediate-sized druse or pigment abnormalities in at least one eye, and visual acuity of 20/32 or better in both eyes (**Figure 11–1**).

Category 3. Absence of advanced AMD in both eyes and at least one eye with visual acuity of 20/32 or better and extensive intermediate drusen, at least one large druse, non-central GA, or any combination of the above in at least one eye (**Figures 11–2, 11–3 and 11–4**).

Category 4. Visual acuity of 20/32 or better and no advanced AMD (GA involving the center of the fovea or CNVM) in the study eye and advanced AMD in the fellow eye (**Figure 11–7**).

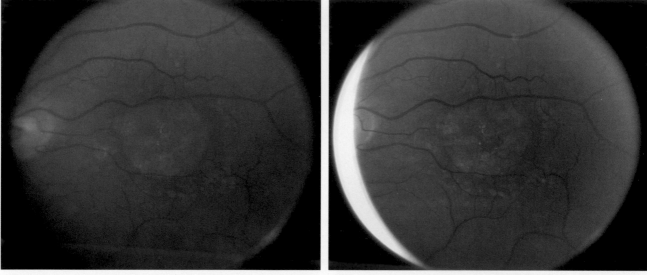

Figure 11–7 *(stereo)* The same eye in **Figure 11–6** is shown here 4 years later. These stereoscopic photographs show a large area of geographic atrophy that has developed in the same area of the pigmentary changes that was present before. Given the central GA, this patient would be classified as having category 4 AMD (assuming that the other eye does not have advanced AMD). This eye would be assigned the maximum of 2 points in the AREDS grading scale.

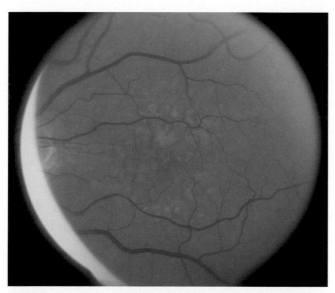

Figure 11–8 Many large and intermediate drusen with significant pigmentary abnormalities including a small area inferior to the fovea that probably represents an early stage of non-central geographic atrophy. This eye would place the patient in AREDS category 3 and would be awarded 2 points in the AREDS grading system.

Another clinically useful scale has been recently proposed by Bressler et al. as part of the AREDS research initiative. It grades AMD using a 4-point scale, in which each eye is scored individually for up to 2 points (**Figures 11–1** to **11–3** and **11–8**). The presence of at least one large druse (≥125 microns) is awarded 1 point. In the absence of large drusen, the presence of multiple intermediate drusen (63 to 124 microns) is awarded ½ point. Definite pigmentary changes (definite hyperpigmentation, hypopigmentation, or non-central GA), if present, account for 1 point. An eye with central GA or neovascular AMD is automatically assigned the maximum 2 points. The points for each eye are added together to determine the risk of clinical progression. The 5-year risk of progression to advanced AMD in a patient with a score of 0 is 0.5%. Scores of 1, 2, 3, and 4 have corresponding risks of 3%, 12%, 25%, and 50%.

11.4 Imaging and Diagnostic Tests

11.4.1 FLUORESCEIN ANGIOGRAPHY

Fluorescein angiography may reveal the presence of more drusen than are apparent ophthalmoscopically. Angiographic findings in drusen are variable and depend upon their size and consistency and the degree of pigmentation of the RPE on their surface (**Figure 11–9**). Most drusen cause a focal well-defined area of hyperfluorescence. The time of appearance of their early fluorescence depends upon the rate of staining of Bruch's membrane and the sub-RPE material and their translucency. The intensity of their later staining with fluorescein depends primarily on their consistency. Smaller nodular ("hard") drusen typically show a peak fluorescence within several minutes after injection and then fade, paralleling the fading of the background choroidal fluorescence. Fluorescence of medium and large drusen may be delayed until the later stages of angiography. This may be caused by the thickness of the drusen as well as the lipid content of the drusen and the underlying Bruch's membrane. GA appears as a well-defined window defect with hyperfluorescence in early transit views and fading in late views (**Figure 11–10**).

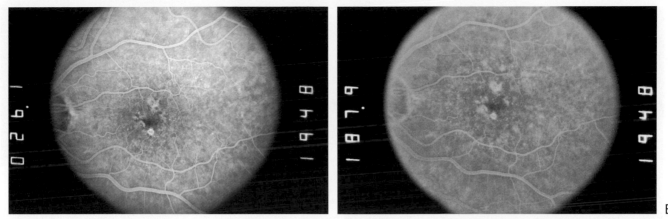

Figure 11–9   Fluorescein angiogram of the eye in **Figure 11–8**. *A:* Early phase showing early hyperfluorescence of small, intermediate, and large drusen and a window defect corresponding to the area of early GA inferior to the center of the foveal avascular zone. *B:* Late frame showing staining of the drusen and fading in the area of geographic atrophy. There is no leakage of dye. Careful comparison of the early and late frames demonstrates that, although the hyperfluorescence from most drusen is fading, there are a few new drusen that appeared late in the angiogram.

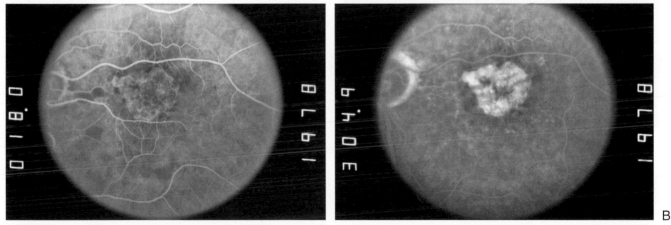

Figure 11–10   An early frame (*A*) of a fluorescein angiogram obtained on the same eye shown in **Figure 11–7** demonstrates a well-demarcated area of hyperfluorescence caused by the window defect that results from the atrophic retina-RPE in the region of geographic atrophy. A late frame (*B*) shows fading of the same well-demarcated area.

11.4.2 OPTICAL COHERENCE TOMOGRAPHY

Optical coherence tomography (OCT) documents drusen as thickenings and deformations of the hyperreflective RPE band without an underlying shadowing effect (**Figure 11–11**). GA (**Figure 11–12**) is seen as a thinning of the sensory retina (including absence of the minimally reflective band that corresponds to the retinal photoreceptor layer). Because of increased penetration of the OCT light through atrophic neurosensory retina and RPE, the choroid exhibits a well-defined area of increased optical reflectivity (a sharply demarcated vertical reflective band).

11.4.3 INDOCYANINE GREEN ANGIOGRAPHY

Indocyanine green angiography has no role in the evaluation of dry AMD.

11.4.4 AUTOFLUORESCENCE

Some chemical compounds and fundus lesions are capable of emitting yellow-green light when irradiated with blue light. Vitamin A and lipofuscin can fluoresce but only very inefficiently. However, calcified drusen of the optic nerve head and large deposits of lipofuscin can autofluoresce enough to expose photographic film. This leads to the phenomenon of *autofluorescence*, or fluorescence before the administration of fluorescein. There is evidence suggesting that in AMD a shift occurs towards the blue-green autofluorescence of Bruch's membrane relative to the yellow-orange autofluorescence of RPE-associated lipofuscin. Patients with AMD show localized areas of high autofluorescence that do not correspond with drusen. Choroidal neovascular membranes show areas of low and high levels of autofluorescence. Autofluorescence is low in areas of GA.

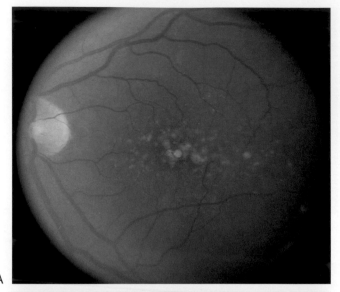

A

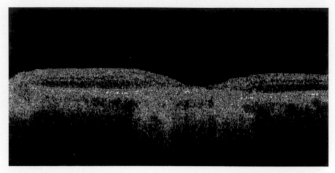

Figure 11–12 An OCT image of the same eye with geographic atrophy shown in **Figure 11–7** demonstrates thinning of the photoreceptor layer. Although it is harder to distinguish, the RPE layer is also thinned. In fact, the increase in light penetration through the atrophic retina and RPE, leads to the underlying sharply demarcated area of increased optical reflectivity observed on OCT.

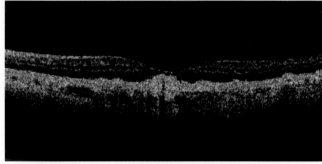

B

Figure 11–11 Many large, intermediate, and small drusen are seen in this eye (A). Significant pigmentary changes are also observed. An OCT image of this eye (B) shows focal thickenings of the hyperreflective RPE/choriocapillaris band. This thickening corresponds to the drusen seen in the fundus photograph. There is no shadowing effect under these areas of thickening.

11.5 Pathology

Clinicopathologic correlation demonstrates that drusen are sub-RPE deposits, which are most commonly discrete, round, and slightly elevated. They are deposits of extracellular material lying between the relatively normal basement membrane of the RPE and the inner collagenous part of Bruch's membrane and thus represent focal detachments of the RPE and its relatively normal thickness basement membrane from Bruch's membrane.

GA is seen clinically as a well-demarcated area of RPE depigmentation. It is seen histopathologically as a sharply demarcated area of loss of photoreceptors and RPE with varying degrees of atrophy of the choriocapillaris.

Basal laminar drusen (**Figure 11–13**) are clinically and histopathologically different from the exudative or

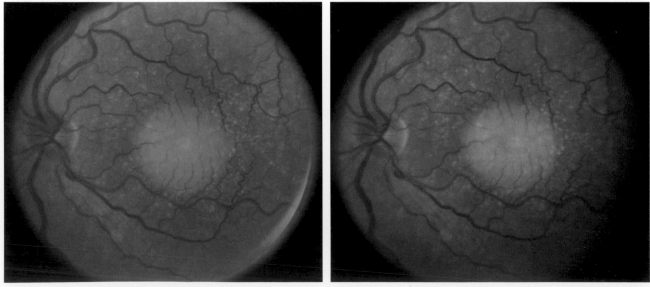

A
B

Figure 11–13 *(stereo)* Extensive basal laminar drusen are scattered throughout the macula in this patient. A vitelliform exudative detachment is seen in the center of the macula.

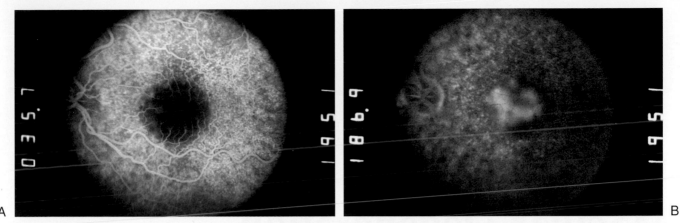

Figure 11–14 The basal laminar drusen create a "stars-in-the-sky" appearance in the early phase of the angiogram (A). The exudative detachment blocks fluorescence in the early phase (A) and leads to pooling of fluorescein in the late phase (B) of the angiogram.

typical drusen characteristic of AMD. They are caused by nodularity of a diffusely thickened RPE basement membrane. They are usually round and 25 to 75 microns in size. They fluoresce discretely during the early arteriovenous phase, sometimes giving a "stars-in-the-sky" or "Milky Way" appearance (**Figure 11–14**). In some cases, patients with basal laminar drusen can develop an unusual vitelliform exudative macular detachment.

SUGGESTED READINGS

Age-Related Eye Disease Study Research Group. A randomized, placebo-controlled, clinical trial of high-dose supplementation with vitamins C and E, beta carotene, and zinc for age-related macular degeneration and vision loss: AREDS report no. 8. Arch Ophthalmol. 2001;119:1417–1436.

Bressler SB, Ferris FL, Davis MD, et al. A simple clinical scale for estimating the risk of age-related macular degeneration progression. Invest Ophthalmol Vis Sci 2005;46:E-Abstract.

Gass JDM. Stereoscopic Atlas of Macular Diseases: Diagnosis and Treatment. 4th ed. St Louis, Mo: Mosby, 1997;3:70–111.

Sarks SH, Sarks JP. Age-related maculopathy: Nonneovascular age-related macular degeneration and the evolution of geographic atrophy. In: Ryan SJ, Schachat AP, eds. Retina. St Louis, Mo: Mosby, 2001:1064–1099.

Seddon JM. Epidemiology of age-related macular degeneration. In: Ryan SJ, Schachat AP, eds. Retina. St Louis, Mo: Mosby, 2001:1039–1050.

Chapter 12

Neovascular Age-Related Macular Degeneration

ADAM H. ROGERS, MD • ANDRE WITKIN, BS

12.1 Introduction

Neovascular age-related macular degeneration (AMD) is the leading cause of blindness in the U.S. population in persons older than 65 years, as well as the most common cause of blindness in the Western world. It is estimated that 6.4% of patients 65 to 74 years old and 19.7% of patients 75 years or older had signs of AMD in the Framingham Eye Study. AMD is more prevalent in Caucasians and has a slight female predilection. Risk factors for AMD include increasing age (75 years of age or older), a positive family history, cigarette smoking, hyperopia, light iris color, hypertension, hyper-cholesterolemia, female gender, genetic factors, and cardiovascular disease.

Imaging is the cornerstone for diagnosing AMD, categorizing lesions, and directing treatment for exudative AMD. The three main imaging modalities are fluorescein angiography (FA), indocyanine green (ICG) angiography, and optical coherence tomography (OCT). Although all three have an active role in evaluation of neovascular AMD, FA remains the gold standard. In three landmark clinical trials over the past 20 years—the Macular Photocoagulation Study (MPS), the Treatment of Age Related Macular Degeneration with Photodynamic Therapy (TAP) Study, and the VEGF Inhibition Study in Ocular Neovascularization (VISION) Clinical Trial Group (which included the use of pegaptanib)—FA was used to qualify eyes for enrollment and retreatment during the study. Although FA, ICG angiography, and OCT each provide different information, they are all valuable in the diagnosis and treatment of exudative AMD.

12.2 Clinical Signs and Symptoms

Patients who develop neovascular AMD will complain of the sudden onset of decreased vision, metamorphopsia, and paracentral scotomas. These early findings are often followed by rapid and permanent central visual loss. The hallmark of the neovascular form of AMD is the presence of choroidal neovascularization (CNV). Signs of exudative AMD include the appearance of a gray-green choroidal neovascular membrane, lipid exudates, subretinal or intraretinal hemorrhage/fluid, pigment epithelial detach-ment (PED), retinal pigment epithelial tears, and in late stages a fibrovascular disciform scar.

12.3 Imaging and Diagnostic Tests

12.3.1 FLUORESCEIN ANGIOGRAPHY

FA is the gold standard for the diagnosis of neovascular AMD. In the normal eye, unbound sodium fluorescein is able to diffuse through the fenestrated vessels in the choriocapillaris but is retained by intact tight junctions of the retinal vascular endothelium as well as the retinal pigment epithelium (RPE). With alterations in these structures, specific patterns of increased fluorescence are imaged in AMD. These patterns include transmission defects, leakage, pooling, and staining (**Figure 12–1**).

Transmission defects result from atrophy of the RPE, allowing normal fluorescence from the underlying choriocapillaris to appear more intense (**Figure 12–2**). They are most commonly seen in nonexudative macular

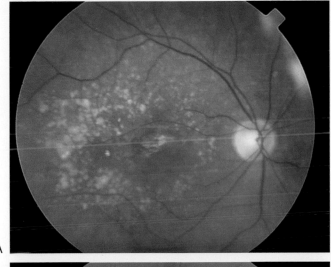

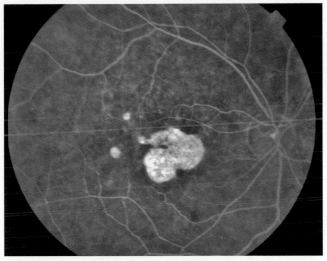

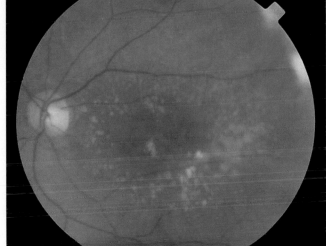

Figure 12–2 Fluorescein angiogram demonstrating a transmission (window) defect in the area of geographic atrophy of the right eye from **Figure 12–1A**. There is also faint staining of the drusen.

Figure 12–1 *A:* Hard drusen, pigmentary changes, and central geographic atrophy in nonexudative AMD. *B:* Same patient, left eye with similar findings including soft confluent drusen in the temporal macula.

degeneration. The timing of this hyperfluorescent pattern follows the filling and emptying of fluorescein from the choriocapillaris. This is characterized by early hyperfluorescence that fades late and maintains a constant size and shape determined by the structural RPE defect. In RPE tears that can occur with occult CNV, the RPE scrolls, leaving an area devoid of RPE cells. This creates an area of window defect on FA (**Figure 12–3**).

Leakage, pooling, and staining occur when fluorescein dye exits the vasculature from abnormalities in endothelial tight junctions. These characteristics are typically seen in exudative AMD (**Figure 12–4**). Pooling and staining are two specific types of leakage. In pooling dye leaks into a distinct anatomic space (**Figure 12–5**), and in staining dye affixes to certain structures such as drusen (**Figure 12–6**) or scar tissue (**Figure 12–7**). In staining of scar tissue, there is fluorescence of the

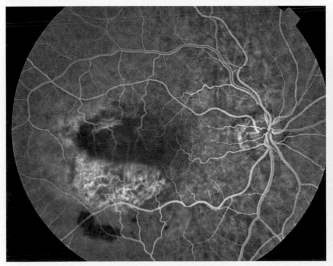

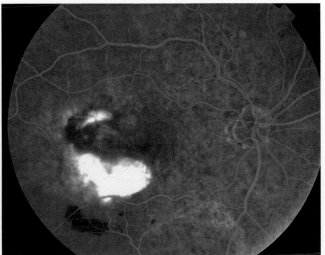

Figure 12–3 *A:* Early view of a window defect from an RPE rip on FA. *B:* Late view of the RPE rip.

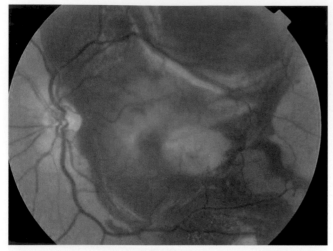

Figure 12–4 Extensive subretinal hemorrhage in an eye with exudative AMD.

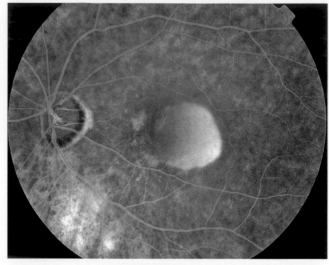

Figure 12–5 Late view of fluorescein pooling into the cavity of a serous PED with the occult CNV seen at the nasal edge of the serous cavity.

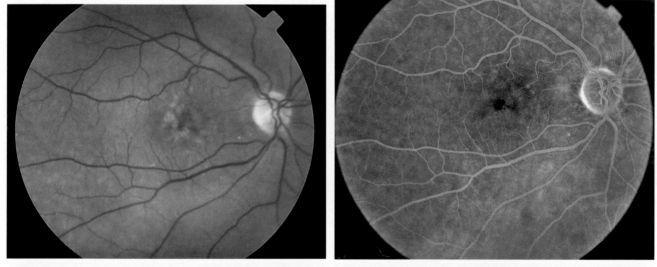

Figure 12–6 Color photograph of drusen (*A*) with staining of the drusen on FA (*B*).

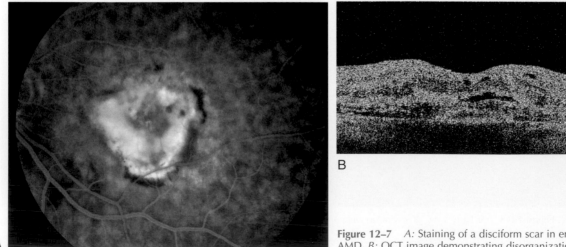

Figure 12–7 *A:* Staining of a disciform scar in end-stage exudative AMD. *B:* OCT image demonstrating disorganization of retinal layers.

lesion, but the borders of the lesion remain fixed without blurring in later frames of the fluorescein angiogram. Staining should not be misinterpreted as active leakage, and this distinction is important when the clinician decides whether to treat or observe CNV.

Interpretation of leakage is important for clinicians to identify CNV lesion location, classification, and size. This information is then converted into the ideal treatment modality for a given CNV lesion.

Location

CNV lesions are found in the following locations:

- *Subfoveal*—CNV under the geometric center of the fovea
- *Juxtafoveal*—CNV between 1 and 199 microns from the foveal center or CNV 200 to 2500 microns from center of the foveal avascular zone with blood or blocked fluorescence within 1 to 199 microns of the foveal center
- *Extrafoveal*—CNV 200 to 2500 microns from the foveal center (**Figure 12–8**)

The classification of CNV into classic, occult, or mixed CNV is based on its appearance on FA. Classic CNV usually appears as a well-defined lesion, occasionally with arborization of fine choroidal vessels extending under the retina. It demonstrates early, bright, uniform hyperfluorescence (**Figure 12–9**). As the angiogram progresses, fluorescein continues to leak out of the vasculature, blurring the margins of the lesion even as fluorescence from the normal choroidal and retinal vasculature fades.

In contrast to classic CNV, occult CNV is typically less well defined and can be further subdivided into two types. These subdivisions include type 1 fibrovascular pigment epithelial detachment (FVPED), which is the most common form of occult CNV, and type 2 occult CNV or late leakage of undetermined origin. An FVPED refers to an irregular elevation of the RPE with stippled or granular irregular fluorescence first seen early in the angiogram, usually by 1 to 2 minutes after dye injection. The irregular elevation of the RPE is best seen with stereo views. The FVPED continues to increase in fluorescence throughout the angiogram with late leakage that is not as diffuse as classic leakage (**Figure 12–10**). Late leakage of undetermined origin demonstrates similar leakage in late views and the level of the RPE, but the source of leakage cannot be ascertained in early views. The terms *poorly defined* or *poorly demarcated* CNV and *well-defined* or *well-demarcated* CNV should not be used as synonyms for classic and occult CNV, respectively. *Classic* and *occult* describe *fluorescein patterns* of CNV. *Poorly defined* and *well-defined* describe how distinct the *boundaries* of the lesion appear.

When determining the classification of a CNV lesion, one must take into account all areas of classic and occult CNV as well as areas of obscuring features including blood, pigment, scar tissue, serous PED, and blocked fluorescence that all count as part of the entire lesion for determining CNV classification.

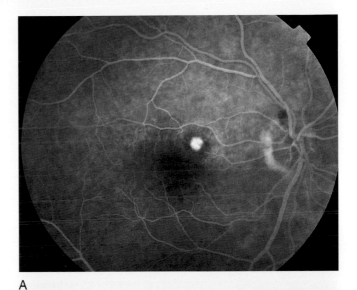

A

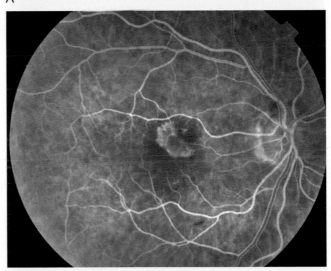

B

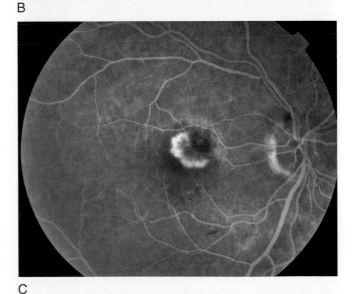

C

Figure 12–8 A small, classic, extrafoveal CNV imaged on FA (*A*) was treated with argon laser photocoagulation. Three months later the patient returned with a recurrent subfoveal, classic CNV extending from the laser scar that appears hypofluorescent (*B* and *C*).

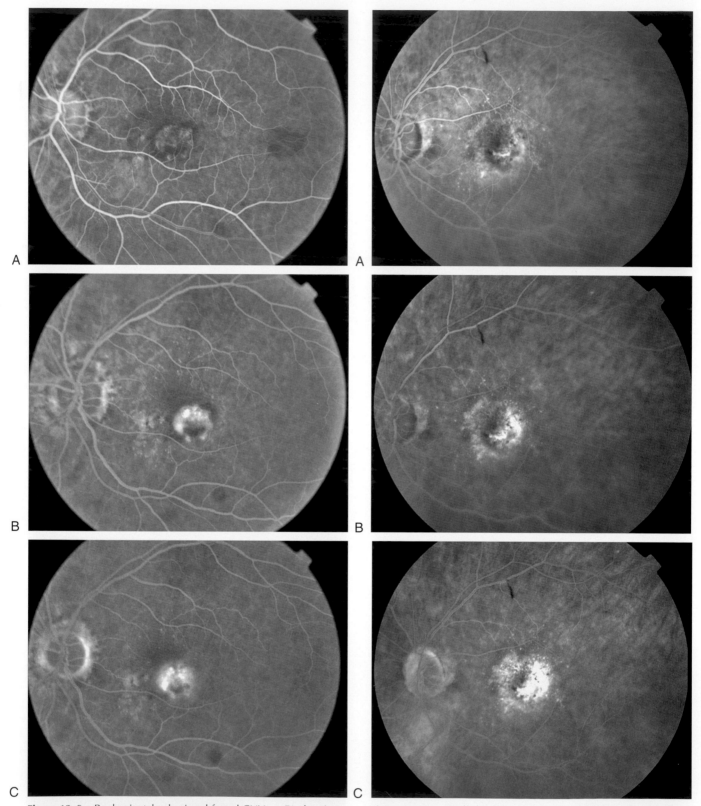

Figure 12–9 Predominately classic subfoveal CNV on FA showing early hyperfluorescence with fine delineation of the vessels (*A*). Increased leakage beyond the border of the CNV is visible in mid (*B*) and late frames (*C*) as fluorescein dye continues to leak beyond the boundaries of the lesion.

Figure 12–10 An ill-defined, subfoveal occult CNV with a small amount of classic CNV. Stippled hyperfluorescence is visible in the early frame of the FA (*A*) with more leakage in the mid (*B*) and late frames (*C*); the classic component leaks more profusely than the occult component.

Classification of CNV

CNV is classified as follows:

- *Predominately classic*—50% of the entire lesion is composed of classic CNV
- *Minimally classic*—1% to 49% of the entire lesion is composed of classic CNV (**Figure 12–11**)
- *Occult only*—no classic CNV in the lesion (**Figure 12–10**)

In a serous PED, an early, rapid, uniform, circular, fluid-filled cavity is formed under and elevates the RPE due to an adjacent area of CNV leakage typically outside of the serous cavity. Pooling of dye into the serous cavity occurs uniformly over the course of the angiogram with the boarders confined by the limits of the RPE detachment (**Figure 12–12**).

A variant of CNV is a lesion recently termed retinal angiomatous proliferation (RAP). In a RAP lesion, there is presumed retinal neovascularization with the eventual formation of a retinal choroidal anastomosis as the retinal vessel grows into the subretinal and choroidal space. On clinical examination, a PED is present with a focal area of intraretinal hemorrhage at the point of neovascularization. Angiographically, the RAP lesions appear as a focal area of fluorescence within the PED. In later frames of the angiogram, there is pooling of dye within the PED (**Figure 12–13**). In more chronic lesions in AMD, the CNV may create a retinal-choroidal anastomosis when the choroidal vessels break through the RPE and neurosensory retina and create a communication with the retinal circulation (**Figure 12–14**).

Hypofluorescence is caused by blockage or a perfusion-related filling defect. Blockage of fluorescence is caused by anything that obstructs the transmission of fluorescence from the fundus to the camera (**Figure 12–15**). Common causes in AMD include hemorrhage, exudate, and pigment. Perfusion-related filling defects

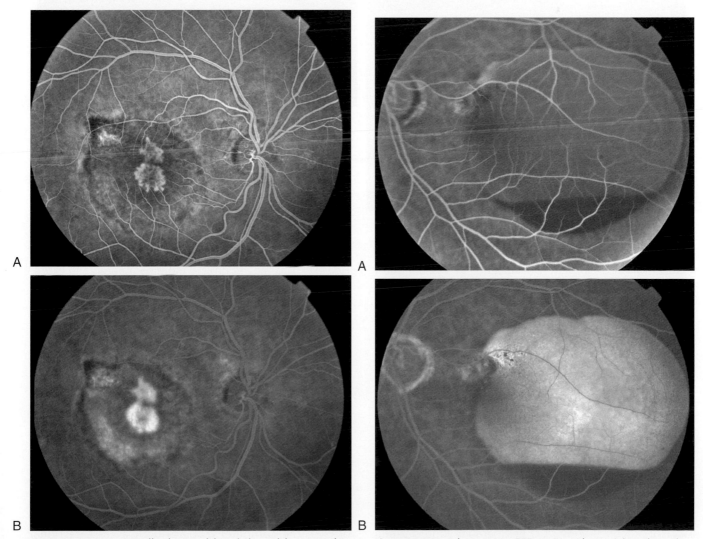

Figure 12–11 A minimally classic subfoveal choroidal neovascular membrane composed of a large, well-defined occult lesion with two smaller, classic lesions. The classic component demonstrates early hyperfluorescence (*A*) with intense late leakage (*B*).

Figure 12–12 A large serous PED on FA with a juxtafoveal occult CNV at the nasal edge of the lesion (*A*). Pooling of fluorescein dye into the serous cavity (*B*) is visible in later frames with a hypofluorescent fluid level from hemorrhage.

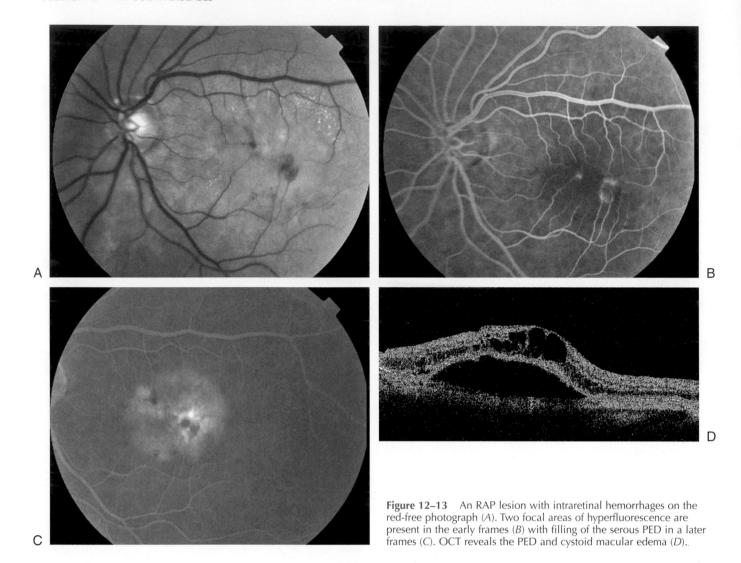

Figure 12–13 An RAP lesion with intraretinal hemorrhages on the red-free photograph (*A*). Two focal areas of hyperfluorescence are present in the early frames (*B*) with filling of the serous PED in a later frames (*C*). OCT reveals the PED and cystoid macular edema (*D*)..

result from an obstruction or absence of vessels. After conventional laser photocoagulation, for example, the choriocapillaris is destroyed in the treated area and cannot fill with fluorescein from the circulation (**Figure 12–16**). Delayed choroidal filling is another source of hypofluorescence immediately after photodynamic therapy (PDT) with Visudyne (**Figure 12–17**).

12.3.2 INDOCYANINE GREEN ANGIOGRAPHY

In AMD, ICG angiography is most useful in eyes with occult or poorly defined CNV. Two forms of fluorescence in ICG are typically seen. In an occult FVPED, placoid hyperfluorescence is visible in later frames of the ICG angiogram (**Figure 12–18**). In more poorly defined occult CNV, a focal area of hyperfluorescence (often referred to as a *hot spot*) may be visible (**Figure 12–19**) and is useful in guiding treatment of the lesion with argon or diode laser photocoagulation. ICG angiography is less useful in imaging classic CNV because placoid staining of the lesion is present, similar to that in occult lesions. In classic CNV, FA remains the dominant imaging modality.

However, ICG may delineate more completely the extent of the lesion compared with FA (**Figure 12–20**). In contrast to FA with pooling into the cavity of a serous PED, the serous detachment on ICG angiography is hypofluorescent. In RAP lesions, ICG angiography is felt to more accurately identify the abnormal vessel. However, this is similar to a focal hot spot (**Figure 12–19**), and differentiating the two lesions may be difficult.

12.3.3 OPTICAL COHERENCE TOMOGRAPHY

OCT has been proven to be useful in aiding the diagnosis of exudative AMD, understanding disease subtypes, and following patients over time. The information provided by OCT is complementary to that provided by FA and ICG angiography and currently should not be used as the sole source to initially diagnose and treat a new case of exudative AMD. When interpreting results of OCT, the computer displays both a cross-sectional image of the retina as well as a topographic map. This topographic map is useful for identifying the location of retinal thickening in the macula in reference to the

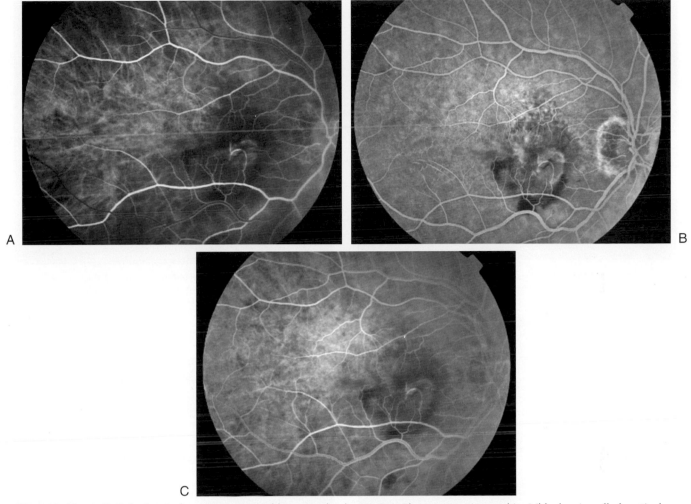

Figure 12–14 *A–C:* A chorioretinal anastomosis is visible on FA of a chronic CNV. The anastomotic vessel is visible, looping off of a retinal arteriole and then making a right-hand turn to connect to the choroidal circulation.

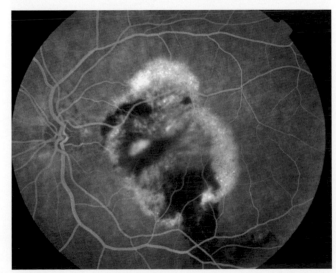

Figure 12–15 A well-defined occult lesion without classic CNV. Blockage of fluorescence occurs from the accompanying subretinal hemorrhage overlying the lesion.

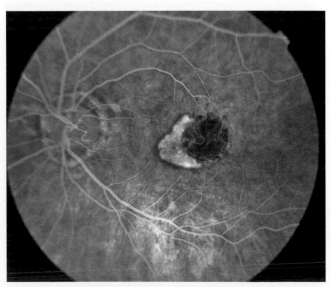

Figure 12–16 Hypofluorescence from a laser treatment. Recurrent subfoveal classic CNV is present from the nasal edge of the scar.

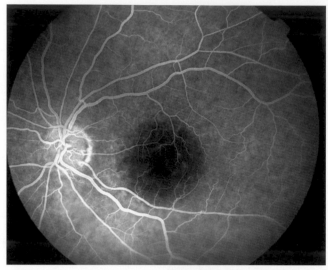

Figure 12–17 Choroidal hypofluorescence corresponding to the treatment spot seen on FA 1 week after verteporfin PDT treatment.

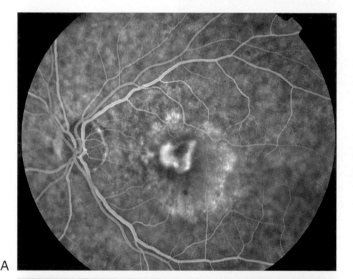

A

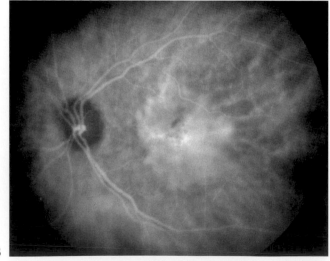

B

Figure 12–18 Minimally classic CNV on FA (A). The late frames of the ICG angiogram show placoid staining of the lesion (B). Little differentiation is seen between the classic and occult component on the ICG angiogram.

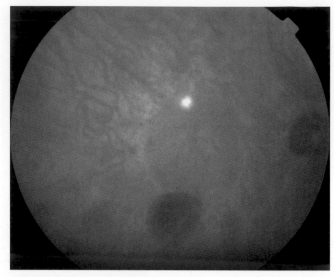

Figure 12–19 Focal area of hyperfluorescence (hot spots) on ICG angiography. The accompanying serous PED is hypofluorescent. A nevus inferior to the serous PED demonstrates greater hypofluorescence than the PED.

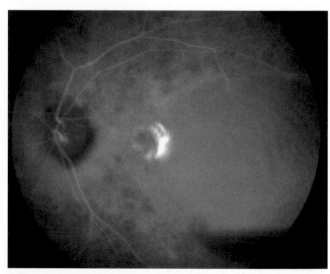

Figure 12–20 ICG angiogram of the serous PED in **Figure 12–12**, showing greater delineation of the causative CNV compared with FA.

fixation point. For the purpose of accurately interpreting what is anatomically occurring in the retina, the cross-sectional scan should be used.

When imaging structures on OCT, one must understand and recognize the reflective properties of the retina (**Figure 12–21**). The OCT signal from any particular tissue layer is a function of its reflectivity and the absorption and scattering properties of the overlying tissue layers. For example, a tissue with a high level of backscatter that lies deep to a tissue with low absorption and low backscatter will produce a high signal. More reflective structures emit a yellow-red signal. Less reflective structures emit a blue-green signal. Non-reflective structures are black. More highly reflective

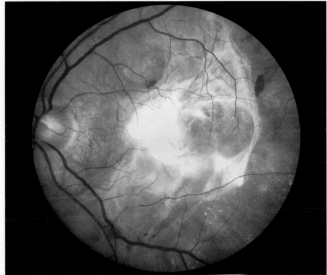

A

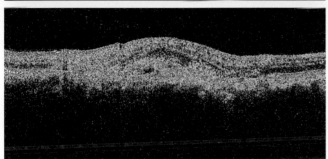

B

Figure 12–21 *A:* Color photograph of a disciform scar. *B:* OCT of same patient showing disorganized retinal layers.

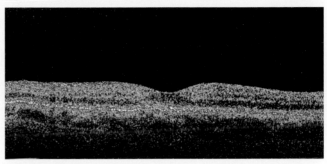

Figure 12–22 OCT of drusen with fine undulation of the RPE layer.

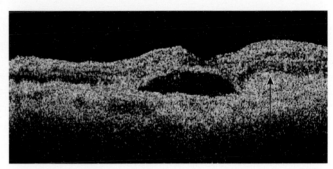

Figure 12–23 OCT of a classic CNV which appears as a thickening of the hyperreflective RPE-Bruch's membrane band. The black space under the retina is subretinal fluid.

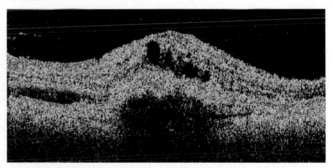

Figure 12–24 OCT scan of an occult FVPED. There is a raised, irregular RPE layer over the occult CNV with shadowed backscattering from the lesion. Subretinal fluid and CME are present.

structures, such as the RPE and epiretinal membranes, scan in the yellow-red spectrum. The retina, with mild to moderate reflectivity, scans in the blue-green spectrum as interpreted by the computer program. The choroid is also poorly imaged with minimal reflectivity and scans primarily in the blue spectrum. Fluid-filled intraretinal spaces (cystoid macular edema [CME]), subretinal fluid, and the vitreous cavity have poorly reflective intrinsic properties with minimal or absent backscatter and are visualized as hyporeflective, black spaces. A normal retina also has a foveal depression that is the center of all scans. Alterations of normal retinal architecture in disease states will lead to loss of the foveal "dimple."

In nonexudative AMD, soft drusen are accumulations of material in the sub-RPE space. OCT interprets these deposits as reflective, small elevations or undulations of the RPE layer (**Figure 12–22**). In geographic atrophy, there is thinning of the retina with a more reflective RPE layer due to a decrease in overlying retinal tissue.

In exudative AMD, OCT may be used to distinguish between occult versus classic forms of CNV. Classic neovascular lesions are highly reflective on OCT, owing to the presence of blood, fibrous tissue, and RPE cells that tend to surround the membrane. Classic lesions are often well defined on OCT and typically appear to grow as an extension of the RPE into the subretinal

space (**Figure 12–23**). Active CNV leak fluid is visualized on OCT as subretinal or intraretinal (CME) hyporeflective black spaces. Occult CNV lesions often occur underneath the RPE and are less accurately imaged than classic lesions. In a FVPED, there is irregular elevation of the RPE layer with blue-green backscattering in the choroid. Subretinal or intraretinal fluid is present from the actively leaking CNV (**Figure 12–24**). In a serous PED, there is a smooth, dome-shaped elevation of the RPE overlying a hyporeflective, black semicircular space with little change in the underlying choroid. The hyporeflective space represents the fluid-filled cavity (**Figure 12–25**). The neovascular portion of the lesion is usually unable to be imaged. In RAP lesions, the OCT image is similar to a serous PED. The intraretinal area of

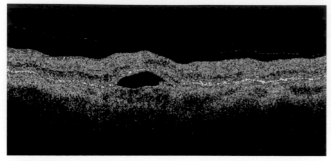

Figure 12–25 A serous PED imaged on OCT. A serous cavity is present elevating the RPE without shadowing of the choroid as seen in an FVPED in **Figure 12–24.**

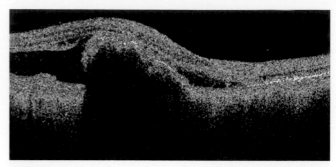

Figure 12–26 OCT of an RPE rip illustrating the discontinuity of the RPE. The accompanying FA image is **Figure 12–3.**

neovascularization may be viewed as a more reflective area within the retina, casting a shadow over the RPE. This creates an image of discontinuity of the RPE in the area of RAP. The RAP lesion is difficult to image because it is small and may be missed by the OCT scanner. In an RPE tear, there is an irregular elevation of the RPE layer similar to an occult membrane with an artifactual break in the RPE layer (**Figure 12–26**).

A particularly useful application of OCT is in the localization, detection, and measurement of retinal fluid. A fluid collection is accurately depicted in its anatomic layer whether it is intraretinal, subretinal, or under the RPE. OCT can provide clinically useful information about

neovascular AMD because it manifests by changing macular thickness or accumulation of fluid in the macula. It also has utility in following the response to PDT and guiding retreatment decisions (**Figure 12–27**), because the presence of fluid implies an actively leaking CNV.

The ability for OCT to follow fluid collections makes it a powerful tool in conjunction with FA in treating and following CNV. Whereas FA can be used initially to categorize a specific lesion, following fluid collections is the most useful piece of information when the clinician decides to retreat or observe CNV. FA alone can provide this information. However, differentiating between staining of scar tissue and an actively leaking CNV that

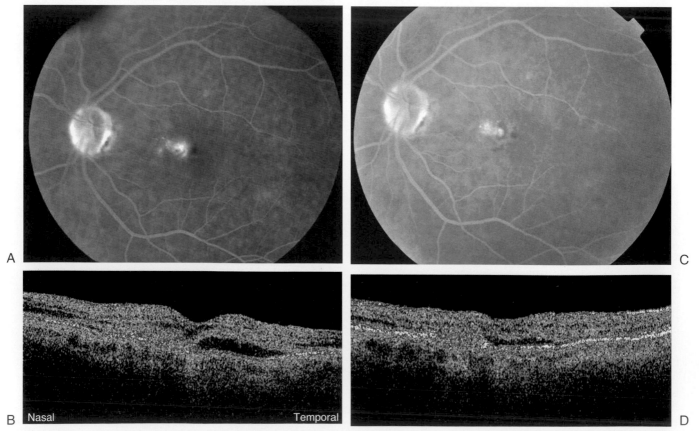

Figure 12–27 Pretreatment (A and B) and 1-month (C and D) FA and OCT images during a single PDT treatment of a classic subfoveal CNV.

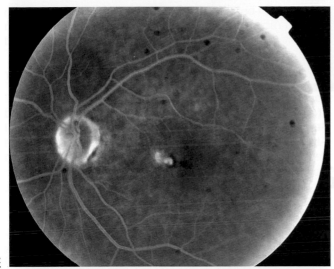

E

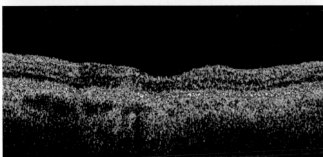

F

Figure 12–27 E and F: 3-month OCT and FA images during a single PDT treatment of a classic subfoveal CNV. At 3 months there is staining of the CNV and resolution of the subretinal fluid on OCT.

would benefit from retreatment on FA is often difficult. The ability to follow fluid collections on the cross-sectional image created by OCT complements the information received from FA and facilitates the ability to analyze CNV. As a result, OCT is gaining popularity with ophthalmologists treating AMD.

12.4 Pathology

Choroidal neovascularization is an ingrowth of new vessels from the choriocapillaris through a break in the outer aspect of Bruch's membrane into the subpigment epithelial space. This neovascularization may be accompanied by fibrous tissue that grows within Bruch's membrane or between the neurosensory retina and the RPE. Eventually, this process results in a disciform fibrovascular scar that replaces the normal architecture of the outer retina and leads to permanent loss of central vision.

SUGGESTED READINGS

Diagnostic imaging for photodynamic therapy: fluorescein angiography and optical coherence tomography. In: Puliafito CA, Rogers AH, Martidis A, Greenberg PG, eds. Ocular Photodynamic Therapy. Thorofare, NJ: Slack, 2003:34–45.

Hee MR, Baumal C, Puliafito CA, et al. Optical coherence tomography of age related macular degeneration and choroidal neovascularization. Ophthalmology. 1996;103:1260–1270.

Puliafito CA, Hee MR, Schuman JS, et al. Optical coherence tomography of ocular diseases.

Rogers AH, Martidis A, Greenberg PB, Puliafito CA. Optical coherence tomography findings following photodynamic therapy of choroidal neovascularization. Am J Ophthalmol. 2002;134:566–576.

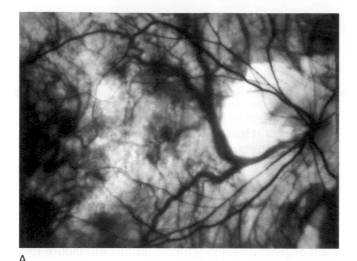

A

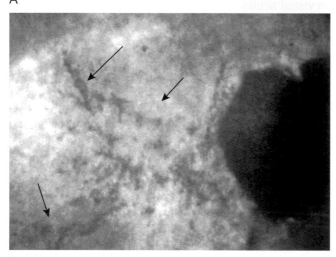

B

Figure 13–3   ICG angiography. Lacquer cracks became clearly identifiable during late stages. They appear as well-defined, hypofluorescent lines, more numerous and longer than on fluorescein angiography.

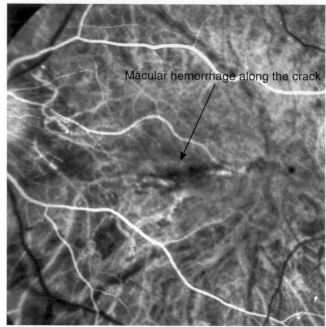

Macular hemorrhage along the crack

A

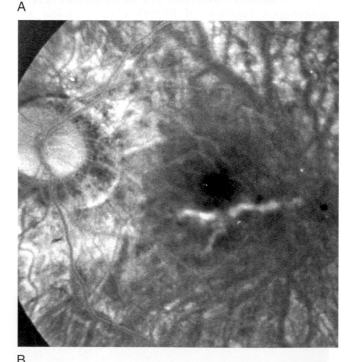

B

Figure 13–4   Macular hemorrhages associated with lacquer cracks, along the crack itself and near the center of the fovea.

hyperfluorescence, even in late ICG angiography. When not associated with CNV, hemorrhages usually resolve in nearly all cases with a good prognosis. Hemorrhages may recur in the same or in another location with extension of the cracks, increasing the risk of CNV development (**Figure 13–5A–C**). Close follow-up with FA and eventually with scanning laser ophthalmoscope ICG angiography is particularly useful for detecting complications. In some cases, the fovea could be partially masked by deep macular hemorrhages (**Figure 13–6**).

13.2.4 FOERSTER-FUCHS' SPOT

Foerster-Fuchs' spot is defined as a dark spot in the posterior pole of patients with pathologic myopia, due to sub- or intraretinal migration and proliferation of RPE cells. The spots are associated with CNV that has been surrounded by hyperplasia of the RPE. Neovascularization extending from the choroid and preceding the development of the Foerster-Fuchs' spot has been

identified with the use of FA. Eventually, the subepithelial hemorrhage organizes and combines with the proliferation of RPE cells, resulting in the dark Foerster-Fuchs' spot (**Figure 13–7A** and **B**). FA will show early hyperfluorescence of the spot with late leakage of the dye that is present mainly in recent lesions and will confirm the presence of new vessels. This leakage is usually limited and does not increase significantly. In addition, leakage is often masked by the pigmented rim (**Figure 13–8A–D**).

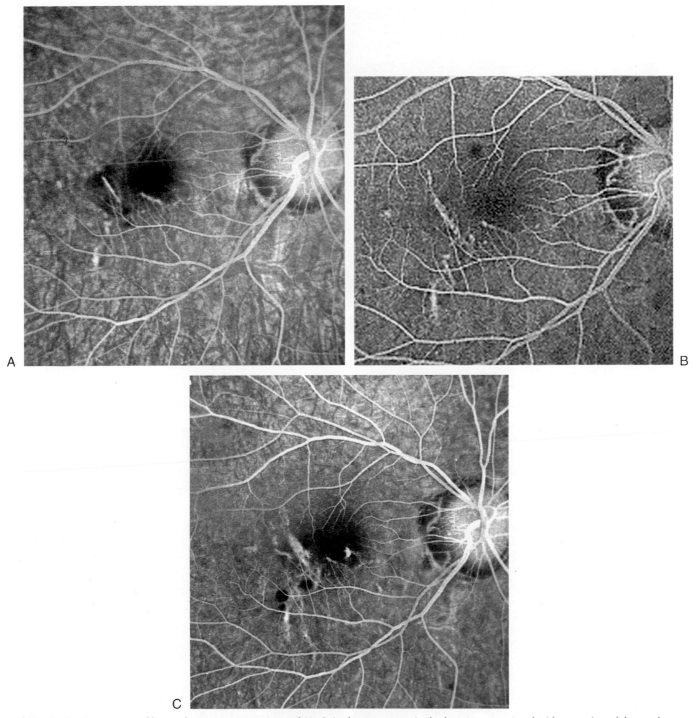

Figure 13–5 Recurrence of hemorrhages at a 1-year interval (A–C) in the same or a similar location, associated with extension of the cracks and high risk of development of CNV.

13.3 Choroidal Neovascularization

CNV is usually subfoveal or very near the center of the fovea at the time of the presentation. A break in Bruch's membrane may precede the development of CNV. On biomicroscopic examination, after the development of CNV, the crack will exhibit a grayish zone, usually juxtafoveal, with a very localized overlying serous detachment. The neovascularization presents as a light grey, roundish, macular lesion, usually small and limited. The lesion is located at or very close to the fovea. A pigmented circle will rapidly outline the lesion, more or less completely. The retinal detachment is absent or shallow and is best detected by stereo photographs

FA

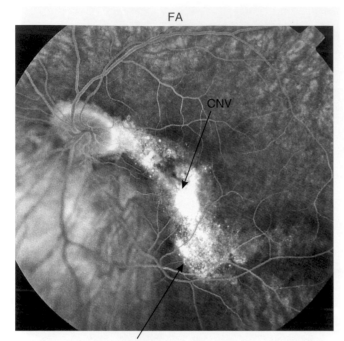

CNV

Border of the crest of the staphyloma

A

ICG

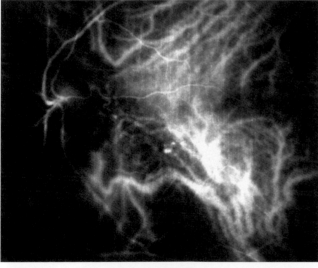

B

Figure 13–9 CNV may be localized to the border of a staphyloma. FA and ICG angiography in this case allow identification and localization of a hyperfluorescent CNV, juxtafoveal, at the border of the crest of a large inferior staphyloma.

lesion with minimal leakage on FA, contrasting with the late hypofluorescence of the RPE atrophy. ICG angiography will easily confirm the presence of CNV (**Figure 13–11A** and **B**). Subretinal hemorrhages may partly or totally obscure all features of CNV. The entire fovea may be masked by a large and deep macular hemorrhage. ICG angiography will then show late and focal hyperfluorescence, with late and limited leakage, suggesting the presence of foveal CNV (**Figure 13–12A–C**).

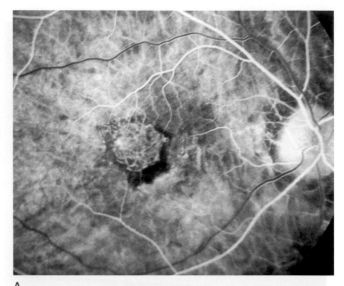

A

B

Figure 13–10 In an elderly patient, neovascularization may be larger and with more active leakage MFA, beyond the boundaries of the initially well-delimited neovascular network, associated with a rim of hypofluorescent hemorrhages inferiorly.

FA can give information related to the age of the lesion. During the first weeks, CNVs show early and rapid hyperfluorescence with relatively active leakage and early central washout. After a few months, the lesion becomes more dense in the center with intense and late staining but with limited, if any, leakage and persistently visible pigmented rim.

13.3.2 ICG ANGIOGRAPHY

ICG angiography may detect, at early stages during the choroidal arterial and venous phases, a localized area of hyperfluorescence and even a neovascular net, that fades progressively because of partial washout of the dye, concomitantly with the diminution of fluorescence from the larger choroidal vessels. In the late phases, CNV will become clearly hyperfluorescent, localized, and

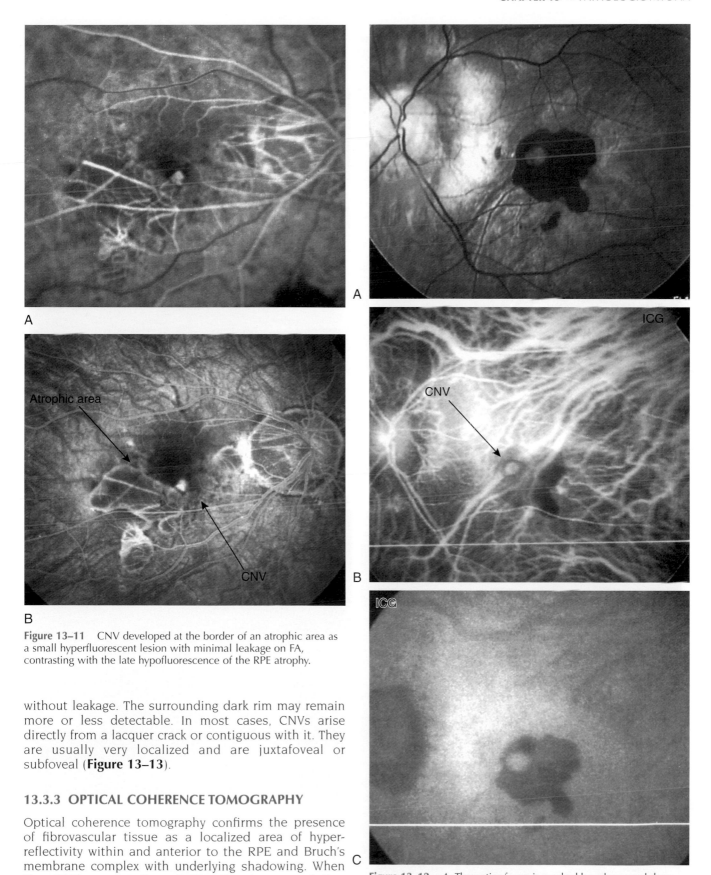

Figure 13–11 CNV developed at the border of an atrophic area as a small hyperfluorescent lesion with minimal leakage on FA, contrasting with the late hypofluorescence of the RPE atrophy.

without leakage. The surrounding dark rim may remain more or less detectable. In most cases, CNVs arise directly from a lacquer crack or contiguous with it. They are usually very localized and are juxtafoveal or subfoveal (**Figure 13–13**).

13.3.3 OPTICAL COHERENCE TOMOGRAPHY

Optical coherence tomography confirms the presence of fibrovascular tissue as a localized area of hyper-reflectivity within and anterior to the RPE and Bruch's membrane complex with underlying shadowing. When the CNVs are active, OCT will show exudation and fluid accumulation as well as a subretinal hyper-reflective band (**Figures 13–14** to **13–17**).

Figure 13–12 *A:* The entire fovea is masked by a large and deep macular hemorrhage (*B* and *C*). ICG angiography shows early and focal hyperfluorescence persisting at the late stage, with limited leakage, suggesting the presence of foveal CNV.

Before PDT

After PDT

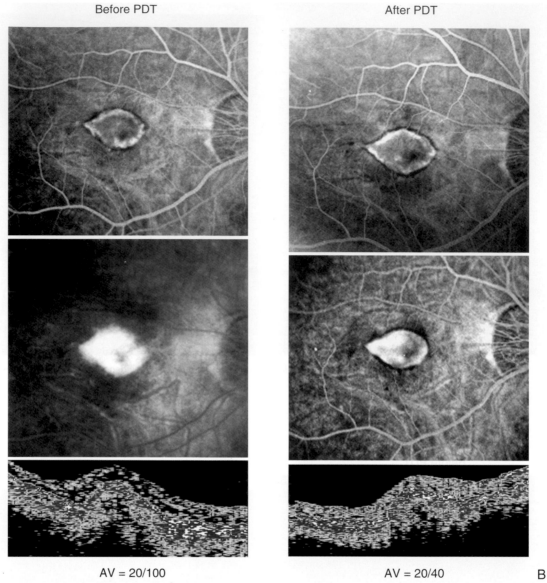

A   AV = 20/100   AV = 20/40   B

Figure 13–17   Subfoveal CNV treated with photodynamic therapy (PDT). *A:* Before treatment. *B:* After PDT, there is absence of leakage, late staining, and flattening of the retinal thickening on OCT.

SUGGESTED READINGS

Binder KJ, Blumenkranz MS, Bressler NM, et al. Verteporfin therapy of subfoveal choroidal neovascularization in pathologic myopia: 2-year results of a randomized clinical trial: VIP report no. 3. Ophthalmology. 2003;110:667–673.

Hamelin N, Glacet-Bernard A, Brindeau C, et al. Surgical treatment of subfoveal neovascularization in myopia: macular translocation vs surgical removal. Am J Ophthalmol. 2002; 133:530–536.

Quaranta M, Arnold J, Coscas G, et al. Indocyanine green angiographic features of pathologic myopia. Am J Ophthalmol. 1996;122:663–671.

Soubrane G, Coscas G. Choroidal neovascularization membranes in degenerative myopia. In: Ryan SJ, Schachat AP, eds. Retina. St Louis, Mo: Mosby, 2002;2:201–215.

Tano Y. Pathologic myopia: Where are we now? Am J Ophthalmol. 2002;134:645–660.

Chapter 14

Central Serous Retinopathy

ANITA LEYS, MD, PhD

14.1 Introduction

Central serous chorioretinopathy (CSC), a common ocular disorder in adults, affects the choroidal circulation and the retinal pigment epithelium (RPE) function with secondary damage to the retina. Acute episodes of visual loss due to subretinal fluid leakage and macular neurosensory detachment occur most often in young male patients and may occasionally occur in pregnant women. Chronic CSC with irreversible visual loss due to widespread RPE damage and retinal atrophy or cystoid macular degeneration is usually seen in patients aged 50 or older or in patients with organ transplants. A special type of CSC is the pigment epithelial detachment (PED) of the young adult with or without neurosensory detachment.

Corticosteroids and catecholamines have been linked with CSC. The condition is often identified in patients with type A personality and psychophysical stress and in patients with high glucocorticoid levels due to endogenous increased production or administration. Possible mechanisms for induction of CSC are choroidal vasoconstriction mediated by catecholamines and thrombotic occlusion of choroidal veins caused by impaired fibrinolysis resulting in decreased choroidal blood flow and hyperpermeability. A link with *Helicobacter* infection has been proposed.

14.2 Clinical Signs and Symptoms

Acute CSC is associated with macular neurosensory detachment due to subretinal leakage. Affected patients experience acute visual loss, micropsia, or metamorphopsia. The clinical diagnosis of acute CSC is based on the history and on careful fundus examination showing the serous elevation of the macula without evidence of inflammation or choroidal neovascularization. During the acute episode, small subretinal exudates or larger serofibrinous exudates may become apparent. Fluorescein angiography (FA) typically shows leaking points at the level of the RPE and confirms the diagnosis of acute CSC (**Figure 14–1A–C;** see also **Figures 14–5** and **14–6**). In many patients, CSC becomes inactive after several weeks to months: the neurosensory detachment flattens, focal leakage points close, and vision returns to normal. However, recurrences are common, and acute episodes may be prolonged in some patients, resulting in chronic damage to the RPE and retina. Rarely, choroidal neovascularization develops as a complication of CSC (**Figure 14–1D–F**).

Chronic CSC or diffuse retinal pigment epitheliopathy is characterized by widespread areas of pigment mottling and atrophic changes of RPE associated with retinal degeneration and atrophy due to chronic serous detachment. FA confirms the diagnosis of chronic CSC and shows large areas of RPE damage with a combination of window defects, atrophic changes, staining, and subtle or manifest leaks (**Figures 14–2** to **14–4**).

The RPE detachment of the young adult only causes visual loss or metamorphopsia when the fovea is overlying the PED or when the PED is associated with subretinal leakage and neurosensory detachment (**Figure 14–5**).

14.3 Imaging and Diagnostic Tests

14.3.1 FLUORESCEIN ANGIOGRAPHY

FA is the most important diagnostic test. In the acute stages of CSC, FA shows RPE lesions with or without

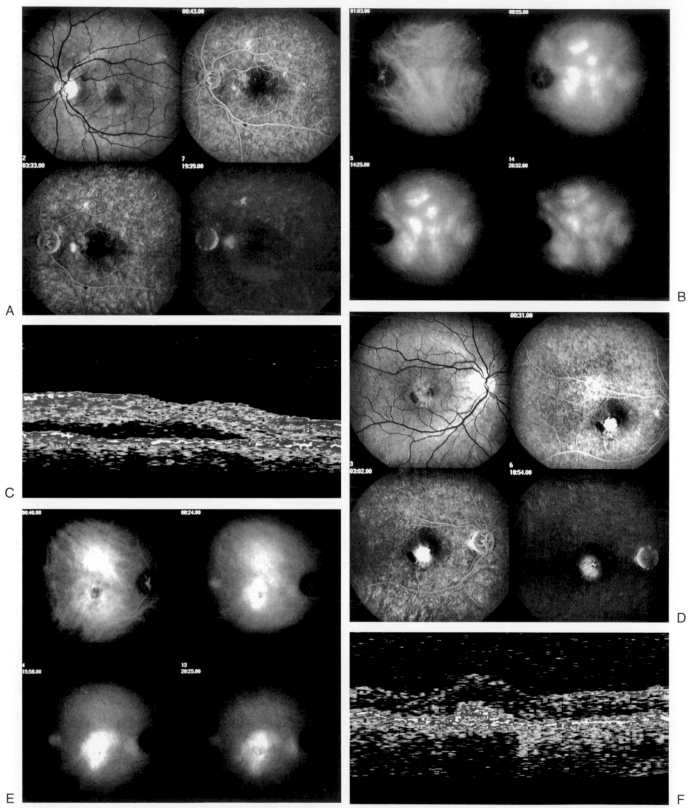

Figure 14–1   Acute CSC in the left eye of a male patient aged 42. *A:* Red-free photograph and fluorescein angiogram demonstrating a macular neurosensory detachment and progressive subretinal leakage from a single papillomacular leak. *B:* ICG angiogram shows hyperfluorescent areas at 8 minutes with progressive washout of the dye. *C:* OCT image demonstrates a large papillomacular and macular neurosensory detachment. *D:* The right eye of the same patient had rapidly progressive visual loss due to CNV. Note on the red-free photograph and fluorescein angiogram a classic CNV with associated hemorrhage. *E:* An ICG angiogram shows the CNV with progressive hyperfluorescence and three hyperfluorescent areas with washout of dye, pointing to CSC as the cause of the CNV and not other causes. *F:* OCT image shows the CNV with overlying retinal edema.

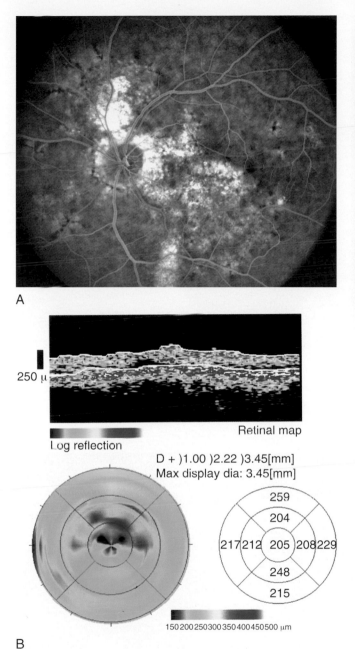

A

B

Figure 14–2 Chronic CSC in a male patient aged 52 years.
A: Fluorescein angiogram shows large areas of RPE damage with staining and subtle leaks and with vertically oriented atrophic tracts. *B:* OCT image shows a subtle neurosensory detachment and retinal atrophic changes with normal thickness map.

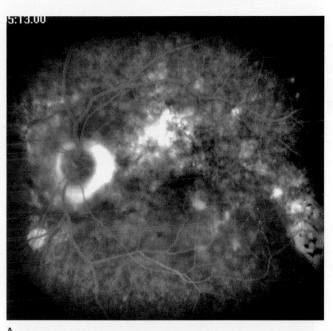

A

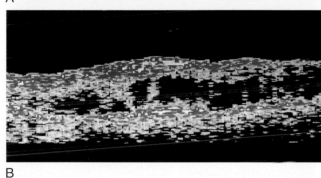

B

Figure 14–3 Chronic CSC in a male patient aged 76. *A:* Fluorescein angiogram shows widespread areas of RPE lesions with leaks, staining, atrophic spots, and tracts. *B:* OCT image shows cystoid retinal degeneration.

RPE detachments and with subretinal leakage from one or more leakage points. Characteristic patterns of the focal leakage points include hyperfluorescence early that leaks in a characteristic smoke-stack pattern in 10% of patients; gradual pooling into a serous retinal detatchment is seen in the other 90% (**Figures 14–5** and **14–6**). After the acute episode, leakage points become subtle or resolve and window defects are left. In patients with repeated episodes of acute CSC or with chronic neurosensory detachment, the RPE and retinal damage increases, and FA typically shows chorioretinal atrophic changes with vertically oriented atrophic tracts. In clinical practice, FA is used to identify subretinal leaking points and to direct laser coagulation. Moreover, FA is useful for excluding or confirming choroidal neovascularization.

14.3.2 INDOCYANINE GREEN ANGIOGRAPHY

Indocyanine green (ICG) angiography has demonstrated choroidal vascular abnormalities in CSC including filling delays in choroidal arteries and choriocapillaris, venous dilatation, focal hypofluorescent and hyperfluorescent areas indicative of poorly perfused choroid and choriocapillaris, and hyperpermeability of the choroidal vessels. Areas of hyperfluorescence or choroidal leakage with rapid diffusion of the dye and a washout pattern is a characteristic finding observed in nearly all patients with CSC even during a clinically inactive phase (**Figure 14–1**). These areas of hyperfluorescence remain unchanged during follow-up of patients with CSC. Moreover, appearance of focal leaks on the fluorescein angiogram has been observed in preexisting areas of

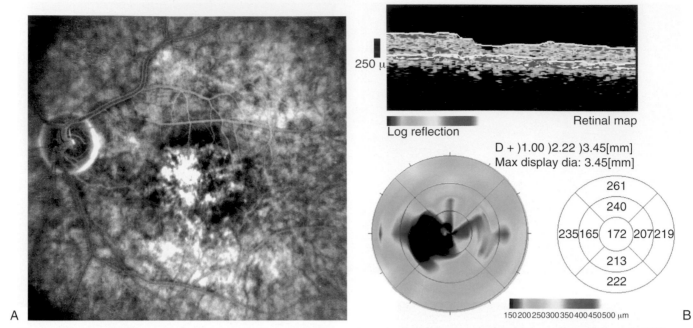

Figure 14–4 Chronic CSC in a male patient aged 53 years. *A:* Fluorescein angiogram shows macular RPE lesions without leakage. *B:* OCT image shows marked atrophy of retina.

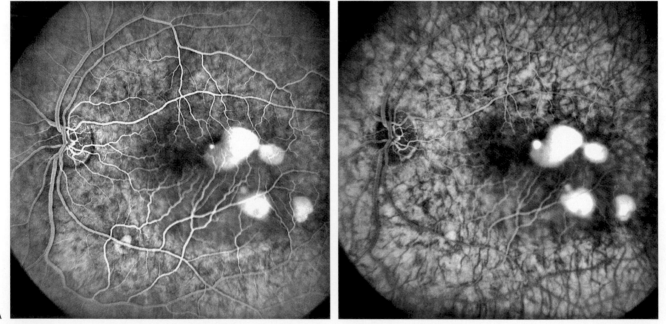

Figure 14–5 A and B (*Continued; legend on following page*)

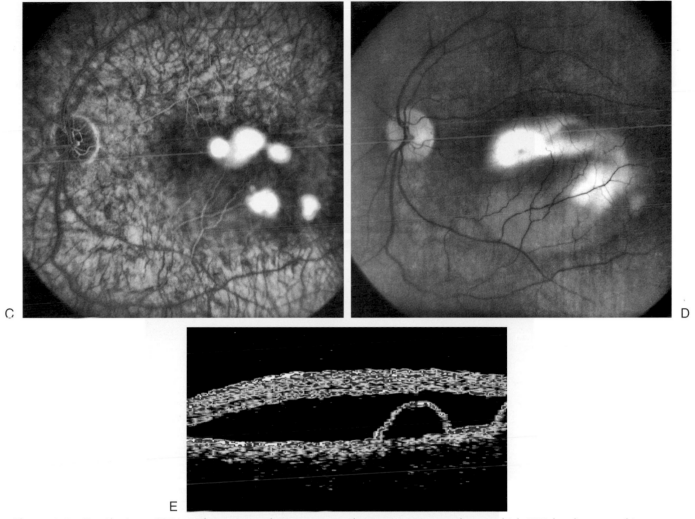

Figure 14–5 *Cont'd* Acute CSC in male patient aged 56 years. *A–D:* Fluorescein angiogram shows multiple RPE detachments and intense subretinal leakage from one leakage point. *E:* OCT image shows RPE and neurosensory detachment.

choroidal leakage. ICG angiography is used in clinical practice for confirmation of CSC and differential diagnosis with age-related macular degeneration–associated pigment epithelial changes, choroidal neovascularization, and polypoidal choroidopathy. Recently, ICG angiography–guided photo-dynamic therapy with a laser applied to areas of choroidal hyperpermeability has been proposed for patients with chronic CSC.

14.3.3 LASER DOPPLER FLOWMETRY

Laser Doppler flowmetry with measurement of the foveal choroidal blood flow has been performed in patients with acute CSC. Decreased flow was demonstrated, with the blood flow in eyes with CSC being 45% lower than in fellow eyes ($p < 0.01$).

14.3.4 OPTICAL COHERENCE TOMOGRAPHY

Optical coherence tomography (OCT) provides diagnostic information on intraretinal morphologic features and allows detection of subclinical serous detachment of

the macula or PEDs (**Figure 14–2**). In the active phase of CSC, OCT allows monitoring of the serous detachments of the RPE and/or the sensory retina (**Figures 14–5** and **14–6**). These data are an excellent guideline for either spontaneous follow-up or institution of therapy. In patients with incomplete recovery of vision after resolution of the detachment, OCT will furnish information on the anatomic anomalies responsible for visual loss being either retinal attenuation with foveal atrophy or cystoid macular degeneration with intraretinal cystoid spaces (**Figures 14–3** and **14–4**).

14.4 Pathology

The limited information available on the pathologic features of CSC indicates no definite abnormality in the choriocapillaris. The presence of fibrin in a lesion that clinically was a white subretinal exudate is indicative of marked changes of permeability of the choriocapillaris with escape of serum proteins as large as fibrinogen.

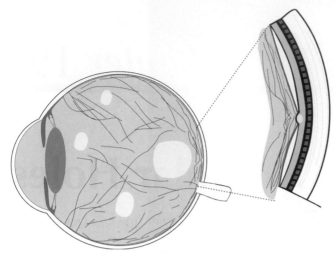

Figure 15–3 Some of the earliest stages of a posterior vitreous detachment start as a separation of the vitreous around the fovea to produce a perifoveal posterior vitreous detachment (*red lines*).

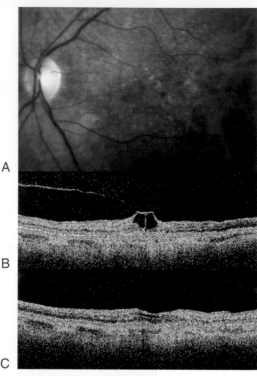

Figure 15–4 A 74-year-old man had a history of nonexudative age macular degeneration in his right eye and a visual acuity of 20/30. The patient had a gradual decrease in acuity to 20/80. *A:* Color photograph reveals typical macular degenerative changes such as drusen and focal hyperpigmentation. *B:* Optical coherence tomography (OCT) imaging shows vitreofoveal traction with cystic change that is not easily seen with biomicroscopy. *C:* OCT image 1 week after pars plana vitrectomy showing improvement of the foveal contour; the visual acuity was 20/30.

form an outer lamellar hole (**Figure 15–6**) and finally dehiscence of the inner retina to produce a full-thickness hole (**Figure 15–7**). If the process is aborted along this progression, the patient may develop an outer lamellar hole. On occasion, patients will have an un-roofing of the pseudocyst, which then develops into a full-thickness hole or only an inner lamellar hole. Rarely macular holes may develop without an intervening pseudocyst, usually in the context of epiretinal membrane formation (**Figure 15–8**). Trauma can lead to macular hole formation also, presumably without the intermediate step of pseudocyst formation (**Figure 15–9**).

In addition to the forces related to a posterior vitreous detachment, other operative forces can lead to macular hole formation (**Figure 15–10**). These forces include epiretinal membranes and residual plaques of cortical vitreous on the surface of the retina. Even after the development of a posterior vitreous detachment, ultrastructural examination of the retina shows remnants of vitreous fibers on the internal limiting membrane in the macular region. During vitreous surgery using triamcinolone, it is common to identify plaques of adherent vitreous even though the patient had the clinical appearance of a posterior vitreous detachment. Once a macular hole forms, the retina bordering the hole begins to elevate and thus separates

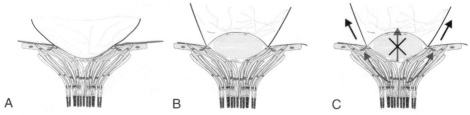

Figure 15–5 *A:* Schematic drawing of the fovea. There are a large number of Müller cells in the fovea, many of which course in an eccentric fashion from the center of the fovea to the perifoveal region. The internal limiting membrane is attenuated centrally, but is quite thick in the perifoveal area. The external limiting membrane is discontinuous in the center of the fovea due to lack of zonulae. *B:* Vitreous traction is thought to lead to a foveal cyst. There is a relative lack of Müller cells coursing perpendicularly through the center of the fovea, which may decrease the tensile strength of the fovea and allow splitting of the tissue and subsequent cyst formation. *C:* Once a cyst forms, there cannot be any direct anterior-posterior force transmitted through the cyst. Any force transmitted posteriorly must come around the cyst. The Müller cells in the foveal region course eccentrically with the cell body being located in the perifoveal region and the cell processes extending toward the center of the fovea. They would act to direct the force vector from the vitreous to the center of the fovea. The foveal center is a potential weak point, because of the lack of zonular attachments there, setting the stage for hole formation. (From Spaide RF. Closure of an outer lamellar macular hole by vitrectomy: Hypothesis for one mechanism of macular hole formation. Retina. 2000;20:587–590.)

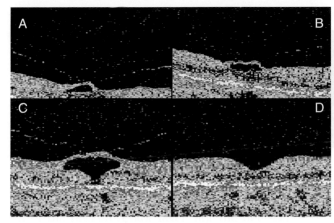

Figure 15–6 *A* and *B*: This patient had a full-thickness macular hole in the fellow eye. She had a tractional pseudocyst in the right eye with a perifoveal posterior vitreous detachment. The perifoveal vitreous detachment was easier to visualize at this stage when the vitreous face was toward the posterior portion of the region scanned (*B*). *C:* Eight months after the scans shown in *A* and *B* were obtained the patient had an acute loss of central visual acuity, an increase in distortion, and a central scotoma. The patient appeared to have an increase in the size of the hole, which was confirmed by OCT. The inner portion of the pseudocyst measured 55 μm in thickness. *D:* Two weeks after vitrectomy with release of the vitreous traction, the patient had a collapse of the pseudocyst, an improvement in visual acuity, and a restoration of a normal foveal contour. Her central foveal thickness was 145 μm.

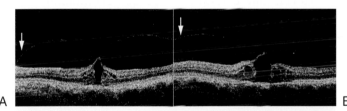

Figure 15–7 Although the patient had an intact internal limiting membrane (*A*) and therefore did not have a "hole," there is almost no functional difference between the image in (*A*) and in (*B*), taken 2 weeks later, when the patient in fact developed a full-thickness hole. The vision-defining event was the division of the photoreceptor layer.

from the pumping effect of the retinal pigment epithelium (RPE); the involved retina may hydrate excessively, leading to edema, cystoid space formation, and further bending moment, lifting the edges of the retina. Successful surgical repair of the macular hole follows general tenets of surgery elsewhere in the body: the forces leading to tissue separation need to be overcome and the tissue should to be immobilized for a period of time for the healing process to begin. Removal of the forces opening the hole include removing the vitreous and potentially removing any forces acting in the plane of the retina, such as those from epiretinal membranes and adherent vitreous plaques. This is often done by just peeling the internal limiting membrane. It was popular to use indocyanine green as a staining agent to improve visualization and decrease the adhesiveness of the internal limiting membrane to the underlying retina, but concerns arose about the potential toxicity of

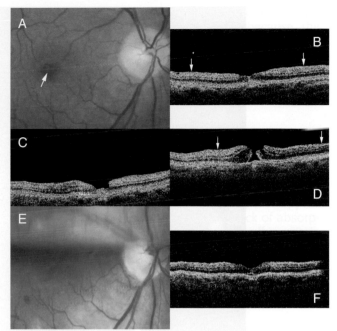

Figure 15–8 On presentation, this 66-year-old man had complaints of distorted vision, and his visual acuity was 20/40 *A:* Color photograph with a yellow spot at the fovea (*arrow*), often referred to as a Stage 1A macular hole. *B:* The corresponding OCT image shows a modest epiretinal membrane (*arrows*) and loss of foveal contour. *C:* One month later, the patient developed an inner lamellar hole, but his acuity remained 20/40. *D:* Six months after presentation he developed a full-thickness macular hole with more prominence of his epiretinal membrane (*arrows*), and his visual acuity was 20/60. *E:* Color photograph 1 week after pars plana vitrectomy with an inner limiting membrane peel. Note the residual gas bubble and the closed macular hole. *F:* OCT image shows a small layer of residual subretinal fluid, a common finding immediately after surgery. His visual acuity was 20/40+.

indocyanine green and the prolonged staining of the intraocular tissue with this dye (**Figure 15–11**). Nearly every patient can have adequate internal limiting membrane peeling without any staining agents by using modern vitrectomy forceps. The removal of the internal limiting membrane probably increases the closure rate as well as decreases the reopening rate after surgery.

15.2 Clinical Signs and Symptoms

A staging system should convey useful information about the severity of disease, potentially offer prognostic information, and be based on pathophysiologically plausible concepts, and its results be accurate, reproducible, and ideally derived from objectively acquired information. OCT is the ideal method to form the basis of staging information. A staging system for macular holes is the following:

- **Stage 0** or **Premacular hole state:** This occurs in patients with a perifoveal posterior vitreous detachment who have no or subtle changes in the macular topography, such as loss of the foveal

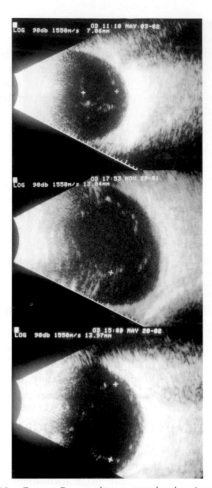

Figure 15–13 Contact B-scan ultrasonography showing various sized posterior premacular vitreous pockets.

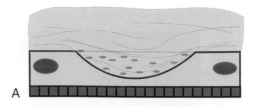

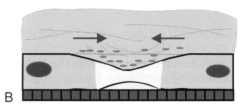

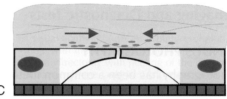

Figure 15–14 *A:* Gass proposed that Müller cells migrated into the prefoveolar vitreous and proliferated there. *B:* They then induced contraction of this vitreous, causing the foveola to become elevated. This stage of macular hole formation, Stage 1A according to Gass, was marked by accumulation of xanthophyll pigment centrally. *C:* With continued contraction of the vitreous more of the central fovea was supposed to have become detached. The yellow pigment was supposed to have migrated laterally to make a ring appearance. Even though the contracture of the vitreous was toward the center of the fovea, a hole was supposed to have formed in the central fovea (an occult hole). This hole was theorized to expand outward, even though the vector of the proposed force was toward the center of the macula.

the pre-foveolar vitreous and then began to multiply (**Figure 15–14**). These cells contributed to a condensation of the vitreous in front of the foveola and allegedly caused a generation of a centripetal contraction of the vitreous with traction toward *the center* of the fovea. It was proposed that in a Stage 1A macular hole, visible as a small yellow dot, there is tractional elevation of the foveola. In Stage 1B, there is an expansion of the tractional detachment to the point that the fovea is elevated and was proposed to have the ophthalmoscopic appearance of a yellow ring centered in the macula. Patients with a Stage 1B hole were thought to have an undetectable (occult) full-thickness hole in the central fovea. How this defect arises in the central fovea when the tangential forces are centripetal toward the center is not addressed in the theory.

OCT has shown that patients with the ophthalmoscopic findings of a Stage 1A or Stage 1B hole actually may have a variety of anatomic configurations, suggesting that these ophthalmoscopic phenotypes are nonspecific (**Figures 15–8** and **15–15** to **15–17**). In addition, OCT can demonstrate partial posterior vitreous detachments, foveal pseudocysts, and outer lamellar holes, features not even considered in older pathogenic theories, better than other techniques. Because of the

high resolution of OCT, the macrophages on the RPE can be imaged to a striking degree (**Figure 15–18**). OCT is repeatable and provides consistent and objective results. The size of the vitreous attachment to the fovea can be measured as can the induced structural deformation, the two of which are correlated. Associated epiretinal membranes can also be seen. Some eyes with macular holes appear to have glial proliferation on the posterior vitreous face (**Figure 15–19**). The preoperative size of the macular hole is inversely correlated to the surgical success rate. Some patients, particularly those with pathologic myopia, may have a relatively large retinal detachment due to a macular hole (**Figure 15–20**). Patients with pathologic myopia often need peeling of the internal limiting membrane to cause macular hole closure (**Figure 15–21**). In the early postoperative period visual acuity can be better than the preoperative acuity, but by ophthalmoscopy the outline of the macular hole can be seen. By OCT a small region of subfoveal fluid

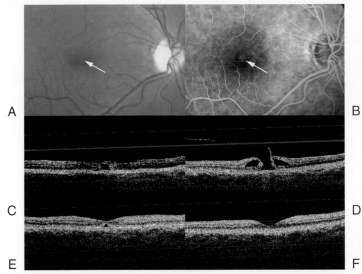

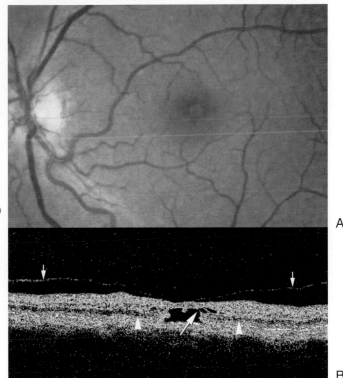

Figure 15–15 This patient presented with a decreased visual acuity of 20/40. *A:* Color photograph demonstrating a yellow spot in fovea (*arrow*) with clinical appearance of a Stage 1A macular hole. *B:* Fluorescein angiography shows a corresponding area of hyperfluorescence (*arrow*). *C:* OCT image shows decreased foveal thickness with absence of the normally hyporeflective outer retinal layer. *D:* Within 2 weeks, the visual acuity decreased to 20/100, and the patient developed a full-thickness macular hole with evident vitreous attachment to the elevated flap. *E:* OCT image 3 months after pars plana vitrectomy and inner limiting membrane peel shows a small amount of subfoveal fluid and a visual acuity of 20/40. *F:* Six months after surgery, the fovea was flat and the visual acuity was 20/30.

Figure 15–16 This patient presented with a visual acuity of 20/400. *A:* Color photograph demonstrates a yellow ring commonly termed a Stage 1B hole. The corresponding OCT image (*B*) shows an outer lamellar hole. The vitreous face is visible (*small arrows*) with attachment at the fovea. There is a disruption of the outer plexiform layer (*arrowheads*) and a cystic communication with the inner plexiform layer (*large arrow*) into the outer lamellar dehiscence.

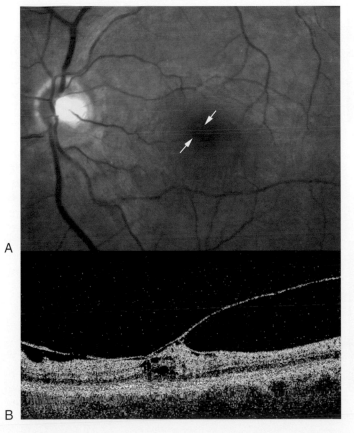

Figure 15–17 *A:* Color photograph of a patient, who had a foveal appearance resembling a Stage 1B hole (*arrows*). The visual acuity was 20/30. *B:* OCT image shows vitreofoveal traction with distortion of the foveal tissue, but no hole or retinal elevation.

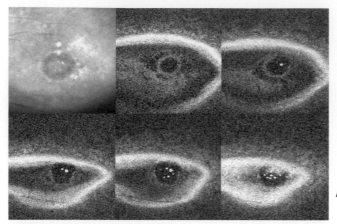

Figure 15–18 En face imaging of a macular hole showing white dots, thought to correspond to macrophages at the base of the hole. (Courtesy of Dennis Orlock.)

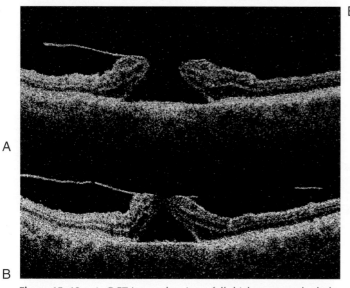

Figure 15–19 *A:* OCT image showing a full-thickness macular hole with vitreofoveal traction. *B:* OCT image slightly temporal to *A*. The intense signal reflectance of the vitreous probably represents glial proliferation along the posterior vitreous face.

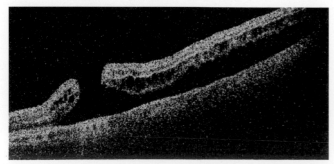

Figure 15–20 Macular holes can be associated with larger retinal detachments, particularly in myopic patients.

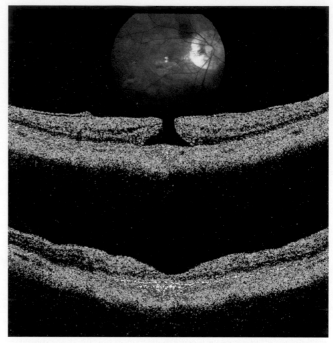

Figure 15–21 This patient presented with pathologic myopia and a visual acuity of 20/200. *A:* OCT image with a full-thickness macular hole and epiretinal membrane. *B:* OCT image 3 months after pars plana vitrectomy and inner limiting membrane peel with a visual acuity of 20/30. The color photograph *inset* of this patient shows some of the challenges in closing macular holes in myopic patients: these patients frequently have attenuated retinal layers and regions of RPE atrophy.

can often be seen, and as this subfoveal fluid resolves the acuity further improves. Hole re-opening is preceded by the formation of cystoid macular edema, particularly after cataract surgery or by a separation of the glial plug holding the retina together at the center of the macula (**Figure 15–22**).

15.3.5 ULTRASONOGRAPHY

The presence of a posterior vitreous detachment usually can be identified by careful contact B-scan ultrasonography. The posterior precortical vitreous pocket can also be visualized and measured (**Figure 15–13**). Fellow eyes of patients with macular holes show larger posterior precortical vitreous pockets than do comparable fellow eyes of patients with just posterior vitreous detachments. This suggests that the posterior precortical vitreous pocket may alter vitreous forces on the macula.

15.4 Inner Lamellar Holes and Pseudoholes

Vitreous traction leading to pseudocyst formation can also result in unroofing of the pseudocyst and tractional elevation of one edge of the inner retinal tissue (**Figure 15–23**). This creates an inner lamellar hole with an

A

B

C

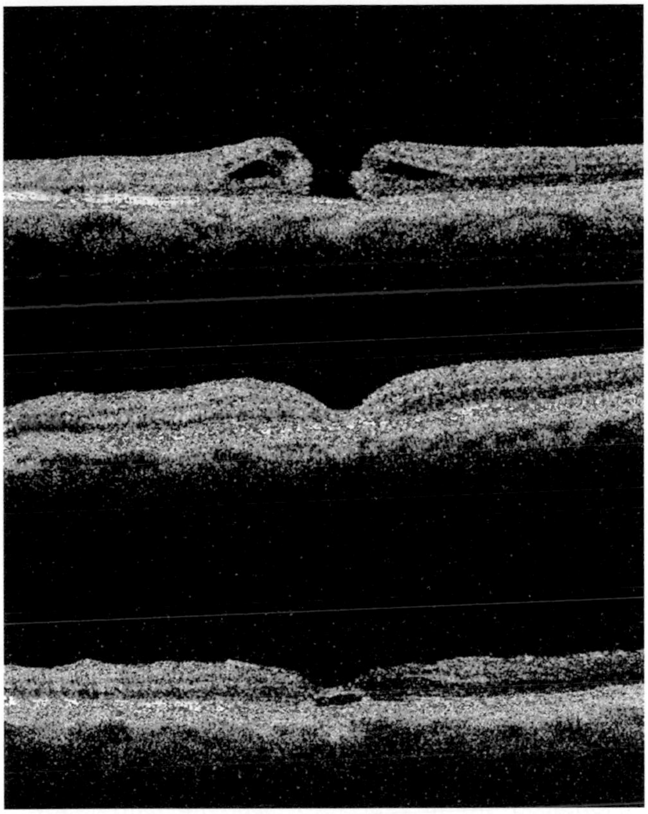

Figure 15–22 *A:* Preoperative OCT image of a patient with a full-thickness macular hole and a visual acuity of 20/200. *B:* Two weeks after vitrectomy without peeling of the internal limiting membrane the macular hole appeared to be closed, but the central fovea was thin. The visual acuity was 20/200. *C:* Image 3 months after surgery shows thinning and elevation of the central fovea. The patient eventually developed a reopening of the hole.

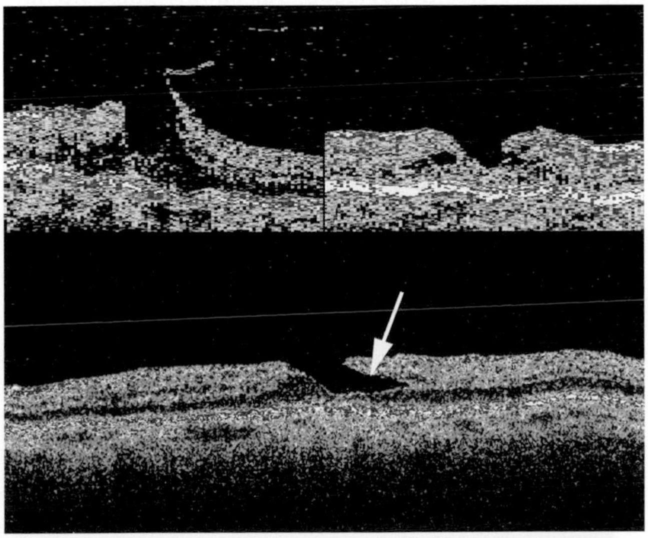

A

B

C

Figure 15–23 A variation on an inner lamellar hole starts with traction and dehiscence of the inner retinal layers (*A*). After release of the vitreous (*B*), there is separation and undermining of the inner retinal layers such that the cross-sectional image shows an obliquely angled defect in the inner retina. *C:* Image from another patient with this configuration showing the extent of the undermining of the inner retinal layers (*arrow*). The visual acuity was 20/30.

undermined edge. Other cases of inner lamellar holes appear to result from a simple unroofing of inner retinal tissue (**Figure 15–24**). Epiretinal proliferation around the fovea, but not including the foveola itself, can lead to the appearance of a macular hole. This is termed a *pseudohole*. OCT has shown that some of these patients have steeply sloping sides to the fovea with a slight thickening of the central foveola (**Figure 15–25**). Some patients may have what appears to be loss of substance

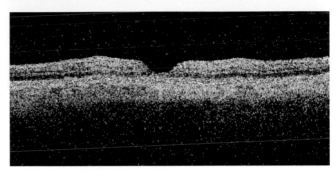

Figure 15–24 This patient had a macular hole in the fellow eye and an inner lamellar hole as demonstrated by OCT. Note the irregular foveal contour and the central thickness of 58 microns.

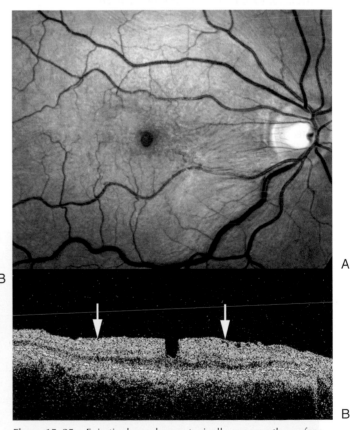

A

B

Figure 15–25 Epiretinal membranes typically grow on the surface of the retina and produce tractional effects. When the membrane growth surrounds, but does not directly involve the fovea, the resultant contraction of the epiretinal membrane causes a bunching of the retina around the fovea. This well-like depression (*A*) can mimic the ophthalmoscopic appearance of a macular hole. OCT image (*B*) demonstrates the epiretinal membrane (*arrows*) and the steeply sloping sides of the fovea (pseudohole).

vascular diseases, retinal detachment, diabetic retinopathy, retinal hemangioma, retinal arteriolar macroaneurysms, uveitis, intraocular inflammation, and hyperpermeable conditions including surgery and trauma. ERMs develop in 3% to 8.5% of eyes after retinal reattachment surgery. Proliferation of cells, including retinal pigment epithelium (RPE) and subsequent fibrous connective tissue formation, can result in secondary ERM.

16.2 Clinical Signs and Symptoms

Most patients with idiopathic ERMs are asymptomatic and have almost normal vision. As an ERM progresses to become opaque or to shrink, metamorphopsia,

distortion, or blurred vision may develop. Less commonly, some patients may describe diplopia, photopsia, or macropsia.

In the initial stage, the membrane is transparent and the tortuosity of vessels is minimal to mild if observed; therefore, the visual acuity is usually well preserved. About 85% of patients with an idiopathic ERM have a visual acuity of 20/70 or better, and 67% have a visual acuity of 20/30 or better. Less than 5% of patients have a visual acuity worse than 20/200. When followed for 2 years, only 10% to 25% of patients have a decrease in visual acuity of one or two lines.

Initially, a simple ERM is visible only as a glinting, irregular reflex (**Figure 16–1**). Although these subtle ERMs usually do not have a distinct edge, as they become more apparent, translucent membranes can be detected that cover the entire macula and even extend anteriorly beyond the vascular arcades. When the membrane contracts more, minimal wrinkling of the ILM is observed (**Figure 16–3**). The membrane also may lift the fovea off the RPE, resulting in disappearance of the foveal reflex. Although this focal detachment of the fovea had been thought to be a characteristic of more advanced cases, optical coherence tomography (OCT) has revealed recently that the focal detachment occurs even at a relatively early stage of ERM development (**Figure 16–4**).

The folds of the ILM are observed in an intermediate case. Traction on the inner retina results in folds

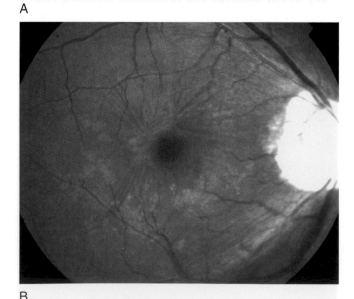

A

B

Figure 16–3 When the membrane contracts, minimal wrinkling of the ILM is observed (*A*). Observation with a red-free filter (*right*) facilitates detection of fine striae (*B*).

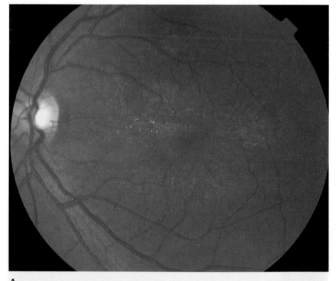

A

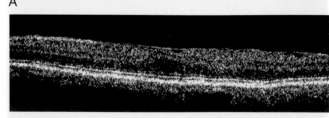

B

Figure 16–4 Color photograph of an ERM (*A*). An OCT image in the same patient shows that blunting of the foveal depression occurs even at a relatively early stage of ERM development (*B*).

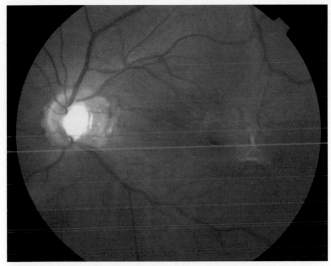

Figure 16–5 Traction on the inner retina results in folds radiating from the center of the ERM.

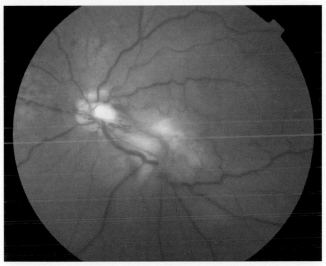

Figure 16–7 Foveal ectopia occurs in a patient with the ERM centering distal to the macula. This case is a secondary FRM (proliferative vitreoretinopathy) associated with retinal detachment.

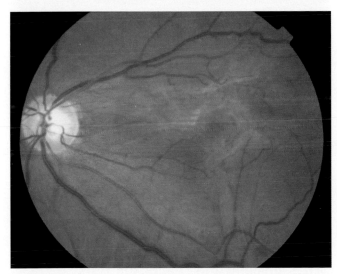

Figure 16–6 As contraction progresses, straightening of the capillaries around the macula and tortuosity of the retinal vessels are observed.

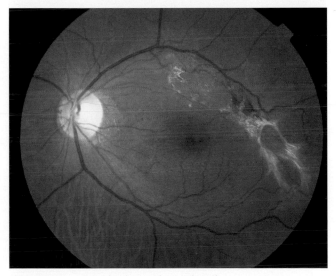

Figure 16–8 Microbleeding and irregular telangiectasis are occasionally observed in the inner retina of an eye with an advanced ERM.

radiating from the center of the ERM (**Figure 16–5**), straightening of the capillaries around the macula, and tortuosity of the retinal vessels (**Figure 16–6**).

A further increase in the tangential traction on the retina causes macular dislocation or macular edema as a result of breakdown of the blood-retinal barrier. If the membrane is centered distal to the macula, a certain degree of foveal ectopia can occur (**Figure 16–7**). These advanced changes cause a further decrease of the visual acuity and diplopia. Microbleeding occasionally is observed in the inner retina (**Figure 16–8**), and microaneurysms and irregular telangiectasis also develop in some patients. Furthermore, cotton-wool spots (**Figure 16–9**) and a secondary retinal detachment (**Figure 16–10**) are induced as the result of retinal traction and

blockage of axoplasmic flow. These findings can resolve when the ERM is removed surgically.

A pseudomacular hole is observed in the following two situations: when the ERM is thinner at the fovea and the color contrast between a darker-red fovea and the relative pallor surrounding the ERM causes a macular hole–like appearance (**Figure 16–11**) and when long-standing macular edema causes a large foveal cyst beneath the ERM (**Figure 16–12**). Most pseudo-macular holes fall into the former category, and the patients usually have good vision; with the latter, occasionally patients have poor vision, usually 20/100 or less.

A full-thickness macular hole occurs in up to 30% of patients with ERM (**Figure 16–13**). It is important to differentiate a true hole from a pseudohole. A detailed

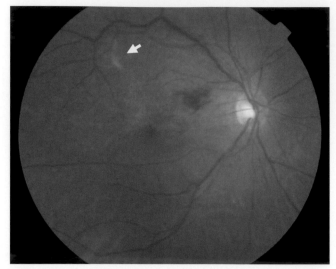

Figure 16–9   A cotton-wool spot (*arrow*) is induced as the result of blockage of axoplasmic flow.

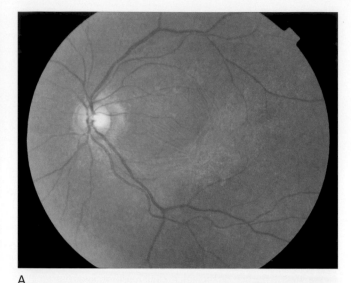

A

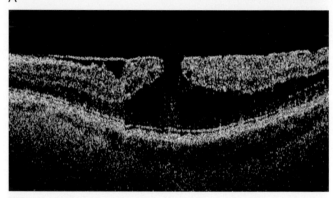

B

Figure 16–11   *A:* A pseudo-macular hole is observed when the ERM is thinner at the fovea. The color contrast between a darker-red fovea and the relative pallor surrounding the ERM causes a macular hole–like appearance. *B:* OCT image demonstrating the pseudohole appearance.

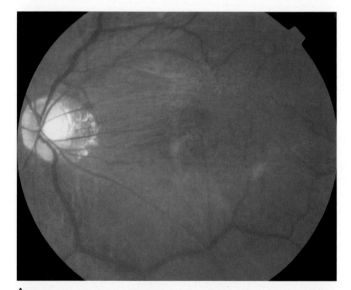

A

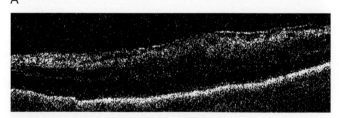

B

Figure 16–10   *A:* Advanced retinal traction from an ERM. *B:* OCT image of the same patient.

history, visual acuity measurement, careful fundus examination, the Watzke-Allen test, and fluorescein angiography are useful when OCT is unavailable. A PVD is observed in 70% to 95% of idiopathic ERMs, but it is not required for the ERM to form. Patients with vitreoretinal traction on the fovea have a higher incidence of cystoid macular edema and lower visual acuity than those with a complete vitreous detachment.

16.3 Imaging and Diagnostic Tests

16.3.1 RED-FREE FUNDUS PHOTOGRAPHY

Red-free fundus photography is a convenient and useful way to diagnose an ERM. Green-blue and blue light do not penetrate beyond the retinal nerve fiber layer and are reflected from the superficial nerve fiber layer back to the observer or the camera. Observing or recording through a short-pass cut-off filter can provide a monochromatic (or black-and-white) image of the retinal surface without disturbing the image from the deeper retina and choroid, resulting in visualization of subtle changes at the vitreoretinal interface (**Figure 16–3**).

16.3.2 OPTICAL COHERENCE TOMOGRAPHY

OCT is a powerful tool for evaluating the status of the vitreoretinal interface. OCT can provide subtle information that cannot be evaluated with a biomicroscope (**Figure 16–14**). An ERM is observed with OCT as a

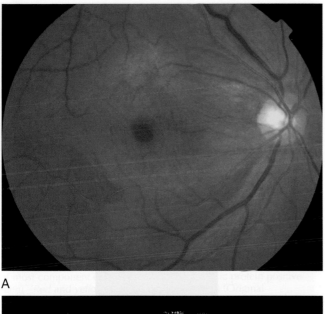

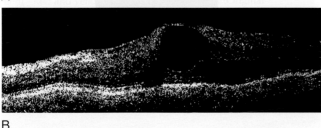

Figure 16–12 *A:* Long-standing macular edema causes a foveal cyst beneath the ERM, resulting in a pseudo-macular hole appearance. *B:* OCT image of same patient showing a large foveal cyst.

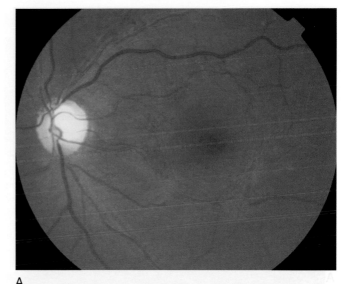

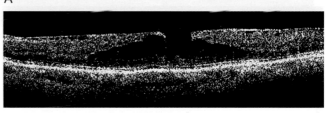

Figure 16–13 *A:* A pseudo-macular hole can be difficult to differentiate from a true macular hole. *B:* It is important to differentiate a true hole from a pseudohole with OCT, which shows that the retinal defect is not full thickness.

highly reflective line on the retinal surface. It mostly adheres to the inner retinal surface (**Figure 16–15**) but sometimes separates from the surface and adheres only at several points (**Figure 16–16**). As the ERM becomes denser, the reflection has a higher and more linear shape, demonstrating a taut membrane. OCT is useful to distinguish a macular pseudohole caused by an ERM (**Figure 16–14**) from a full-thickness secondary macular hole (**Figure 16–13**). OCT is also useful for determining an indication for surgery and monitoring the therapeutic response. An OCT ophthalmoscope can provide a series of images, slicing the tissue at orientations parallel to the retinal surface. The OCT ophthalmoscopic examination shows the extent of retinal distortion (**Figure 16–17**).

16.3.3 FLUORESCEIN ANGIOGRAPHY

Fluorescein angiography is also useful for diagnosing an ERM. The severity of vessel damage and macular edema by leakage and pooling of fluorescein as well as retinal wrinkling by retinal vascular tortuosity and straightening can be evaluated by fluorescein angiography (**Figure 16–18**). When vessel damage progresses, irregular fluorescein leakage is observed at the area covered by the ERM.

Fluorescein angiography is also useful for distinguishing ERM from other diseases. The differential diagnosis of ERM includes a full-thickness macular hole, cystoid macular edema associated with diabetic retinopathy or retinal vein occlusion, age-related macular degeneration (AMD), and other macular diseases. Whereas an ERM shows diffuse, irregular, and weak hyperfluorescence, a full-thickness macular hole shows a central window defect, cystoid macular edema shows "flower petal" pooling of fluorescence, and AMD shows leakage from choroidal neovascularization.

16.4 Pathology

Pathologically, an ERM is a fibrous hypocellular avascular sheet that forms on the ILM. Roth et al. first reported that retinal glial cells might migrate through a gap in the ILM and proliferate as a membrane on the retina. Bellhorn et al. reported that glial cells of the neural retina might migrate through a break in the ILM that is associated with a PVD and proliferate. Glial cells can proliferate into the vitreous cortex in eyes in which an ERM forms before vitreous detachment occurs.

Cell types that contribute to the development of an ERM vary according to the original diseases. The cell types include fibrous astrocytes, fibrocytes, myofibroblasts, macrophages, inflammatory cells, hyalocytes, RPE cells, and vascular endothelial cells (**Figure 16–19**).

Chapter 17

Macular Dystrophies

ELIAS I. TRABOULSI, MD

17.1 Central Areolar Choroidal Dystrophy (also called *central areolar choroidal atrophy* and *central areolar choroidal sclerosis*)

17.1.1 GENETICS

Inheritance: Autosomal dominant

OMIM (Online Mendelian Inheritance in Man) Number: 215500

Symbol: CACD

Genetic Locus: 17p13

17.1.2 CLINICAL SIGNS AND SYMPTOMS

Symptoms appear in the third to fifth decades. There is decreased central vision (20/25 to 20/200). Mild nonspecific foveal granularity is present early and later develops into a circumscribed zone of neurosensory retina, retinal pigment epithelium (RPE), and choriocapillaris atrophy within the central macula and between the arcades.

17.1.3 ANCILLARY TESTING

On fluorescein angiography, early lesions may show faint RPE transmission defects within the fovea. Later, a well-circumscribed zone of choriocapillaris atrophy appears within the central macula. The photopic electro-retinogram (ERG) is normal to slightly subnormal, and results of the scotopic ERG are normal. The electro-oculogram (EOG) is normal to slightly subnormal. Color vision testing reveals a moderate protan-deutan defect. A large central scotoma is present in advanced cases.

17.1.4 HISTOPATHOLOGY

Histopathologic studies show well-demarcated areas of RPE and choriocapillaris atrophy, with no evidence of choroidal sclerosis.

17.2 Dominant Cystoid Macular Dystrophy

17.2.1 GENETICS

Inheritance: Autosomal dominant

OMIM Number: 153880

Gene Locus: 7p21-p15

17.2.2 CLINICAL SIGNS AND SYMPTOMS

The disease has its onset in the first and second decades. Patients present with decreased central vision (20/25 to 20/80) that progresses to 20/200 to count fingers.

Ophthalmoscopy reveals early cystoid macular edema. Macular RPE changes and atrophy set in late. Some patients may have RPE changes in a bull's-eye configuration that progress to atrophy. Whitish punctate deposits may be present in the vitreous. There is moderate-to-high hypermetropia.

17.2.3 ANCILLARY TESTING

Fluorescein angiography shows cystoid macular edema and increased retinal capillary permeability in the posterior pole. The ERG is normal. The EOG may be subnormal. Dark adaptation may also be subnormal. There may be a mild-to-moderate deutan-tritan color vision defect. A central scotoma may be present.

17.3 Dominant Progressive Foveal Dystrophy (also called *autosomal dominant Stargardt's disease*)

17.3.1 GENETICS

Inheritance: Autosomal dominant
OMIM Number: 600110
Gene: ELOVL4
Gene Locus: 6q14

17.3.2 CLINICAL SIGNS AND SYMPTOMS

Onset is the in second to fourth decades. Patients present with decreased central vision. There are mild color and night vision changes. There is no photophobia. This condition is differentiated from juvenile-onset Stargardt's disease by its autosomal dominant inheritance pattern, later onset, and generally less severe clinical course. The fundus may be normal early in the disease, with later occurrence of macular dystrophic changes, with or without flecks in the posterior pole and midperipheral retina.

17.3.3 ANCILLARY TESTING

Fluorescein angiography shows irregular RPE transmission defects within the fovea. The photopic ERG is normal to subnormal whereas the scotopic ERG is normal. The EOG may be slightly subnormal. Dark adaptation is generally normal. Color vision shows a mild-to-moderate deutan-tritan defect. There is a central scotoma in advanced cases.

17.4 Enhanced S-Cone Syndrome (includes Goldmann-Favre syndrome and clumped pigmentary retinopathy)

17.4.1 GENETICS

Inheritance: Autosomal recessive
OMIM Numbers: 268100 and 604485
Gene: NR2E3 or PNR
Gene Locus: 15q23

17.4.2 CLINICAL SIGNS AND SYMPTOMS

Night blindness is present from early childhood and reduced visual acuity becomes evident toward the end of the first decade. The severe end-of-disease spectrum is referred to as *Goldmann-Favre syndrome*. Fundus findings include round, clumped, and bony spicule pigmentary changes (**Figure 17–1**) and subretinal dot-like flecks in the posterior pole and peripheral retina (**Figure 17–2**) and cystic lesions similar to those of juvenile retinoschisis in the fovea of some patients (**Figures 17–3**

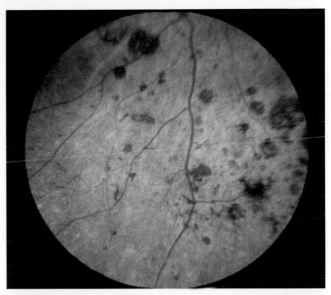

Figure 17–1 Peripheral pigmentary changes in a patient with clumped pigmentary retinopathy. There are round, irregular, and bony spicule pigment intra- and subretinal deposits.

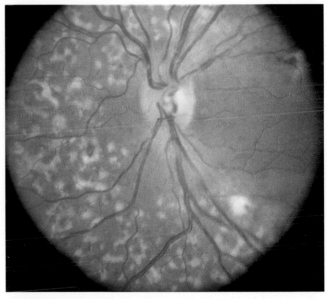

Figure 17–2 Peripapillary area in a patient with Goldmann-Favre syndrome and a mutation in the *NR2E3* gene. Deep, irregular whitish lesions are sometimes associated with pigmentary changes forming what look like scars.

and **17–4**). The vitreous is liquefied with veils in some patients. Errors of refraction vary from hypermetropic to myopic.

17.4.3 ANCILLARY TESTS

Angiographic findings depend on the type and severity of retinal dystrophic changes and on the stage of the disease. The scotopic ERG does not reveal any rod-driven responses; large, slow waveforms are detected in response to bright flashes and the photopic ERG shows

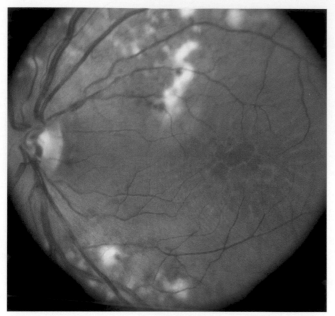

Figure 17–3 Same patient as in **Figure 17–2.** A net-like pattern is present in the macular area. More subretinal lesions/scars are located under the vascular arcades.

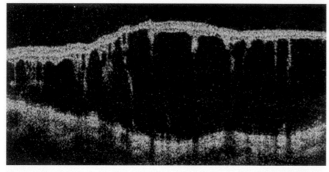

Figure 17–4 Optical coherence tomography image of the macula in the same patient showing a schisis cavity.

more sensitivity to blue than to red or white stimuli, hence the term *enhanced S-cone syndrome*. The EOG has a reduced light peak.

17.5 Familial Radial Drusen (also called Doyne Honeycomb Choroiditis, Holthouse-Batten Superficial Choroiditis, Hutchinson-Tays Central Guttate Choroiditis, and Malattia Leventinese)

17.5.1 GENETICS

Inheritance: Autosomal dominant

OMIM Number: 126600

Gene: EFEMP1

Gene Locus: 2p16-p21

17.5.2 CLINICAL SIGNS AND SYMPTOMS

Onset of drusen is in the first to fourth decades with rare congenital cases. Patients are asymptomatic, unless degenerative or neovascular changes occur in the macula. Ophthalmoscopy shows round, yellow-white deposits within the posterior pole and radially into the fundus midperiphery. Some drusen are associated with pigmentary changes and tend to enlarge and coalesce with time (**Figure 17–5**). In later stages of the disease there may be degenerative changes within macula in the form of RPE pigmentary disturbance, RPE detachment, or subretinal neovascularization (**Figure 17–6**).

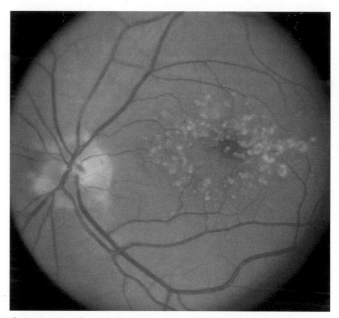

Figure 17–5 This North-American patient has dominant radial drusen and a mutation in the *EFEMP1* gene. Some of the drusen are associated with fine pigment changes. Note the drusen at the edge of the disc.

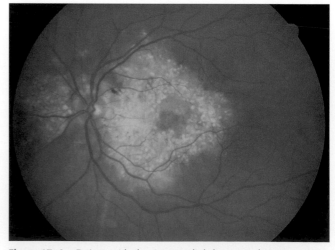

Figure 17–6 Patient with dominant radial drusen and more extensive drusen than his sister in **Figure 17–5.**

17.5.3 ANCILLARY TESTS

Fluorescein angiography shows early blockage of transmission and possible late staining. There may be irregular dye transmission, leakage, and pooling within the macula, depending on the degree of associated degenerative change. The ERG is normal. The EOG may be slightly subnormal. There are no abnormalities of dark adaptation or of color vision perception. A central scotoma may be present if there is macular degeneration.

17.6 Fundus Flavimaculatus (subtype of Stargardt's disease)

17.6.1 GENETICS

Inheritance: Autosomal Recessive
OMIM Number: 248200
Gene: ABCA4
Gene Locus: 1p21-p13

17.6.2 CLINICAL SIGNS AND SYMPTOMS

Loss of vision starts in the first up to the sixth decades. The disease is asymptomatic if there are no flecks in the fovea; otherwise, there is a slow and progressive reduction of vision. Angulated (pisciform) yellow-white flecks are present in the posterior pole and midperipheral retina (**Figure 17–7**).

17.6.3 ANCILLARY TESTS

There is a characteristic generalized decrease in choroidal fluorescence (dark choroid sign) on fluorescein angiography in most, but not all, patients (**Figure 17–8**); subretinal flecks demonstrate early blockage and late hyperfluorescent staining. The photopic ERG may be

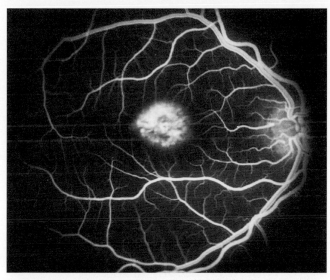

Figure 17–8 A dark choroid sign on a fluorescein angiogram from a patient with Stargardt's disease/fundus flavimaculatus. Confluent transmission defects are present in the macular area.

slightly subnormal, whereas the scotopic ERG is normal. The EOG is subnormal. Dark adaptation is normal. Color vision may become abnormal as the disease progresses. Visual field testing is generally normal or shows central scotomata if there is macular involvement.

17.6.4 HISTOPATHOLOGY

Histopathologic studies show that yellow flecks are groups of enlarged RPE cells packed with granular substance with ultrastructural, autofluorescent, and histochemical properties consistent with lipofuscin.

17.7 North Carolina Macular Dystrophy (also called *Lefler-Wadsworth-Sidbury dystrophy*)

17.7.1 GENETICS

Inheritance: Autosomal dominant
OMIM Numbers: 136550 and 600790
Symbol: MCDR1
Gene Locus: 6q14-q16.2

17.7.2 CLINICAL SIGNS AND SYMPTOMS

The disease is of presumed congenital onset. Central vision is normal early in life, unless atrophic macular "colobomas" are present. Possible late progression to 20/200 visual acuity or worse is seen in some patients with choroidal neovascular membranes. The disease is, however, typically nonprogressive. Initial reports of associated aminoaciduria have been later refuted. Grade I refers to drusen-like lesions and pigment dispersion in

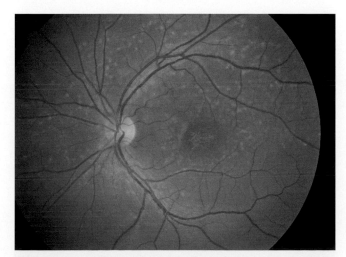

Figure 17–7 This patient has fundus flavimaculatus with macular involvement. The subretinal flecks have the classic fishtail appearance and extend into the retinal midperiphery.

fovea; in Grade II there are confluent drusen-like lesions in fovea, whereas in Grade III there is atrophy of RPE and choriocapillaris within the central macula. Visual acuity is normal in patients with Grade I lesions; Grade III lesions may resemble chorioretinal colobomas (**Figure 17–9**).

17.7.3 ANCILLARY TESTS

On fluorescein angiography, in Grades I and II, there are RPE transmission defects and late staining of drusen-like lesions. In Grade III, there is nonperfusion of the choriocapillaris in the central lesion. The ERG and EOG, dark adaptation, and color vision are normal. Visual field testing may show a central scotoma.

17.8 Pattern Dystrophy (also called *reticular, macroreticular,* and *butterfly-shaped pigment dystrophies*)

17.8.1 GENETICS

Inheritance: Autosomal dominant
OMIM Number: 169150
Gene: *Peripherin*/RDS
Gene Locus: 6p21.1-cen

17.8.2 CLINICAL SIGNS AND SYMPTOMS

The onset of the maculopathy is in the second to fifth decades. Patients are generally asymptomatic or have a slight decrease in central vision (20/25 to 20/40) until late in the disease. Ophthalmoscopy shows subtle RPE mottling in younger patients and a butterfly or net-like pigment pattern in the macular area of older patients.

17.8.3 ANCILLARY TESTS

Angiography shows an ovoid area of hyperfluorescence and late staining surrounding a central hypofluorescent spot, with or without hyperfluorescence of posterior pole flecks. The photopic and scotopic ERG tracings may be subnormal. The EOG is usually normal. Color vision is normal. There may be a relative central scotoma with normal peripheral fields.

17.9 Stargardt's Disease (also called *juvenile macular degeneration*)

17.9.1 GENETICS

Inheritance: Autosomal recessive
OMIM Numbers: 248200 and 601691 and 601718
Gene: ABCA4
Gene Locus: 1p21-p22

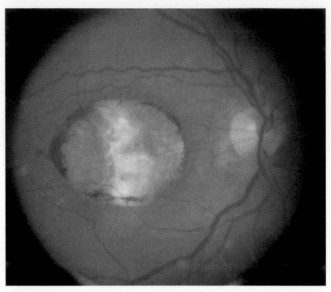

Figure 17–9 Large macular "coloboma" in a patient with North Carolina macular dystrophy Grade III. A few drusen are also present on the temporal edge of the lesion as well as two small hemorrhages.

17.9.2 CLINICAL SIGNS AND SYMPTOMS

The onset of visual loss is usually in the first or second decade. Many children are dismissed as having functional visual loss because of reduced central vision (+20/200) out of proportion to macular changes. Color vision is moderately defective. There is no photophobia. Ophthalmoscopy may not show any macular changes very early in the disease. Later, a beaten-bronze appearance to the macula is followed by an oval zone of RPE and choriocapillaris atrophy or a bull's-eye maculopathy (**Figures 17–10** and **17–11**). There may or may not be flecks in the posterior pole and midperiphery of the fundus.

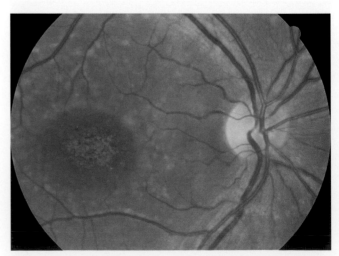

Figure 17–10 A patient with Stargardt's disease and subretinal flecks in the macula and posterior pole.

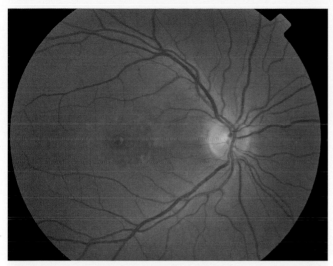

Figure 17–11 A patient with Stargardt's disease and a subtle bull's-eye lesion. The center of the fovea is dark, and there is a ring of faint flecks around the fovea.

17.9.3 ANCILLARY TESTS

Fluorescein angiography is extremely helpful in the diagnosis. Irregular RPE transmission defects are seen in the fovea, with an occasional bull's-eye pattern of transmission. Nonperfusion of the choriocapillaris is seen in advanced cases. When flecks are present, the angiographic pattern is similar to that of fundus flavimaculatus (**Figure 17–12**).

The photopic ERG may be subnormal, whereas the scotopic ERG is normal. The multifocal ERG is subnormal in the macular region. The EOG may be subnormal, as may be dark adaptation and color vision. There is a central scotoma.

17.10 Vitelliform Dystrophy (also called *Best's disease, polymorphic macular degeneration of Braley, vitelliruptive macular dystrophy*)

17.10.1 GENETICS

Inheritance: Autosomal dominant
OMIM Number: 153700
Gene: VMD2, *bestrophin*
Gene Locus: 11q13

17.10.2 CLINICAL SIGNS AND SYMPTOMS

Onset of the disease is in the first decade of life. Decreased central vision (20/30 to 20/50) occurs at a variable age, and vision may remain relatively stable for many years. The fundus appearance is variable: an egg-yolk lesion is present in the fovea in classic cases (**Figure 17–13**), but these are seen infrequently. When the inside of the lesion is irregular, it is called "scrambled," and sometimes there is a pseudohypopyon (**Figure 17–14**). Some patients have multifocal irregular-shaped whitish lesions in the posterior pole (**Figure 17–15**). Lesions eventually degenerate with associated RPE disturbance and pigment clumping (**Figure 17–16**). Subretinal neovascularization and scarring may also occur.

17.10.3 ANCILLARY TESTS

Fluorescein angiography reveals blockage of fluorescence by vitelliform lesions. Transmission of fluorescence occurs when the cyst ruptures. There is otherwise

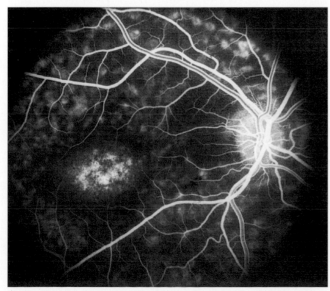

Figure 17–12 Transmission defects from diffuse flecks in the macula and posterior pole of this patient with Stargardt's disease. The rest of the choroid is dark.

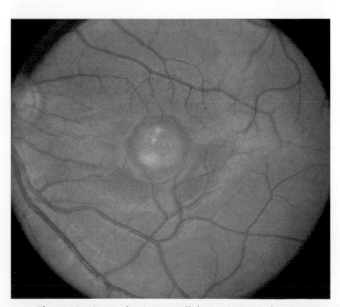

Figure 17–13 A classic egg-yolk lesion in Best's disease.

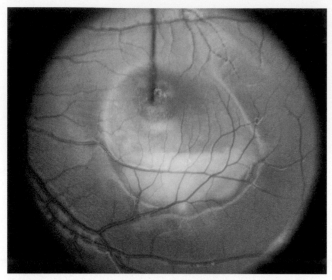

Figure 17–14   Pseudohypopyon in this scrambled large Best's disease lesion.

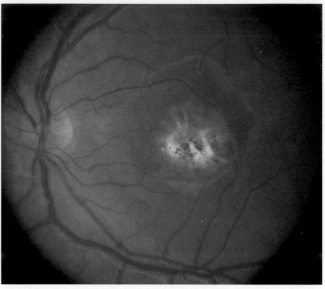

Figure 17–16   Scarred central vitelliform lesion in this patient with Best's disease.

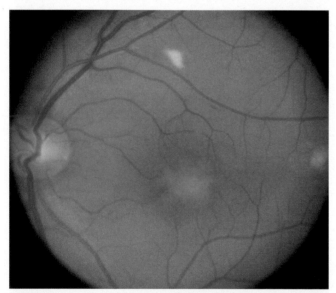

Figure 17–15   Multiple posterior pole lesions in this patient with Best's disease. The macular lesion is faint and round. Two whitish lesions are also present as a manifestation of the disease process.

17.11 X-Linked Juvenile Retinoschisis

17.11.1 GENETICS

Inheritance: X-linked recessing
OMIM Number: 312700
Gene: RS1, *Retinoschisin*
Gene Locus: Xp22.2

17.11.2 CLINICAL SIGNS AND SYMPTOMS

Onset occurs generally in the first decade, and cases have been noted shortly after birth. Patients generally present with decreased central vision (20/25 to 20/50 or worse). The disease is slowly progressive. Ophthalmoscopically, foveal retinoschisis is present in all patients (**Figure 17–17**) and peripheral retinoschisis ("vitreous veils") in half (**Figure 17–18**). Histopathologic studies show splitting of the retina in the nerve fiber layer.

17.11.3 ANCILLARY TESTS

Fluorescein angiography does not reveal any abnormality in the posterior pole until late in the disease, when transmission defects appear within the central macula. The photopic and scotopic ERGs reveal selective decrease in B-wave amplitude (Schubert-Bornsheim tracing or electronegative ERG). The EOG is normal in mild disease and may become subnormal in advanced disease. Dark adaptation examination may show abnormal cone and rod curve segments. There may be an initial tritan defect followed by deutan-tritan color vision defects. Absolute scotomas can be mapped that correspond to areas of schisis.

irregular RPE transmission and staining, depending on the presence of pigmentary disturbances, subretinal neovascularization, and scarring. The combination of a normal ERG and an abnormal EOG is almost pathognomonic and necessary for the diagnosis. The EOG is abnormal even in otherwise normal-appearing "carriers." Rare instances of a normal EOG have been observed in very young individuals. Dark adaptation and color vision are normal. There is a relative central scotoma early, and denser scotomas may occur after degeneration and organization of the vitelliform lesion.

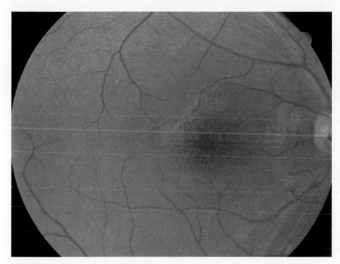

Figure 17–17   Star-shaped foveal schisis lesion in a patient with X-linked juvenile retinoschisis.

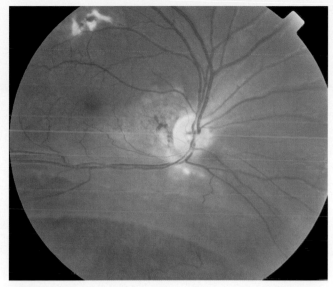

Figure 17–18   Inferior schisis cavity with large internal break in a patient with X-linked juvenile retinoschisis. Two scars are present; one at the inferior edge of the optic nerve head and another along the superotemporal arcade.

SUGGESTED READINGS

Michaelides M, Hunt DM, Moore AT. The genetics of inherited macular dystrophies. J Med Genet. 2003;40:641–650.

Sieving PA. Diagnostic issues with inherited retinal and macular dystrophies. Semin Ophthalmol. 1995;10:279–294.

Tantri A, Vrabec TR, Cu-Unjieng A, Frost A, Annesley WH Jr, Donoso LA. X-linked retinoschisis: a clinical and molecular genetic review. Surv Ophthalmol. 2004;49:214–230.

Chapter 18

Cystoid Macular Edema

GLENN J. JAFFE, MD • MARK T. CAHILL, FRCSI (OPHTH), FRCO

18.1 Introduction

Cystoid macular edema (CME), a common end-point for a wide variety of ocular diseases, is characterized by accumulation of fluid in the extracellular space of the retina, particularly in the macula, with subsequent thickening of the parafoveal retina (**Figure 18–1**). This fluid accumulation is a consequence of disruption of the blood-retinal barrier, which normally restricts movement of plasma constituents into the retina. Any disease that disrupts the blood-retinal barrier can cause CME, including vasculopathies such as diabetes mellitus, retinal vascular occlusions, hypertensive retinopathy, choroidal neovascularization, vascular malformations and tumors, and radiation retinopathy. Intraocular inflammation such as that seen in uveitis or after intraocular surgery can also produce CME, can direct traction on macular vessels resulting from vitreoretinal interface abnormalities. Hereditary retinal degenerations can result in CME just as some chemicals including epinephrine, betaxolol, and latanoprost can also cause CME.

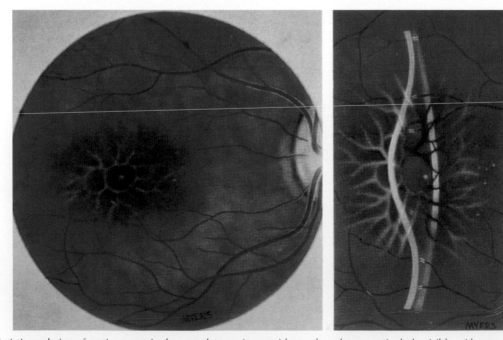

Figure 18–1   Artist's rendering of cystic spaces in the macula seen in cystoid macular edema, particularly visible with retro illumination using a narrow beam of light. (From Gass JD, Norton EW: Cystoid macular edema and papilledema following cataract extraction: A fluorescein fundoscopic and angiographic study. Arch Ophthalmol. 1966;77:647.)

18.2 Clinical Signs and Symptoms

The main symptom of CME is visual loss and in some cases metamorphopsia, although patients may have other symptoms attributable to the etiologic diseases. For example, a patient with uveitis may have floaters associated with the visual loss, whereas a patient with retinal degeneration could have concurrent nyctalopia and visual field restriction. Eliciting a history of previous intraocular surgery, medications, family history, and details of underlying systemic illness that are known to cause CME is also important.

CME is typically associated with reduced visual acuity. Other clinical signs may indicate the etiologic disease such as a recent cataract wound, vitreous in a surgical wound or a peaked pupil, a ruptured posterior capsule, or anterior chamber lens. There may be evidence of intraocular inflammation including keratitic precipitates, anterior chamber cells and flare, posterior synechiae, and iris nodules. Biomicroscopic examination of the macula with a contact lens and retroillumination may allow visualization of the retinal cysts (**Figure 18–2**). Ophthalmoscopy may also show other signs of possible etiologic diseases such as vitreous opacities in uveitis, vitreomacular traction, vascular abnormalities, vascular tumors, or evidence of retinal degeneration.

18.3 Imaging and Diagnostic Tests

18.3.1 FLUORESCEIN ANGIOGRAPHY

Fluorescein angiography can demonstrate the breakdown of the blood-retinal barrier. Normally, there is no leakage of fluorescein into the retina. In CME, sources of

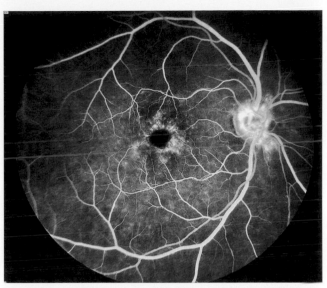

Figure 18–3   Mid phase fluorescein angiogram of the patient in **Figure 18–2** showing punctate hyperfluorescence at fovea with some associated hyperfluorescence of the optic disc. (Courtesy of Dr. Travis Meredith.)

leakage may be seen as early hyperfluorescence, which increases during the middle phase of the angiogram (**Figure 18–3**). The more typical appearance of CME is petaloid hyperfluorescence seen at the fovea in late frames of the angiogram (**Figure 18–4**). This is a result of the accumulation of fluorescein in the cystic retinal spaces. CME is also associated with late staining of the optic disc that is seen as disc hyperfluorescence (**Figure 18–4**). Fluorescein angiography may also define the underlying disease causing the CME (**Figures 18–5** to **18–7**) and may be used to monitor progression of treatments (**Figure 18–8**).

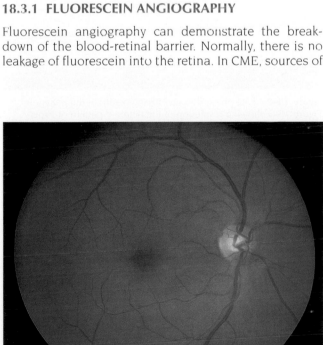

Figure 18–2   Color fundus photograph showing yellowish discoloration of macula associated with cystoid macular edema. (Courtesy of Dr. Travis Meredith.)

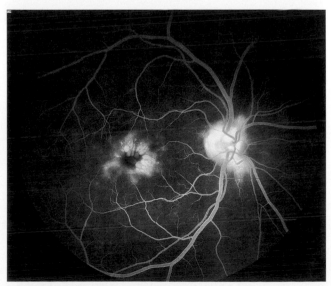

Figure 18–4   Late-phase fluorescein angiogram of the patient in **Figure 18–2** showing foveal hyperfluorescence in a petaloid pattern. The previously noted optic disc hyperfluorescence has also increased. (Courtesy of Dr. Travis Meredith.)

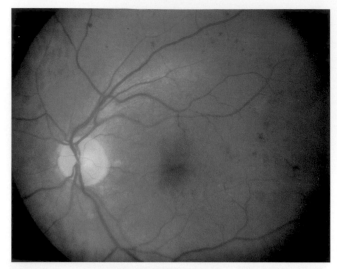

Figure 18–5 Color fundus photograph showing clinical signs of nonproliferative diabetic retinopathy with associated yellowish discoloration of the macula due to CME.

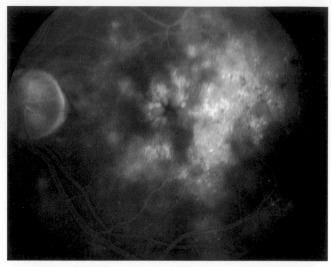

Figure 18–7 Late-phase fluorescein angiogram of the patient in **Figure 18–5** showing a petaloid pattern of foveal hyperfluorescence due to CME. More diffuse hyperfluorescence caused by leakage from microaneurysms is also seen.

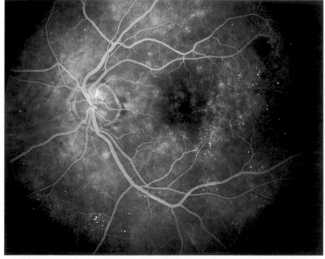

Figure 18–6 Mid-phase fluorescein angiogram of the patient in **Figure 18–5** showing punctate hyperfluorescence caused by numerous microaneurysms. There is also some mild punctate hyperfluorescence at the fovea due to CME.

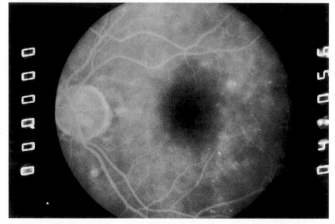

Figure 18–8 Late-phase fluorescein angiogram of the patient in **Figure 18–5** showing resolution of the petaloid pattern of hyperfluorescence as well as the more diffuse pattern of hyperfluorescence after an intravitreal injection of triamcinolone acetonide.

18.3.2 INDOCYANINE GREEN ANGIOGRAPHY

Indocyanine green angiography is not useful in the diagnosis or management of CME.

18.3.3 OPTICAL COHERENCE TOMOGRAPHY

Optical coherence tomography (OCT) can demonstrate retinal thickening that may not be evident on fluorescein angiography (**Figures 18–9** to **18–13**). Different patterns of CME can be distinguished using OCT including intra-retinal cysts only (**Figure 18–14**) or intraretinal cysts with associated with subretinal fluid (**Figure 18–15**). OCT can also demonstrate abnormalities of the vitreoretinal interface that may result in CME, including epiretinal membrane and vitreomacular traction (**Figure 18–16**).

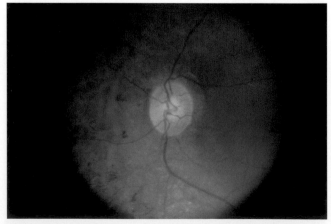

Figure 18–9 Color fundus photograph showing clinical signs of retinitis pigmentosa including retinal pigment clumping, attenuation of retinal vessels, and waxy pallor of the optic disc. A yellowish discoloration of the macula due to CME can also be seen.

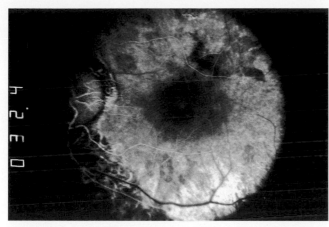

Figure 18–10 Early-phase fluorescein angiogram of the patient in **Figure 18–9** showing very mild punctate hyperfluorescence at the fovea.

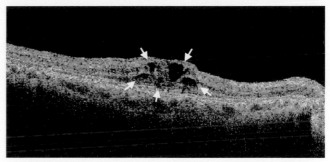

Figure 18–13 OCT image of the same eye as in **Figures 18–8 to 18–12** showing hyporeflective cystic spaces in the retina consistent with CME (*arrows*).

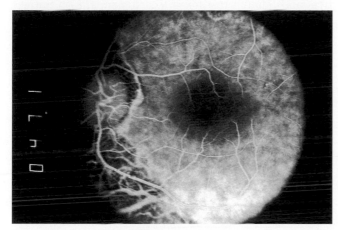

Figure 18–11 Mid-phase fluorescein angiogram of the patient in **Figure 18–9** showing no change in the amount of foveal hyperfluorescence seen in **Figure 18–9.** There is also no hyperfluorescence of the optic disc.

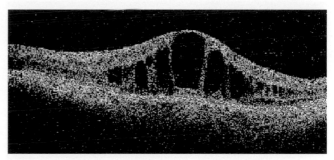

Figure 18–14 OCT image showing cystic retinal changes due to macular edema with intraretinal cysts only.

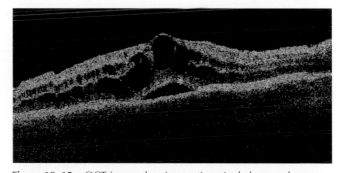

Figure 18–15 OCT image showing cystic retinal changes due to macular edema with intraretinal cysts and subretinal fluid.

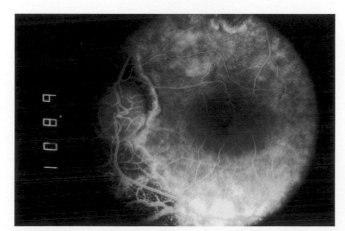

Figure 18–12 Late-phase fluorescein angiogram of the patient in **Figure 18–9** showing no change in the amount of foveal hyperfluorescence seen in the previous two figures.

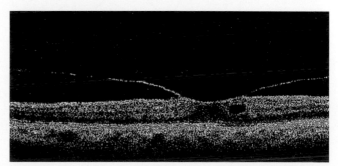

Figure 18–16 OCT image showing CME due to vitreomacular traction.

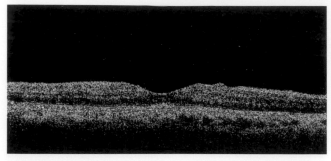

Figure 18–17 OCT image showing resolution of CME after pars plana vitrectomy to relieve the vitreomacular traction seen in **Figure 18–16.**

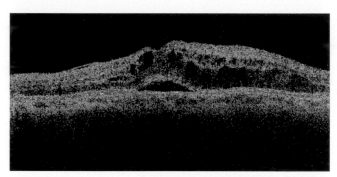

Figure 18–18 OCT image of an eye with nonproliferative diabetic retinopathy and CME seen in **Figures 18–5 to 18–8**, showing intraretinal cysts and subretinal fluid.

Serial OCT images, particularly volumetric OCT images that allow objective measurement of central retinal thickening, can demonstrate regression of CME after treatment (**Figures 18–17** to **18–21**).

18.3.4 RETINAL THICKNESS ANALYSIS

Retinal thickness analysis (RTA) can also demonstrate retinal thickening associated with CME and allows construction of three-dimensional retinal images (**Figures 18–22** to **18–24**). A recent study has demonstrated that there is excellent agreement between RTA and OCT measurements of foveal thickness. However, it was also demonstrated that media opacities created less interference for OCT than for RTA.

18.3.5 ULTRASONOGRAPHY

Ultrasonography has the advantage of reliably imaging the posterior segment regardless of ocular media opacities, and reliable testing is less dependent on patient cooperation than other techniques. Both A-scan and B-scan ultrasonography have been used to detect macular thickening (**Figure 18–25**). Macular thickening determined with B-scan ultrasonography correlates with findings on slit lamp examination, fluorescein angiography, and OCT (**Figures 18–26** to **18–31**). However, ultrasonography has lower resolution than OCT and does not give precise, qualitative retinal thickness measurements.

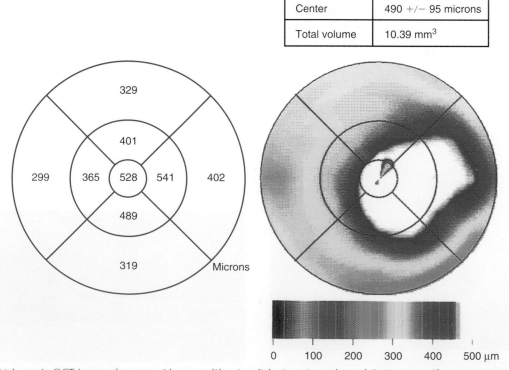

Center	490 +/− 95 microns
Total volume	10.39 mm³

Figure 18–19 Volumetric OCT image of an eye with nonproliferative diabetic retinopathy and CME seen in **Figures 18–5 to 18–8**, showing increased central retinal thickness measurements.

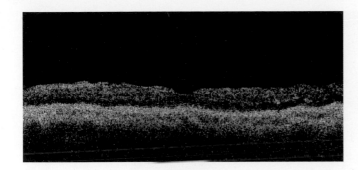

Figure 18–20   OCT image of an eye with nonproliferative diabetic retinopathy and CME seen in **Figures 18–5 to 18–8** after treatment with intravitreal triamcinolone, showing resolution of intraretinal cysts and subretinal fluid.

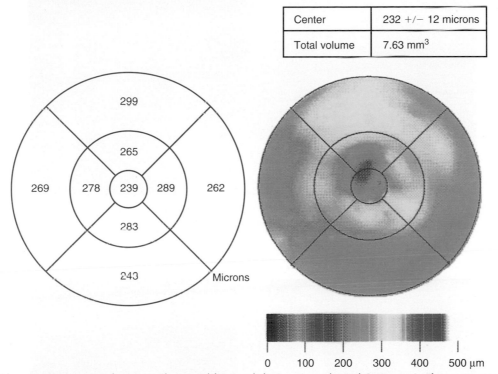

Center	232 +/− 12 microns
Total volume	7.63 mm³

Figure 18–21   Volumetric OCT image of an eye with nonproliferative diabetic retinopathy and CME seen in **Figures 18–5 to 18–8**, showing a reduction in central retinal thickness.

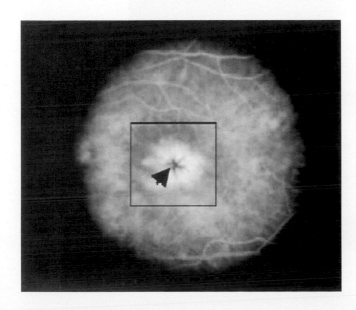

Figure 18–22   Late-phase fluorescein angiogram showing a petaloid pattern of foveal hyperfluorescence due to CME. (From Polito A, Shah SM, Haller JA, et al. Comparison between retinal thickness analyzer and optical coherence tomography for assessment of foveal thickness in eyes with macular disease. Am J Ophthalmol. 2002;134:240–251.)

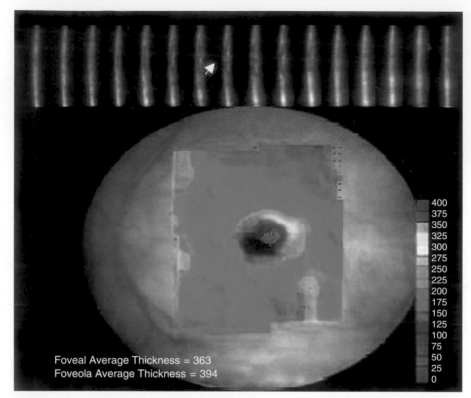

Foveal Average Thickness = 363
Foveola Average Thickness = 394

Figure 18–23   *Top:* A composite of retinal thickness analyzer optical images shows clear elevation and large cystoid spaces across the foveal center (*arrow*). *Bottom:* Retinal thickness analyzer two-dimensional map shows degree and size of the thickened area. (From Polito A, Shah SM, Haller JA, et al. Comparison between retinal thickness analyzer and optical coherence tomography for assessment of foveal thickness in eyes with macular disease. Am J Ophthalmol. 2002;134:240–251.)

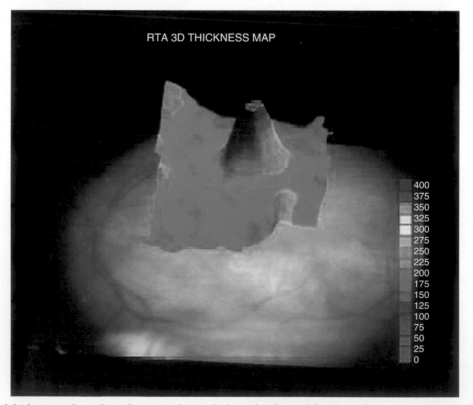

Figure 18–24   Retinal thickness analyzer three-dimensional map discloses the shape of the elevated area. (From Polito A, Shah SM, Haller JA, et al. Comparison between retinal thickness analyzer and optical coherence tomography for assessment of foveal thickness in eyes with macular disease. Am J Ophthalmol. 2002;134:240–251.)

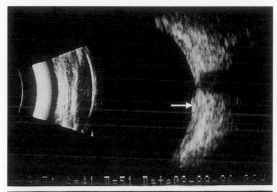

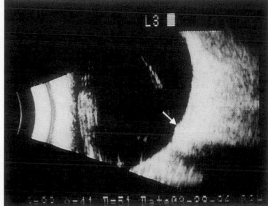

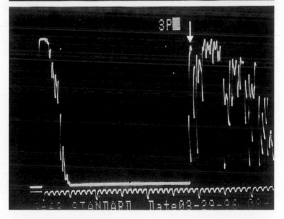

Figure 18–25 Ultrasound images of the eye. *Top:* Horizontal axial B-scan showing mild macular thickening (*arrow*). *Middle:* Longitudinal B-scan showing mild macular edema (*arrow*). *Bottom:* A-scan with the sound directed toward the macula (*arrow*) showing slight thickening. (From DiBernardo C, Schachat A, Fekrat S. Ophthalmic Ultrasound: A Diagnostic Atlas. New York, NY: Thieme, 1988. Reprinted by permission.)

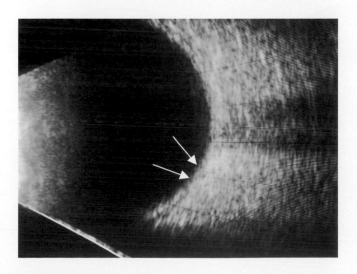

Figure 18–26 B-scan ultrasound of the eye showing a normal macula (*arrows*) (grade 0 thickening). (From Lai JC, Stinnett SS, Jaffe GJ. B-scan ultrasonography for the detection of macular thickening. Am J Ophthalmol. 2003;136:55–61.)

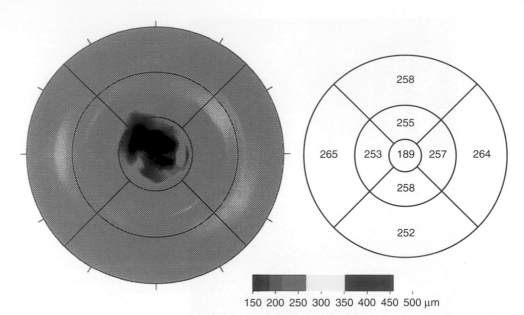

Figure 18–27 Volumetric OCT image of same eye as in **Figure 18–26**, showing no macular thickening. Brighter colors (*red to white*) correspond to areas of increased retinal thickness; dimmer colors (*blue to black*) correspond to areas of decreased retinal thickness. (From Lai JC, Stinnett SS, Jaffe GJ. B-scan ultrasonography for the detection of macular thickening. Am J Ophthalmol. 2003;136:55–61.)

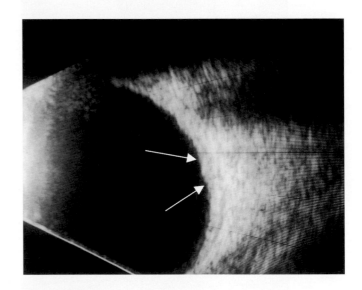

Figure 18–28 B-scan ultrasound of the eye showing subtle macular thickening (*arrows*) (Grade 1 thickening). (From Lai JC, Stinnett SS, Jaffe GJ. B-scan ultrasonography for the detection of macular thickening. Am J Ophthalmol. 2003;136:55–61).

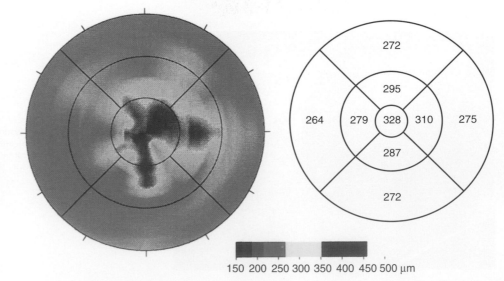

Figure 18–29 Volumetric OCT of the same eye as in **Figure 18–28**, showing moderate macular thickening. (From Lai JC, Stinnett SS, Jaffe GJ. B-scan ultrasonography for the detection of macular thickening. Am J Ophthalmol. 2003;136:55–61.)

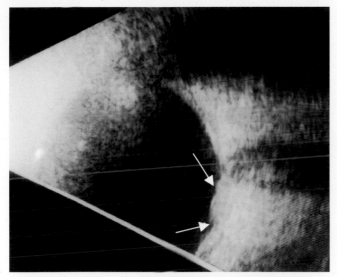

Figure 18–30 B-scan ultrasound of the eye showing prominent macular thickening (*arrows*) (Grade 2 thickening). (From Lai JC, Stinnett SS, Jaffe GJ. B-scan ultrasonography for the detection of macular thickening. Am J Ophthalmol. 2003;136:55–61.)

18.3.6 MICROPERIMETRY

Microperimetry allows simultaneous visualization of the fundus and measurement of retinal function by assessing retinal sensitivity to a light stimulus (**Figures 18–32** to **18–35**). This ability to correlate reduced retinal function with retinal structure abnormalities is an advantage that other tests of central retinal function do not have. A previous study demonstrated that microperimetry can map areas of reduced retinal function that correspond to areas of macular edema.

18.4 Pathology

There are contrasting reports regarding the pathologic changes seen in CME. Light microscopy demonstrates accumulation of eosinophilic material in the outer plexiform and inner nuclear layers of the retina with cyst formation that has been attributed to fluid accumulation in the retinal extracellular space (**Figure 18–36**). The fluid accumulation is a result of a breakdown in the

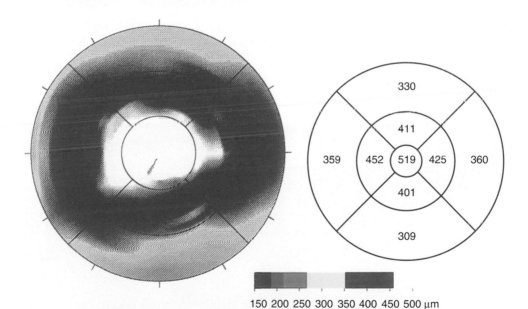

150 200 250 300 350 400 450 500 µm

Figure 18–31 Volumetric OCT image of the same eye as in **Figure 18–30**, showing marked macular thickening. (From Lai JC, Stinnett SS, Jaffe GJ. B-scan ultrasonography for the detection of macular thickening. Am J Ophthalmol. 2003;136:55–61.)

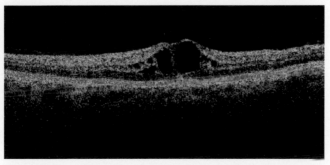

Figure 18–32 OCT image of an eye with CME showing prominent intraretinal cysts.

Center	396 +/− 7 microns
Total volume	8.08 mm³

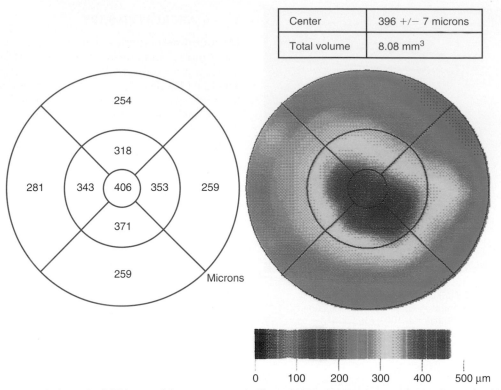

Figure 18–33   Volumetric OCT image of the same eye as in **Figure 18–32**, showing increased central macular thickness.

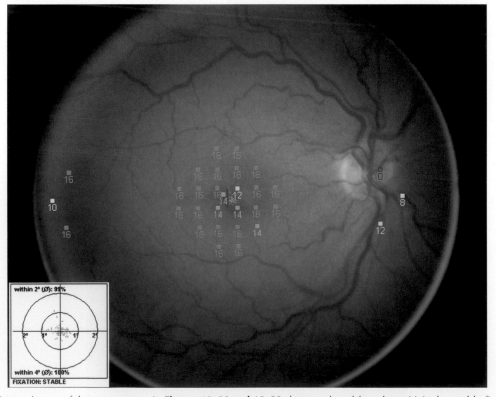

Figure 18–34   Microperimetry of the same eye as in **Figures 18–32 and 18–33** shows reduced foveal sensitivity but stable fixation (*inset*). Zero signifies the highest-intensity stimulus and 16 the lowest, using a Goldmann III equivalent target and 4-2 threshold testing strategy. An *open square* equals no response; a *filled square* equals a response to a stimulus.

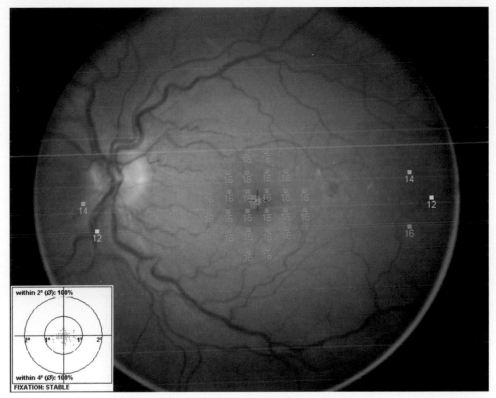

Figure 18–35   Microperimetry of the patient's other eye using the same test strategy as in **Figure 18–34,** showing good foveal sensitivity and stable fixation.

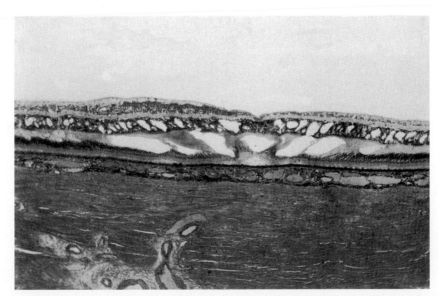

Figure 18–36   Photomicrograph of histology specimen using light microscopy and hematoxylin and eosin stain, showing accumulation of amorphous material in the outer plexiform and inner nuclear layer of the retina with cyst formation.

blood-retinal barrier that has an inner and an outer component. The inner blood-retinal barrier consists of the tight junctions between the endothelial cells of the retinal blood vessels, whereas the outer blood-retinal barrier comprises tight junctions between retinal pigment epithelial cells. Enlargement of the cysts may result in lamellar or full-thickness retinal defects. Other studies have demonstrated that CME is a result of swelling and degeneration of Müller cells without expansion of the extracellular space, which may explain why CME is seen in association with ischemic conditions of the eye. However, it may also be that CME is a clinical finding that results from a number of pathologic processes.

SUGGESTED READINGS

Dick JS, Jampol LM, Haller JA. Macular edema. In: Ryan SJ, Schachat AP, eds. Retina. St Louis, Mo: Mosby, 2001:967–981.

Lai JC, Stinnett SS, Jaffe GJ. B-scan ultrasonography for the detection of macular thickening. Am J Ophthalmol. 2003;136:55–61.

Polito A, Shah SM, Haller JA, et al. Comparison between retinal thickness analyzer and optical coherence tomography for assessment of foveal thickness in eyes with macular disease. Am J Ophthalmol. 2002;134:240–251.

Rohrschneider K, Bultmann S, Gluck R, Kruse FE, Fendrich T, Volcker HE. Scanning laser ophthalmoscope fundus perimetry before and after laser photocoagulation for clinically significant diabetic macular edema. Am J Ophthalmol. 2000;129:27–32.

Chapter 19

Angioid Streaks

ALAIN GAUDRIC, MD • S. YVES COHEN, MD, PhD

19.1 Introduction

Angioid streaks are irregular linear ruptures of Bruch's membrane that mostly occur in patients with pseudoxanthoma elasticum (PXE), of which they may be the only sign for many years (**Figure 19–1**). PXE is an autosomic recessive inherited disease, which mainly affects the skin, blood vessels, and eyes and which is due to a mutation of the ABCC6 gene located on chromosome 16p 13-1. Autosomic dominant transmission has also been reported rarely. Angioid streaks may occur, although rarely, in other diseases such as Paget's disease, sickle cell disease, β-thalassemia, and Ehlers-Danlos syndrome. Their association with many other diseases has also occasionally been reported.

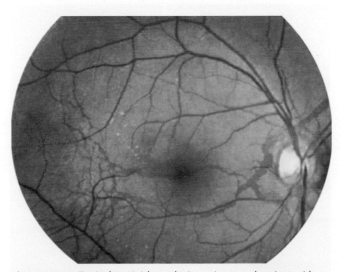

Figure 19–1 Typical angioid streaks in a pigmented patient with PXE. The streaks form a ring around the optic disc, cross the macula, and form a network temporal to the macula. Some drusen-like deposits are present in the posterior pole.

19.2 Clinical Signs and Symptoms

Angioid streaks remain asymptomatic for a long time. Vision disturbance may occur if a streak opens under the macula, resulting in small subretinal hemorrhages, blurred vision, and metamorphopsia, which may resolve spontaneously. More often, however, vision loss is due to macular choroidal neovascularization, which proliferates in the subretinal space through angioid streaks, especially those close to the macula.

On the fundus examination angioid streaks appear as slightly dark lines, radiating from the disc to the mid-periphery, irregular in direction and width, and tapering at their distal end (**Figure 19–1**). Some of them frequently cross the posterior pole and macula. These streaks are often connected to one or several rings of circumpapillary streaks (**Figure 19–2**). They may appear in childhood and progress with time. They tend to widen and lengthen, and in older patients they may merge with the atrophy of the retinal pigment epithelium of the posterior pole, which makes diagnosis harder (**Figure 19–3**).

In PXE, angioid streaks may be associated with several other anomalies of the fundus, including the following:

- A "peau d'orange" appearance, which is a pigmentary change of the fundus characterized by subretinal yellowish small punctuate deposits, mainly temporal to the posterior pole and in the mid-periphery (**Figure 19–4**). This feature is more marked in young patients and may precede the occurrence of angioid streaks.

- Small round subretinal depigmented dots, known as crystalline spots, also frequently seen in the mid-periphery, especially in angioid streaks associated with PXE. They may be combined with a depigmented "comet tail" (**Figure 19–5A**).

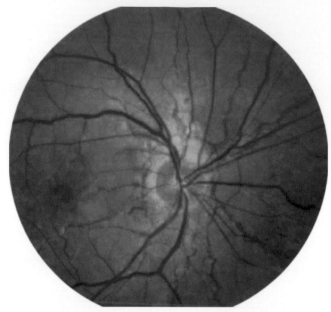

Figure 19–2 Peripapillary ring and radial angioid streaks.

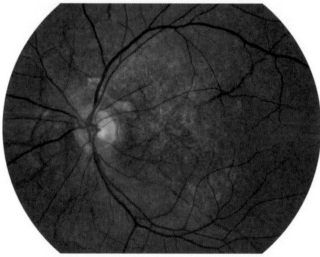

Figure 19–3 In this patient with PXE, long-standing angioid streaks have disappeared into the retinal pigment epithelium atrophy of the posterior pole.

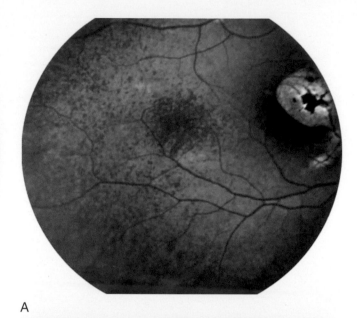

A

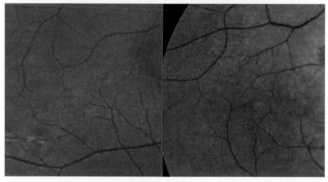

B

Figure 19–4 *A:* Peau d'orange in the temporal part of the posterior pole, associated with angioid streaks and an atrophic scar in the macula. *B:* Two other examples of more subtle peau d'orange.

- Other peripheral round atrophic scars of the retinal pigment epithelium known as "salmon spots" (**Figure 19–5B**).
- Drusen of the optic disc, which may be associated with angioid streaks in PXE (**Figure 19–6**).
- Drusen-like deposits at the posterior pole and pigmentary pattern dystrophy, which may also occur bilaterally. The dystrophy is more clearly visible on fluorescein angiography.

Different kinds of complications may occur:

- Small subretinal hemorrhages may occur during the opening of new streaks and are not due to choroidal neovascularization. Extensive subretinal

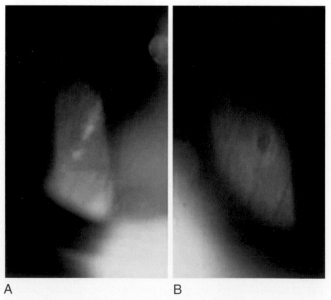

A   B

Figure 19–5 Peripheral anomalies, seen in a three-mirror lens. *A:* Crystalline body with comet tail; *B:* Salmon spot. (Courtesy of Dr. S. Y. Cohen.)

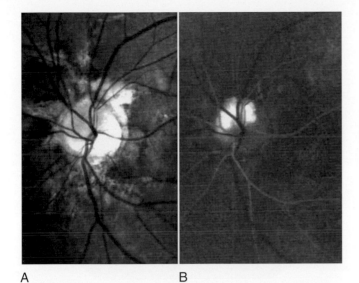

Figure 19–6 Drusen of the optic disc. *A:* On a red-free photograph, the superotemporal quadrant of the disc is elevated. Angioid streaks are present around the disc. *B:* On the very early phase of a fluorescein angiogram, the autofluorescence of the optic disc drusen is still visible.

hemorrhages sometimes occur along the angioid streaks after a minor trauma of the eye (**Figure 19–7A**).

- The most frequent and severe complication is choroidal neovascularization, the frequency of which increases with age. Most patients will have lost their central vision by their sixth decade due to choroidal neovascularization (**Figure 19–7B** and **C**).

- Progressive retinal pigment epithelium atrophy at the posterior pole and subretinal fibrosis are other possible evolutions (**Figure 19–3**).

19.3 Imaging and Diagnostic Tests

19.3.1 FLUORESCEIN ANGIOGRAPHY

Fluorescein angiography is not necessary for the diagnosis of angioid streaks but is useful to detect early choroidal neovascularization. When fluorescein angiography is performed, angioid streaks are usually hyperfluorescent on the early phases of the angiogram, and hyperfluorescence persists on the late phase, with some degree of staining, making the streaks more clearly

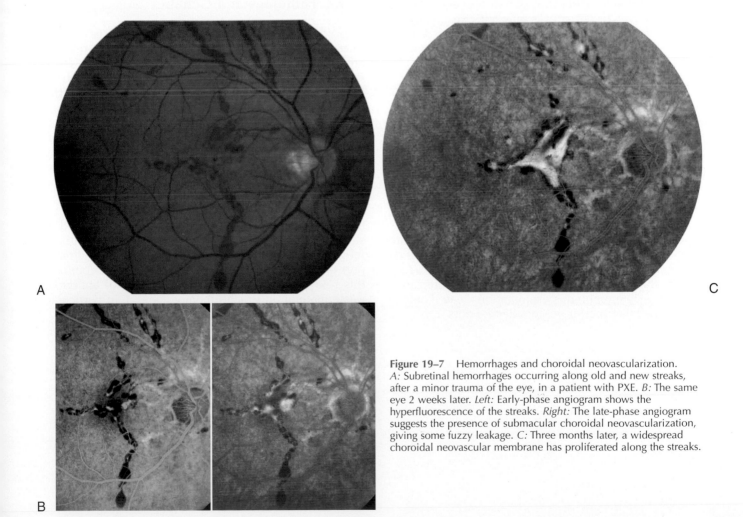

Figure 19–7 Hemorrhages and choroidal neovascularization. *A:* Subretinal hemorrhages occurring along old and new streaks, after a minor trauma of the eye, in a patient with PXE. *B:* The same eye 2 weeks later. *Left:* Early-phase angiogram shows the hyperfluorescence of the streaks. *Right:* The late-phase angiogram suggests the presence of submacular choroidal neovascularization, giving some fuzzy leakage. *C:* Three months later, a widespread choroidal neovascular membrane has proliferated along the streaks.

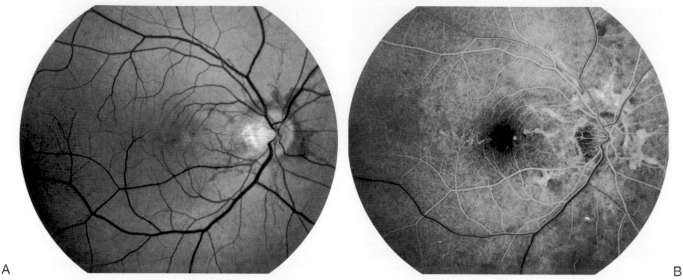

A   B

Figure 19–8   Angioid streaks around the disc and across the macula in the right eye of a 52-year-old man with PXE (fluorescein angiography). *A:* Red-free photograph shows an angioid streak crossing the macula and the "peau d'orange" temporal to the macula. *B:* On the early phase of a fluorescein angiogram, all the angioid streaks are hyperfluorescent, although their fluorescence is discontinuous in the macula.

visible. The contour of the streaks is sharply delineated, but their fluorescence may not be homogeneous (**Figure 19–8**). However, recent streaks may not give any abnormal fluorescence and remain more visible on fundus examination than on fluorescein angiography (**Figure 19–9A** and **B**). There is no leakage, unless choroidal neovascularization have started to proliferate, giving a focal fuzzy hyperfluorescence that masks the contours of the streak (**Figure 19–7B**). In other patients, early occult neovascularization may not be seen on fluorescein angiography.

19.3.2 INDOCYANINE GREEN ANGIOGRAPHY

Indocyanine green angiography is not a routine examination for angioid streaks but can be used to detect any occult choroidal neovascularization. Typically, angioid streaks appear hyperfluorescent on the late phase of the angiogram and are more clearly visible than on funduscopy or fluorescein angiography. However, some of them may be hypofluorescent or undetectable, although visible on fundus examination. Peau d'orange also appears as hyperfluorescent flecked dots.

19.4 Pathology and Genetics

Angioid streaks (**Figure 19–10**) are ruptures in the thickened and calcified Bruch's membrane, features that are similar to those noted in the skin in PXE. Once Bruch's membrane is ruptured, the overlying retinal pigment epithelium and photoreceptors, as well as the underlying choriocapillaris, evolve to progressive atrophy. Choroidal neovascularization may proliferate and obtain access to the subretinal space, through the streaks, especially in the macular region. In Paget's disease, calcification of Bruch's membrane is particularly extensive, whereas in sickle cell disease, Bruch's membrane thickening may be due to iron-calcium deposition.

The mechanisms by which calcification of the elastic fibers of Bruch's membrane occurs are not well understood. The PXE gene, ABCC6, is expressed in neuronal retinal cells and is assumed to play a role in the transport of organic anions in the retina. Failure to perform this role might lead to the accumulation of abnormal waste material in Bruch's membrane and, in particular, affect its elasticity.

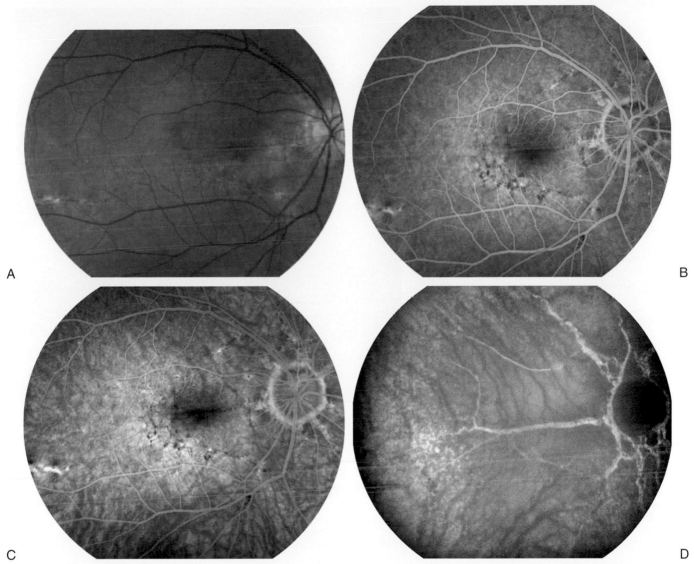

Figure 19–9   Angioid streaks in a 48-year-old woman with PXE (fluorescein and indocyanine green angiography). *A:* Angioid streak runs across the macula. Another streak inferotemporal to the macula has no connection with the disc. Subretinal reticular pigmentation is present inferior to the macula. A subtle "peau d'orange" is also visible temporally (see detail in **Figure 19–B,** *left*). *B:* Early-phase fluorescein angiogram shows irregular hyperfluorescence of the streaks: the macular streak remains hypofluorescent whereas the streaks around the disc and inferotemporal to the macula are hyperfluorescent. Note the presence of reticular retinal pigment epithelium dystrophy in the macula. *C:* On the late phase of the angiogram, the macular streak is still hypofluorescent. *D:* On the late phase of an indocyanine green angiogram, angioid streaks are much more visible than on funduscopy or on fluorescein angiography, but the temporal streak is hypofluorescent. Note the fluorescence of the "peau d'orange" temporal to the macula.

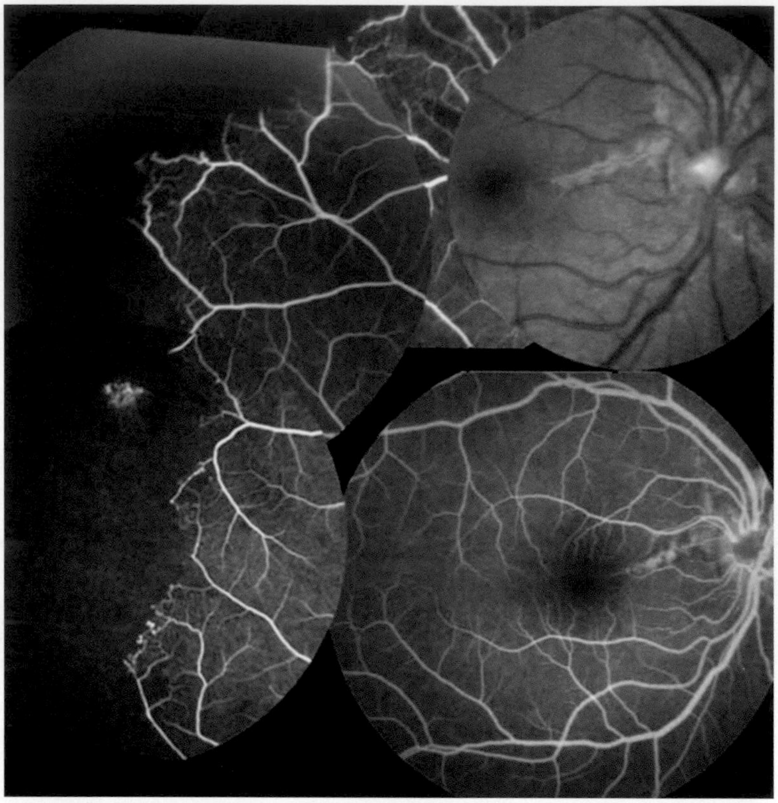

Figure 19–10 Angioid streaks in sickle cell disease. Angioid streaks around the disc in the right eye of a 42-year-old woman with double heterozygous SC sickle cell disease. Fluorescein angiography montage, showing angioid streaks and peripheral ischemia.

SUGGESTED READINGS

Clarkson JG. Paget's disease and angioid streaks: one complication less? Br J Ophthalmol. 1991;75:511.

Gass JDM: Angioid streaks and associated diseases. In: Stereoscopic Atlas of Macular Diseases. St Louis, Mo: Mosby, 1999:118–125.

Hu X, Plomp AS, van Soest S, Wijnholds J, de Jong PT, Bergen AA. Pseudoxanthoma elasticum: A clinical, histopathological, and molecular update. Surv Ophthalmol. 2003;48:424–438.

Mansour AM, Annesley WH. Comet-tailed drusen of the retinal pigment epithelium in angioid streaks. Eye. 1998;12:943–944.

Quaranta M, Cohen SY, Krott R, Sterkers M, Soubrane G, Coscas GJ. Indocyanine green videoangiography of angioid streaks. Am J Ophthalmol. 1995;119:136–142.

Chapter 20

Chorioretinal Folds

ALAIN GAUDRIC, MD • ALI ERGINAY, MD

20.1 Introduction

Chorioretinal folds are usually a benign asymptomatic condition associated with hyperopia but may also be associated with various ocular and systemic diseases. The term *chorioretinal fold* refers to a situation in which the retinal pigment epithelium (RPE), Bruch's membrane, and choriocapillaris are pleated, forming parallel folds, running mostly in the temporal part of the fundus. Other arrangements are possible, depending on the etiology of the folds.

Idiopathic chorioretinal folds are usually bilateral and symmetrical and typically exhibit an oblique orientation in the temporal quadrants of the fundus. Orbital masses and inflammation may also result in chorioretinal folds, although they are not usually the main feature in these diseases. In such cases, the folds are unilateral, especially in orbital tumors, but may involve both eyes in bilateral inflammatory diseases of the orbit.

20.2 Clinical Signs and Symptoms

Typical idiopathic chorioretinal folds are asymptomatic. They may be revealed by routine fundus examination for decreased vision due to the progression of hyperopia. In secondary chorioretinal folds, visual symptoms are not usually due to the folds themselves but to their cause (tumor, inflammation, or hypotony) or to their accidental association with another fundus disease.

On fundus examination, idiopathic chorioretinal folds are located in the temporal quadrants of the fundus, where they run in an oblique direction, from above the optic disc to the horizontal line, temporally. The folds are parallel, and their course is slightly curved. They may be more pronounced in the superior than in the inferior quadrant. The crest of the fold is pale and relatively broad, whereas the trough between two folds is narrow and darker (**Figures 20–1A** and **B**). In other eyes the folds may irradiate horizontally through the posterior pole (**Figure 20–2**).

The course of secondary chorioretinal folds may be less typical on fundus examination. For instance, their pattern may be determined by the location and shape of an extraocular tumor. They may also be associated with true superficial retinal folds and disc edema, which makes their diagnosis more difficult.

20.3 Imaging and Diagnostic Tests

20.3.1 FLUORESCEIN ANGIOGRAPHY

Fluorescein angiography is not essential for diagnosis but makes its easier, allows better appreciation of the pattern of the folds, and facilitates the detection of associated signs. It also allows differentiation between chorioretinal folds and pure retinal folds. On the early phase of the angiogram, the crest of the folds exhibits moderate hyperfluorescence, which persists on the late phase. The troughs between crests appear as dark lines between the folds, probably due to compression of the retinal pigment epithelium between two folds (**Figure 20–2C**).

Fluorescein angiography may also reveal features associated with chronic chorioretinal folds, including changes in the retinal pigment epithelium, which are frequent (**Figure 20–2C**), as well as focal leaks similar to those occurring in central serous choroidopathy and choroidal neovascularization, a rare complication of chorioretinal folds.

20.3.2 INDOCYANINE GREEN ANGIOGRAPHY

There is no need for indocyanine green angiography for the diagnosis of chorioretinal folds.

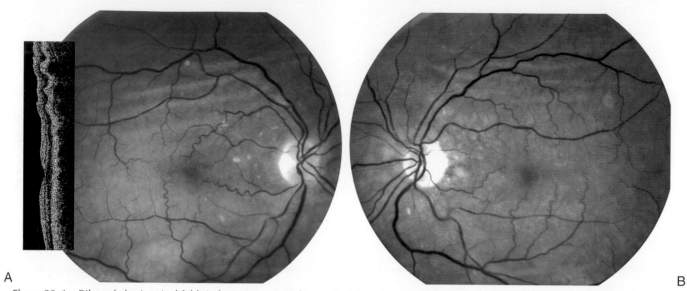

Figure 20–1 Bilateral chorioretinal folds in hyperopia. *A:* Right eye. Red-free photograph showing curved temporal chorioretinal folds with large pale crests. An 8-mm vertical OCT scan passing through the macula shows the folding of choriocapillaris and retinal pigment epithelium. This folding is attenuated at the retinal surface. *B:* Left eye. Chorioretinal folds symmetrical to those of the right eye.

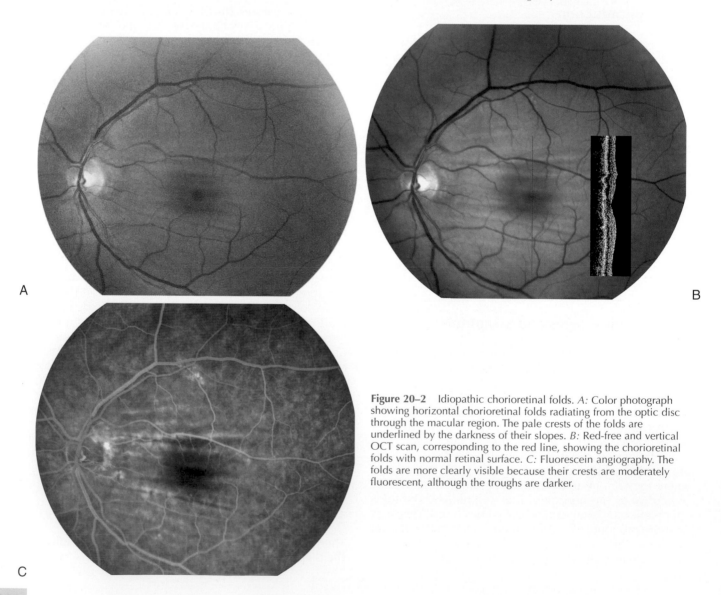

Figure 20–2 Idiopathic chorioretinal folds. *A:* Color photograph showing horizontal chorioretinal folds radiating from the optic disc through the macular region. The pale crests of the folds are underlined by the darkness of their slopes. *B:* Red-free and vertical OCT scan, corresponding to the red line, showing the chorioretinal folds with normal retinal surface. *C:* Fluorescein angiography. The folds are more clearly visible because their crests are moderately fluorescent, although the troughs are darker.

20.3.3 ULTRASOUND

The main reason for performing ultrasonography is to detect any inflammatory or tumoral cause of the chorioretinal folds. However, even eyes with idiopathic chorioretinal folds may exhibit abnormal features, including flattening of the posterior pole and sclerochoroidal thickening, as well as shortened axial length due to hyperopia.

20.3.4 OPTICAL COHERENCE TOMOGRAPHY

The usefulness of optical coherence tomography (OCT) is only anecdotal, but in some eyes, scans perpendicular to the direction of the chorioretinal folds show the hollows and bulges formed by the folds at the bright level of the RPE. This contrasts with normal pattern of the OCT on the retinal surface (**Figures 20–1, 20–2,** and **20–3**).

20.3.5 DIFFERENTIAL DIAGNOSIS

Fundus examination and imaging will allow differentiation between chorioretinal folds and retinal folds. Retinal folds due to the contraction of an epiretinal membrane are attracted by the foci of membrane contraction, clearly visible on blue filter fundus photographs (**Figure 20–4A**). Retinal folds due to shallow retinal detachment are thin and have a radial pattern centered on the macula (**Figure 20–6A**).

20.4 Causes

Although most chorioretinal folds are idiopathic and are only related to hyperopia, they may, in a few cases, be associated with various orbital and ocular diseases.

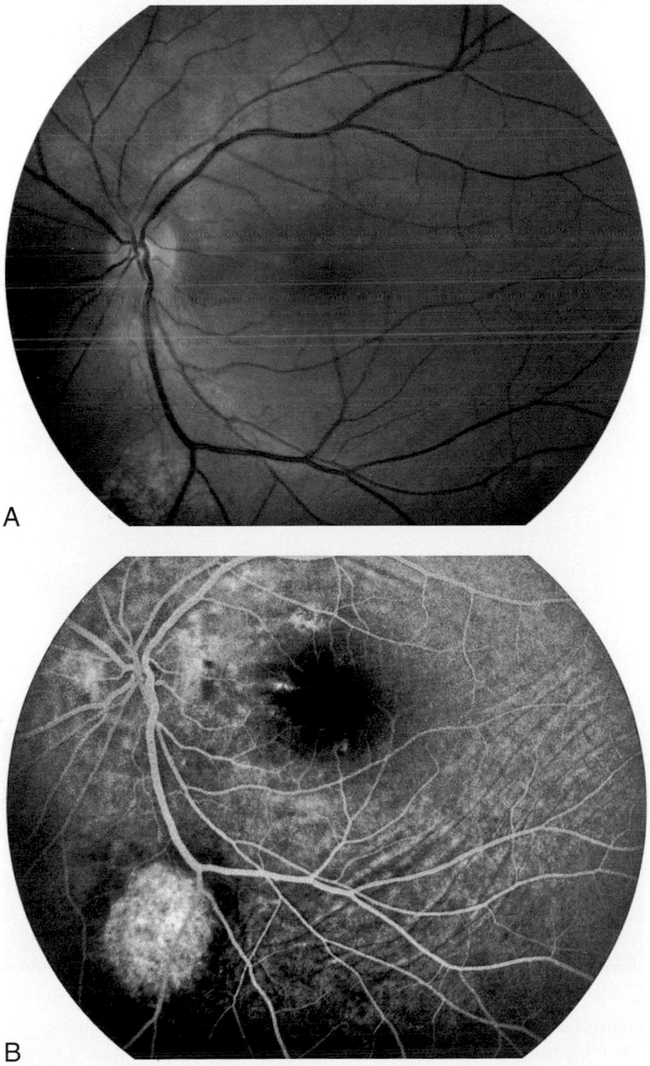

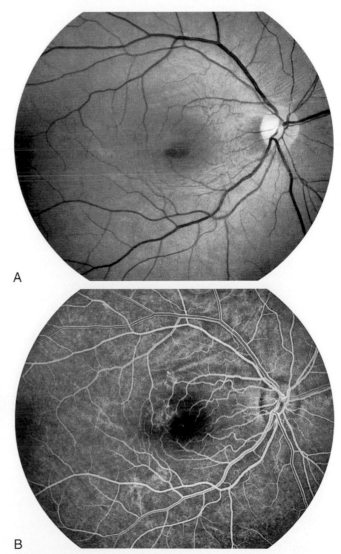

Figure 20–3 Chorioretinal folds and choroidal nevus. *A:* Thin chorioretinal folds, mainly visible inferotemporally. A choroidal nevus is present inferior to the disc. *B:* Fluorescein angiography. More chorioretinal folds are visible. Those near the disc are horizontal.

Figure 20–4 Inner retinal folds and retinochoroidal folds in an epiretinal membrane. *A:* Blue filter photograph showing retinal folds converging onto a contracted epiretinal membrane. *B:* Fluorescein angiography shows several slightly fluorescent chorioretinal folds, whereas the retinal folds are not visible.

20.4.1 HYPEROPIA

Idiopathic chorioretinal folds are often related to relative hyperopia and are mostly bilateral in this setting, although the second eye may be involved later. They have the typical oblique curved course and may be associated with some degree of retinal pigment epithelium disturbance (**Figure 20–1**).

20.4.2 ORBITAL COMPRESSION

Orbital tumors, orbital inflammation, or Grave's ophthalmopathy may be the cause of chorioretinal folds, which are unilateral or bilateral depending on the causative disease. Folds radiating from the disc are more likely to indicate an intraconal tumor (**Figure 20–5**), whereas extraconal tumors are supposed to yield concentric folds.

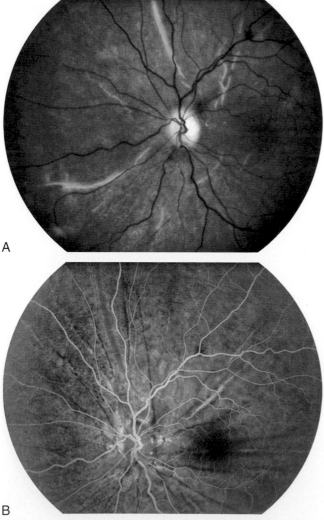

Figure 20–5 Chorioretinal folds and orbital lymphoma with choroidal infiltration. *A:* Red-free photograph. Full-thickness retinal folds around the disc. *B:* Fluorescein angiography. Retinal folds are not fluorescent. Numerous radial chorioretinal folds, dark or fluorescent, irradiate from the disc and are evocative of intraconal compression.

20.4.3 POSTERIOR SCLERITIS

The diagnosis of posterior scleritis is not easy and is based on a number of clues. It may be facilitated by the presence of chorioretinal folds on fluorescein angiography.

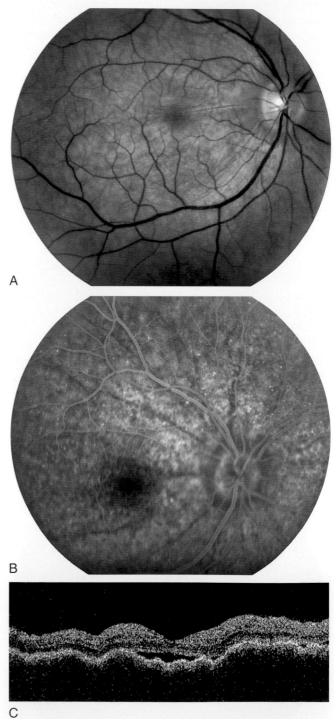

Figure 20–6 Harada's disease. *A:* Red-free photograph showing some superficial retinal folds converging onto the macula. *B:* Late-phase fluorescein angiogram shows diffuse subretinal leakage, numerous small bright spots, and several dark chorioretinal folds radiating from the disc, which are due to severe chorioretinal thickening. *C:* Vertical OCT scan through the macula shows shallow macular detachment and more choroidal folds than are visible on angiography.

20.4.4 CHOROIDAL INFLAMMATION

Diffuse choroidal inflammation, as is seen in Harada's or Whipple's disease, may induce chorioretinal folds, which are often pigmented, and are mainly visible on fluorescein angiography (**Figure 20–6**).

20.4.5 HYPOTONY

Chronic hypotony after filtration surgery or ocular blunt trauma causing an iridocyclodialysis cleft, may be the cause of marked chorioretinal folds. They often form square arrays and may be combined with optic disc swelling, retinal folds, and macular edema. There is no subretinal leakage on fluorescein angiography, but optic disc staining may be present (**Figure 20–7**).

20.4.6 OPTIC NERVE EDEMA

Many causes of optic disc edema may be associated with chorioretinal folds (**Figure 20–8**). The most typical is their association with the disc edema that occurs in pseudotumor cerebri. The association of chorioretinal folds and the pseudopapilledema of the "crowded disc" has also been described.

20.4.7 CHOROIDAL NEOVASCULAR MEMBRANES

Particular radial chorioretinal folds due to the retraction of a submacular neovascular choroidal membrane have been described in age-related macular degeneration (**Figure 20–9**).

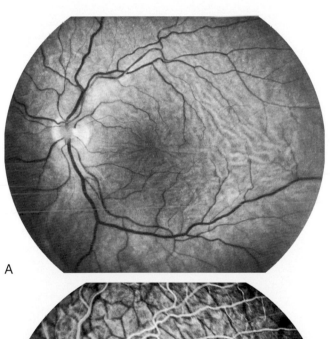
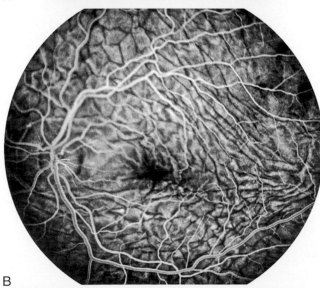

Figure 20–7 Chronic hypotony after traumatic iridocyclodialysis. *A:* Red-free photograph. Many choroidal folds are visible in the posterior pole. *B:* Fluorescein angiography shows numerous chorioretinal folds forming dark square arrays and occupying all of the posterior pole. (Courtesy of Dr. S. Y. Cohen.)

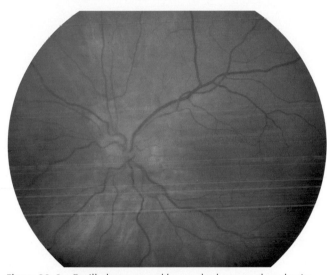

Figure 20–8 Papilledema caused by cerebral venous thrombosis: horizontal chorioretinal folds.

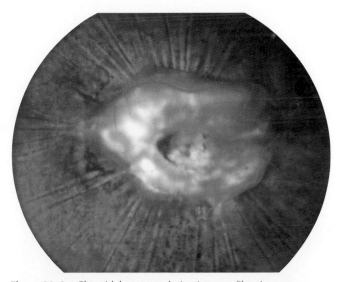

Figure 20–9 Choroidal neovascularization at a fibrotic stage, causing retraction of the choroid and radial choroidal folds. (Courtesy of Dr. S. Y. Cohen.)

SUGGESTED READINGS

Cassidy LM, Sanders MD. Choroidal folds and papilledema. Br J Ophthalmol. 1999;83:1139–1143.

Gass JDM. Chorioretinal folds. In: Stereoscopic Atlas of Macular Diseases. 4th ed. St Louis, Mo: Mosby:288–297.

Griebel SR, Kosmorsky GS. Choroidal folds associated with increased intracranial pressure. Am J Ophthalmol. 2000;129:513–516.

Kokame GT, de Leon MD, Tanji T. Serous retinal detachment and cystoid macular edema in hypotony maculopathy. Am J Ophthalmol. 2001;131:384–386.

Leahey AB, Brucker AJ, Wyszynski RE, Shaman P. Chorioretinal folds: A comparison of unilateral and bilateral cases. Arch Ophthalmol. 1993;111:357–359.

Sarraf D, Schwartz SD. Bilateral choroidal folds and optic neuropathy: A variant of the crowded disk syndrome? Ophthalmology. 2003;110:1047–1052.

Suner IJ, Greenfield DS, Miller MP, Nicolela MT, Palmberg PF. Hypotony maculopathy after filtering surgery with mitomycin C: Incidence and treatment. Ophthalmology. 1997;104:207–214; discussion 214–215.

Weissgold DJ, Brucker AJ. Chorioretinal and retinal folds. In: Guyer DR, Yannuzzi LA, et al., eds. Retina-Macula-Vitreous. Philadelphia, Pa: Saunders, 1999:256–263.

Retinal Vascular Diseases

Chapter 21

Diabetic Retinopathy

SOPHIE J. BAKRI, MD • PETER K. KAISER, MD

21.1 Introduction

Diabetic retinopathy is the leading cause of blindness in the United States in people aged 20 to 74 years. The risk of developing diabetic retinopathy depends on the duration and type of diabetes mellitus. In patients with type 1 diabetes of 15 years or greater duration, the risk is 98%, and in those with type 2 diabetes of 15 years or greater duration the risk is 78%.

Depending on the presence or absence of ocular neovascularization, diabetic retinopathy is classified into nonproliferative and proliferative forms. Nonproliferative diabetic retinopathy (NPDR) is characterized by abnormalities of the retinal vasculature, including microaneurysms, intraretinal hemorrhages, venous beading, cotton wool spots, hard exudates, capillary nonperfusion and macular edema. In addition to these signs, proliferative diabetic retinopathy (PDR) includes the presence of neovascularization of the optic nerve, retina, or iris.

21.2 Nonproliferative Diabetic Retinopathy

21.2.1 CLINICAL SIGNS AND SYMPTOMS

Microaneurysms

The first identifiable sign of diabetic retinopathy is the presence of microaneurysms. Microaneurysms are saccular outpouchings of the walls of the retinal capillaries and occur after loss of pericytes from the capillary wall. They appear clinically as tiny red dots, 15 to 60 microns in diameter, most often in the posterior pole (**Figure 21–1**), and are seen in the early phases of the fluorescein angiogram as pinpoint areas of hyperfluorescence (**Figure 21–2**) that leak in late views.

Intraretinal Hemorrhages

Intraretinal hemorrhages may take on variable appearances depending on their location within the retina. Flame-shaped hemorrhages are splinter-shaped because they occur in the retinal nerve fiber layer (**Figure 21–3**). "Dot and blot" hemorrhages are located deeper in the retina, in the outer plexiform layer (**Figures 21–2** and **21–4**). In contrast to microaneurysms, dot and blot hemorrhages appear larger and may also be located in the periphery as well as the posterior pole. On fluorescein angiography, microaneurysms hyperfluoresce, and dot and blot hemorrhages appear as areas of blocked fluorescence (**Figure 21–2**).

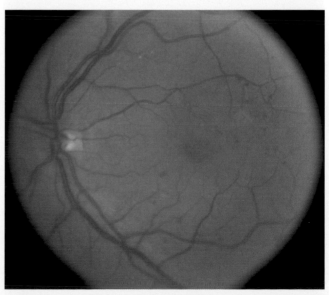

Figure 21–1 Color fundus photograph left eye (OS). Several microaneurysms can be seen in the posterior pole as small red dots.

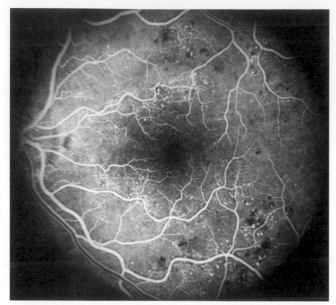

Figure 21–2 Early-phase fluorescein angiogram OS of the patient shown in Figure 21–1 shows microaneurysms as multiple pinpoint areas of hyperfluorescence. In addition, areas of blockage representing dot and blot hemorrhages are seen.

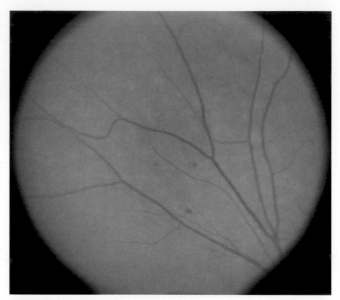

Figure 21–4 Color fundus photograph shows dot and blot hemorrhages in the superior fundus.

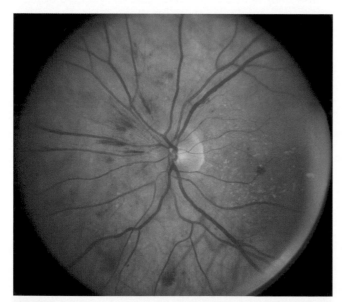

Figure 21–3 Color fundus photograph shows multiple flame-shaped nerve fiber layer hemorrhages radiating superonasally from the optic nerve. Hard exudates are present in the macula.

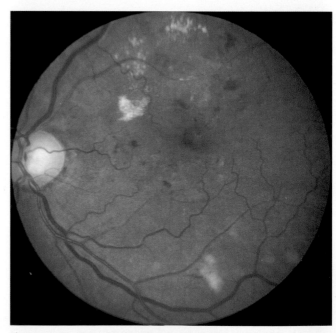

Figure 21–5 Color fundus photograph OS shows cotton wool spots seen as fluffy white areas in the inferotemporal macula. These are in contrast to the yellow hard exudates seen in the superior macula.

Cotton Wool Spots

Cotton wool spots appear clinically as fluffy white lesions usually located in the posterior pole (**Figure 21–5**). Pathologically, they are areas of nerve fiber infarction with axoplasmic stasis. Their presence is not a predictor of progression of diabetic retinopathy.

Capillary Nonperfusion

As pericytes are lost and microaneurysms form, capillary closure ensues, leading to the development of acellular capillaries. The terminal arterioles that supply these capillaries then become occluded, and subsequently the veins develop sausage-shaped dilated segments (venous beading). Areas of capillary nonperfusion appear clinically as a "featureless" retina and are seen angiographically as areas devoid of capillaries (**Figure 21–6**). Adjacent to areas of capillary nonperfusion, tortuous vessels are often found, which are referred to as *intraretinal microvascular abnormalities* (IRMAs) (**Figure 21–7**). There is some debate as to whether these represent dilated capillaries or whether they are areas of

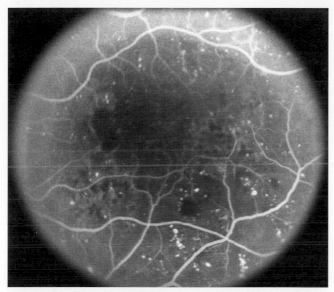

Figure 21–6 Fluorescein angiogram shows areas of hypoperfusion representing capillary nonperfusion and resulting macular ischemia.

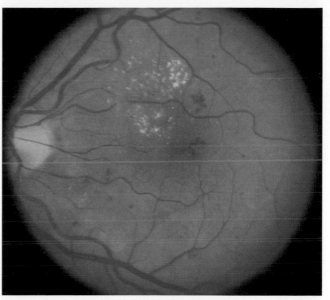

Figure 21–8 Color fundus photograph shows a cluster of hard exudates in the superior macula. Microaneurysms and dot and blot hemorrhages are seen scattered throughout the macula.

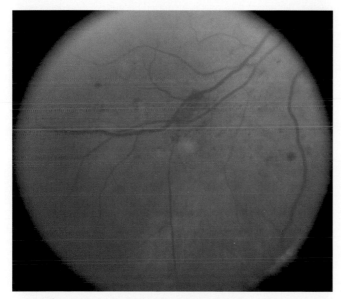

Figure 21–7 Color fundus photograph shows IRMAs.

retinal neovascularization that have not broken through the internal limiting membrane.

Diabetic Macular Edema

Macular edema is the most common cause of visual loss in patients with diabetic retinopathy and can be associated with both forms of diabetic retinopathy. Increased vascular permeability from breakdown of the blood-retinal barrier results in transudation of plasma and its constituents into the retina. This is seen clinically as hard exudates (**Figure 21–8**) and thickening of the

retina that can be recognized stereoscopically. The Early Treatment Diabetic Retinopathy Study (ETDRS) defined *clinically significant macular edema* (CSME) requiring focal laser treatment as a condition meeting any of the following criteria:

- Retinal thickening within 500 microns of the fovea
- Hard exudates within 500 microns of the fovea, if associated with adjacent retinal thickening
- Retinal thickening of 1 disc area or greater, any part of which is within 1 disc diameter of the fovea

Note: Visual acuity is not part of the definition of CSME, and patients with CSME may have 20/20 visual acuity. CSME is a clinical not a fluorescein angiographic diagnosis.

More recently, several patterns of diabetic macular edema have been identified on optical coherence tomography (OCT) (see later). Patients may have posterior hyaloidal traction contributing to macular edema; in this case, pars plana vitrectomy with peeling of the posterior hyaloid is the treatment of choice.

Classification of Nonproliferative Diabetic Retinopathy

NPDR is classified according to its severity: mild, moderate, severe, and very severe. Mild NPDR is defined as microaneurysms plus retinal hemorrhages only; moderate NPDR includes cotton wool spots and/or IRMAs. Severe NPDR is defined by the 4:2:1 rule: either hemorrhages and microaneurysms in 4 quadrants or venous beading in 2 quadrants, or IRMA in 1 quadrant. Very severe NPDR requires two of the features of severe NPDR.

21.2.2 IMAGING AND DIAGNOSTIC TESTS

Fluorescein Angiography

Fluorescein angiography is most commonly done after the diagnosis of macular edema is made clinically. It is performed to rule out macular ischemia (**Figure 21–6**) before focal or grid laser photocoagulation is initiated because areas of macular ischemia should be avoided in focal photocoagulation. It also helps identify focal areas of leakage from microaneurysms. **Figure 21–9** is a late-phase angiogram showing cystoid macular edema, seen angiographically as petaloid leakage around the fovea; there is also diffuse macular edema. **Figure 21–10**

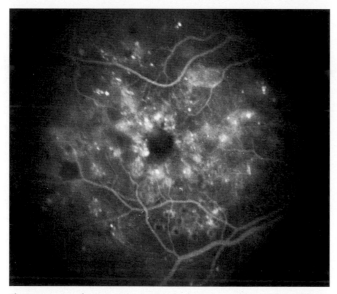

Figure 21–9 Fluorescein angiogram shows cystoid macular edema, with diffuse macular edema.

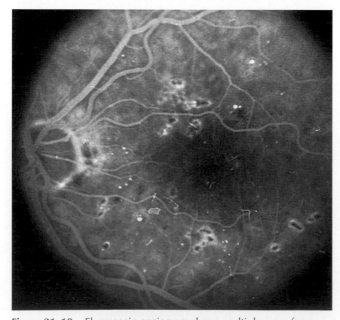

Figure 21–10 Fluorescein angiogram shows multiple scars from prior laser photocoagulation to microaneurysms; macular edema has resolved.

shows the presence of focal laser scars and resolved macular edema.

Optical Coherence Tomography

OCT reveals several patterns of diabetic macular edema:

- Diffuse retinal thickening (**Figure 21–11**)
- Cystoid macular edema (**Figure 21–12**)
- Subretinal fluid (**Figure 21–13**)

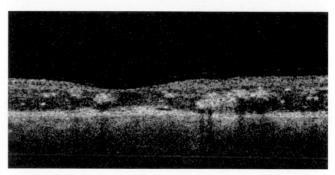

Figure 21–11 OCT shows multiple hard exudates as hyperreflective lesions with shadowing beyond the lesion, with diffuse macular edema. The retinal thickness is increased because of the edema and intraretinal swelling.

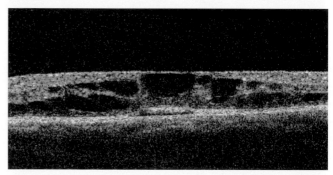

Figure 21–12 OCT shows cystoid macular edema with hyporeflective cystic spaces separated by thin hyperreflective septae. There is also a hyperreflective epiretinal membrane present on the surface of the retina.

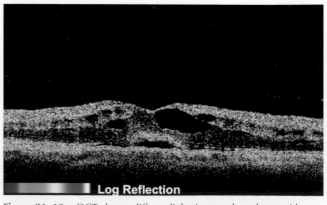

Figure 21–13 OCT shows diffuse diabetic macular edema with thickening of the retina and underlying subretinal fluid with no posterior hyaloidal traction evident.

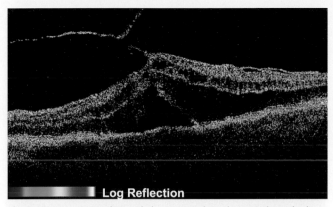

Figure 21–14 OCT shows diabetic macular edema with peaked, tractional retinal detachment due to posterior hyaloidal traction.

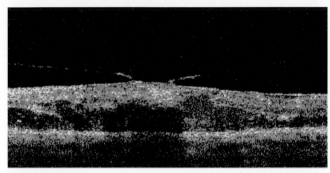

Figure 21–15 OCT shows diabetic macular edema with a fine epiretinal membrane. The posterior hyaloid is evident, but no traction is seen and there is no tractional retinal detachment.

- Posterior hyaloidal traction with traction retinal detachment (**Figure 21–14**)
- Posterior hyaloidal traction without traction retinal detachment (**Figure 21–15**)

Hard exudates (**Figure 21–11**) can also be identified on OCT, as well as epiretinal membranes (**Figure 21–12**). These patterns often appear together and only the diffuse retinal thickening pattern is seen alone.

21.2.3 PATHOLOGY

Intraretinal hemorrhages can be seen in the nerve fiber layer as flame-shaped hemorrhages or in the outer plexiform layer as dot and blot hemorrhages.

Cystoid macular edema can be seen pathologically as cystoid spaces in the inner nuclear and outer plexiform layers. Hard exudates are seen as eosinophilic spaces within the retina, are located in the outer plexiform layer of the macula (Henle's layer), and may produce a star figure because of the orientation of nerve fibers in this layer.

2.3 Proliferative Diabetic Retinopathy

The risk of development of PDR in patients with NPDR depends on the severity of the NPDR. According to the ETDRS, the risk of progression of severe NPDR to PDR is 15% in 1 year. The chance of progression of very severe NPDR to PDR in 1 year is 45%.

PDR is defined as the presence of newly formed blood vessels, fibrous tissue, or both, arising from the retina or optic disc and extending along the inner surface of the retina or disc or into the vitreous cavity. In the Diabetic Retinopathy Study, 15% of eyes had new vessels on or within 1 disc diameter of the optic disc (NVD), 40% had new vessels elsewhere (NVE), and 45% had both NVD and NVE. Eyes with PDR also have the features of NPDR, such as microaneurysms, intraretinal hemorrhages, venous beading, and intraretinal microvascular abnormalities.

21.3.1 CLINICAL SIGNS

New vessels on the disc (**Figure 21–16** and **Figure 21–17**) are usually easily identified, but occasionally can be difficult to distinguish from normal vessels, especially

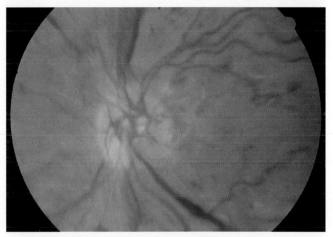

Figure 21–16 Color photograph OD. NVD can be seen as fine, lacy vessels on the optic nerve.

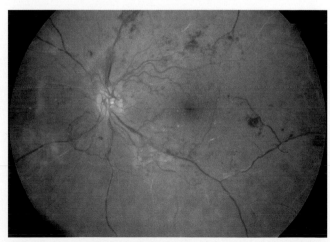

Figure 21–17 Color photograph OS shows NVD and extensive NVE along the arcades. There is an early fibrous component to the NVE along the inferotemporal arcade.

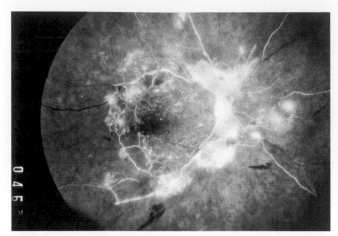

Figure 21–18 Fluorescein angiogram OD shows extensive leakage from both NVD and NVE and capillary nonperfusion.

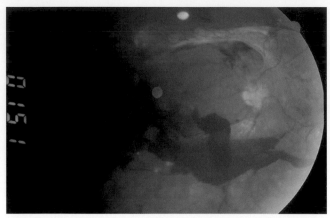

Figure 21–20 Color photograph showing a boat-shaped subhyaloid hemorrhage inferiorly, as well as a vitreous hemorrhage temporally.

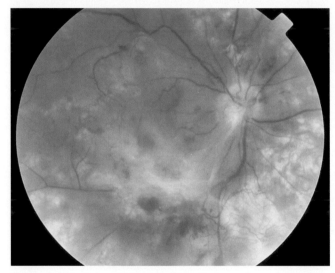

Figure 21–19 Color photograph shows fibrovascular proliferation extending from the optic nerve and along the inferotemporal arcade.

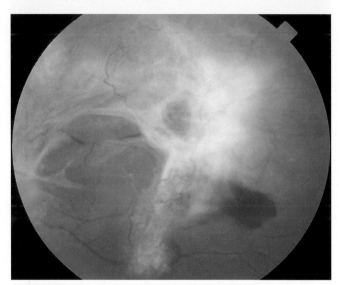

Figure 21–21 Color photograph shows a traction retinal detachment involving the macula.

on monocular viewing. Fluorescein angiography shows leakage of NVD (**Figure 21–18**).

New vessels elsewhere should be distinguished from IRMAs. The classic features of NVE are the formation of cartwheel-like networks (**Figure 21–17**); NVEs are also more superficial than IRMAs on stereoscopic viewing and may have a fibrous component (**Figures 21–17** and **21–19**). Borderline cases can be distinguished by the profuse leakage of NVE in late views on fluorescein angiography (**Figure 21–18**).

New vessels are usually asymptomatic until a posterior vitreous detachment occurs. Traction exerted on the new vessels may cause a vitreous hemorrhage (**Figure 21–20**). A subhyaloid hemorrhage may form in an area of detached vitreous between two areas of vitreous attachment (**Figure 21–20**).

Retinal detachment may result from contraction of the vitreous or of fibrovascular proliferations. These traction retinal detachments (**Figure 21–21**) usually have a concave anterior surface. If retinal holes are present, a combined traction-rhegmatogenous detachment may occur. These are usually more extensive and have a flat or convex anterior surface. Distortion of the macula may occur, particularly nasally, due to traction from fibrovascular proliferation at the optic disc.

New vessels may also occur on the iris (NVI) (rubeosis iridis). They typically start in the papillary area and may also involve the anterior chamber angle, when they can be diagnosed by gonioscopy (**Figure 21–22**). Hyphema may result from bleeding of NVI.

Classification of Proliferative Diabetic Retinopathy

The Diabetic Retinopathy Study classified PDR as "high-risk" PDR, necessitating prompt panretinal scatter

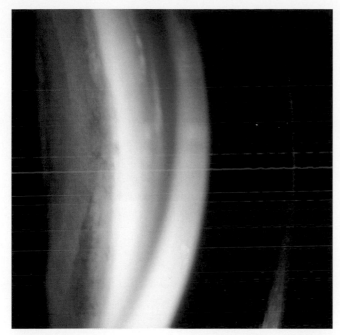

Figure 21–22 Color photograph of the anterior chamber angle seen by gonioscopy. Fine new vessels can be seen in the angle. Peripheral anterior synechiae are present due to the traction exerted by the new vessels.

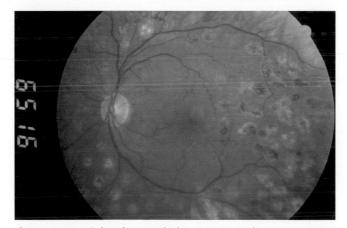

Figure 21–23 Color photograph shows an eye with quiescent PDR, after being treated with panretinal scatter photocoagulation.

photocoagulation (**Figure 21–23**), in the following circumstances:

- NVD greater than ¹/₃ disc diameter
- Vitreous or preretinal hemorrhage associated with any amount of NVD or associated with NVE of ¹/₂ disc diameter or greater.

Macular edema (see preceding section on NPDR) may be present at any stage of diabetic retinopathy, whether proliferative or not (**Figure 21–24**). According to the ETDRS, in eyes with high-risk PDR, macular edema should receive focal laser treatment before scatter panretinal photocoagulation is performed.

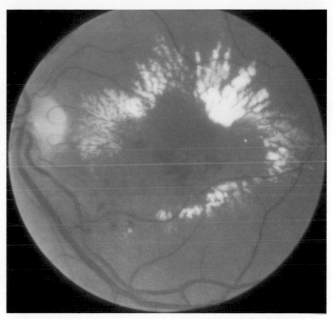

Figure 21–24 Color photograph shows macular edema, with microaneurysms, and extensive hard exudates in a circinate pattern.

21.3.2 IMAGING AND DIAGNOSTIC TESTS

Color Fundus Photography

Color fundus photography is seldom necessary for diagnostic purposes. It may be used to document disease status, progression, and response to treatment. Stereo fundus photography may be useful to document neovascularization and areas of traction and fibrovascular proliferation (**Figures 21–16, 21–17, 21–19** to **21–21, 21–23,** and **21–24**).

Fluorescein Angiography

Fluorescein angiography is indicated for evaluating unexplained vision loss in eyes with diabetic retinopathy: it shows areas of capillary nonperfusion (**Figure 21–25**)

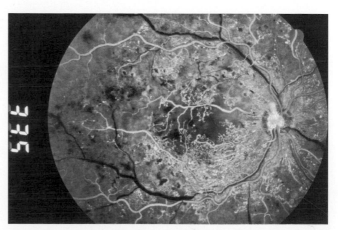

Figure 21–25 Fluorescein angiogram shows extensive capillary nonperfusion in the macula.

as well as leakage from macular edema. It is also used as a guide for focal laser treatment of microaneurysms in diabetic macular edema. However, angiography is not necessary for the diagnosis of clinically significant macular edema or PDR, both of which can be diagnosed on clinical examination.

Ultrasonography

B-scan ultrasonography is indicated when a vitreous hemorrhage or media opacity obscures a view of the fundus, and retinal detachment cannot be ruled out by indirect ophthalmoscopy (**Figure 21–26**).

Optical Coherence Tomography

OCT is used for imaging macular edema and its response to treatment. It may also be used to identify vitreomacular traction contributing to a taut posterior hyaloid face in eyes being considered for vitrectomy for persistent macular edema (**Figure 21–27**).

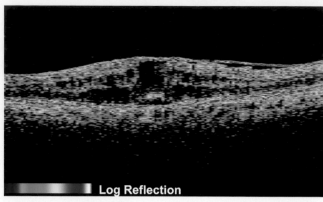

Figure 21–27   OCT shows macular edema with a taut posterior hyaloid.

SUGGESTED READINGS

Classification of diabetic retinopathy from fluorescein angiograms. ETDRS report number 11. Early Treatment Diabetic Retinopathy Study Research Group. Ophthalmology. 1991; May;98(5 suppl): 807–822.

Early vitrectomy for severe vitreous hemorrhage in diabetic retinopathy. Four-year results of a randomized trial: Diabetic Retinopathy Vitrectomy Study report 5. Arch Ophthalmol. 1990;108:958–964

Early photocoagulation for diabetic retinopathy. ETDRS report number 9. Early Treatment Diabetic Retinopathy Study Research Group. Ophthalmology. 1991;98(5 suppl):766–785.

Grading diabetic retinopathy from stereoscopic color fundus photographs—An extension of the modified Airlie House classification. ETDRS report number 10. Early Treatment Diabetic Retinopathy Study Research Group. Ophthalmology. 1991 May;98(5 Suppl):786–806.

Kinyoun J, Barton F, Fisher M, Hubbard L, Aiello L, Ferris F 3rd. Detection of diabetic macular edema. Ophthalmoscopy versus photography—Early Treatment Diabetic Retinopathy Study report number 5. The ETDRS Research Group. Ophthalmology. 1989; 96:746–750; discussion 750–751.

Photocoagulation treatment of proliferative diabetic retinopathy: The second report of diabetic retinopathy study findings. Ophthalmology. 1978;85:82–106.

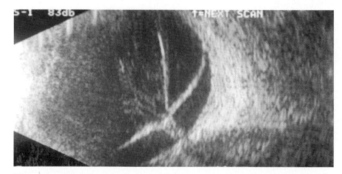

Figure 21–26   B-scan ultrasound shows a vitreous hemorrhage with a traction retinal detachment and a partially closed funnel configuration.

Chapter 22

Arterial Obstructive Disease

SUNIR J. GARG, MD • ALLEN C. HO, MD

22.1 Introduction

Retinal artery obstructions usually occur in individuals older than age 65 but may occur in any age group. They may affect the large vessels leading to the eye as well as the arteriole system within the eye. The clinical appearance of these occlusions varies, depending on which portion of the vascular tree is obstructed.

Ocular ischemic syndrome (OIS) is the term given to the ocular manifestations of carotid artery obstruction. Most cases of OIS develop when there is at least 70% obstruction of the ipsilateral carotid artery, with most cases occurring with at least 90% obstruction. Because most cases of OIS are due to atherosclerosis, men are affected twice as often as women. In addition, a high mortality rate is associated with this condition; individuals with OIS have a 5-year mortality rate of 40%, usually dying of coronary disease or stroke.

Ophthalmic, central retinal artery, and branch retinal artery occlusions also cause vision loss. Central retinal artery occlusions (CRAOs) generally affect the portion of the artery that lies within the optic nerve itself; thus, the site of the occlusion is often not visible clinically. In contrast, branch retinal artery occlusions (BRAOs) affect a part of the vascular system that is distal to the optic nerve head and an embolus may be identified. Although there are numerous causes for these occlusions, most BRAOs are due to emboli, whereas the majority of CRAOs are caused by thrombosis. Both BRAOs and CRAOs can cause immediate, permanent, and significant visual loss. Importantly, arterial occlusions may be the first sign of significant medical problems, thus all patients with an artery obstruction must have a systemic evaluation for an underlying cause.

22.2 Clinical Signs and Symptoms

The clinical presentation varies, depending on the location of the obstruction. In OIS, more than 90% of patients have vision loss at presentation. Most patients experience slow vision loss, but sudden vision loss can occur. Approximately one-third of patients have vision better than 20/40, one-third have vision of count fingers or worse, and one-third have vision in between these. A number of patients may also present with "ocular angina," which is a dull ache around the eye. Prolonged recovery from bright light may also be noted.

OIS presents with a number of clinical findings. Two-thirds of patients have iris neovascularization at presentation. However, neovascular glaucoma is present in only one-half of patients with iris neovascularization; even with a completely closed angle, the intraocular pressure may be normal because of ciliary body hypoperfusion. Mid-peripheral hemorrhages are the most common retinal finding. There is often arteriolar narrowing with dilated retinal veins. In contrast to central retinal vein obstruction, there is no retinal tortuosity. Cotton wool spots, retinal neovascularization, and a cherry-red spot occasionally may also be seen. An uncommon but helpful retinal sign is retinal arterial pulsations, which can be elicited by minimal pressure on the globe.

CRAO usually causes sudden, catastrophic, painless loss of vision. An afferent pupillary defect is usually present. Immediately after occlusion, the retina may appear normal, but within a few hours, a cherry-red spot often appears (**Figure 22–1**). Splinter hemorrhages on the disc are common. One to 2 months later, the optic nerve becomes pale, disc collaterals form, the retinal

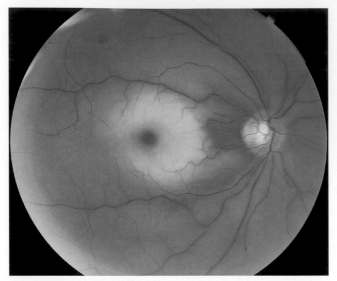

Figure 22–1 As much of the retina is edematous, the normal choroidal flow is visible as a cherry-red spot through the thinner retina overlying the fovea in this patient with a CRAD.

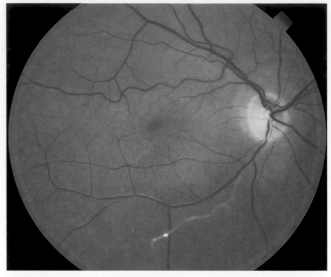

Figure 22–3 A chronic BRAO leading to attenuation and sclerosis of the involved vessel.

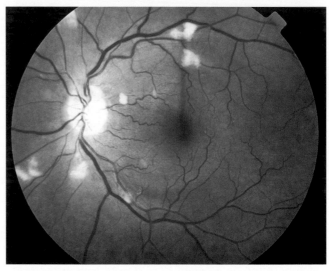

Figure 22–4 Cotton wool spots due to interferon use. Cotton wool spots are infarctions of the nerve fiber layer.

whitening resolves, and the retina may appear atrophic. In 15% of people a cilioretinal artery supplies the retina; in the setting of CRAO the portion of the retina supplied by the cilioretinal artery may be spared. Conversely, the cilioretinal artery may be obstructed with a patent central retinal artery. Although disc neovascularization is uncommon, iris neovascularization occurs in about 20% of eyes.

BRAOs also present with sudden, painless vision loss in the area corresponding to the site of obstruction. Approximately one-half of patients have unaffected visual acuity. Depending upon the extent of the retinal involvement, an afferent pupillary defect may be present. Triangle-shaped retinal whitening is the most characteristic finding. Flame-shaped hemorrhages may be present in the area of ischemia. Emboli are seen in

two-thirds of the eyes at the apex of the triangle (**Figure 22–2**). Over time, the retinal whitening resolves and a normal or atrophic appearing retina may be apparent (**Figure 22–3**). Cotton-wool spots indicate infarction involving capillaries. A myriad of conditions can cause them; diabetes, radiation retinopathy, human immunodeficiency virus (HIV) infection, vasculitis, and interferon treatment are a few (**Figure 22–4**).

22.3 Imaging and Diagnostic Tests

22.3.1 FLUORESCEIN ANGIOGRAPHY

With OIS delayed arm-to-retina and arteriovenous transit time is seen (**Figures 22–5** to **22–7**). A leading

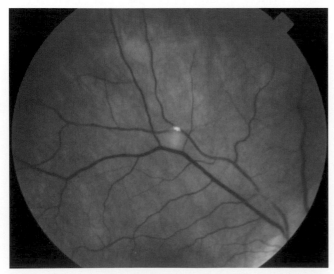

Figure 22–2 An embolus is lodged at a bifurcation point causing a BRAO.

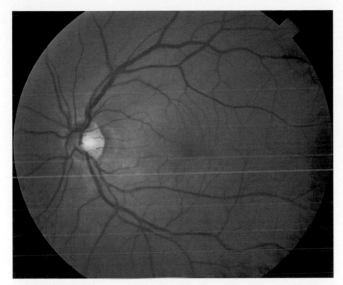

Figure 22–5 The fundus photograph of a patient with OIS shows only mild attenuation of the arterioles and no venous tortuosity.

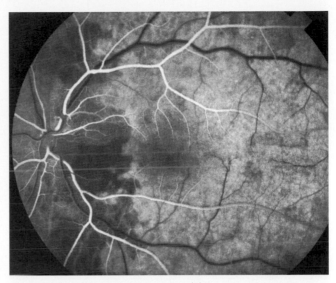

Figure 22–7 Fluorescein angiogram of the same patient at 44 seconds shows delayed and patchy choroidal filling pattern.

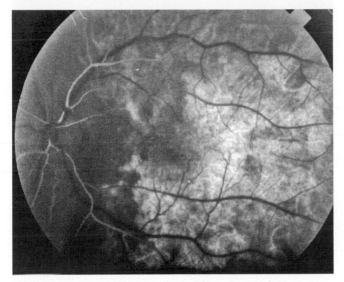

Figure 22–6 Fluorescein angiogram of the same eye shown in **Figure 22–5** at 35 seconds shows slightly delayed arm-to-retina transit time.

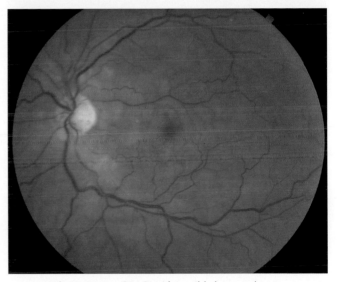

Figure 22–8 CRAO with a mild cherry-red spot.

edge of dye occasionally can be seen. Patchy choroidal filling, segmentation of flow, microaneurysms, late staining of the retinal vessels, and capillary nonperfusion may also be present.

Delayed arm-to-retina and arteriovenous transit time, retrograde filling of the arterioles, and a leading edge of dye may also be seen with central retinal artery occlusion (**Figures 22–8 to 22–11**). There may be late staining of the optic disc. A patent cilioretinal artery may cause sparing of the retina that gives a striking appearance (**Figures 22–12 to 22–17**). A cilioretinal artery obstruction often looks similar to a BRAO (**Figures 22–18 to 22–20**).

Fluorescein angiography in BRAOs shows absent or delayed arteriole filling in the area of obstruction with

late staining in the area around the embolus. Retinal thickening may cause a ground-glass appearance (**Figures 22–21 to 22–23**).

22.3.2 INDOCYANINE GREEN ANGIOGRAPHY

Indocyanine green angiography does not aid in diagnosis.

22.3.3 OPTICAL COHERENCE TOMOGRAPHY

During the acute injury, optical coherence tomography may show intraretinal edema in the areas of infarct. Months afterwards, the retinal thickness may be attenuated, consistent with retinal atrophy.

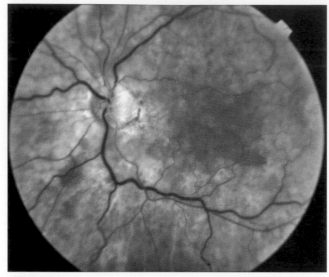

Figure 22–9   Fluorescein angiogram of the same patient showing normal arm-to-retina transit time of 21 seconds.

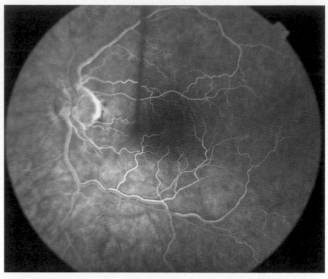

Figure 22–11   Fluorescein angiogram at 63 seconds shows delayed arteriovenous transit time.

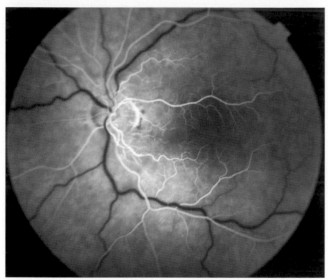

Figure 22–10   Fluorescein angiogram at 33 seconds shows delayed arteriovenous transit time.

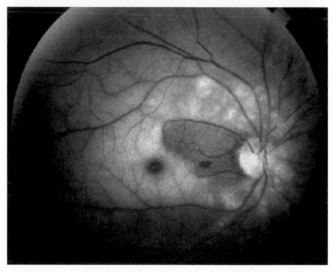

Figure 22–12   Color photograph of CRAO (whitened retina) with sparing of the cilioretinal artery (temporal to the optic nerve).

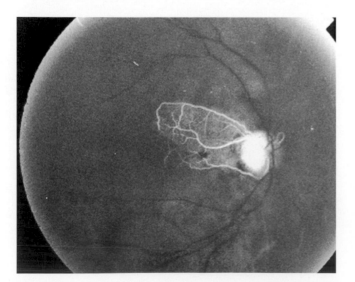

Figure 22–13   Fluorescein angiogram of the same eye shown in **Figure 22–12** showing cilioretinal artery sparing with CRAO. Image taken at 23 seconds.

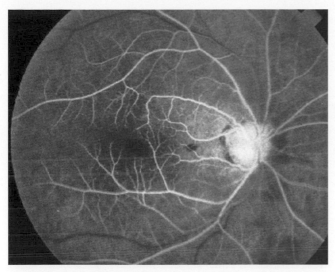

Figure 22–14 Angiogram taken at 57 seconds. Note delayed arteriovenous transit time.

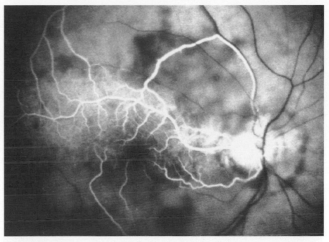

Figure 22–17 Fluorescein angiogram of the same eye shown in **Figure 22–16** at 52 seconds shows delayed arteriovenous transit time.

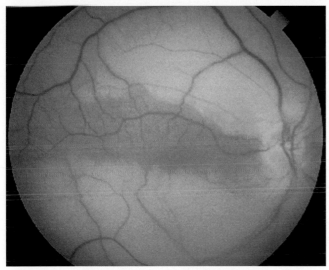

Figure 22–15 Color picture of a patent cilioretinal artery with a central retinal artery occlusion. A central band of orange-perfused retina is surrounded by white edematous retina.

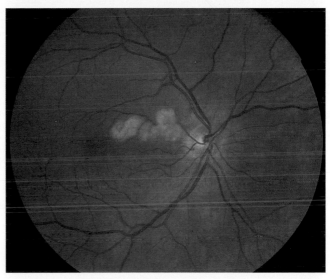

Figure 22–18 Color photograph of a cilioretinal artery obstruction. Patient has 20/25 visual acuity. (Photograph courtesy of Kent A. Blade, MD.)

22.3.4 ULTRASONOGRAPHY

In OIS, carotid Doppler testing usually reveals obstruction of the ipsilateral carotid artery. In eyes in which the ultrasonography does not reveal significant obstruction, magnetic resonance arteriography or conventional angiography may be useful to demonstrate more distal obstruction. Orbital Doppler testing may reveal decreased blood flow velocities in the retrobulbar circulation in both OIS and CRAOs.

Carotid Doppler and cardiac echography studies should be ordered to find a potential cause for a presumed embolus for both CRAOs and BRAOs.

22.3.5 ELECTRORETINOGRAPHIC STUDY

Electroretinography shows diminished a and b waves in OIS. In contrast, a CRAO demonstrates an intact a wave with a diminished b wave.

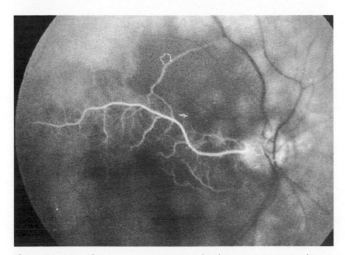

Figure 22–16 Fluorescein angiogram of right eye at 34 seconds shows a patent cilioretinal artery.

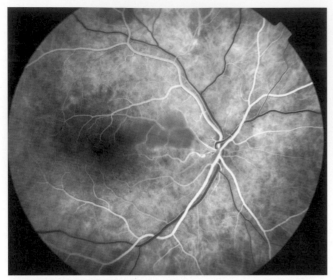

Figure 22–19 Fluorescein angiogram at 21 seconds shows early ground-glass appearance in the involved area of the same eye shown in **Figure 22–18**. (Photograph courtesy of Kent A. Blade, MD.)

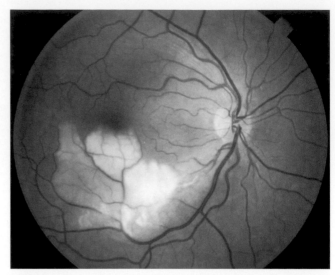

Figure 22–21 Branch retinal artery occlusion with marked retinal ischemia and whitening.

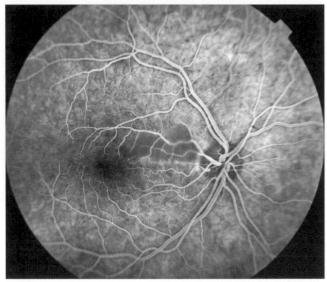

Figure 22–20 More prominent ground-glass appearance in the later frames of the fluorescein angiogram of the same patient shown in **Figure 22–18**. (Photograph courtesy of Kent A. Blade, MD.)

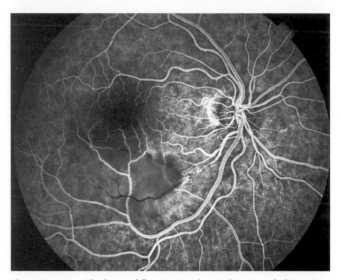

Figure 22–22 Blockage of fluorescein dye in the area of obstruction of the same eye shown in **Figure 22–21**.

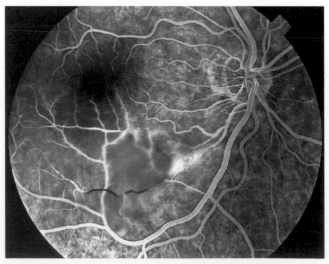

Figure 22–23 Prominent ground-glass appearance of ischemic retina in later views of the same eye shown in **Figure 22–21**.

22.3.6 MISCELLANEOUS LABORATORY TESTS

Patients with arterial obstruction should be evaluated for hypertension, diabetes mellitus, and atherosclerosis. In addition, patients with CRAOs should be evaluated for temporal arteritis. An erythrocyte sedimentation rate and possibly a C-reactive protein measurement should be ordered immediately. A temporal artery biopsy should be considered.

BRAOs (and to a lesser extent, CRAOs) should be evaluated for an embolic source. In younger patients, a search for an underlying cause may include evaluation for coagulopathies, including protein C, protein S,

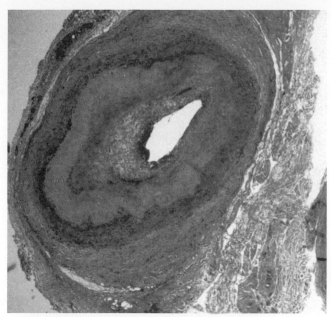

Figure 22-24 Temporal artery biopsy from a patient with a CRAO. Disruption of the internal elastic lamina is seen, and a few giant cells are present.

antithrombin III, and factor V Leiden deficiency. In addition, patients may have elevated homocysteine levels. Underlying vasculitis, pancreatitis, Kawasaki disease, and bone or amniotic embolism should also be considered in appropriate circumstances. Carotid and cardiac echography should also be ordered.

22.4 Pathology

In all forms of retinal artery obstructions, cytoid bodies may be present. Corresponding to an acute ischemic infarct (or cotton wool spot), a cytoid body represents a swollen axon. The inner retina also demonstrates edema in the acute stages, followed by necrosis and atrophy in the chronic stages. Giant cell arteritis shows giant cells and disruption of the internal elastic lamina (**Figure 22-24**).

SUGGESTED READINGS

Brown GC, Magargal LE. Central retinal artery obstruction and visual acuity. Ophthalmology. 1982;89:14–21

Brown GC, Magargal LE. The ocular ischemic syndrome: Clinical, fluorescein angiographic and carotid angiographic features. Int Ophthal. 1988;11:239–242.

Duker JS, Brown GC. Iris neovascularization associated with obstruction of the central retinal artery. Ophthalmology. 1988;95:1244–1250.

McLeod D, Marshall J, Kohner EM, Bird AC. The role of axoplasmic transport in the pathogenesis of retinal cotton-wool spots. Br J Ophthalmol. 1977;61:177–191.

Weger M, Stanger O, Deutschmann H, et al. The role of hyperhomocysteinemia and methylenetetrahydrofolate reductase (MTHFR) C677T mutation in patients with retinal artery occlusion. Am J Ophthalmol. 2002;134:57–61.

Chapter 23

Venous Obstructive Disease

SUNIL K. SRIVASTAVA, MD • SHARON FEKRAT, MD

23.1 Introduction

Retinal venous occlusive disease, which includes central retinal vein occlusions (CVOs), hemiretinal vein occlusions (HVOs), and branch retinal vein occlusions (BVOs), is the second most common retinal vascular disorder after diabetic retinopathy. Vein occlusions typically affect persons older than 50 years of age. Individuals who develop a CVO typically have associated hypertension, cardiovascular disease, diabetes mellitus, and/or glaucoma. An increased risk of BVO has been reported in those with hypertension, cardiovascular disease, and/or glaucoma.

In two major clinical trials, the Central Vein Occlusion Study (CVOS) and the Branch Vein Occlusion Study (BVOS), the natural history and the clinical effectiveness of laser photocoagulation have been described.

23.2 Clinical Signs and Symptoms

A person with venous occlusive disease presents with a sudden change in visual acuity or visual field in one eye. The severity of the visual loss depends on the area of involvement and the perfusion status as determined by fluorescein angiography.

23.2.1 BRANCH RETINAL VEIN OCCLUSION

Ophthalmoscopy discloses a segmental area of intra-retinal hemorrhage, dilated branch retinal veins, and, sometimes, cotton wool spots (**Figure 23–1**). A BVO usually occurs at an arteriovenous crossing, where the artery overlies the vein. Proximal obstructions (optic nerve head or first-order crossings) will lead to more

extensive involvement and intraretinal hemorrhages than obstructions at more distal crossings (**Figure 23–2**). More severe visual loss occurs with those BVOs that involve the macula than those that do not.

Visual loss in eyes with a BVO may be due to one or more factors including foveal intraretinal hemorrhage (**Figure 23–3**), cystoid macular edema, macular ischemia, vitreous hemorrhage, traction retinal detachment, and, rarely, subretinal hemorrhage. Cystoid macular edema develops in most eyes with a BVO and may be further assessed by fluorescein angiography and optical coherence tomography (see later). The BVOS demonstrated

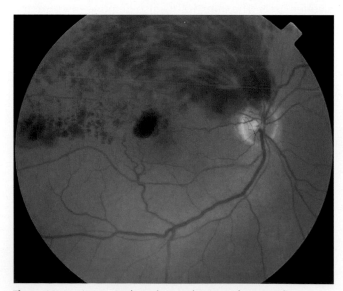

Figure 23–1 A superior branch retinal vein occlusion with intraretinal hemorrhage and dilated retinal veins. There is an extensive area of involvement due to a proximal obstruction.

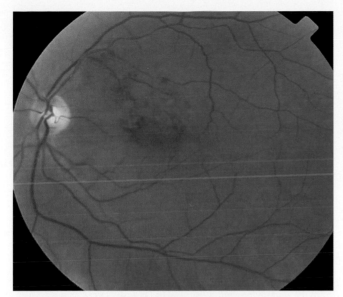

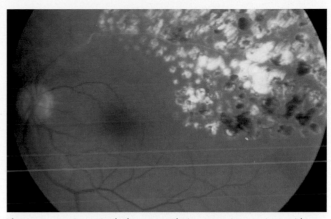

Figure 23–4 Panretinal photocoagulation scars in a patient with a history of a branch retinal vein occlusion and retinal neovascularization.

Figure 23–2 In comparison to **Figure 23–1,** the obstruction in this branch retinal vein occlusion occurs at a more distal crossing, leading to a more restricted area of involvement.

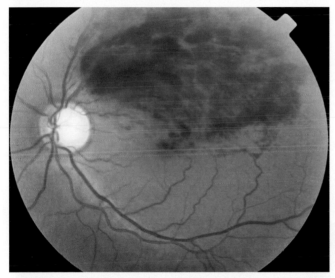

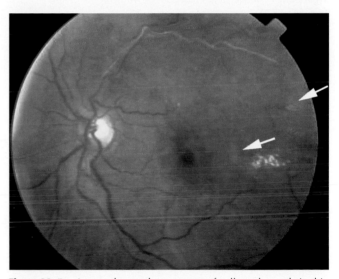

Figure 23–5 *Arrows* denote the presence of collateral vessels in this patient with a chronic branch retinal vein occlusion.

Figure 23–3 A branch retinal vein occlusion with foveal intraretinal hemorrhage. The patient's visual acuity was 20/200.

the benefit of grid pattern laser photocoagulation in the treatment of macular edema associated with a recent (3 to 18 months) BVO in those eyes with a visual acuity of 20/40. Macular capillary nonperfusion can also contribute to visual loss in eyes with a BVO. This is evaluated best by fluorescein angiography (see later). Grid pattern laser photocoagulation is not recommended for ischemic macular edema.

Retinal neovascularization develops in approximately 40% of eyes with greater than 5 disc diameters in diameter of capillary nonperfusion. Vitreous hemorrhage occurs in about 60% of these eyes. The BVOS demonstrated that sectoral peripheral scatter laser photocoagulation (**Figure 23–4**) was effective in reducing the

risk of vitreous hemorrhage once neovascularization had developed.

Over time, the intraretinal hemorrhage slowly reabsorbs, leaving less ophthalmoscopic evidence of the BVO. Ophthalmoscopy in the chronic phase (>6 months) discloses collateral vessel formation across the horizontal raphe (**Figure 23–5**), cystoid macular edema, capillary dilation, and retinal pigment epithelium changes in the fovea due to chronic cystoid macular edema (**Figure 23–6**).

Treatment modalities under investigation include pars plana vitrectomy with arteriovenous sheathotomy. In this procedure, a pars plana vitrectomy is performed followed by sectioning of the common adventital sheath of the branch vein and artery (**Figure 23–7**). Relieving the compression on the retinal vein, in theory, could restore normal flow through the vein. The reported effectiveness of this therapy has been variable, and a randomized clinical trial is needed to truly evaluate its value.

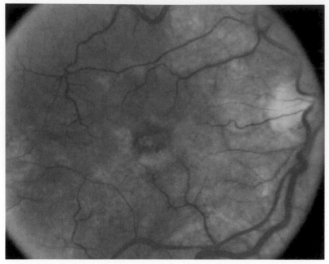

Figure 23–6 RPE changes in the fovea with chronic cystoid macular edema.

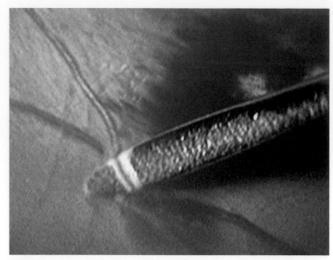

Figure 23–7 Intraoperative photograph of an arteriovenous sheathotomy. Here the adventitial sheath of the artery is separated from the underlying vein. (Courtesy of Dr. Jose Garcia Arumi.)

Intravitreal injection of triamcinolone acetonide is also under investigation for the treatment of macular edema associated with BVO. Recent articles report improvement on optical coherence tomography and fluorescein angiography (see later). The NEI collaborative SCORE (Standard of Care versus COrticosteroid for REtinal Vein Occlusion) study is currently underway to evaluate the effectiveness of this modality to the standard of care.

23.2.2 CENTRAL RETINAL VEIN OCCLUSION

The ophthalmoscopic appearance of eyes with a recent CVO consists of intraretinal hemorrhages in all four quadrants with dilated and tortuous veins (**Figure 23–8**).

Other findings include optic nerve edema and hyperemia, macular edema, and cotton wool spots. Breakthrough vitreous or subretinal hemorrhage can occur in some eyes. At presentation, patients with a CVO can have ciliary injection and dilation of normal iris vessels.

Visual acuity can range from 20/20 to hand motion. Presenting visual acuity less than 20/200 is an important risk factor for the development of anterior segment neovascularization. Decreased visual acuity usually is attributed to foveal hemorrhage, macular edema, and capillary nonperfusion, but sometimes can be due to vitreous hemorrhage, tractional retinal detachment, and subretinal hemorrhage.

Monthly follow-up is recommended for the first 4 to 6 months after the onset of a CVO to monitor for the

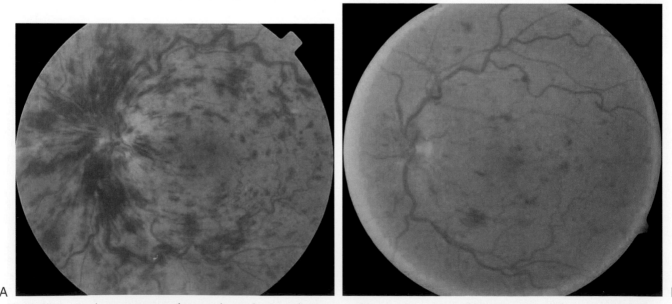

Figure 23–8 Fundus appearances of a central retinal vein occlusion. Note the extensive intraretinal hemorrhage in all four quadrants with dilated retinal veins (*A*) and with less involvement (*B*). Some blurring of the optic disc margin is also present in *A*.

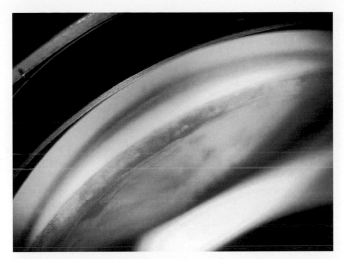

Figure 23–9 Gonioscopy photograph reveals extensive neovascularization of the angle in this patient with a history of a central retinal vein occlusion. (Courtesy of Dr. John Halabis.)

development of anterior segment neovascularization. Eyes at greatest risk include those with greater than 10 disc diameters of capillary nonperfusion as documented by fluorescein angiography, visual acuity of 20/200, or a relative afferent pupillary defect. According to the CVOS, 35% of eyes with a nonperfused or indeterminate CVO develop iris or angle neovascularization (**Figure 23–9**), compared with just 10% of perfused eyes. Once iris or angle neovascularization develops, panretinal photocoagulation is recommended to promote regression.

Cystoid macular edema commonly occurs in eyes with CVO, leading to a decrease in central vision. The CVOS found that macular grid pattern laser photocoagulation reduced angiographic leakage but did not have a statistically significant effect on visual acuity.

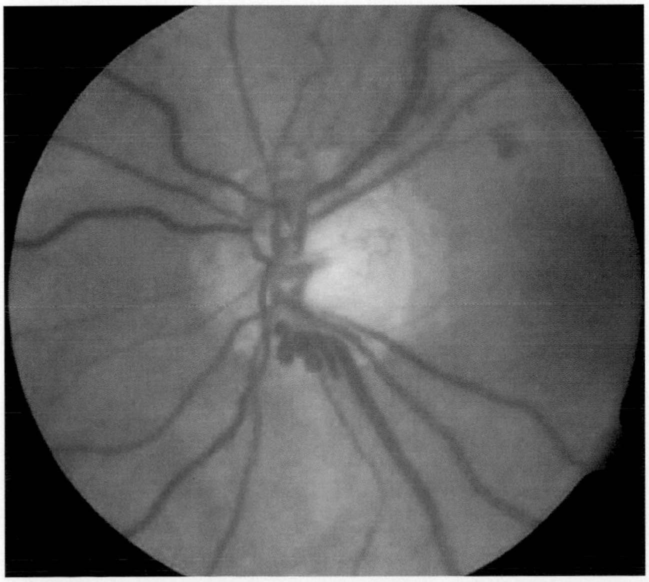

Over time, the intraretinal hemorrhage will resolve. Collateral vessels typically develop on the optic nerve (**Figure 23–10**). Retinal or disc neovascularization (**Figure 23–11**) can develop and may require panretinal laser photocoagulation.

The poor visual outcome of eyes with an initial visual acuity <20/200 has led to the investigation of various therapeutic modalities. These include radial optic neurotomy (**Figure 23–12**), chorioretinal laser anastomosis (**Figures 23–13** and **23–14**), and intravitreal injection of triamcinolone acetonide. These treatments are currently under investigation for their efficacy.

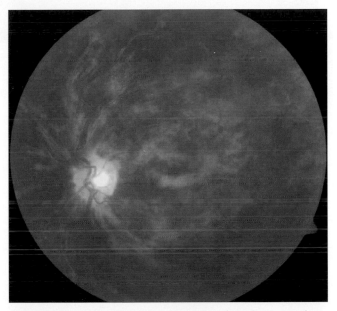

Figure 23–11 Optic disc neovascularization along the temporal margin of the nerve.

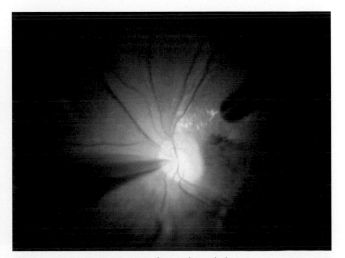

Figure 23–10 Collateral vessels on the optic nerve in a patient with a history of a central retinal vein occlusion. Note the larger collaterals along the inferior margin and the smaller collateral temporally.

Figure 23–12 Intraoperative photo of a radial optic neurotomy. Here a microvitreoretinal blade is placed through the nasal optic disc margin to relieve compression on the central retinal vein.

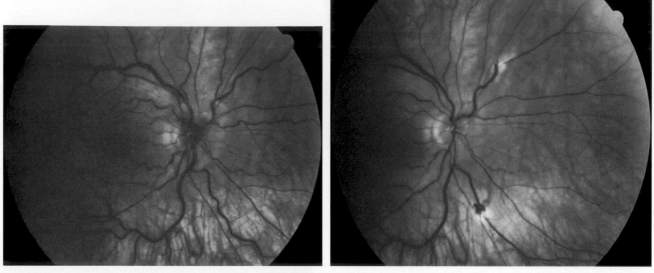

Figure 23–13   Laser-induced chorioretinal anastomosis is used to create venous anastomoses between the retinal and choroidal circulation. In these photographs, a patient with a CVO (*A*) has two anastomoses created (*B*).

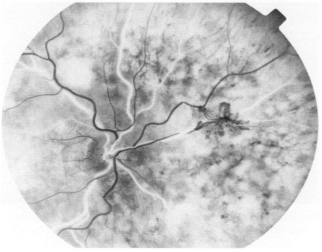

Figure 23–14   Fluorescein negative of a patient who developed choroid-vitreal neovascularization through a laser anastomosis site.

23.2.3 HEMIRETINAL VEIN OCCLUSION

Ophthalmoscopy reveals intraretinal hemorrhage, dilated retinal veins, and occasionally cotton wool spots distributed in either the superior or inferior hemisphere (**Figure 23–15**). The visual acuity depends on the amount of macular ischemia, macular edema, and intra-retinal hemorrhage. Hemiretinal vein occlusion is a variant of both CVO and BVO (**Figure 23–16**) and can develop many of the same sequelae including retinal neovascularization, anterior segment neovascularization, and collateral vessel formation. Eyes that develop neovascularization require panretinal photocoagulation.

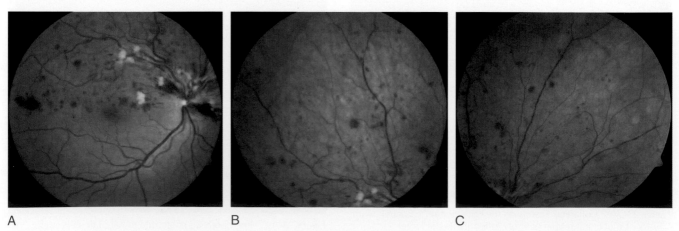

Figure 23–15   Posterior pole (*A*) and peripheral (*B* and *C*) photographs of a superior hemiretinal vein occlusion with dilated veins, intraretinal hemorrhages, and cotton wool spots involving the superior retina.

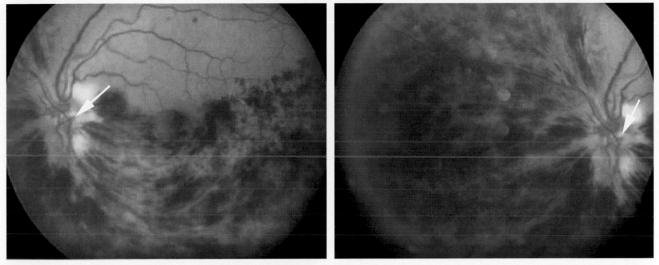

Figure 23–16   Fundus photograph of a vein occlusion involving three-quarters of the retina. The inferior hemiretina is involved (*A*), as is the superior-nasal quadrant (*B*). Note the common proximal vein (*arrow*), which drains these quadrants.

23.3 Imaging and Diagnostic Tests

23.3.1 FLUORESCEIN ANGIOGRAPHY

Branch Retinal Vein Occlusion

In eyes with BVO, the early frames of a fluorescein angiogram usually reveal a segmental area of fluorescein blockage due to the intraretinal hemorrhage, which is present throughout the angiogram (**Figure 23–17**). With clearing of the intraretinal hemorrhage, there is an improved view of the retinal vasculature. In the early-phase frames, capillary dilation and capillary nonperfusion may also be observed.

Mid-phase frames of the angiogram demonstrate dilated, tortuous veins with delayed venous filling proximal to the area of blockage (**Figure 23–18**). In eyes with a chronic (>6 months) BVO, collateral vessels (**Figure 23–19A**) can be observed during the mid-phase frames, as can retinal neovascularization (**Figure 23–19B**). These are differentiated from each other by the lack of dye leakage in the former.

Cystoid macular edema with parafoveal capillary leakage is commonly seen in the late-phase frames in both the acute (<6 months) and chronic stage of a BVO (**Figure 23–20**). Staining of retinal veins is also present in many eyes (**Figure 23–21**).

Fluorescein angiography can be used to monitor the effectiveness of treatment. Focal laser photocoagulation can decrease the amount of capillary leakage (**Figure 23–22**). Intravitreal triamcinolone acetonide injections can lessen the amount of capillary leakage in both CVOs and BVOs (**Figure 23–23**).

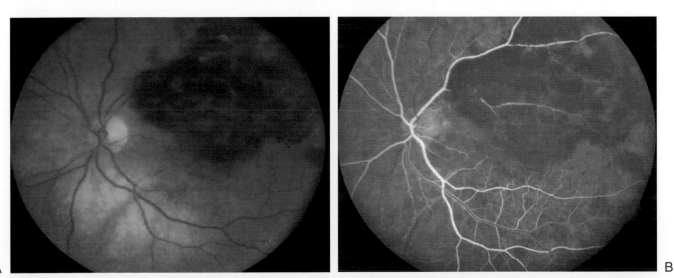

Figure 23–17   Color fundus photograph (*A*) and corresponding early-phase fluorescein angiogram frame (*B*) revealing blockage due to intraretinal hemorrhage and delayed filling of the involved vein.

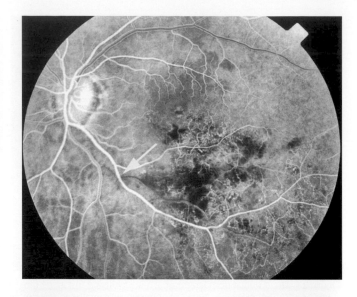

Figure 23–18 Mid-phase angiogram frame with a delay in venous filling along the blocked vein (*arrow*). Also note the scattered pinpoint hyperfluorescence in the macula due to capillary dilatation.

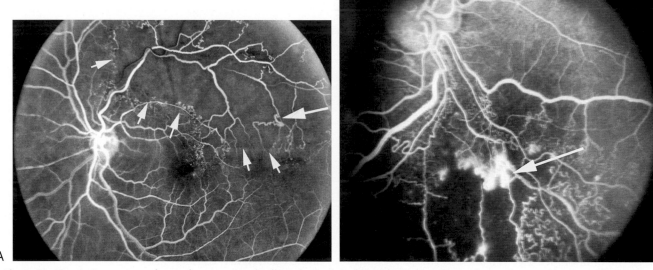

A

B

Figure 23–19 *A: Large arrows* denote the presence of collateral vessels in this mid-phase angiogram frame. There is a large area of capillary nonperfusion present as well (*small arrows*). *B:* Mid- to late-phase frame revealing areas of retinal neovascularization with extensive dye leakage (*large arrow*).

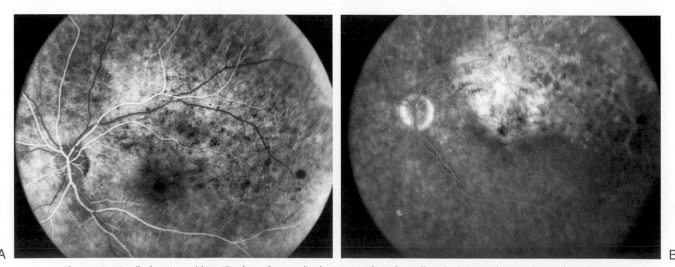

A

B

Figure 23–20 Early (*A*)- and late (*B*)-phase frames displaying parafoveal capillary leakage and cystoid macular edema.

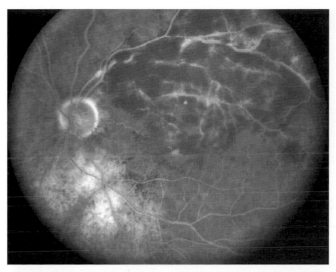

Figure 23–21 Late-phase frame with staining of retinal vein walls.

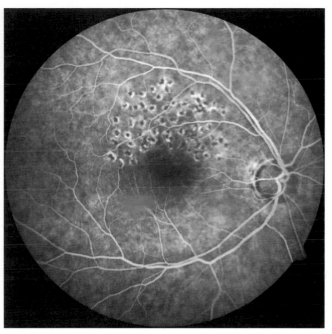

Figure 23–22 Late-phase frame of a patient with a branch retinal vein occlusion after grid laser photocoagulation. Note the absence of parafoveal leakage.

Central Retinal Vein Occlusion

In the acute phase (<6 months) of a CVO, scattered intraretinal hemorrhage produces blockage in the early frames of the fluorescein angiogram, which continues through the duration of the angiogram. The degree of blockage tends to be greater in nonperfused than in perfused occlusions. Retinal capillary nonperfusion is also present, the degree of which can be used to distinguish between a perfused and a nonperfused CVO (**Figure 23–24**). Other findings during the early phase include retinal capillary dilation and early disc hyperfluorescence (**Figure 23–25**).

Dilated tortuous veins with marked delay in filling are characteristic of mid-phase frames (**Figure 23–26**). Areas of blocked fluorescence due to intraretinal hemorrhage and hypofluorescence due to capillary non-

perfusion continue to appear during mid-phase frames. In eyes with a long-standing CVO, optic disc shunt vessels or neovascularization, if present, can be observed during the mid-phase or late-phase frames (**Figure 23–27**).

Late-phase frames in CVO demonstrate marked macular leakage from parafoveal capillary vessels (**Figure 23–28**). Other areas of retinal vascular leakage of fluorescein may be present in the mid-periphery and optic nerve. Additionally, hyperfluorescence of retinal venous walls can occur, which is more often present in nonperfused eyes (**Figure 23–29**).

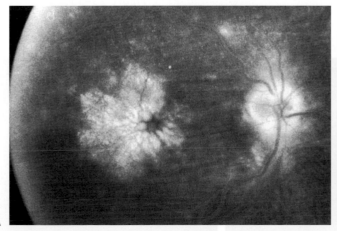
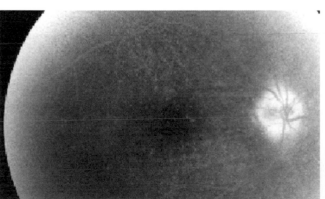

A   B

Figure 23–23 Late angiogram frames revealing cystoid macular edema (*A*) with resolution of the edema after intravitreal injection of triamcinolone acetonide (*B*).

however, treatment is difficult because the lesion is often very close to the foveal avascular zone. More recently, photodynamic therapy for choroidal neovascular membranes due to IPT has been suggested. In addition, the use of intravitreal triamcinolone has also been reported to be successful in decreasing macular edema due to IPT. Initial success with these treatments warrants further research to ascertain whether these newer modalities will be useful in treating certain subsets of patients with IPT.

24.2 Clinical Signs and Symptoms

Patients typically present with a minimal decrease in visual acuity to the level of 20/30 or better when they develop serous exudation, macular edema, or hard exudates in areas adjacent to the telangiectasia. There is evidence of occult telangiectasis smaller than 1 disc diameter, confined to the temporal macula, although larger zones of capillary abnormality may be present. There is minimal intraretinal serous exudation and intraretinal hemorrhages. Clinical features and progression of the disease severity are best understood by staging. Stage 1 is characterized by mild staining in the outer retina of the temporal macula but often also of a small wedge-shaped area of nasal macula on fluorescein angiography. There is no biomicroscopic or angiographic evidence of telangiectasis. In Stage 2, there is graying of the involved area and the onset of biomicroscopic and angiographic evidence of telangiectasis. Right-angle venules diving deep into the outer retinal plexus are characteristic of Stage 3 (**Figure 24–2**). Stage 4 is associated with stellate retinal pigment epithelium (RPE) plaques due to a RPE hyperplastic response in the distribution of the right-angle venules (**Figures 24–2, 24–3,** and **24–4**). Finally, Stage 5 is associated with choroidal neovascularization and peculiar retinochoroidal anastomoses often with a clinical picture similar to retinal angiomatous proliferation.

The Gass classification (**Table 24–1**) subdivides the disease into three groups: Group 1 may be congenital or acquired and typically occurs in males. It is usually

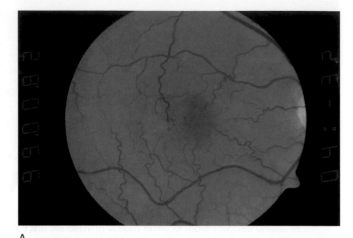

A

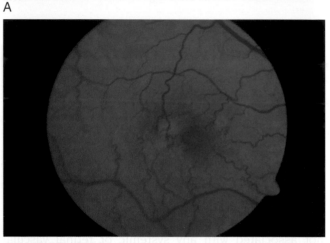

B

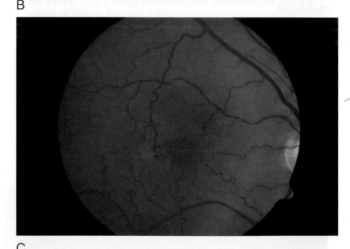

C

Figure 24–2   IPT. Prominent right-angle venule with progression of retinal pigment epithelial changes from 1999 (*A*), 2001 (*B*), and 2002 (*C*).

TABLE 24–1 ▮
Perifoveal Retinal Telangiectasis (Gass Classification)

Group	Description
Group 1A	Unilateral, congenital parafoveolar telangiectasis
Group 1B	Unilateral, idiopathic, focal juxtafoveolar telangiectasis
Group 2A	Bilateral, idiopathic, acquired perifoveolar telangiectasis
Group 3A	Occlusive idiopathic juxtafoveolar retinal telangiectasis
Group 3B	Occlusive idiopathic juxtafoveolar retinal telangiectasis associated with central nervous system vasculopathy

unilateral and presents with yellow, lipid-rich exudation at the outer margins of the area of telangiectasis forming circinate-type exudates. It is thought to be a variant of Coats' disease; Group 2 occurs in both males and females and is bilateral. Blunted right-angle venules, superficial retinal crystals, intraretinal pigment plaques, and subretinal neovascularization are common findings.

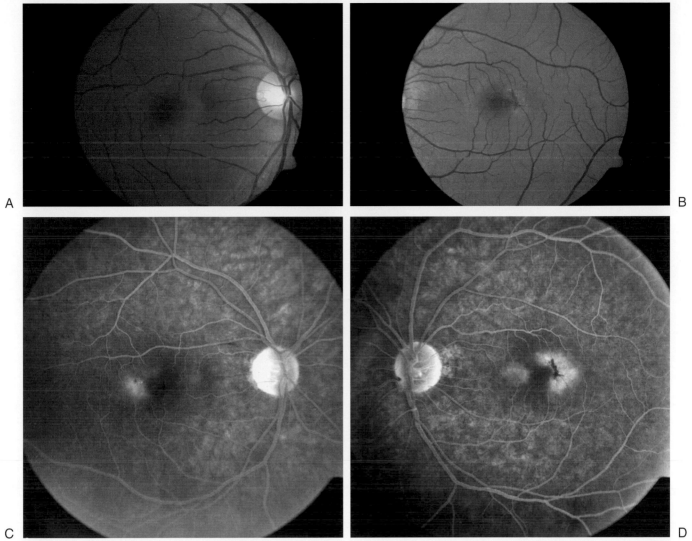

Figure 24–3   IPT, Group 2. *A:* Mild retinal pigment epithelial hyperplasia temporal to the right macula. *B:* Prominent pigment clump temporal to the left macula of the same patient. *C* and *D:* Corresponding late-phase fluorescein angiogram shows intraretinal leakage of dye surrounding the pigment clump.

Finally, Group 3 consists of bilateral perifoveal telangiectasis with retinal capillary obliteration. The capillary nonperfusion often leads to progressive loss of vision. This group is associated with a variety of systemic diseases including polycythemia, hypoglycemia, ulcerative colitis, multiple myeloma, and chronic lymphatic leukemia. The very rare variant, Group 3B, is also associated with central nervous system findings including optic atrophy, decreased deep tendon reflexes, or other findings.

Other clinical findings can include superficial glistening white dots (Singerman spots) and small, refractile, golden crystalline deposits, seen in approximately one half of patients with worse than Stage 2 disease. Also, in 5% of affected patients, a yellow foveal lesion develops in one or both eyes. This lesion may appear similar to a lamellar macular hole due to progressive atrophy of the outer retina (**Figure 24–5**). Finally, cystoid macular edema, more prominent in the temporal fovea, may occur.

24.3   Imaging and Diagnostic Tests

The diagnosis of IPT can be difficult because its principle features are also seen in other disease processes. Telangiectatic vascular changes are seen in diabetic retinopathy, venous occlusive disease, radiation retinopathy, Coats' disease, cystoid macular edema, and Eales' disease. The most distinguishing feature of IPT is the limitation of the disease process to the perifoveal region.

24.3.1   FLUORESCEIN ANGIOGRAPHY

Fluorescein angiography is the most useful diagnostic test and is very helpful in obtaining the correct diagnosis, particularly in Stage 1 disease in which there is no biomicroscopic evidence of telangiectasis. In early views, the telangiectatic vessels hyperfluoresce quickly. The late phase of the fluorescein angiogram shows intraretinal

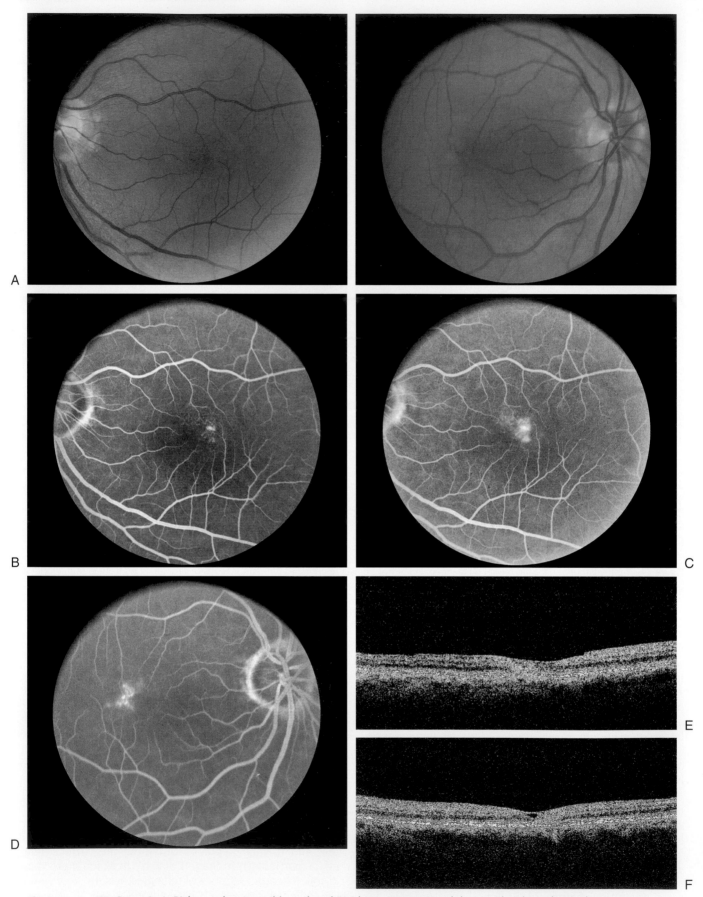

Figure 24–4   IPT, Group 2. *A:* Right eye showing mild, perifoveal RPE hyperpigmentation; left eye with right angle venules. *B:* Fluorescein angiogram of the same patient demonstrating hyperfluorescence of the telangiectatic vessels of the left eye in early views. *C and D:* Perifoveal leakage in both eyes in late views. *E:* Optical coherence tomography image of the same patient illustrating a hyperechogenic lesion in the perifoveal region with hyperplasia of RPE in the right eye and (*F*) a small cyst in the left eye.

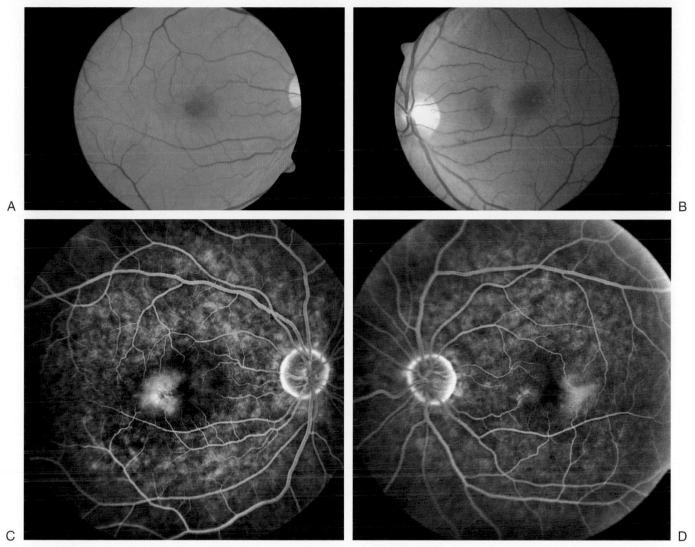

Figure 24–5 IPT. Appearance of bilateral lamellar macular holes in the right eye (*A*) and left eye (*B*). *C* and *D*: Corresponding intravenous fluorescein angiograms showing late temporal staining in both eyes.

leakage of dye with staining. RPE hyperplasia and intraretinal hemorrhages appear as blocking defects. It may be difficult to differentiate intraretinal leakage from IPT and leakage from a choroidal neovascular membrane. Group 3 patients have characteristic capillary nonperfusion.

24.3.2 OPTICAL COHERENCE TOMOGRAPHY

Optical coherence tomography (OCT) illustrates RPE changes as deformations of the hyperreflective retinal pigment epithelium band. In some cases the actual telangiectatic vessel can be imaged. It will be hyper-reflective and have mild shadowing beyond the vessel. It is useful for differentiating CNV from intraretinal leakage from the telangiectatic vessels.

24.4 Pathology

Gass contended that retinal capillary invasion of the retinal receptor layer and accumulation of extracellular fluid within the retina are seen in IPT. In addition, the angiographic staining pattern typical of IPT is due to nutritional deprivation of the middle retina, which leads to cellular damage. Eventually, degeneration of outer retinal cell layers leads to outer retinal atrophy that may simulate a lamellar macular hole. Loss of photoreceptor cells is responsible for the gradual decline in visual acuity and allows for retinal pigment epithelial cells to migrate into the overlying retina, particularly along right-angle venules. The etiology of the inner retinal crystals is unknown.

SUGGESTED READINGS

Alldredge CD, Garretson BR. Intravitreal triamcinolone for the treatment of idiopathic juxtafoveal telangiectasis. Retina. 2003; 23:113–116.

Gass JDM. Stereoscopic Atlas of Macular Diseases: Diagnosis and Treatment. 4th ed. St Louis, Mo: Mosby-Year Book, 1997:506–510.

Maberley DAL, Yannuzzi LA, Gitter K, et al. Radiation exposure: A new risk factor for idiopathic perifoveal telangiectasis. Ophthalmology. 1999;106:2248–2253.

Park DW, Schatz H, McDonald HR, Johnson RN. Grid laser photocoagulation for macular edema in bilateral juxtafoveal telangiectasis. Ophthalmology. 1997;104:1838–1846.

Potter MJ, Szabo SM, Chan EY, Morris AHC. Photodynamic therapy of a subretinal neovascular membrane in type 2a idiopathic juxtafoveolar retinal telangiectasis. Am J Ophthalmol. 2002; 133:149–151.

Chapter 25

Coats' Disease

ALEX MELAMUD, MD, MA • ELIAS I. TRABOULSI, MD • JONATHAN SEARS, M.D.

25.1 Introduction

Coats' disease was initially described by George Coats in 1908 and is an idiopathic condition characterized by retinal vascular telangiectasia and exudative retinopathy. It is one cause of nonrhegmatogenous or transudative or exudative retinal detachment. It can begin in early childhood with a mean age at diagnosis of 10 years and is generally unilateral (95%) and more frequent in male patients, often without hereditary or familial linkage. There are no systemic manifestations. The most common referral diagnoses are Coats' disease in 41% of patients, retinoblastoma (RB) in 27%, retinal detachment in 8%, retinal hemorrhage in 4%, toxocariasis in 3%, and unknown in 11%.

25.2 Clinical Signs and Symptoms

Patients with Coats' disease can present with leukocoria, strabismus, or poor vision in one eye or the abnormality may be discovered on a routine eye examination. Rarely, patients present with iris neovascularization and glaucoma. Coats' disease begins with excessive arborization and dilation of retinal vessels and capillary nonperfusion, usually on the temporal side of the peripheral fundus (**Figure 25–1A** and **B**). Abnormal arteriovenous communication can be seen early, which develops into tortuous, sheathed vessels with beading and aneurysm dilatations (**Figure 25–2**). Perivascular sheathing, circinate exudate, and subretinal exudate are commonly seen. Often perifoveal telangiectasia (**Figure 25–3A**)

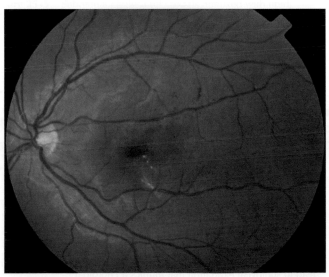
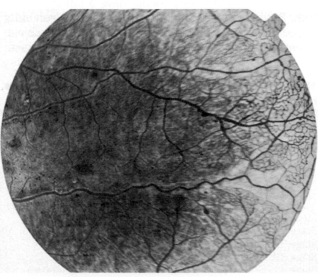

A   B

Figure 25–1   *A:* Telangiectatic vessels and aneurysms can be subtle but are often noted temporally. *B:* The extent of capillary nonperfusion is determined by fluorescein angiography to define the need for treatment.

25.3 Imaging and Diagnostic Tests

Fluorescein angiography is extremely helpful in differentiating Coats' disease from RB by highlighting the characteristic saccular aneurysms.

Ultrasonography does not show any evidence of calcification, which also helps in the differentiation from RB.

Computed tomography and magnetic resonance imaging scans can help in evaluation for calcium.

25.4 Pathology

Large saccular aneurysms with hypocellular vessels are seen as a result of an absent endothelium. Plasmoid and fibrinous transudates are found within and outside the vessel coat.

SUGGESTED READINGS

Chang MM, McLean IW, Merritt JC. Coats' disease: A study of 62 histologically confirmed cases. J Pediatr Ophthalmol. 1984;21:163–168.

Char DH. Coats' syndrome: Long term follow up. Br J Ophthalmol. 2000;84:37–39.

O'Brien JM, Char DH, Tucker N, et al. Efficacy of unanesthetized spiral computed tomography scanning in initial evaluation of childhood leukocoria. Ophthalmology. 1995;102:1345–1348.

Shields JA, Shields CL, Honavar S, Demirci H, Carter J. Classification and management of Coats disease. The 2000 Proctor Lecture. Am J Ophthalmol. 2001;131:572–583.

Shields JA, Shields CL, Honovar S, Demirci H, Coats disease: Clinical variations and complications of Coats disease in 150 cases. The 2000 Sanford Gifford Memorial Lecture. Am J Opthalmol. 2001; 31:561–571.

Chapter 26

Retinopathy of Prematurity

JONATHAN SEARS, MD

26.1 Introduction

Retinopathy of prematurity (ROP) is a disorder of low-birth-weight premature infants that features abnormal proliferation of developing blood vessels at the junction of vascular and avascular retina. First described in 1942, the relationship between oxygen supplementation and ROP became apparent after nearly 10,000 infants developed severe visual loss from intensive oxygen therapy, which was proven to increase the risk of ROP by three-fold in a subsequent multicenter randomized trial. The incidence of ROP fell as the use of supplemental oxygen was reduced, but a rebound in disease incidence has recently reflected the improved ability of neonatologists to decrease the mortality of extremely premature infants. Diagnosis and management of ROP offers insight into vasoproliferative retinal disease and the privilege of preserving vision in neonates. Today, ROP causes visual loss in 1300 children and severe visual loss in 500 children born each year in the United States.

26.2 Clinical Signs and Symptoms

The natural history of ROP has been clearly defined by the Cryotherapy for Retinopathy of Prematurity trial that demonstrated the relationship between low birth weight and early gestational age in a prospective cohort of 4009 infants with birth weight less than 1251 g. ROP occurred in 47% of infants weighing 1000 to 1251 g, 78% of infants weighing 750 to 999 g, and 90% of infants weighing less than 750 g. Eighty percent of infants born before 28 weeks of gestation develop ROP, whereas 60% of infants born between 28 and 31 weeks develop ROP. Low birth weight and young gestational age increase the likelihood of a larger area of avascular disease, which is related directly to unfavorable outcome. Approximately 50% of all premature infants develop ROP, 85% of whom demonstrate spontaneous regression. Although cryoretinopexy of avascular retina produced a favorable outcome in 50% of these infants in the original study, the rate of good anatomic outcome today has improved to better than 85% through the use of laser indirect ophthalmoscopy with a decrease in induced myopia compared with cryoretinopexy.

The International Classification of Retinopathy of Prematurity was created in 1984 and revised in 1987. The stages of ROP as described in this system begin with the development of a thin flat white demarcation between avascular and vascular retina, called Stage 1 (**Figure 26–1**). Stage 2 ROP occurs as the demarcation develops into an elevated thickened ridge or mesenchymal shunt (**Figure 26–2**). Stage 3 (**Figure 26–3**) is defined as extraretinal fibrovascular proliferation on the ridge, which may develop into a place of traction retinal detachment sparing the fovea, as in Stage 4A (**Figure 26–4A**), or including the fovea, as in Stage 4B (**Figure 26–4B**). Stage 5 describes a total, funnel-shaped retinal detachment that can be open or closed anteriorly and open or closed posteriorly (**Figure 26–5**). "Plus disease" is a critical sign of worsening disease and is seen as venous engorgement and arterial tortuosity at the disc and in the posterior pole (**Figure 26–6**). The ratio of the total area of vascularized versus avascular retina is an important prognostic feature of ROP because the avascular retina secretes growth factors such as vascular endothelial growth factor that promote normal vascularization in the nondisease state and abnormal vascularization in the disease state. Therefore, classification of ROP by location is a critical part of the examination for ROP as it is important for prognosis (**Figure 26–7**). Zone I is a circle the center of which is the disc with a radius twice

incorporating digital imaging into ROP screening, mostly because vasodilatation is probably the most important finding on an examination for ROP. Digital imaging is also useful for identifying high-risk Zone I eyes. Ultrasonography is useful for the diagnosis of retinal detachment in eyes with cataract and to help classify the shape and extent of detachment.

26.4 Treatment

Threshold ROP (the minimal extent of disease beyond which treatment with cryotherapy significantly improves vision) is defined as 5 contiguous or 8 noncontiguous clock hours of Stage 3 in Zone II or less with four of four quadrants plus disease, but the timing of laser therapy is open to debate, especially in Zone I eyes. Perhaps the most significant indicator of disease progression is plus disease, and often the extent of Stage 3 is under-

estimated because it may be difficult to visualize in its early development. The Early Treatment of Retinopathy of Prematurity Study has preliminarily shown a reduction in unfavorable outcome by modifying the threshold definition. At best, the definition of threshold is a synthesis of eye findings, gestational age and birth weight, systemic ongoing disease, and social situation with regard to follow-up. Cryotherapy has largely been replaced by argon or diode laser indirect ophthalmoscopy. Laser therapy may be easier to apply than cryotherapy, especially in posterior disease, at least as long as there is a good view of the retina (**Figure 26–8A** and **B**). Laser therapy has been shown to be superior to cryotherapy because of better structural and functional outcomes with laser indirect ophthalmoscopy. Lasered eyes are 5.2 times more likely to have 20/50 best-corrected visual acuity. Cryotherapy-treated eyes are 7.2 times more likely to have retinal dragging. Laser-treated eyes demonstrate a refraction of –4.48 D versus –7.65 D

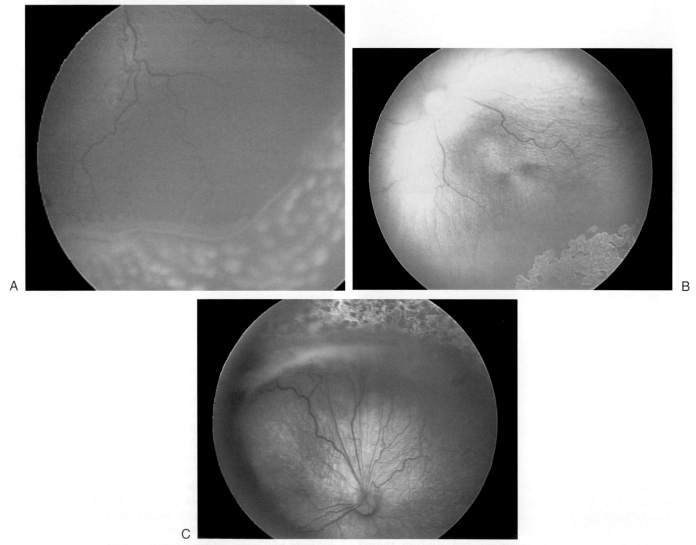

A

B

C

Figure 26–8 Laser indirect ophthalmoscopy. *A:* Laser burns become confluent acutely after laser use, indicating the need to maintain one burn width between spots. Typical settings for a diode laser include 250-mW power and 200-msec duration. *B:* Excellent regression after laser therapy can occur as early at 7 to 10 days. *C:* Active proliferation in the vitreous even after laser therapy indicates early Stage 4A detachment.

for cryotherapy-treated eyes. General anesthesia is usually used after dilation for laser treatment. A lid speculum is placed between the lids and topical methylcellulose is applied to preserve corneal clarity. Burns are placed 1 burn width apart beginning close to the ridge and covering all avascular retina. Small skip areas can lead to detachment with persistent disease; therefore, double-checking of the laser treatment is vital, as is meticulous scleral depression. Postlaser examination is performed at 1 to 2 weeks, and persistent plus disease or neovascular proliferation is an indications for segmental retreatment. Complications of laser treatment include cataract, burns of the iris and cornea, vitreous hemorrhage, and choroidal rupture. Hypotony is possible if the laser is applied too heavily at the horizontal meridians because of ischemia to the ciliary body from ablation of the long posterior ciliary artery and nerve. After laser use, 1 drop each of topical prednisolone acetate 1% 4 times per day and 0.5% cyclopentolate 2 times per day are administered for 1 week. Acutely elevating the head 30 degrees or more may help prevent pooling of edema in the macula after a particularly heavy laser treatment.

Surgical repair of ROP retinal detachment can involve scleral buckle, lens-sparing vitrectomy (LSV), or limbal lensectomy and vitrectomy. Success largely depends on stage: Stage 4A detachments are successfully repaired in more than 90% of infants by LSV, Stage 4B detachments are repaired successfully in 80% to 90% by LSV or limbal lensectomy and vitrectomy, and Stage 5 detachments are repaired successfully in less than 50% by either limbal lensectomy or vitrectomy with or without scleral buckle. There is some debate as to the validity of scleral buckle for 4A detachment when excellent results have been reported for LSV alone.

26.5 Pathology

Stage 1 ROP is characterized by hyperplasia of primitive spindle-shaped cells of the advancing mesenchymal tissue at the intersection of the avascular and vascular retina. Stage 2 consists of proliferating endothelial cells at the vascular retina side of the ridge. Stage 3 shows extraretinal vascular tissue that emanates from the ridge. Critically, condensation of vitreous sheets and strands become oriented anteriorly toward the lens. These tractional forces draw the retina anteriorly and centrally.

26.6 Controversies in Retinopathy of Prematurity

Controversial issues in the management of ROP include screening, neonatal intensive care unit (NICU) practice, the definition of threshold disease, and the treatment of threshold disease. Currently, screening recommendations at the Cleveland Clinic include examination for any infant of less than 1500-g birth weight or less than 31 weeks' gestation or use of oxygen for longer than 24 hours. The initial eye examination is performed at

5 to 7 weeks of age. Examinations are discontinued when any one of three "minimal risk" signs is present: 45 weeks' postmenstrual age without prethreshold ROP or worse, Zone III without previous Zone II, or full retinal vascularization. Screening using telemedicine is currently under clinical study. Trained technician and certified graders using digital fundus imaging achieve a sensitivity of 60% to 80% in detecting and grading. Ophthalmoscopy at present is still necessary.

NICU practice has changed to conform to the findings that vitamin E, light, and steroids do not contribute to the development or regression of ROP. The use of supplemental oxygen with saturation maintained at greater than 94% did not cause progression of prethreshold ROP and did not reduce the number of threshold cases, although avoidance of hyperoxia-hypoxia changes has resulted in a 10% reduction in Stage 3 ROP and a reduction in threshold ROP from 4.5% to 0%. Although these may be modest results, they confirm findings in the animal model of ROP and the paradoxical nature of oxygen therapy.

Treatment of threshold eyes and eyes with retinal detachment are perhaps the last areas of controversy. A reevaluation of the definition of threshold disease is necessary because (1) the Cryotherapy for Retinopathy of Prematurity study dealt mainly with Zone II eyes, (2) 44% of treated eyes had unfavorable outcome, and (3) untreated Zone I threshold eyes have a 90% chance of an unfavorable outcome. Therefore, Zone I eyes may behave differently than anterior Zone II eyes. For example, there may be direct progression to Stage 3 without a ridge. Finally, the concept of early treatment of retinal detachment in Stage 4A deserves evaluation. Recent data have shown that Stage 4A detachment is easier to fix than 4B and especially Stage 5 detachments. In addition, scleral buckle may or may not be helpful in Stage 4A because greater than 90% success with lens-sparing vitrectomy alone has been reported for Stage 4A detachment. Despite the controversial issues regarding the diagnosis and management of ROP, success depends on sustained diligence and vigilance.

SUGGESTED READINGS

Capone A Jr, Diaz-Rohena R, Sternberg P Jr, Mandell B, Lambert HM, Lopez PF. Diode-laser photocoagulation for zone 1 threshold retinopathy of prematurity. Am J Ophthalmol. 1993;116:444–450.
Capone A Jr, Trese M. Lens sparing vitreous surgery for tractional stage 4A retinopathy of prematurity retinal detachments. Ophthalmology. 2001; 108:2068–2070.
International Committee for the Classification of the Late Stages of Retinopathy of Prematurity. An international classification of retinopathy of prematurity: The classification of retinal detachment. Arch Ophthalmol. 1987;104:905–912.
Nagata M, Kobayashi Y, Fukuda H, et al. Photocoagulation for the treatment of retinopathy of prematurity. Jpn J Clin Ophthalmol. 1968;22:419–427.
Patz A, Hoeck LE, DeLacruz E. Studies on the effect of high oxygen concentration on retrolental fibroplasias: Nursery observations. Am J Ophthalmol. 1952;35:1248–1253.
Phelps DL. Retinopathy of prematurity. N Engl J Med. 1995; 326;1078–1080.
Terry TL. Extreme prematurity and fibroblastic overgrowth of persistent vascular sheath behind each crystalline lens: I. Preliminary report. Am J Ophthalmol. 1942;25:203–204.

Chapter 27

Ocular Ischemic Syndrome

PETER G. HOVLAND, MD, PhD • MICHAEL S. IP, MD

27.1 Introduction

Ocular ischemic syndrome (OIS) results from significantly reduced blood flow to the eye and orbit, most often as a consequence of ipsilateral internal carotid artery atherosclerotic stenosis or obstruction. The reduction of normal blood flow to the eye may result in a variety of signs and symptoms depending on the severity of the compromise, as well as the degree to which anastomotic sources of perfusion are present. Although the majority of patients with OIS have severe occlusive carotid artery disease, a significant minority do not, with the ocular ischemic condition resulting from occlusive disease of the ophthalmic, central retinal, or ciliary arteries. Anterior and posterior segments may be affected with differing degrees of severity. Other causes of impaired ocular blood flow and consequent OIS include vasculitides, such as giant cell arteritis, Takayasu's arteritis, or carotid artery dissection. Not all patients with significant carotid artery occlusion have OIS.

The major source of blood flow to the eye and orbital structures is the ophthalmic artery, which is the first major intracranial branch of the internal carotid artery. With significant stenosis of the internal carotid artery—usually at the level of the carotid bifurcation—the supply of blood to the ipsilateral eye becomes compromised. Anastomotic perfusion of the affected orbit can come from the circle of Willis via retrograde flow inferiorly in the patent superior portion of the internal carotid artery to the ipsilateral ophthalmic artery. In the event of an imperforate anterior communicating artery, or other compromise to the communications of the circle of Willis, the blood flow to the ischemic eye may come from alternative anastomoses from the ipsilateral external carotid artery. The anastomotic pathway may be via the angular artery or, alternatively, via the recurrent meningeal artery to the lacrimal artery. Either anastomotic pathway leads to the ophthalmic artery. A pathognomonic finding of OIS is detection of retrograde blood flow in the ophthalmic artery.

The average age of a patient with OIS is approximately 65 years. There is an approximate twofold predilection for males, with no known racial bias. Whereas the disease is usually unilateral in presentation, there is no associated right-left laterality. The prevalence has been estimated at 7.5 per 1 million. The systemic associations found in OIS include diabetes mellitus (56%), hypertension (50% to 73%), ischemic heart disease (38% to 48%), and cerebrovascular disease (27% to 31%). The 5-year mortality of patients with OIS has been estimated to be 40%, with the majority of deaths occurring as a consequence of cardiovascular disease. The differential diagnosis of OIS includes central retinal artery occlusion, central retinal vein occlusion, giant cell arteritis, and hyperviscosity syndromes such as leukemia.

27.2 Clinical Signs and Symptoms

Decreased flow of blood to the eye may cause an array of effects, with findings in both the anterior and posterior segments, depending on the degree of which specific tissues are affected. A right-left asymmetry of signs or symptoms should raise suspicion of ocular ischemia.

Intraocular pressure (IOP) is elevated in approximately one third of patients with OIS, whereas it is normal or low IOP in approximately two thirds of patients. Pressure elevation may be due to neovascularization of the angle, whereas reduced IOP may result from decreased perfusion of the ciliary body. Anterior segment

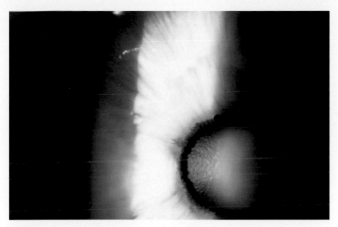

Figure 27–1 Neovascularization of the iris in a patient with OIS. (Courtesy of Matthew Johnson.)

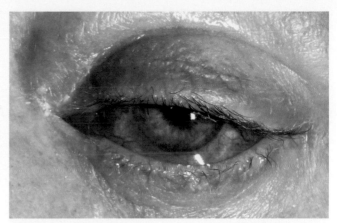

Figure 27–3 External photo of a patient with OIS demonstrating episcleral injection. (Courtesy of Barbara Blodi, MD.)

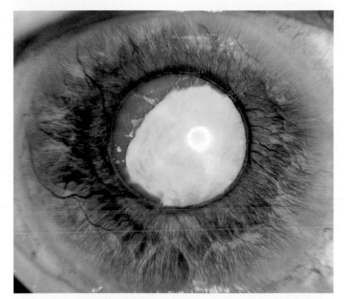

Figure 27–2 Advanced neovascularization of the iris in a patient with chronic OIS. Note the cataractous lens. (Courtesy of Celeste Jend, OD.)

findings include neovascularization of the iris (NVI) (**Figures 27–1** and **27–2**), occurring in 67% to 90% of patients with OIS. The stimulus driving NVI is probably impairment of either retinal or uveal circulation. NVI is commonly associated with an anterior chamber inflammatory response. Another characteristic sign of OIS in the anterior segment is episcleral vessel dilation (**Figure 27–3**), which is thought to be due to increased anastomotic blood flow from the branches of the ipsilateral external carotid artery. Other OIS-associated signs include a mid-dilated, poorly reactive pupil, corneal edema due to elevated IOP, iris atrophy, and cataract.

Posterior segment findings primarily involve the retinal vasculature. The majority—estimated to be 80%—of patients with OIS have unilateral retinal involvement. A characteristic finding in OIS is patchy, mid-peripheral retinal hemorrhages (**Figure 27–4A–C**).

The distribution of retinal hemorrhages in OIS may be distinguished from that found in CRVO in that they are less commonly found in the posterior pole. Retinal venous dilation with or without tortuosity is a common feature. Retinal arterial pulsation may be easily induced with light digital pressure to the eye during funduscopy, indicative of poor ocular perfusion pressure. Spontaneous retinal arterial pulsations occur when the diastolic retinal arterial pressure falls below the IOP. This finding is highly suggestive of OIS. Retinal arteriolar narrowing as a consequence of ischemia may also be seen. Retinal capillary nonperfusion may be noted on fluorescein angiography. The macula may have a cherry red spot in the center indicative of ischemia (12%). Neovascularization of the disc (NVD) is common (35%), and neovascularization elsewhere occurs less commonly (5%) and usually in the setting of concurrent NVD. Macular edema may occur, thought to be a consequence of damaged vascular endothelium, with subsequent leakage of fluid from vessel walls.

The main symptom of OIS is visual loss. Typically, patients experience an onset of visual loss over a period of weeks to months. However, the visual loss may be sudden or transient or associated with positional changes or even light-evoked amaurosis. A significant proportion of patients, estimated to be 20%, will be asymptomatic. Additionally, approximately 40% of patients with OIS may report an ipsilateral brow ache, sometimes termed *ocular angina*. Patients suspected of having OIS need to have a careful review of their neurologic history to identify any signs of concurrent cerebral ischemia. Patient history questions should be directed to elicit occurrences of sensory or motor deficits, headaches, dizziness, numbness, tingling, and memory loss. The risk factors for ocular ischemia (hypertension, diabetes, and carotid stenosis) predispose patients for an increased probability of stroke. If OIS is suspected urgent referral to a neurologist, neurosurgeon, or vascular surgeon is indicated for management of stroke risk factors. Definitive treatment of the patient's condition may require further medical or surgical intervention.

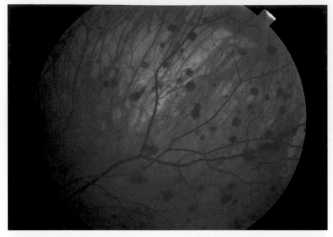

A

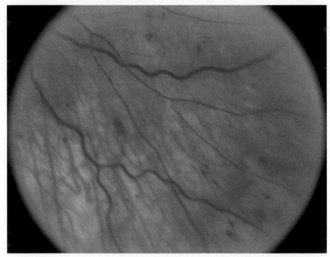

B

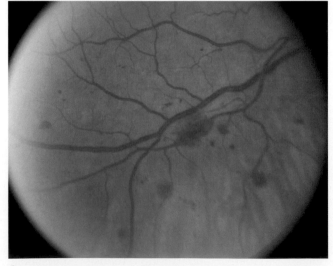

C

Figure 27–4 *A–C:* Mid-peripheral hemorrhages of two patients with complete ipsilateral internal carotid artery occlusion. (Courtesy of Thomas Stevens, MD.)

27.3 Imaging and Diagnostic Tests

27.3.1 FLUORESCEIN ANGIOGRAPHY

OIS is characterized by delayed arterial filling and delayed arteriovenous transit time (**Figures 27–5** and **27–6A–D**), found in 95% of patients with OIS. Capillary nonperfusion may be noted more in the periphery, in a diffuse distribution, in contrast to the sharp border seen more commonly in branch retinal vein occlusions. The areas of nonperfused retina, if present, are important to identify carefully for targeted scatter laser treatment. Delayed or patchy choroidal filling may also be found. Late leakage from retinal arterioles and veins is a common finding (85%), as is macular edema.

27.3.2 OPHTHALMODYNAMOMETRY

This technique allows measurement of the force applied externally to the globe to cause retinal arterial pulsations and obstruction. As a diagnostic tool, it may detect, by inference, obstructions of greater than 90% of the ipsilateral internal carotid artery.

27.3.3 ORBITAL DOPPLER/COLOR DOPPLER IMAGING

This ultrasound technology may be used to examine blood flow in orbital arteries and to establish the presence of retrograde flow in the ophthalmic artery. Use of this technique is not commonplace clinically, but it has been used to establish the association of reduced retrobulbar blood flow with OIS.

27.3.4 PHOTOPIC STRESS TEST

Patients with OIS may experience increased sensation of afterimages, with prolonged recovery of visual acuity after temporary exposure to bright illumination. This phenomenon is thought to be due to impaired regeneration of photopigments within the photoreceptors as a consequence of reduced blood flow. Asymmetric, prolonged recovery of visual acuity is suggestive of OIS.

27.3.5 ELECTRORETINOGRAPHY

Electroretinography testing shows depressed a and b waves indicative of both inner and outer retinal ischemia, as a consequence of the comorbid retinal and choroidal ischemia found in OIS.

27.3.6 VISUAL FIELD TESTING

A variety of visual field defects have been described in OIS, including central scotoma, temporal island only, and central and nasal defects.

27.3.7 CAROTID DOPPLER DUPLEX ULTRASOUND

This noninvasive study is a common preliminary screening test to evaluate internal carotid artery stenosis and

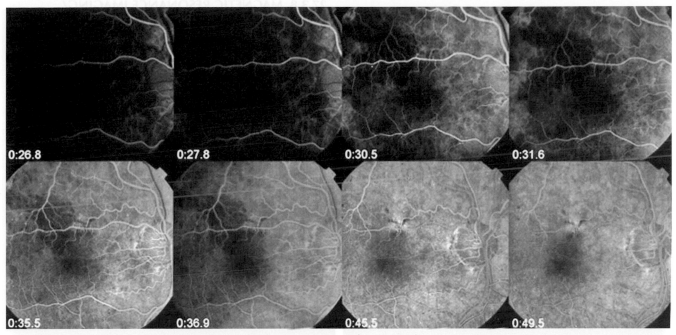

Figure 27–5 Fluorescein angiography demonstrating delayed arteriolar filling and late arteriolar leakage.

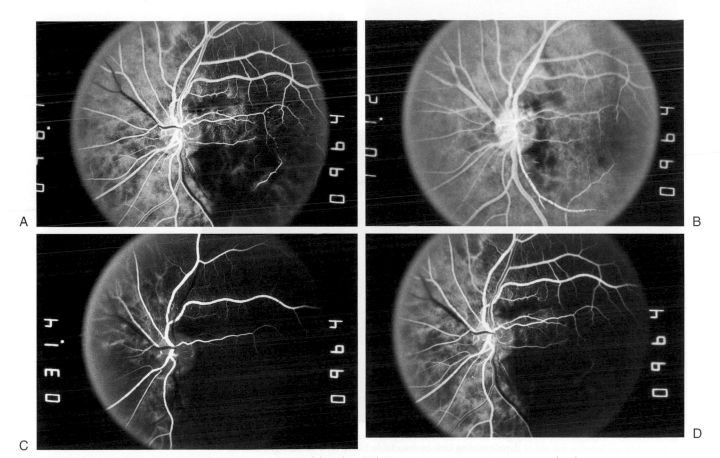

Figure 27–6 *A–D:* Fluorescein angiography demonstrating delayed arterial-venous transition time in a patient with Takayasu's arteritis. (Courtesy of Barbara Blodi, MD.)

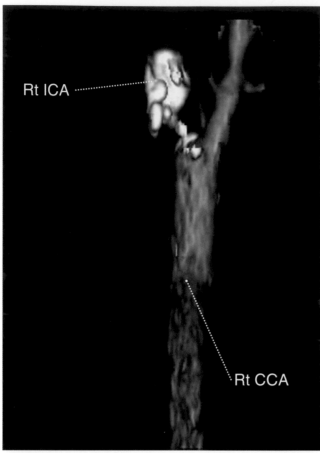

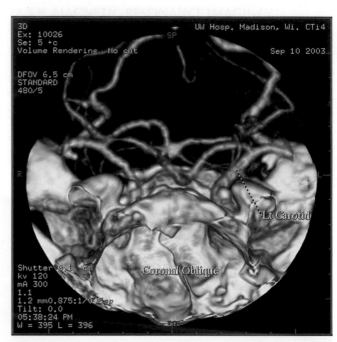

Figure 27–14 Computed tomography arteriography anatomic reconstruction showing complete lack of perfusion to the circle of Willis from an obstructed right internal carotid artery.

Figure 27–12 Computed tomography arteriography demonstrating complete obstruction of the right internal carotid artery (Rt ICA). Rt CCA, right common carotid artery.

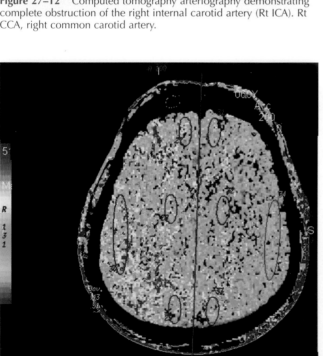

Figure 27–13 Computed tomography arteriography demonstrating complete delayed cerebral perfusion of the right cerebral hemisphere as a consequence of a right internal carotid artery obstruction in a patient with OIS.

27.4 Pathology

Intraretinal hemorrhages and microaneurysms have been found in the midperipheral retina by histologic examination and are probably a consequence of loss of pericytes due to chronic ischemia of the vessels.

SUGGESTED READINGS

Atebara NH, Brown GC. Ocular ischemic syndrome. In: Tasman W, Jaeger EA, eds. Duane's Clinical Ophthalmology. Philadelphia, Pa: Lippincott Williams & Wilkins, 1998;3 (chap 12):1–19.

Brown GC, Magargal LE. The ocular ischemic syndrome: Clinical, fluorescein angiographic and carotid angiographic features. Int Ophthalmol. 1988;11:239–251.

Fox, GM, Sivalingham A, Brown GC. Ocular ischemic syndrome. In: Yanoff M, Duker J, eds. Ophthalmology. St Louis, Mo: Mosby, 1999.

Mizener JB, Podhajsky P, Hayreh SS. Ocular ischemic syndrome. Ophthalmology. 1997;104:859–864.

Ryan SJ, Schachat AP, Murphy RP, Patz A. The ocular ischemic syndrome. In: Ryan SJ, ed. Retina. 1989;II:547–559.

Chapter 28

Hypertensive Retinopathy

ALEX MELAMUD, MA, MD • PETER K. KAISER, MD

28.1 Introduction

Hypertension is defined as blood pressure greater than 140 mm Hg systolic or 90 mm Hg diastolic. It is estimated that 60 million Americans older than 18 years of age have hypertension, with a higher prevalence in African Americans. Vascular changes related to high blood pressure were first described in the mid-1800s. Uncontrolled hypertension can cause vascular changes in many organ systems. In the eye, vascular changes related to high blood pressure can be observed under direct visualization. Specific attention should be focused on a careful examination of the fundus with particular emphasis on the retina, the choroid, and the optic nerve.

28.2 Clinical Signs and Symptoms

Two systems of classification are most widely used today. The Keith-Wagener-Barker classification groups findings based on the severity of changes observed on ophthalmoscopy (**Table 28–1**). A more recent classification scheme proposed by Scheie organizes hypertensive and arteriolar sclerosis findings separately (**Table 28–2**).

TABLE 28–1 ▰
Keith-Wagener-Barker Classification

Group	Description
I	Minimal constriction and tortuosity of arterioles
II	Moderate constriction of arterioles; focal narrowing and arteriovenous nicking
III	Arteriolar constriction and focal narrowing; cotton-wool spots, hemorrhages and exudates
IV	Similar findings to group III, plus papilledema

Arteriolar narrowing is a hallmark of hypertensive retinopathy (**Figure 28–1**). Narrowing can be focal or diffuse and is probably the most reliable sign of systemic hypertension. In a normal fundus, the arteriole-to-venule ratio is 2:3. This ratio is proportionately reduced at each stage of hypertension-induced retinopathy.

Hypertensive retinopathy manifests as a change in the light reflex of the arterioles observed under ophthalmoscopy. Chronic hypertension induces a hypertrophy of the intima and muscular layers of the arteriole with luminal narrowing (**Figure 28–2**). As the walls of the blood vessels thicken, the light reflex from the arterioles becomes duller and more diffuse. In early hypertension these changes are subtle. With advanced retinopathy, the light reflex takes on a dull reddish hue resembling a "copper wire." Severe chronic hypertension is

TABLE 28–2 ▰
Scheie Classification

Grade	Description
Hypertension Changes	
0	No visible changes
I	Diffuse arteriolar narrowing
II	Pronounced arteriolar narrowing and focal constriction
III	Grade II plus retinal hemorrhages
IV	Grade III plus optic disc edema
Arteriolar Sclerosis Changes	
0	No visible changes
I	Minimal light reflex changes of arterioles
II	Moderate light reflex changes of arterioles
III	Copper-wire appearance of arterioles
IV	Silver-wire appearance of arterioles

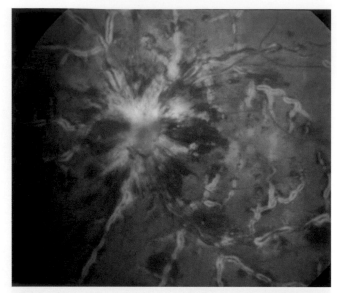

Figure 28–9 Central retinal vein occlusion in a patient with uncontrolled hypertension.

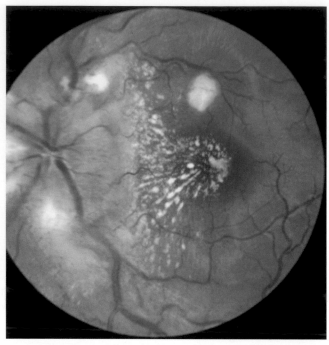

Figure 28–11 Same patient as in **Figure 28–10** (left eye).

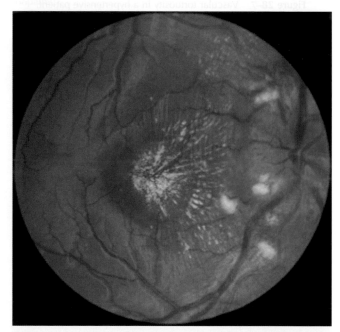

Figure 28–10 Patient with malignant hypertension due to a pheochromocytoma (right eye). Notice the papilledema, cotton-wool spots, and macular exudates due to breakdown of the blood-retina barrier. The patient promptly underwent surgery for removal of the pheochromocytoma.

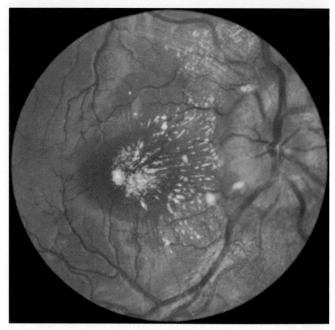

Figure 28–12 After surgery, the patient's blood pressure returned to normal. On ophthalmic examination 1 week later there is minimal improvement (compare with **Figure 28–11**), but already there are fewer cotton-wool spots around the optic nerve (right eye).

patchy yellow lesions (**Figure 28–15**). With time, the RPE becomes hyperpigmented with a surrounding halo of hypopigmentation (Elschnig's spots). These changes are most prominent in the mid-periphery and around the optic nerve. In chronic hypertension, RPE overlying choroidal vessels undergoes hypertrophy and hyperpigmentation, leading to linear configurations known as Siegrist's streaks. Leakage from incompetent choroidal vessels accumulates under the neurosensory retina and

RPE, producing localized bullous serous detachments (**Figures 28–16** and **28–17**).

28.2.3 HYPERTENSIVE OPTIC NEUROPATHY

Malignant hypertension causes acute optic nerve swelling with surrounding capillary dilation and stasis of axoplasmic flow (**Figure 28–18**).

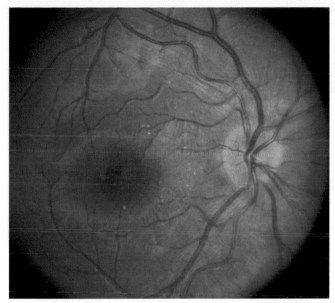

Figure 28–13 At 6 months follow-up after surgery (compare to **Figure 28–12**), there is dramatic improvement in the appearance of the fundus (right eye). The papilledema has resolved along with the macular exudates.

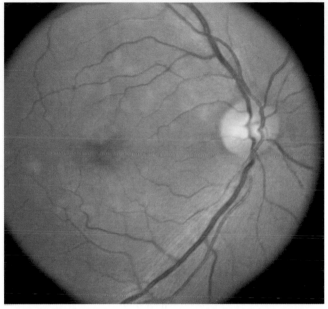

Figure 28–15 Deep patchy hypopigmented lesions in the posterior pole corresponding to areas of choroidal ischemia.

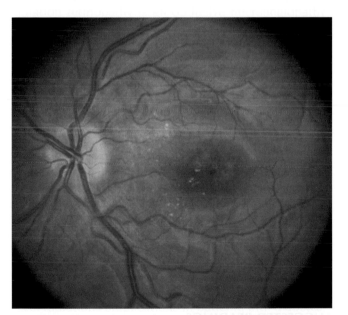

Figure 28–14 Same patient as in **Figure 28–15** (left eye).

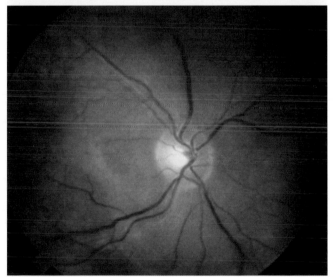

Figure 28–16 Leakage from incompetent choroidal vessels accumulates under the neurosensory retina, producing a localized serous detachment inferior and temporal to the optic nerve.

28.3 Imaging and Diagnostic Tests

28.3.1 COLOR PHOTOGRAPHS

Color photography is a useful way to document findings and monitor progression of the disease. Signs of hypertensive retinopathy include superficial, flame-shaped hemorrhages, arteriovenous crossing changes (nicking), retinal arteriole narrowing/straightening, copper- or silver-wire arteriole changes (arteriolosclerosis), cotton-wool spots, microaneurysms, hard exudates (may be in a circinate or macular star pattern), Elschnig's spots (yellow [early] or hyperpigmented [late] patches of retinal pigment epithelium overlying infarcted choriocapillaris lobules), Siegrist streaks (linear hyperpigmented areas over choroidal vessels), arterial macroaneurysms, and disc hyperemia or edema with dilated tortuous vessels (in malignant hypertension).

28.3.2 FLUORESCEIN ANGIOGRAPHY

Fluorescein angiography can aid in the evaluation of vascular pathologic changes including aneurysms, leaking capillaries, and areas of ischemia (**Figure 28–19**). Areas

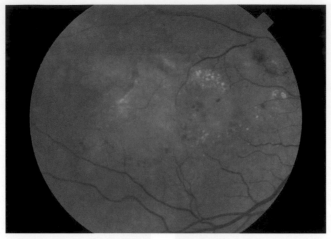

Figure 29–1   Radiation retinopathy after proton beam irradiation for choroidal melanoma with hard exudates, retinal hemorrhages, and macular edema.

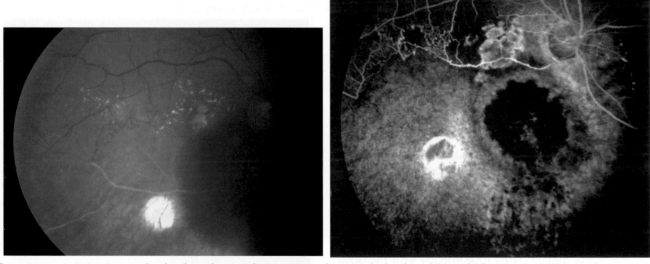

A   B

Figure 29–2   *A:* Extensive vascular sheathing due to radiation retinopathy. Note the hard exudates and telangiectatic retinal vessels. *B:* Fluorescein angiogram of the same eye demonstrating the extensive capillary nonperfusion in the area of the treated melanoma.

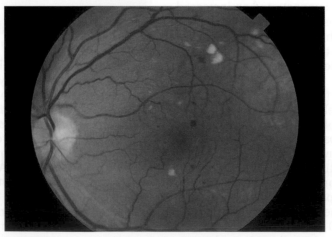

Figure 29–3   Mild radiation retinopathy with a few retinal hemorrhages and cotton-wool spots adjacent to the irradiated area.

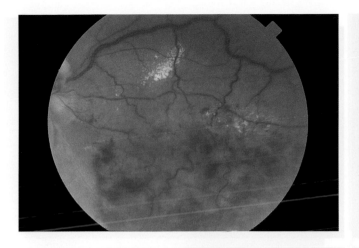
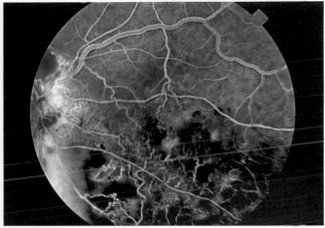

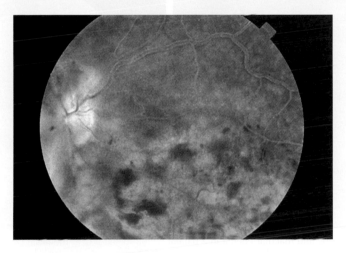

Figure 29–4 *A:* Radiation maculopathy after treatment of a peripapillary melanoma leading to branch vein occlusion with extensive retinal hemorrhages, exudates, and macular edema. *B* and *C:* Fluorescein angiogram of the same patient demonstrating the vein occlusion and prominent telangiectasis of retinal vessels with leakage into the macula.

choroidal melanoma. Similarly, retinal neovascularization occurred in 6% of patients after proton beam irradiation for choroidal melanoma in the series reported by Guyer and co-authors (**Figure 29–6A** and **B**). A higher rate of posterior segment neovascularization (44%) was observed in the group of patients reported by Brown and colleagues who received external beam irradiation, mostly for orbital and other intracranial malignancies. This difference may have been related to the larger retinal area affected with external beam treatment or to the significant proportion of patients in this group who received chemotherapy. Subretinal neovascularization and central retinal artery or vein occlusion have also been described as rare associations with ocular radiation exposure.

Manifestations of radiation papillopathy include disc edema associated with exudates, hemorrhages, cotton-wool spots, microvascular changes, and neovascularization. Radiation-induced optic neuropathy may lead to optic atrophy and loss of light perception, but in a small number of patients, the papillopathy may improve (**Figure 29–7A–C** and **29–8A–C**). Most patients develop some degree of disc pallor. In patients treated with proton beam irradiation, 5 years after the onset of papillopathy, 69% had lost three lines of vision, 31% had visual improvement of three lines, and 17% had lost light perception.

29.3 Imaging and Diagnostic Tests

29.3.1 FLUORESCEIN ANGIOGRAPHY

The hallmark of radiation retinopathy demonstrated on fluorescein angiography is capillary nonperfusion (**Figures 29–9** to **29–11**). Other common findings include telangiectasias, microaneurysms, and macular edema. Leakage from the disc or retinal neovascularization may also be observed.

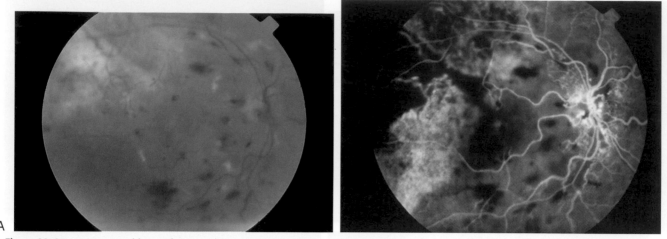

Figure 29–9   *A:* Intraretinal hemorrhages and cotton-wool spots seen after proton beam irradiation for choroidal melanoma. *B:* Extensive capillary nonperfusion seen on fluorescein angiography involving the entire macula in addition to the area overlying the tumor.

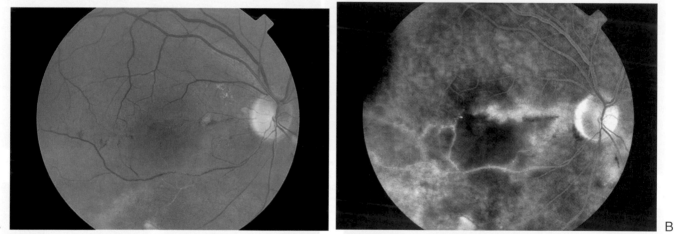

Figure 29–10   *A:* Sheathing and telangiectasis of retinal vessels adjacent to a paramacular melanoma after radiation treatment. A cotton-wool spot and mild exudates are also seen. *B:* Fluorescein angiogram reveals capillary nonperfusion in the foveal area.

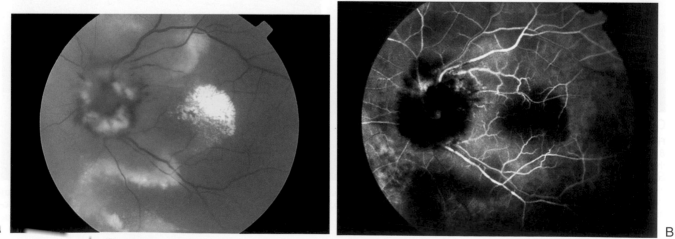

Figure 29–11   *A:* Severe radiation papillopathy with nerve fiber layer infarction surrounding the nerve head, subretinal fluid, and extensive exudation in the macula. *B:* Fluorescein angiogram of the same eye demonstrating severe ischemia of the optic nerve.

29.4 Pathology

Histopathologic analysis of human eyes after radiation exposure has revealed retinal capillary changes including microaneurysms and fusiform dilations. Endothelial cell loss appeared to predominate in contrast to the pericyte loss typically seen in diabetic retinopathy. Thickening of the walls of larger retinal vessels from deposition of fibrillar or hyaline material has also been observed. The vascular damage is presumed to cause secondary changes in the inner retina. Loss of ganglion cells and cystic changes in the outer plexiform and inner nuclear layers have been seen in the setting of neovascular glaucoma. Photoreceptors appear relatively resistant to irradiation.

SUGGESTED READINGS

Brown GC, Shields JA, Sanborn G, Augsburger JJ, Savino PJ, Schatz NJ. Radiation retinopathy. Ophthalmology. 1982;89:1294–1501.

Gragoudas ES, Li W, Lane AM, Munzenrider J, Egan KM. Risk factors for radiation maculopathy and papillopathy after intraocular irradiation. Ophthalmology. 1999;106:1571–1578.

Gündüz K, Shields CL, Shields JA, Cater J, Freire JE, Brady LW. Radiation retinopathy following plaque radiotherapy for posterior uveal melanoma. Arch Ophthalmol. 1999;117:609–614.

Guyer DR, Mukai S, Egan KM, Seddon JM, Walsh SM, Gragoudas ES. Radiation maculopathy after proton beam irradiation for choroidal melanoma. Ophthalmology. 1992;99:1278–1285.

Parsons JT, Bova FJ, Fitzgerald CR, Mendenhall WM, Million RR. Radiation retinopathy after external beam irradiation: Analysis of time-dose factors. Int J Radiat Oncol Biol Phys. 1994;30:765–773.

Chapter 30

Retinal Artery Macroaneurysm

CARL D. REGILLO, MD • NICHOLAS G. ANDERSON, MD

30.1 Introduction

Retinal artery macroaneurysms are acquired focal dilatations of the retinal arterioles. They are typically located at arterial bifurcations or arteriovenous crossings within the first three divisions of arteriolar branching. Involvement of the superotemporal and inferotemporal arcades is most commonly reported. Macroaneurysms have also rarely been reported arising from the optic disc and from a cilioretinal artery. Multiple aneurysms are often found in different arteries of the same eye, but bilateral involvement is seen only in 10% of occurrences.

Affected patients are typically older than 60 years of age. Women comprise approximately three quarters of patients. Systemic hypertension is the most frequently associated condition and is found in two thirds of patients. Generalized arteriosclerotic cardiovascular disease is also commonly seen.

No ocular risk factors for retinal artery macroaneurysms have been identified, although they have been found in patients with branch retinal artery and vein occlusion, angiomatosis retinae, Eale's disease, Leber's military aneurysms, and Coats' disease.

30.2 Clinical Signs and Symptoms

Although patients with retinal artery macroaneurysms may be asymptomatic, the most common presenting symptom is acute or insidious loss of vision due to hemorrhage, retinal edema, or exudation involving the central macular region. On funduscopic examination, macroaneurysms are round or fusiform dilations of the arterial wall (**Figure 30–1**). One third to two thirds of patients have an associated hemorrhage, which may

be located in the subretinal space, within the retina, beneath the internal limiting membrane, or in the vitreous cavity. A hemorrhage involving more than one of these locations is characteristic of retinal arterial macroaneurysm, and the term *hourglass hemorrhage* has been suggested to describe the simultaneous collection of preretinal and subretinal heme (**Figure 30–2**). The aneurysm may be visible within the hemorrhage as a

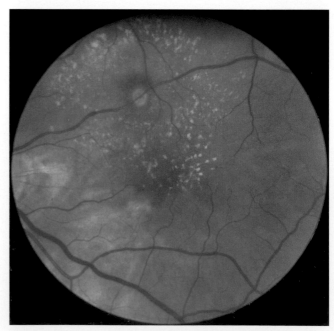

Figure 30–1 On funduscopy, a retinal artery macroaneurysm is visualized as a focal dilation of the artery. Note the surrounding circinate lipid. (Courtesy of William E. Benson, MD.)

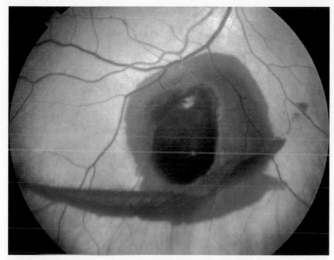

Figure 30–2 Typical hourglass hemorrhage consisting of simultaneous preretinal and subretinal as well as subhyaloid hemorrhage.

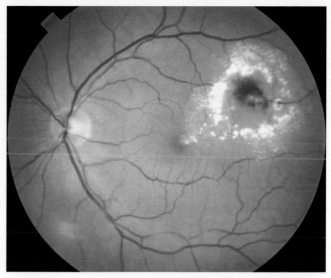

Figure 30–4 Macroaneurysm with chronic exudation leading to circinate lipid deposition. (Courtesy of Alfred Lucier, MD.)

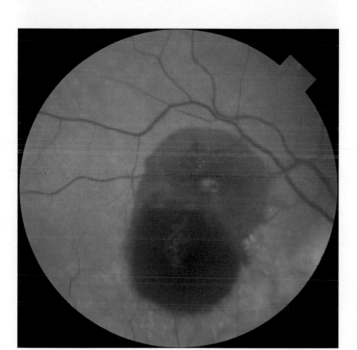

Figure 30–3 Retinal artery macroaneurysm is visible as a white spot within the surrounding intraretinal and subretinal hemorrhage. (Courtesy of William E. Benson, MD.)

30.3 Imaging and Diagnostic Tests

30.3.1 FLUORESCEIN ANGIOGRAPHY

Early phases of the fluorescein angiogram usually demonstrate immediate, uniform filling of the macroaneurysm (**Figure 30–5**). Partial filling may occur due to obliteration of the lumen resulting from thrombosis or spontaneous involution. The involved artery is typically patent but may be narrowed and irregular proximal and distal to the lesion. Surrounding microvascular abnormalities, including capillary microaneurysms, telangiectasias, and nonperfusion, are often seen. The late

white or yellow spot (**Figure 30–3**). A subretinal hemorrhage may simulate a choroidal melanoma or choroidal neovascularization. Occasionally, patients present with dense vitreous hemorrhage from a retinal artery macroaneurysm.

Chronic exudation from the macroaneurysm often leads to intraretinal edema and lipid deposition. These deposits may adopt a circinate pattern, prompting the observer to search for a macroaneurysm in the center of the lesion (**Figure 30–4**). Subretinal fluid accumulation may lead to a neurosensory retinal detachment.

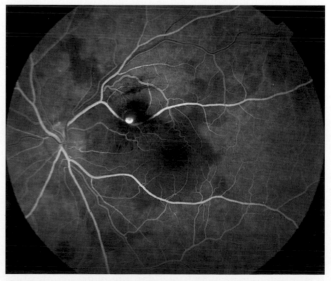

Figure 30–5 Uniform filling of a macroaneurysm during the early phase of a fluorescein angiogram. Note the adjacent preretinal and subretinal hemorrhage that block fluorescein.

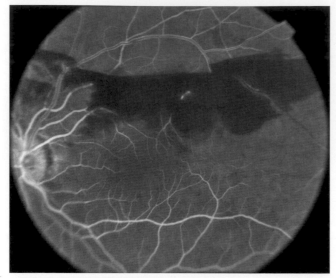

Figure 30–6 Blockage due to a preretinal hemorrhage obscures the underlying macroaneurysm.

phases of the angiogram may demonstrate only faint staining of the involved vessel or may demonstrate marked leakage resulting in cystoid or diffuse retinal edema. Intraretinal and preretinal hemorrhage may block background retinal and choroidal fluorescence or may obscure the macroaneurysm itself (**Figure 30–6**).

30.3.2 INDOCYANINE GREEN ANGIOGRAPHY

With relatively dense intraretinal or preretinal hemorrhages, ophthalmoscopy and fluorescein angiography may not be able to demonstrate the macroaneurysm due to the blocking effect of the overlying blood. Indocyanine green (ICG) angiography can be useful in these cases because the increased penetrance of ICG fluorescent light through blood may allow visualization of the macroaneurysm as a discrete hyperfluorescent lesion (**Figure 30–7A** and **B**).

30.3.3 OPTICAL COHERENCE TOMOGRAPHY

Macular thickness can be accurately measured by optical coherence tomography (OCT) because of the well-defined boundaries in optical reflectivity at the inner and outer margins of the neurosensory retina. The high longitudinal resolution of OCT permits measurement of retinal thickness to within 10 microns. OCT can therefore be useful to demonstrate associated macular edema due to leakage from retinal arterial macroaneurysms (**Figure 30–8**). Sequential tomograms can be used to track spontaneous resolution of macular edema or response to therapy.

30.3.4 ULTRASOUND

If vitreous hemorrhage precludes adequate visualization of the retina by ophthalmoscopy, standard B-scan ultrasonography may be useful in making the diagnosis

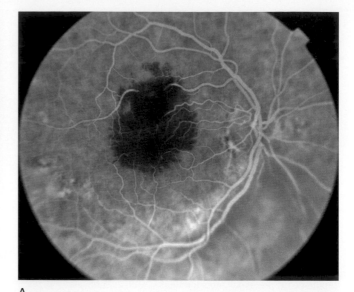

A

B

Figure 30–7 *A:* On a fluorescein angiogram, the macroaneurysm is obscured by overlying hemorrhage. (Courtesy of Sunir Garg, MD.) *B:* Using ICG angiography, the macroaneurysm is visible as a hyperfluorescent lesion beneath the hemorrhage. (Courtesy of Sunir Garg, MD.)

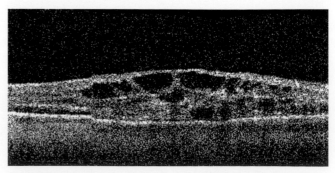

Figure 30–8 OCT image demonstrates cystoid macular edema resulting from chronic macroaneurysm leakage.

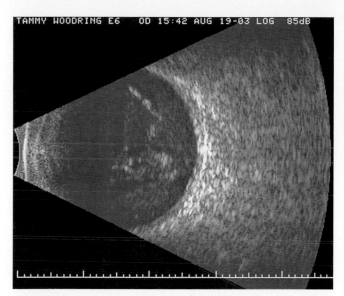

Figure 30–9 Dense vitreous hemorrhage resulting from a ruptured macroaneurysm is visualized on B-scan ultrasonography.

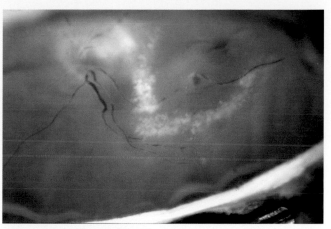

Figure 30–10 Gross pathology of a macroaneurysm with surrounding circinate lipid discovered on routine examination of an eye bank specimen. (Courtesy of Hans E. Grossniklaus, MD.)

of retinal arterial macroaneurysm. Echographic features characteristic of macroaneurysms include an irregular internal reflectivity, a rapid change in the size of the lesion over several months, and a pulsatile vascular structure at the anterior aspect of the lesion (**Figure 30–9**). Ultrasound is also useful in ruling out other diagnoses, such as retinal tears or detachment, in the setting of dense vitreous hemorrhage.

30.4 Pathology

Histopathologic examination of retinal artery macroaneurysms demonstrates thickening of the vessel walls with hyaline, fibrin, and foamy macrophages (**Figure 30–10**). Fresh or organized thrombus may fill the aneurysm. Thickened, hyalinized arterial walls are found in adjacent arterioles. The adjacent retina may show dilation of the capillary bed, edema, lipid exudates, and photoreceptor degeneration (**Figure 30–11**).

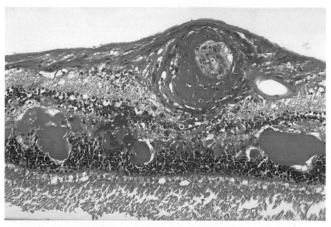

Figure 30–11 Photomicrograph of a partially thrombosed macroaneurysm in the inner retina surrounded by proteinaceous material. Accumulations of proteinaceous material consistent with hard exudates are seen in the outer nuclear and outer plexiform layers. Hematoxylin and eosin, ×100. (Courtesy of Ralph Eagle, MD.)

SUGGESTED READINGS

Fichte C, Friedman, AH. A histopathologic study of retinal arterial aneurysms. Am J Ophthalmol. 1978;85:509–518.

Gass JDM. A fluorescein angiographic study of macular dysfunction secondary to retinal vascular disease: V. Retinal telangiectasis. Arch Ophthalmol. 1968;80:592–605.

Levin MR, Gragoudas ES. Retinal arterial macroaneurysms. In: Albert DM, Jakobiec FA, eds. Principles and Practice of Ophthalmology. Philadelphia, Pa: Saunders, 1994.

Rabb MF, Gagliano DA, Teske MP. Retinal arterial macroaneurysms. Surv Ophthalmol. 1988;33:73–96.

Vander J. Retinal arterial macroaneurysms. In: Tasman WS, ed. Clinical Decisions in Medical Retinal Disease. St Louis, Mo: Mosby, 1994:253–260.

Inflammatory and Infectious Diseases

Chapter 31

Posterior Scleritis

WICO W. LAI, MD, FACS • DEBRA A. GOLDSTEIN, MD, FRCSC •
HOWARD H. TESSLER, MD

31.1 Introduction

Posterior scleritis is an uncommon inflammatory condition of the sclera in which the posterior portion of the eye is primarily affected. It accounts for 2% to 12% of all cases of scleritis. However, Benson pointed out that the actual incidence may be higher, as posterior involvement may be overlooked especially when there is severe anterior involvement. In several series 66% to 83% of the patients who developed posterior scleritis were women. However, at the University of Illinois Uveitis Clinic, of the 54 patients who presented with posterior scleritis, 28 were female and 26 were male (unpublished data). Most cases of posterior scleritis are unilateral. Bilateral disease has been reported to occur in approximately 10% to 33% of patients. The latter is more likely to be associated with an underlying systemic inflammatory condition. Most patients are middle aged, with a mean age of 47 to 58 years on presentation. However, the presenting age can range from 8 to 75 years.

31.2 Clinical Signs and Symptoms

Patients with posterior scleritis most commonly present with pain, redness, and decreased vision. With involvement of the adjacent tissues, diplopia, proptosis, or both may occur. Anterior scleritis may be present, and the pain is often proportional to the degree of anterior involvement. However, some patients may have none or only a few of these symptoms. Vision may be reduced from exudative retinal detachment, from cystoid macular edema, or from a circumscribed choroidal mass due to localized choroidal thickening.

The anterior segment may be quiet. However, anterior scleritis and iridocyclitis may develop. The orbit may be involved and signs of orbital inflammatory syndrome

(orbital pseudotumor) including ptosis, proptosis, and decreased ocular motility may be seen.

On fundus examination, vitreous cells may be present. Inflammation of the sclera adjacent to the optic nerve may produce optic disc edema. Serous retinal detachment (**Figure 31–1**) often with shifting subretinal fluid, chorioretinal folds (**Figures 31–2 and 31–3**), retinal pigment epithelial (RPE) detachment, choroidal detachment, or an orange circumscribed choroidal mass due to a localized area of scleral inflammation (**Figure 31–2**) may be observed. Angle-closure glaucoma may develop from annular choroidal detachment. Cystoid macular

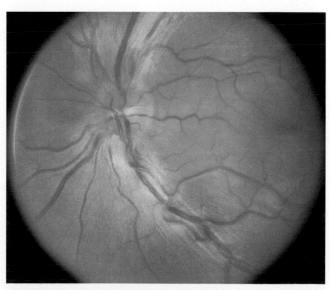

Figure 31–1 Fundus photograph of the left eye showing serous retinal detachment with prominence of the nerve fiber layer along the temporal arcades in a patient with posterior scleritis.

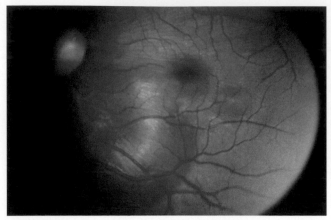

Figure 31–2   Fundus photograph of the left eye showing a circumscribed choroidal mass with adjacent chorioretinal folds in a patient with posterior scleritis.

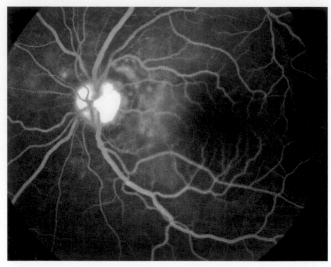

Figure 31–4   B-scan ultrasonogram showing a classic T sign due to edema of the sclerouveal complex and the Tenon's space in a patient with posterior scleritis.

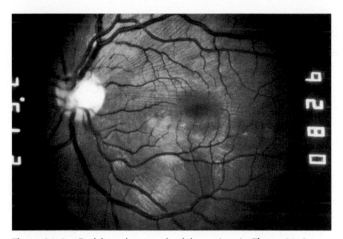

Figure 31–3   Red-free photograph of the patient in **Figure 31–2** accentuating the chorioretinal folds.

31.3.1 FLUORESCEIN ANGIOGRAPHY

Multiple pinpoint areas of hyperfluorescence at the level of the retinal pigment epithelium that leak in the later frames of the angiogram are classically seen (**Figure 31–4**). A similar pattern may be observed in patients with Vogt-Koyanagi-Harada syndrome, except that posterior scleritis is more often a unilateral disease. Inflammation involving the optic nerve may cause leakage around the nerve. Cystoid macular edema with accumulation of dye in a petaloid pattern and staining of the retinal vessels may also be present.

31.3.2 INDOCYANINE GREEN ANGIOGRAPHY

Several patterns have been observed in patients with posterior scleritis using indocyanine green angiography. Diffuse zonal hyperfluorescence in the intermediate and late phases of the angiogram may be seen. Pinpoint areas of hyperfluorescence may also been observed in the areas of zonal hyperfluorescence in the later phases. Delayed choroidal perfusion and hypofluorescent spots present up to the intermediate phase and faded in the late phase of the angiogram may also be visualized. These spots are noted to be smaller and more irregular in size than those observed in Vogt-Koyanagi-Harada syndrome.

edema has been reported due to the spread of the inflammation to the retina.

The most common underlying systemic disease in patients who develop posterior scleritis is rheumatoid arthritis. At the University of Illinois Uveitis Service, posterior scleritis is idiopathic in 82% of patients, and 18% have an associated underlying disease; 7% of patients have rheumatoid arthritis (unpublished data). The condition may also be associated with other inflammatory and vasculitic disorders such as systemic lupus erythematosus, relapsing polychondritis, Wegener's granulomatosis, and sarcoidosis.

31.3 Imaging and Diagnostic Tests

The diagnosis of posterior scleritis can be elusive. Results of imaging and diagnostic tests can be negative or equivocal and yet posterior scleritis can be present.

31.3.3 ULTRASONOGRAPHY

Ultrasonography is very helpful in the diagnosis of posterior scleritis. Scleral and choroidal edema result in moderately high reflective echoes. If the edema accumulates in Tenon's space, an echolucent area around the optic nerve results and the classic "T" sign is seen (**Figure 31–5**). This finding is diagnostic of posterior scleritis. Choroidal detachment may also be identified with ultrasonography (**Figure 31–6**).

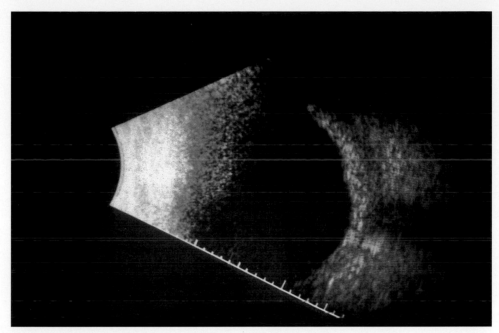

Figure 31–5 Late-phase fluorescein angiogram of the patient depicted in **Figure 31–1** showing pinpoint areas of leakage of the dye adjacent to the optic nerve in an area of exudative retinal detachment.

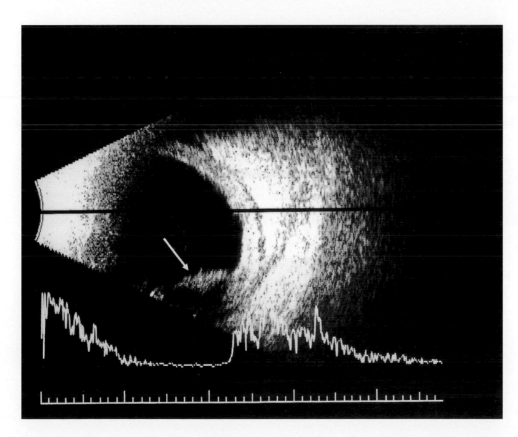

Figure 31–6 B-scan ultrasonogram reveals thickening of the sclerouveal complex and fluid accumulation in the Tenon's space as well as a choroidal detachment (*arrow*).

31.3.4 OPTICAL COHERENCE TOMOGRAPHY

There have been no reports on the use of optical coherence tomography in the diagnosis of posterior scleritis.

31.3.5 COMPUTED TOMOGRAPHY

Computed tomography (CT) may reveal thickening of the posterior sclera (**Figure 31–7**), which is enhanced upon administration of contrast material. Edema of

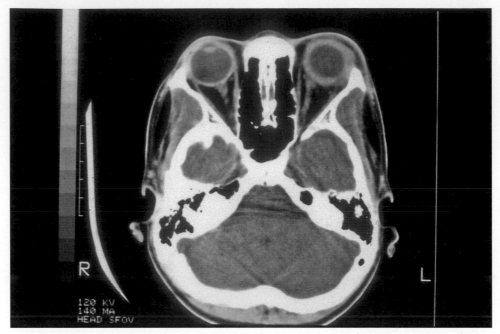

Figure 31–7   CT scan reveals thickening of the posterior sclera in the left eye.

the retrobulbar tissues may also be seen. Similar findings have been reported in a patient with orbital inflammatory syndrome.

31.3.6 MAGNETIC RESONANCE IMAGING

Magnetic resonance imaging has been reported to be less sensitive in diagnosing posterior scleritis than CT. It is reserved for cases in which the ultrasound and CT studies are normal.

31.4 Pathology

The choroid has been reported to be thickened with inflammatory infiltrates in enucleated eyes with posterior scleritis. Choroidal vasculitis, onion skin thickening

with occlusion of vessels, focal absence of the RPE with inflammation in the surrounding RPE, and subretinal exudates are also seen.

SUGGESTED READINGS

Auer C, Herbort CP. Indocyanine green angiographic features in posterior scleritis. Am J Ophthalmol. 1998;126:471–476.

Benson WE. Posterior scleritis. Surv Ophthalmol. 1988;32:297–316.

Calthorpe CM, Watson PG, McCartney ACE. Posterior scleritis: A clinical and histological survey. Eye. 1988;2:267–277.

Chaques VJ, Lam S, Tessler HH, Mafee MF. Computed tomography and magnetic resonance imaging in the diagnosis of posterior scleritis. Ann Ophthalmol. 1993;25:89–94.

Rootman J, Nugent R. The classification and management of acute orbital pseudotumors. Ophthalmology. 1982;89:1040–1048.

Watson PG. The diagnosis and management of scleritis. Ophthalmology. 1980;87:716–720.

Watson PG, Hayreh SS. Scleritis and episcleritis. Br J Ophthalmol. 1976;60:163–191.

Chapter 32

Pars Planitis

LOURDES ARELLANES-GARCÍA, MD • MATILDE RUIZ-CRUZ, MD

32.1 Introduction

Pars planitis (PP) refers to the idiopathic subset of intermediate uveitis in which the vitreous is the major site of inflammation and in which there are pars plana exudates ("snowbanks") or vitreous condensations ("snowball" formation) in the absence of an associated infectious or systemic disease. If there is associated infection or systemic disease, then the term *intermediate uveitis* is used.

Multiple sclerosis, sarcoidosis, Lyme disease, toxocariasis, and intraocular lymphoma, among others, are examples of syndromes associated with intermediate uveitis. Intermediate uveitis has a worldwide distribution. The only survey to determine the epidemiology of intermediate uveitis was conducted in France. The authors found a prevalence of 1 in 15,000 inhabitants, with an annual incidence of 1.4 per 100,000. The frequency of intermediate uveitis in a referral uveitis practice is 8% to 18% of all uveitis diagnoses.

Pars planitis is more often seen in children and young adults with a bimodal age distribution of 5 to 15 years and 25 to 35 years.

The etiology of pars planitis remains unknown, although some clinical, immunogenetic, and histopathologic studies have suggested an autoimmune process with a genetic predisposition.

32.2 Clinical Signs and Symptoms

The onset of symptoms is typically insidious; they often increase and decrease over many months. Most patients complain of blurred vision and floaters. The disease is bilateral at presentation in 70% to 80% of patients. In a series of patients with pars planitis, the primary symptom was decreased visual acuity in 66.2%; in 18 patients (11.2%) parents or teachers noticed a "white dot" in the affected eye, and exotropia was observed in 15 patients (9.4%). A "red eye" and photophobia were less common symptoms.

In adult patients the external eye is usually white, and there is little or no anterior chamber inflammation. Children with classic pars planitis may present with more severe anterior inflammation and with band keratopathy (**Figure 32–1**), posterior synechiae (**Figure 32–2**), and peripheral corneal endotheliopathy of affected eyes.

Inflammatory manifestations of pars planitis are more prominent in the vitreous and retina. Snowballs are white or yellowish aggregates of inflammatory cells. Snowbanks are exudates found on the pars plana or ora serrata. Although usually inferior in location, they may extend 360 degrees. Vitreous cells and strands are often observed. In one study of patients with classic pars planitis, vitreitis was noted in 294 of 295 affected eyes (99.7%) and snowballs in 99.3%. In the same group of patients, the characteristic peripheral retina and pars plana exudates (snowbanks) were found in 63.1%.

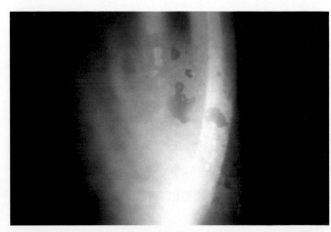

Figure 32–1 Band keratopathy due to calcium deposits in Bowman's membrane.

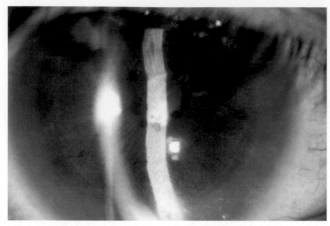

Figure 32–2 Posterior synechiae and fibrous membrane on the anterior lens capsule.

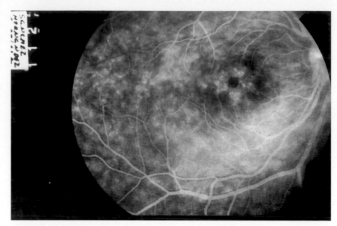

Figure 32–3 Late arteriovenous phase of the fluorescein angiogram shows petaloid perifoveal leakage and cystoid macular edema.

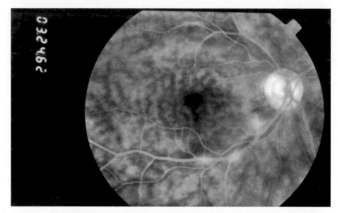

Figure 32–4 Full venous phase of the fluorescein angiogram reveals the characteristic "fern pattern."

Children can develop exuberant exudates, extending behind the crystalline lens to form a cyclitic membrane; these are seen in 15% of eyes.

Clinically detectable peripheral retinal vasculitis occurs in 10% to 32% of patients with intermediate uveitis. In pars planitis it has been found in 89.2% of affected eyes. Arterioles are rarely involved.

Cystoid macular edema occurs in 63% to 88% of eyes with intermediate uveitis or pars planitis. Optic disc edema is present in a similar proportion of eyes.

The most common complications are posterior subcapsular cataract, recorded in 13% to 61% of affected eyes and glaucoma in 3% to 8.2% of eyes. Neovascularization of peripheral pars plana exudates, optic disc, or retina are less common complications. Vitreous hemorrhage has been found in 3% to 5% of eyes. The rate of reported rhegmatogenous retinal detachment varies from 1.7% to 17%.

32.3 Imaging and Diagnostic Tests

32.3.1 FLUORESCEIN ANGIOGRAPHY

This study is very useful because of the high rate of vascular abnormalities found in pars planitis. Segmental hyperfluorescence and leakage from retinal veins have been reported. In a group of 105 patients with pars planitis, the most frequent findings were capillary hyperfluorescence exhibiting a "fern pattern" (65% to 88%), optic disc hyperfluorescence (44% to 69%), and petaloid macular hyperfluorescence (37% to 63%) (**Figures 32–3 to 32–5**).

32.3.2 INDOCYANINE GREEN ANGIOGRAPHY

Indocyanine green angiography is not useful in the diagnosis or management of pars planitis.

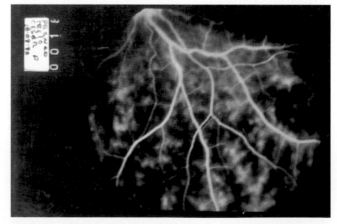

Figure 32–5 Fluorescein angiogram reveals peripheral venous leakage.

32.3.3 OPTICAL COHERENCE TOMOGRAPHY

Optical coherence tomography (OCT) is a very helpful study in the diagnosis and follow up of cystoid macular edema, the most important cause of decreased vision in these patients. OCT reveals intraretinal cystic spaces

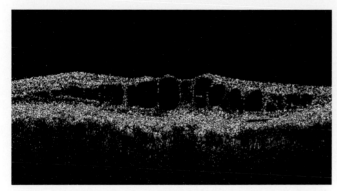

Figure 32–6 OCT image of the fovea showing multiple cysts in the sensory retina.

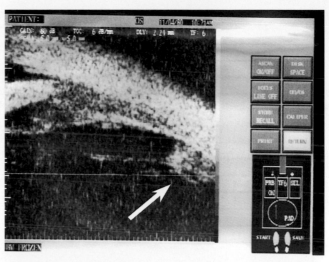

Figure 32–7 Ultrasound biomicroscopy. Snowbank associated with a cyclitic membrane (*arrow*).

(**Figure 32–6**). Macular holes occur in eyes with more severe and chronic disease.

32.3.4 ULTRASOUND BIOMICROSCOPY

In eyes with posterior synechiae, cataract, or vitreous opacities that prevent visualization of the pars plana and peripheral retina, ultrasound biomicroscopy is very helpful in detecting snowbanks (**Figure 32–7**), cyclitic membranes, vitreous membranes, vitreoretinal adhesions, and traction.

32.3.5 B-SCAN ULTRASOUND

In eyes with media opacities, ultrasonography can demonstrate vitreous bands and traction retinal detachments (**Figure 32–8**).

32.4 Pathology

Histopathologic studies in pars planitis are limited to studies performed in eyes enucleated because of complications of advanced disease or to vitrectomy specimens and may not be representative of active disease. Reported histopathologic features include mononuclear inflammatory cells infiltrating the vitreous, fibroglial material over the peripheral retina and pars plana, and lymphocytic infiltration of retinal veins with arteriolar sparing. A low-grade, chronic inflammation of the ciliary body and patchy peripheral choroiditis have also been described.

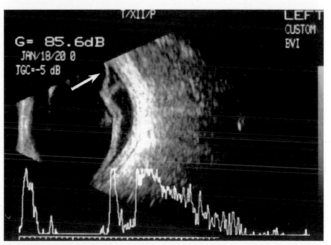

Figure 32–8 B-scan ultrasound reveals a tractional retinal detachment with a superior tractional membrane (*arrow*). (Courtesy of Eduardo Moragrega, MD.)

SUGGESTED READINGS

Arellanes-García L, Navarro-López P, Recillas-Gispert C. Pars planitis in the Mexican Mestizo population: Ocular findings, treatment and visual outcome. Ocul Immunol Inflam. 2003;11:53–60.

Davis JL, Bloch-Michael E. Intermediate uveitis. In: Pepose JS, Holland GN, Wilhelmus KR, eds. Ocular Infection and Immunity. St Louis, Mo: Mosby, 1996:676–693.

Kaplan HJ, Tessler H, Goldstein DA. Classification of intermediate uveitis. Minutes of the First Symposium American Uveitis Society, Breckenridge, Co, January 1997. Ocul Immunol Inflam 1997; 5:283–288.

McCluskey PJ, Lightman S. Intermediate uveitis and pars planitis. In: Ben Ezra D, ed. Ocular Inflammation: Basic and Clinical Concepts. London, England: Martin Dunitz, 1999:227–238.

Smith RE, Godfrey WA, Kimura SJ. Chronic cyclitis: I. Course and visual prognosis. Trans Am Acad Ophthalmol Otolaryngol. 1973;77:760–768.

Chapter 33

Sarcoidosis

CAREEN Y. LOWDER, MD, PhD

33.1 Introduction

Sarcoidosis is a granulomatous multisystem disease that may affect every ocular structure. The incidence is 82 per 100,000 in African Americans and 8 per 100,000 in Caucasians and shows geographic variations: 64 per 100,000 in Sweden and 4 per 100,000 in Spain. The disease has a bimodal distribution: 20 to 30 and 50 to 60. The etiology is unknown, but an infectious agent is suggested by development of sarcoid in husband-wife pairs, in individuals who live in close proximity, and in recipients of organ transplants from patients with sarcoidosis.

33.2 Clinical Signs and Symptoms

The clinical presentation and course of disease vary from patient to patient. Acute anterior uveitis presents with redness, pain, and photophobia. Examination reveals granulomatous keratic precipitates or "mutton fat" on the corneal endothelium (**Figures 33–1** and **33–2**) and nodules may also be seen on the iris surface (Busacca) or at the pupillary margin (Koeppe). Posterior synechiae tend to form in areas of Koeppe nodules. Chronic anterior uveitis may be only mildly symptomatic, and patients may have anterior synechiae at presentation. Chronic anterior uveitis is more commonly seen than acute uveitis in patients with sarcoidosis. Floaters and blurred vision are the most common symptoms of posterior uveitis due to vitreitis and macular edema. Isolated posterior uveitis can be the only presentation in 14% to 43% of patients. Posterior uveitis can involve every structure in the posterior segment. The vitreous can be heavily infiltrated with inflammatory cells, which may be found in clumps or "snowballs." Inflammatory cells may be present on the pars plana and mimic pars planitis and other intermediate uveitis syndromes. Periphlebitis appears as yellowish infiltrates along the walls of venules, which are commonly known as "candle

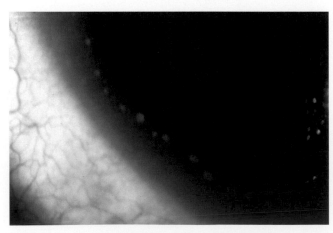

Figure 33–1   Keratic precipitates on the inferior corneal endothelium.

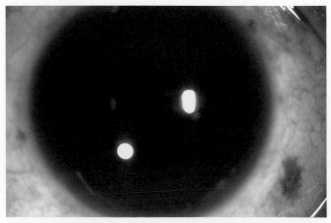

Figure 33–2   Keratic precipitates may also lead to thickening of the inferior cornea.

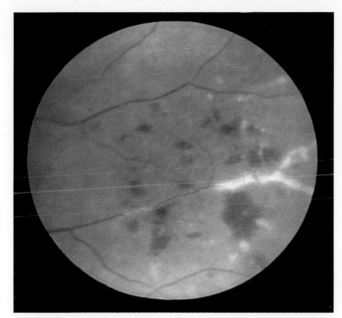

Figure 33–3 Periphlebitis and occlusive vasculitis associated with intraretinal hemorrhages.

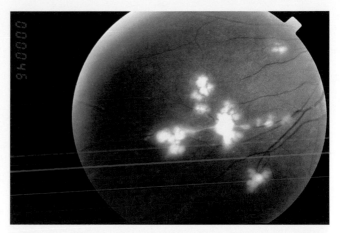

Figure 33–5 Granulomas in the retina appear as white, grape-like lesions.

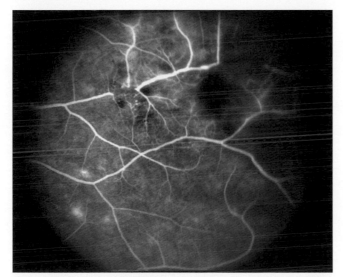

Figure 33–4 Fluorescein angiogram reveals capillary nonperfusion and staining of the blood vessel walls.

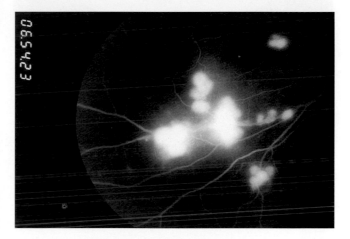

Figure 33–6 Fluorescein angiogram reveals marked hyperfluorescence and leakage of the retinal granulomas.

wax drippings." Focal or occlusive vasculitis (**Figures 33–3** and **33–4**) due to arteritis can lead to intraretinal hemorrhages. Granulomas may be found in the retina, where they appear as white, grape-like lesions (**Figures 33–5** and **33–6**), and in the choroid. Active choroidal granulomas can present as small yellowish lesions with poorly defined borders (**Figure 33–7**); they are multifocal and are found predominantly inferiorly (**Figure 33–8**). Large, single choroidal granulomas can have an overlying serous retinal detachment. Chorioretinal atrophy results from previous choroidal granulomatous inflammation. The optic nerve may be involved and appear edematous due to intraocular inflammation

or granulomatous infiltration (**Figure 33–9**). Isolated granulomas of the optic nerve are rarely seen and present as a yellowish lesion on the optic nerve head. In addition, neovascularization of the optic nerve head can develop in patients with chronic inflammation. Of patients with known sarcoidosis, 25% to 75% develop ocular lesions and 4% to 6% of patients with uveitis will develop clinical sarcoidosis.

33.3 Imaging and Diagnostic Tests

33.3.1 FLUORESCEIN ANGIOGRAPHY

Early phases of the angiogram will show hyperfluorescence of active choroidal granulomas as well as late hyperfluorescence and leakage. In occlusive vasculitis, capillary nonperfusion is clearly demonstrated. Periphlebitis is characterized by staining of the vessel walls. In the late phases, macular edema is demonstrated by perifoveal capillary leakage of fluorescein and optic nerve inflammation by marked hyperfluorescence

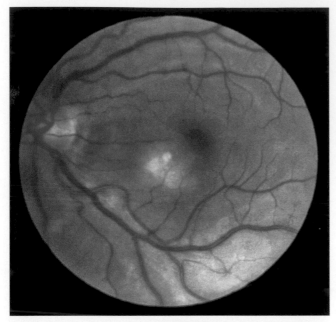

A

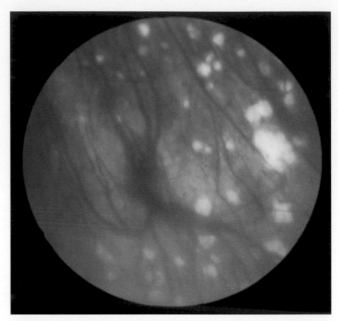

Figure 33–8 Atrophic chorioretinal lesions result from previous choroidal granulomatous inflammation and are most commonly found inferiorly.

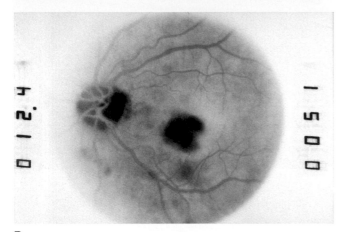

B

Figure 33–7 *A:* Choroidal granuloma with an overlying serous retinal detachment. *B:* Hyperfluorescence of the choroidal granuloma.

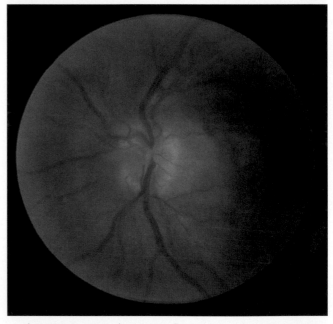

Figure 33–9 Granulomatous inflammation of the optic nerve.

of the optic nerve. In patients with neovascularization of the optic nerve head, the abnormal vessels leak fluorescein in the late phases.

33.3.2 INDOCYANINE GREEN ANGIOGRAPHY

Indocyanine green angiography is not useful in the diagnosis of sarcoidosis.

33.3.3 OPTICAL COHERENCE TOMOGRAPHY

Optical coherence tomography (OCT) reveals several patterns of macular edema: (1) intraretinal cysts; (2) intraretinal cysts with subretinal fluid (**Figure 33–10**); and (3) intraretinal cysts with subretinal and subretinal pigment epithelium fluid. Epiretinal membranes are variably

reflective and can be seen overlying the retina or exerting traction on the retina, leading to intraretinal cysts.

33.3.4 CHEST RADIOGRAPH

A chest radiograph demonstrates a hilar of parenchymal adenopathy, but mediastinal lymphadenopathy is obscured by the trachea and large mediastinal blood vessels.

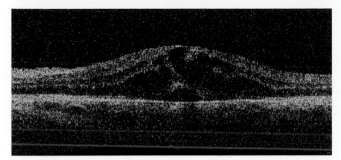

Figure 33–10 OCT image demonstrates macular edema with intraretinal cysts and subretinal fluid.

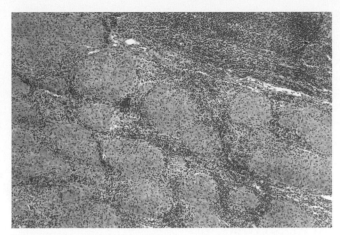

Figure 33–12 Photomicrograph of a mediastinal lymph node stained with hematoxylin and eosin reveals noncaseating granulomas.

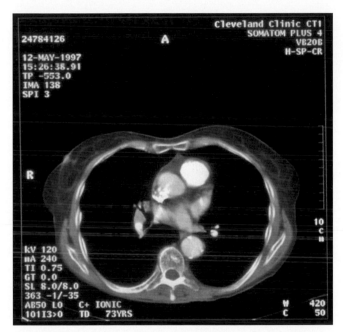

Figure 33–11 Mediastinal lymphadenopathy seen on the chest CT scan. (Reprinted with permission from Kaiser PK, Lowder CY, Sullivan P, et al. Chest computerized tomography in the evaluation of uveitis in elderly women. Am J Ophthalmol. 2002;133:499–505.)

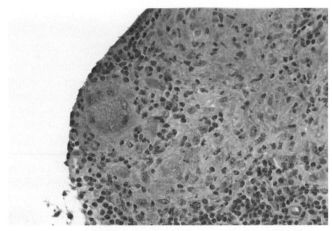

Figure 33–13 High-power photomicrograph reveals a Langhans giant cell.

33.3.5 COMPUTED TOMOGRAPHY

Computed tomography (CT) of the chest is the most sensitive test to demonstrate lymphadenopathy associated with sarcoidosis. Lymph nodes can be found in the paratracheal, periaortic, and subcarinal regions (**Figure 33–11**). Diagnosis is made by finding noncaseating granulomas in specimens obtained by CT-guided mediastinoscopy.

33.3.6 OTHER TESTS

Serum angiotensin-converting enzyme levels and gallium scans have low sensitivity and specificity individually, but when combined, specificity increases to 99%. Serum lysozyme levels are nonspecific and have been reported in 40% of patients with sarcoidosis.

33.4 Pathology

Sarcoid granulomas consist of noncaseating granulomas characterized by epithelioid cells, monocytes, fibroblasts, and Langhans giant cells (**Figures 33–12 and 33–13**).

SUGGESTED READINGS

Chatzistefanou K, Markomichelakis NN, Christen W, Soheilian M, Foster CS. Characteristics of uveitis presenting for the first time in the elderly. Ophthalmology. 1998;105:347–352.

Hershey JM, Pulido JS, Folberg R, Folk JC, Massicotte SJ. Non-caseating conjunctival granulomas in patients with multifocal choroiditis and panuveitis. Ophthalmology 1994;101.

Kosmorsky GS, Meisler DM, Rice TW, Meziane MA, Lowder CY. Chest computerized tomography and mediastinoscopy in the diagnosis of sarcoidosis-associated uveitis. Am J Ophthalmol. 1998;126:132–134.

Lardenoye CWTA, Van der Lelij A, de Loos WS, Treffers WF, Rothova A. Peripheral multifocal chorioretinitis. Ophthalmology. 1997; 104:1820–1826.

Newman LS, Rose CS, Maier LA. Sarcoidosis. N Engl J Med. 1997, 336:1224–1234.

Chapter 34

Uveal Effusion Syndrome

JAY M. STEWART, MD

34.1 Introduction

Idiopathic uveal effusion syndrome (IUES) consists primarily of serous choroidal and retinal detachments associated with abnormalities of the sclera. The condition was first described as a syndrome in 1963, when Schepens and Brockhurst identified an association of exudative retinal detachment and shifting subretinal fluid, choroidal detachment, elevated cerebrospinal fluid protein, and unusually thick sclera predominantly in male patients. Subsequently Gass and Jallow proposed that these changes could result from impaired venous outflow of the uveal tract due to pathologic alterations in the sclera. Their hypothesis has been validated by more recent studies.

Incidence and prevalence figures are unavailable, but the syndrome occurs with sufficient frequency to be well characterized and recognized by many clinicians. It is seen mostly in middle-aged men. IUES can be diagnosed after excluding other causes of uveal effusion, such as nanophthalmos, orbital inflammation, trauma- or surgery-induced serous effusions, primary pulmonary hypertension, carotid-cavernous fistulas, dural sinus fistulas, choroidal inflammation, Hunter's syndrome, disseminated intravascular coagulation, eclampsia, uveal neoplasms or lymphoid hyperplasia, and carotid artery obstruction.

Histologically, sclera from patients with IUES has been found to contain irregularly arranged collagen fibers and increased extracellular matrix deposition. The fibers also have varying diameters and are spaced further apart than normal. Histochemical staining has confirmed the presence of glycosaminoglycans in these spaces. All of these changes result in thickening and impermeability of the sclera, creating a major barrier to transscleral flow of fluid and protein. The accumulation of protein in the suprachoroidal space furthers the cycle of fluid buildup via an oncotic effect, leading to choroidal and retinal detachment. Compression of

vortex veins by the thickened sclera also contributes. The mechanism of effusion in IUES by obstruction of transscleral fluid flow is also suggested by the occurrence of uveal effusion in Hunter's syndrome, in which mucopolysaccharide deposition causes thickening of the sclera. Another proposed cause of IUES is ocular hypotony, in which it has been suggested that effusions can occur due to a pressure gradient effect when pressure in the globe drops below that in the suprachoroidal space.

34.2 Clinical Signs and Symptoms

Patients present with loss of vision, sometimes bilaterally. Inferior retinal and choroidal detachments can result in a superior scotoma before the central acuity drops. Metamorphopsia has also been reported.

On examination, patients often have dilated episcleral veins. Anterior chamber flare, but usually not cells, may be present. Gonioscopy may reveal blood in Schlemm's canal. Nonpigmented vitreous cells are commonly seen. Retinal detachment may either be limited to the macula or may involve mainly the inferior retina when the patient is upright. In the latter instance, the detachment can be bullous with markedly shifting fluid. In longstanding disease, leopard-spot pigment changes may be visible in the fundus (**Figure 34–1**). Choroidal detachments may be detectable on ophthalmoscopy. They often have an annular configuration, which can cause them to be mistaken for ring melanoma. In many eyes, though, the serous choroidal detachment may be detectable only on imaging studies such as ultrasonography. Intraocular pressure may be normal or low. Spontaneous remissions and exacerbations may occur.

Anterior ischemic optic neuropathy as a secondary effect in IUES has been described. This is presumed to result from compression of posterior ciliary arteries as they pass through the thickened sclera.

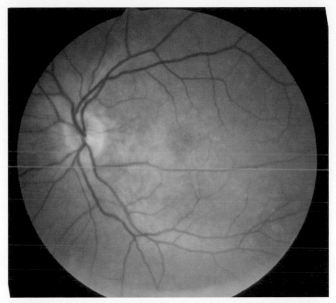

Figure 34–1 Leopard-spot pattern pigment changes in the fundus of a patient with IUES. A shallow inferior retinal detachment is also present. (Courtesy of Christina J. Flaxel, MD.)

34.3 Imaging and Diagnostic Tests

34.3.1 FLUORESCEIN ANGIOGRAPHY

Early frames can show a delay in choroidal filling and prolongation of the background choroidal fluorescence. Generally, no focal leak into the subretinal space will be identified. In the late frames, leopard-spot pattern hyperfluorescence is often present, even in eyes in which the changes are not detectable ophthalmoscopically (**Figure 34–2**). Retinochoroidal folds may also be noted.

34.3.2 INDOCYANINE GREEN ANGIOGRAPHY

Late frames may show choroidal hyperfluorescence and perivascular leakage from dilated choroidal vessels. These findings can persist even after surgery with resolution of the retinal detachment.

34.3.3 OPTICAL COHERENCE TOMOGRAPHY

Retinal detachment can be identified by optical coherence tomography.

34.3.4 ULTRASOUND

Thickening of the retinochoroid layer and the sclera are typically demonstrated on ultrasonography. Choroidal, ciliary body, and retinal detachments can also be identified (**Figures 34–3** and **34–4**). Nanophthalmos is ruled out by using ultrasonography to demonstrate a normal, instead of a shortened, axial length. The anterior chamber angle may be narrowed due to the choroidal and ciliary body detachment. Finally, optic nerve sheath dilation can be seen on ultrasonography in patients with IUES from increased fluid and protein accumulating secondarily in the subarachnoid space.

34.3.5 COMPUTED TOMOGRAPHY AND MAGNETIC RESONANCE IMAGING

These modalities can demonstrate the thickened sclera and choroid as well as associated serous detachments. Dilated optic nerve sheaths can also be identified.

34.3.6 LABORATORY TESTS

Lumbar puncture can show elevated protein levels in the cerebrospinal fluid (up to 2 to 3 times) in the presence of normal cell counts.

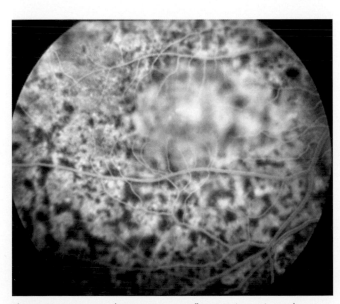

Figure 34–2 Leopard-spot pattern on fluorescein angiography. (Courtesy of Christina J. Flaxel, MD.)

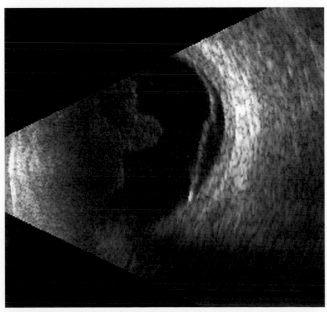

Figure 34–3 Thickened sclera and serous retinal detachment in a patient with IUES. (Courtesy of Ronald L. Green, MD.)

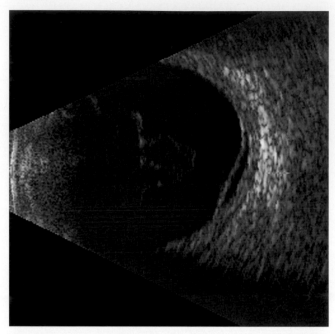

Figure 34–4 After scleral-window surgery to facilitate transscleral fluid flow, the retinal detachment is shallower. (Courtesy of Ronald L. Green, MD.)

34.4 Pathology

As described earlier, disarray of collagen fibers in the sclera can be observed in IUES, along with variation in the diameter of the fibers. Increased extracellular matrix, consisting primarily of accumulated glycosaminoglycans, is also present between the fibers. Electron microscopy of scleral cell cultures from patients with IUES shows intracellular glycogen granules.

SUGGESTED READINGS

Byrne SF, Green RL. Vitreoretinal disease. In: Ultrasound of the Eye and Orbit, 2nd ed. St Louis, Mo: Mosby, 2002:82–84.

Forrester JV, Lee WR, Kerr PR, Dua HS. The uveal effusion syndrome and trans-scleral flow. Eye. 1990;4:354–365.

Gass JDM. Idiopathic uveal effusion syndrome. In: Stereoscopic Atlas of Macular Diseases: Diagnosis and Treatment, 4th ed. St Louis, Mo: Mosby, 1997:200–205.

Schepens CL, Brockhurst RJ. Uveal effusion: I. Clinical picture. Arch Ophthalmol. 1963;70:189–201.

Uyama M, Takahashi K, Kozaki J, et al. Uveal effusion syndrome: clinical features, surgical treatment, histologic examination of the sclera, and pathophysiology. Ophthalmology. 2000;107:441–449.

Ward RC, Gragoudas ES, Pon DM, Albert DM. Abnormal scleral findings in uveal effusion syndrome. Am J Ophthalmol. 1988;106:139–146.

Chapter 35

White Dot Syndromes

EMILIO M. DODDS, MD

35.1 Multiple Evanescent White Dot Syndrome

35.1.1 INTRODUCTION

Multiple evanescent white dot syndrome (MEWDS) is a multifocal retinopathy first described in 1984 that involves mainly the retinal pigment epithelium (RPE). This disease affects mostly young women, and the mean age at time of diagnosis is 28 with a reported age range of 10 to 67 years. Although it is usually a unilateral disease, it can be bilateral with asymmetrical involvement. The cause is not known, but a viral etiology is suspected because many patients have a history of a preceding viral illness. In two patients, the disease developed after vaccination for hepatitis.

35.1.2 CLINICAL SIGNS AND SYMPTOMS

Patients present with decreased vision, scotomas, or photopsias without associated external ocular signs of inflammation. Initially, vision may be only mildly reduced but may be as low as 20/200. Slit-lamp examination reveals no external or anterior segment signs of inflammation except in rare instances. Ophthalmoscopy reveals deep retinal lesions in only one eye, which can be associated with vitreous cells and vascular sheathing in some patients. The multifocal lesions are white and range in size from 200 to 500 microns. They are located at the level of the RPE and the retinal vessels can be clearly seen crossing over them (**Figure 35–1**). Each lesion is made up of a multitude of smaller white dots (**Figure 35–2**). The lesions are distributed in the

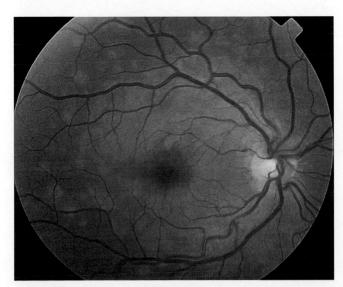

Figure 35–1 Fundus photograph shows a clear view of a retina with the typical white dots of MEWDS.

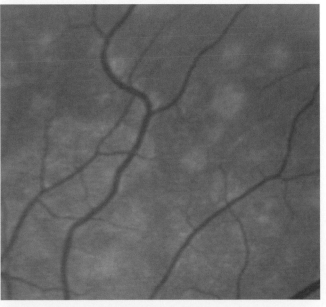

Figure 35–2 White dots areas in the deeper layers of the retina.

317

posterior pole and extend to the mid-periphery of the fundus. They rarely involve the fovea (**Figure 35–3**).

Another typical manifestation of the disease is a macular granularity that consists of white or orange specks smaller than the white dots seen elsewhere (**Figure 35–4**).

The third clinical sign of MEWDS is a neuropathy characterized by optic nerve hyperemia, mild blurring of the optic disc or even frank disc edema and an afferent pupillary defect, dyschromatopsia, and visual field defects (**Figure 35–5A** and **B**). Optic neuritis should

be considered as one of the differential diagnoses of MEWDS.

The white dots disappear without therapy, and visual acuity improves after about 7 weeks. The macular granularity and optic nerve inflammation may persist. In most patients, vision returns to normal. (**Figure 35–6A** and **B**).

Although MEWDS is usually a unilateral and self-limited disease, it can recur multiple times in both eyes, but the visual prognosis remains good.

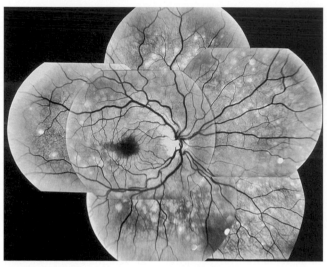

Figure 35–3 This photograph shows the distribution of the white dots posterior to the equator.

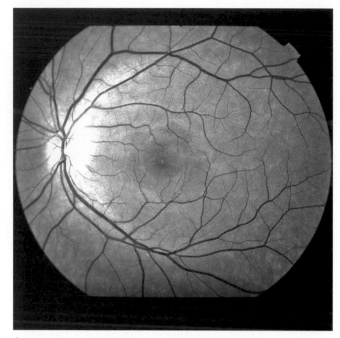

A

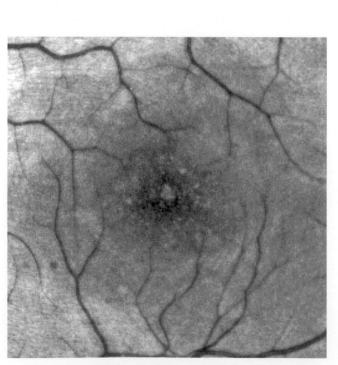

Figure 35–4 Macular granularity present in the affected eye.

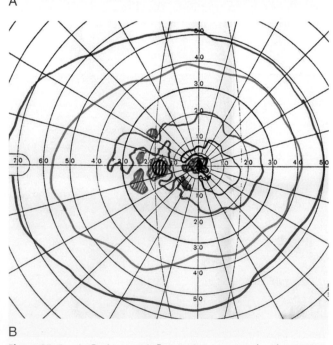

B

Figure 35–5 *A:* Optic nerve inflammation associated with MEWDS. *B:* Visual field defect simulating optic neuritis.

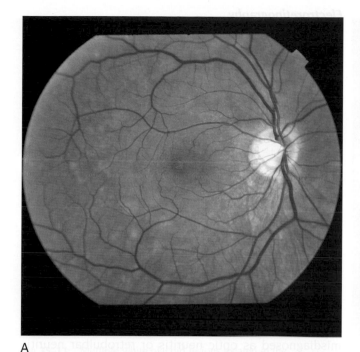

A

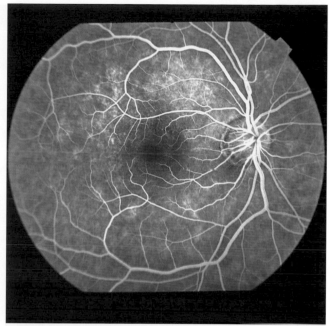

Figure 35–7 Fluorescein angiogram during the acute phase reveals mild hyperfluorescence of the retinal lesions.

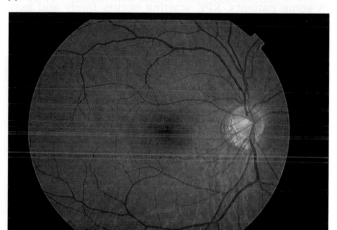

B

Figure 35–6 *A:* Photograph of a young woman with white dots limited to the posterior pole. *B:* Fundus appearance of the same patient 1 year later.

35.1.3 IMAGING AND DIAGNOSTIC TESTS

Fluorescein Angiography

Fluorescein angiography during the acute phases shows "wreath-like" collections of punctate hyperfluorescence at the site of the lesions and also in areas where the lesions are not clinically apparent. There is late staining of the retinal lesions and of the optic disc in some patients (**Figures 35–7** and **35–8**).

Indocyanine Green Angiography

Indocyanine green (ICG) angiography reveals hypofluorescent lesions throughout the whole angiogram,

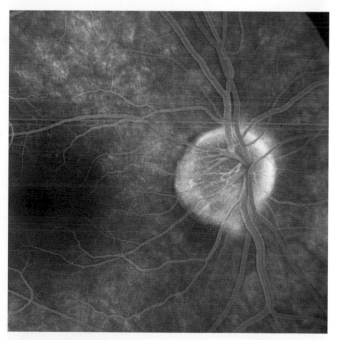

Figure 35–8 Late staining of the optic disc.

which are better visualized in the late phases. ICG angiography shows better demarcation of the lesions than clinical examination or fluorescein angiography. Occasionally more lesions are apparent on the ICG angiogram than on the fluorescein angiogram. Although MEWDS is considered a primary disease of the RPE, it is very unlikely that a single layer of dysfunctional RPE would block ICG dye. Based on the hypofluorescence of these lesions on ICG angiography, it has been

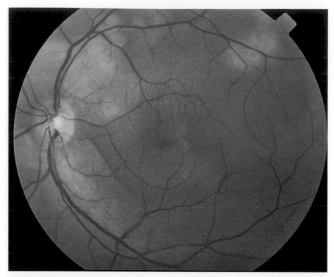

Figure 35–15 Placoid lesions associated with subretinal fluid mimicking VKH syndrome.

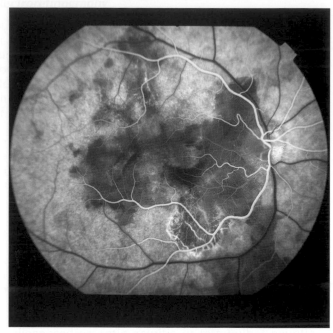

Figure 35–17 Fluorescein angiogram reveals mainly hypofluorescent lesions and an area of atrophy inferiorly.

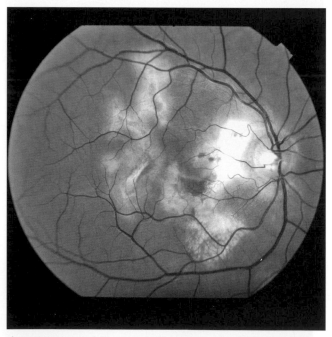

Figure 35–16 Red-free image of a patient with 20/20 vision and placoid lesions.

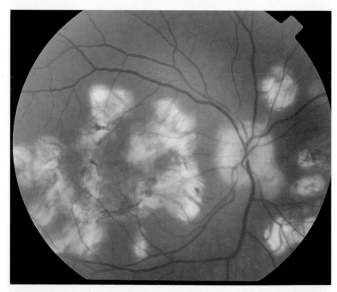

Figure 35–18 Photograph of the right eye of a patient with good visual acuity shows placoid and atrophic lesions resembling serpiginous choroidopathy.

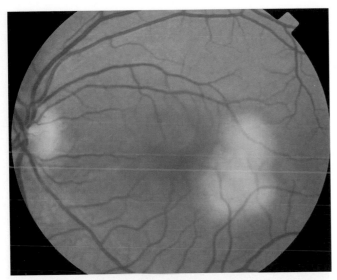

Figure 35–19 Left eye of the patient in **Figure 35–18** reveals a single plaque resembling APMPPE.

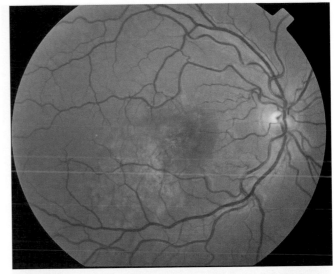

Figure 35–21 Permanent RPE damage due to APMPPE.

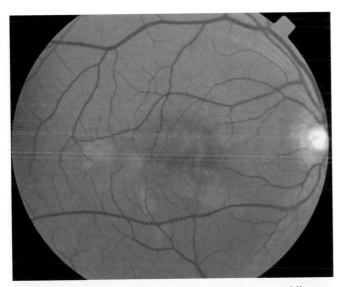

Figure 35–20 Photograph shows small placoid lesions at different stages of resolution.

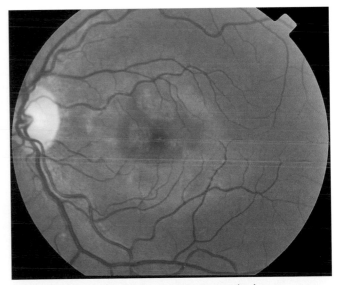

Figure 35–22 RPE mottling sparing the fovea.

35.2.3 IMAGING AND DIAGNOSTIC TESTS

Fluorescein Angiography

APMPPE has a characteristic fluorescein angiographic appearance. The placoid lesions are hypofluorescent in the early phases and stain late (**Figures 35–24** to **35–26**). This early hypofluorescence was initially thought to be due to blockage of the fluorescein by edematous RPE. It is more likely to result from a delayed hypersensitivity reaction that causes obstruction of the precapillary choroidal arterioles feeding the lobules of the choriocapillaris.

Indocyanine Green Angiography

ICG angiography also shows hypofluorescent lesions throughout the entire angiogram, suggesting a primary choroidal vascular disease rather than an inflammatory disease of the RPE (**Figures 35–27** to **35–29**).

Visual Field Testing

In one report 70% of the eyes with APMPPE had significant central visual field defects on follow-up examination. The scotomas correspond to the areas of RPE disturbance. Absolute scotomas seldom occur even in the presence of chorioretinal atrophy.

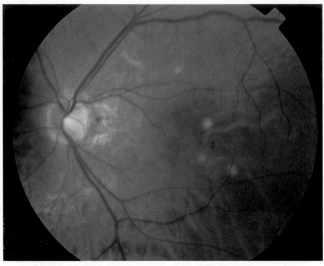

Figure 35–44   Fundus photograph of a myopic patient with macular lesions.

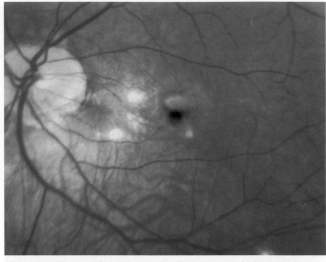

Figure 35–47   Fundus photograph of a patient with decreased vision in a later stage of disease showing enlarged lesions and a CNVM.

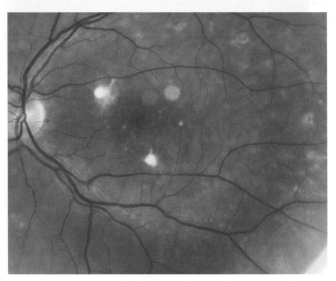

Figure 35–45   Atrophic lesions with residual retinal exudates.

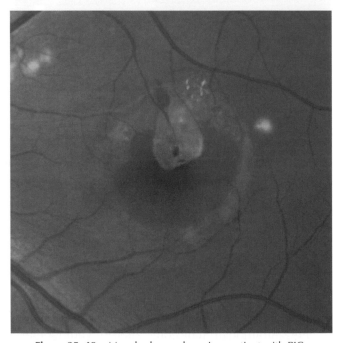

Figure 35–48   Macular hemorrhage in a patient with PIC.

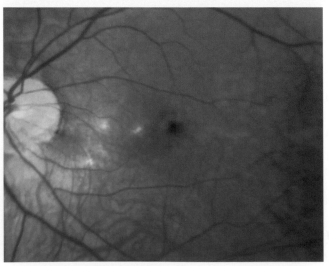

Figure 35–46   Fundus photograph of small lesions present in the initial stages of PIC in a patient who has no visual limitations.

have a type II choroidal neovascular growth pattern (**Figures 35–51** and **35–52**).

Indocyanine Green Angiography

Choroidal neovascular membranes and the typical lesions of punctate inner choroidopathy are better detected with ICG angiography than with indirect ophthalmoscopy or fluorescein angiography (**Figures 35–52** to **35–54**).

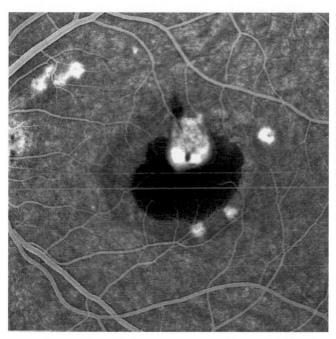

Figure 35–49 Fluorescein angiogram shows a CNVM.

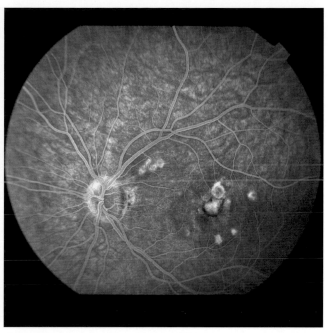

Figure 35–51 Fluorescein angiogram shows staining of the chorioretinal lesions and a CNVM.

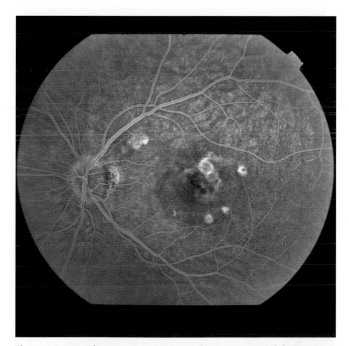

Figure 35–50 Fluorescein angiogram shows staining of the chorioretinal lesions.

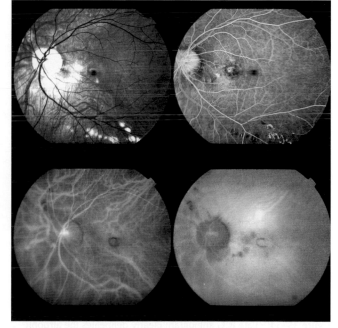

Figure 35–52 Red-free, fluorescein angiogram (*top*) and ICG angiogram (*bottom*) of a patient with PIC.

35.5 Multifocal Choroiditis and Panuveitis

35.5.1 INTRODUCTION

Nozik and Dorsch first described this syndrome as anterior uveitis and vitreitis associated with fundus lesions that resembled those of presumed ocular histo-plasmosis syndrome. Later, Dryer and Gass described a series of 28 patients with similar findings and renamed this constellation of findings multifocal choroiditis and panuveitis (MCP).

MCP is bilateral in 78% of patients and affects women in their third decade of life with a mean age of onset of 36 years and a range of 9 to 69 years.

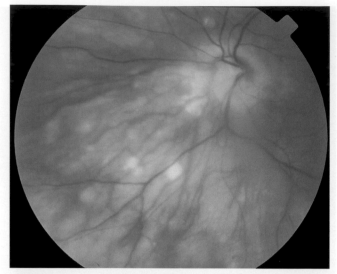

Figure 35–59 Whitish lesions associated with vitreitis in a 70 -year-old man.

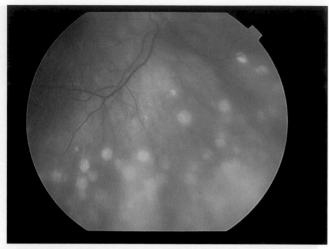

Figure 35–61 Inferior location of punched-out lesions.

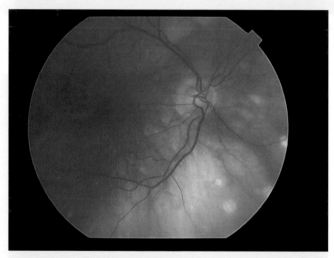

Figure 35–60 A 60-year-old woman with mild vitreitis and chorioretinal lesions sparing the fovea.

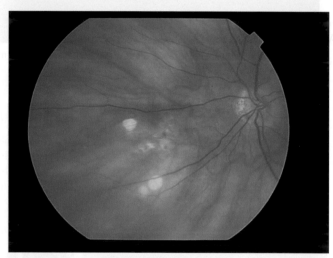

Figure 35–62 Asymmetric distribution of these chorioretinal lesions in both eyes of the same patient.

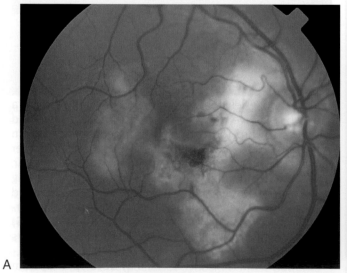

A

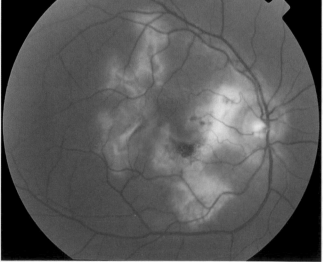

B

Figure 35–63 *A:* Acute lesion of serpiginous choroidopathy temporal to the macula. *B:* Same patient with a reactivation of the disease.

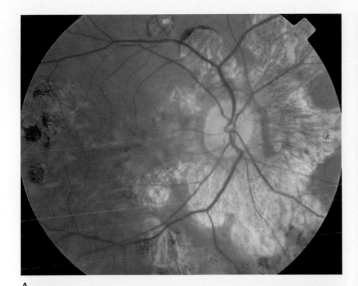

A

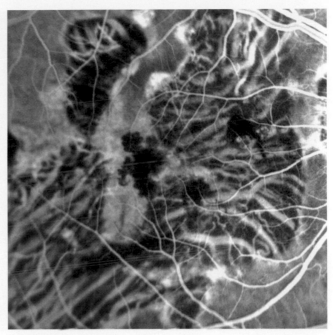

Figure 35–65 Clear view of choroidal vessels due to atrophy of choriocapillaris and RPE.

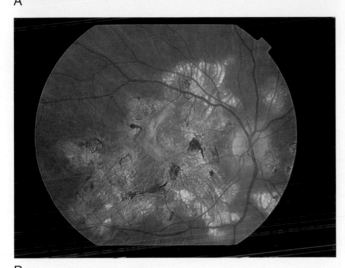

B

Figure 35–64 *A:* Atrophic lesion with well-demarcated borders. *B:* Atrophic lesion with areas of hyperpigmentation.

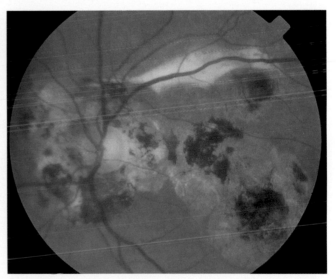

Figure 35–66 Subretinal fibrosis in a patient with serpiginous choroidopathy.

difficult (**Figure 35–67A** and **B**). Placoid lesions may occur with very little choriocapillaris and RPE atrophy, which may be indistinguishable from APMPPE. This condition has been called APMPPiginous choroidopathy (**Figure 35–68A** and **B**). The latter patients may have recurrent disease as in serpiginous choroidopathy, but have fundus lesions typical of APMPPE, even retaining good visual acuity despite macular involvement.

Choroidal neovascularization can complicate serpiginous choroidopathy and develops in 10% to 25% of patients. Neovascularization usually develops at the border of an old scar (**Figure 35–69A** and **B**).

35.6.3 IMAGING AND DIAGNOSTIC TESTS

Fluorescein Angiography

Acute lesions block fluorescence early and stain late. Atrophic lesions show early hypofluorescence due to absence of choriocapillaris and show progressive staining of the borders of the lesion (**Figure 35–70A** and **B**).

Indocyanine Green Angiography

The lesions are well demarcated on ICG angiography and remain hypofluorescent throughout the study. ICG angiography is helpful in detecting the leading edges of minimally active inflammation (**Figure 35–71**).

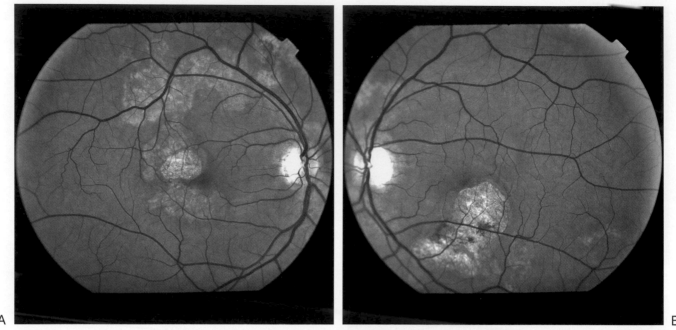

Figure 35–67 *A* and *B:* Placoid lesions located away from the optic disc.

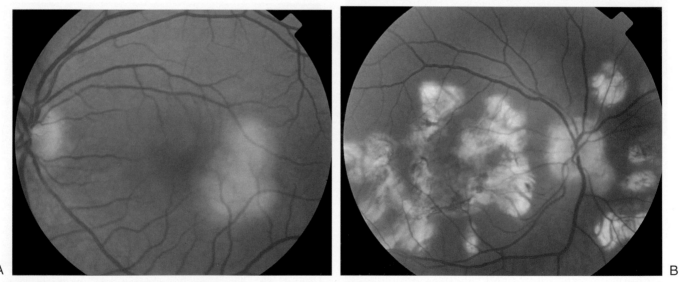

Figure 35–68 *A* and *B:* APMPPiginous: photographs of the same patient. The right eye reveals lesions that resemble serpiginous choroidopathy and the left eye APMPPE.

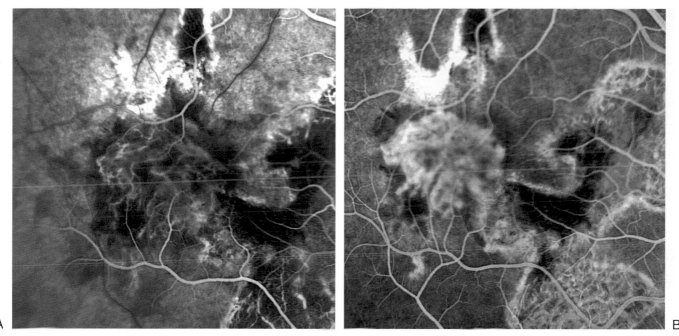

Figure 35–69   *A* and *B:* Fluorescein angiograms of a CNVM in a patient with serpiginous choroidopathy.

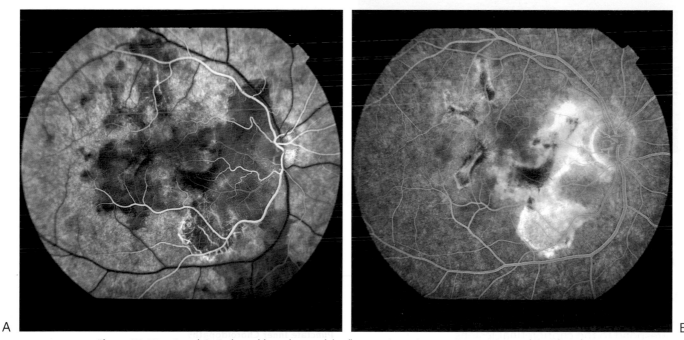

Figure 35–70   *A* and *B:* Early and late phases of the fluorescein angiograms in serpiginous choroidopathy.

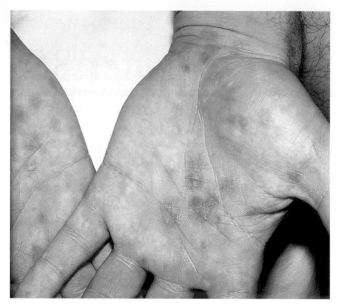

Figure 38–2 Secondary syphilis. Maculopapular rash located on the palms.

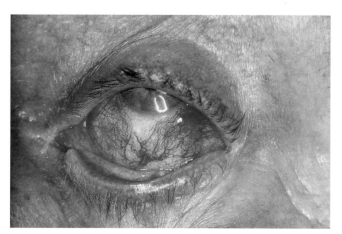

Figure 38–3 Diffuse syphilitic scleritis.

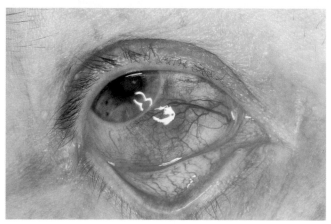

Figure 38–4 Nodular scleritis associated with anterior uveitis (sclerouveitis).

detected (**Figure 38–5**). A necrotizing retinitis, which varies in severity, may be seen in some affected patients (**Figure 38–6**).

Retinal vasculitis is commonly found in active ocular syphilis (**Figure 38–7**) and, in rare instances, may obstruct normal retinal blood flow and lead to retinal hemorrhage (**Figure 38–8**), retinal neovascularization, and vitreous hemorrhage. Migration of retinal pigment epithelium (RPE) into the overlying retina in a bone-spiculed pattern simulating retinitis pigmentosa (**Figure 38–9**) and choroidal neovascularization developing at the edge of a chorioretinal scar are less commonly observed ocular features. The optic nerve may appear edematous due to intraocular inflammation (**Figures 38–10** and **38–11**) or granulomatous infiltration, as well as during a Jarisch-Herxheimer reaction (constitutional symptoms due to penicillin-induced spirochete death). Optic atrophy may be due to syphilitic chorioretinitis or may be the presenting sign of tabes dorsalis (late neurosyphilis).

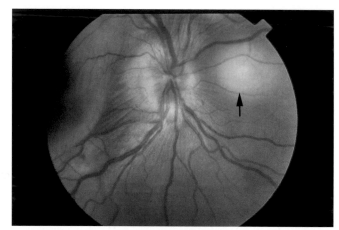

Figure 38–5 Syphilitic choroidal granuloma (*arrow*).

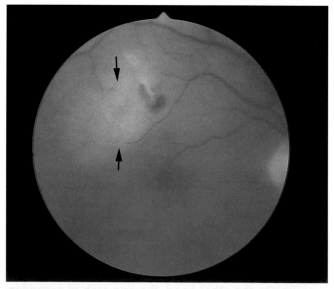

Figure 38–6 Severe necrotizing retinitis in a patient with HIV infection. (Courtesy of Drs. A. and L. Muralha.)

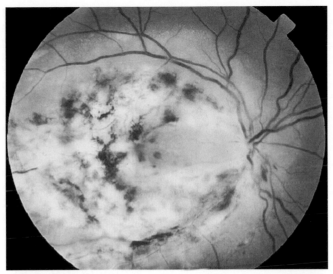

Figure 38-7 Vitreitis and retinal vasculitis due to syphilis.

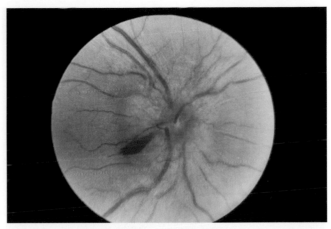

Figure 38-10 Syphilitic papillitis.

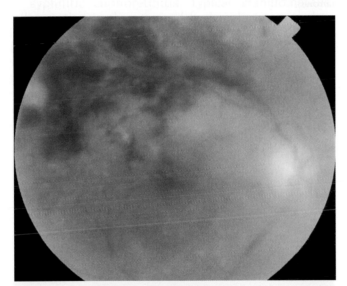

Figure 38-8 Acute temporal superior branch retinal vein obstruction due to syphilitic vasculitis in an immunocompetent patient. (Courtesy of Drs. A and L. Muralha.)

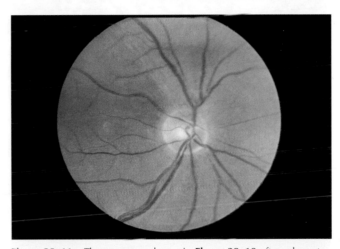

Figure 38-11 The same eye shown in **Figure 38-10** after adequate neurosyphilis therapy.

38.3 Imaging and Diagnostic Tests

38.3.1 FLUORESCEIN ANGIOGRAPHY

Fluorescein staining of the optic discs and major retinal veins is often observed in patients with syphilitic involvement of the posterior pole (**Figures 38-12** and **38-13**). In syphilitic acute posterior placoid chorioretinitis, fluorescein angiography shows hypofluorescence of the active yellow-white chorioretinal lesions, followed by late staining at the level of the RPE. Some placoid lesions may be mistaken for those seen in acute placoid multifocal pigment epitheliopathy and serpiginous choroiditis. Posterior chorioretinitis with serous retinal detachment may also be observed in syphilitic patients (**Figure 38-14**). In these patients, the late phases of the angiogram show hyperfluorescence of the lesion due to pooling of the dye (**Figure 38-15**).

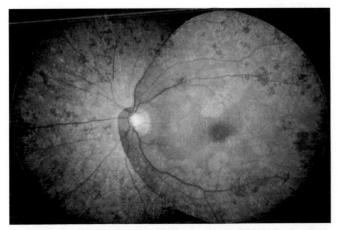

Figure 38-9 Pseudo-retinitis pigmentosa in a patient with acquired immunodeficiency syndrome (AIDS) and neurosyphilis.

351

Chapter 39

Tuberculosis

HAROLDO VIEIRA DE MORAES, JR., MD, PhD

39.1 Introduction

Documentation of the existence of tuberculosis dates back to 3,000 BC. Three *Mycobacteria* species can cause human disease: *Mycobacterium tuberculosis, Mycobacterium bovis, and Mycobacterium africanum.* Any part of the body can be affected, including the eyes. The World Health Organization estimates that 20 million people have active tuberculosis, with an incidence of 8 million cases per year. Tuberculosis is the cause of mortality in one third of affected patients.

The pathogenicity of M. *tuberculosis* is the result of its ability to resist the natural defense mechanisms or immune response of the infected host. Recrudescence of tuberculosis has been seen in patients with the acquired immunodeficiency syndrome (AIDS), because the human immunodeficiency virus (HIV) depletes cell-mediated immunity by eliminating the CD4+ T-lymphocyte cells required for protection against tuberculosis.

Lesions in different parts of the eye cause a variety of clinical presentations and are characterized by a significant inflammatory reaction with subsequent granuloma formation and tissue necrosis. These lesions develop because the proliferation of acid-fast bacilli leads to a delayed-type hypersensitivity reaction to the M. *tuberculosis* antigens.

39.2 Clinical Signs and Symptoms

The most frequent ocular manifestation of tuberculosis is uveitis. Ocular disease may be present without systemic involvement. Active disease may be caused by direct inoculation of the bacilli into the eye, leading to a primary ocular infection, or more often, by hematologic dissemination from primary sites (nose and meninges). Granulomas may form in the conjunctiva, cornea, sclera, uveal tract, optic nerve, orbit, or lids (**Figure 39–1**).

The prevalence of tuberculous uveitis ranges from 1% to 6% in developing countries and is approximately 1% in developed nations. The uveitis is characterized by "mutton-fat" keratic precipitates, Koeppe and Busacca iris nodules (**Figure 39–2**), inflammatory pupillary membranes, and posterior synechiae. Patients with chronic ocular tuberculosis affecting the anterior segment of the eye experience a waxing and waning course of iridocyclitis.

Because of the extensive blood supply to the choroid, choroidal tubercles are the most common manifestation of hematogenous infection. Choroidal granulomas occur commonly in ocular tuberculosis. They may be single or multiple and appear as whitish-yellowish lesions, ranging from 0.5 to 2.0 mm in size. Most lesion are present in the posterior pole of the eye and may occur even in the absence of systemic disease (**Figure 39–3**).

Exudative retinochoroiditis, vasculitis (periphlebitis), vitreitis, and papillitis are less common manifestations of tuberculosis. Tuberculous chorioretinal scars are often misdiagnosed as sequelae of toxoplasmosis,

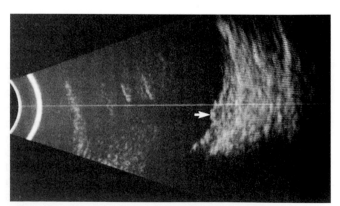

Figure 39–1 B-scan ultrasound demonstrates a mildly elevated lesion with an irregular surface.

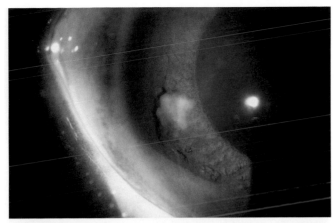

Figure 39–2   Iris nodules usually seen in tuberculous uveitis.

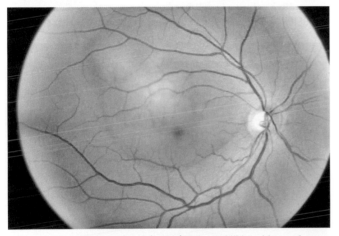

Figure 39–3   Tuberculous choroiditis in an HIV-positive patient.

sarcoidosis, histoplasmosis, syphilis, toxocariasis, or retinoblastoma.

Tuberculous choroiditis is the most common ocular manifestation in patients with AIDS and in severely immunocompromised individuals. It is important to rule out *Pneumocystis carinii*, atypical mycobacterial infections, syphilis, lymphoma, and metastatic cancer. Patients usually present with unilateral involvement. Bilateral ocular tuberculous involvement may occur in patients with miliary tuberculosis. Serous retinal detachment overlying areas of tuberculous choroiditis are frequently observed in these patients (**Figure 39–4**).

The orbit can be affected by dacryoadenitis, orbital cellulitis, or periostitis. Bony erosions may be observed on orbital x-ray films. Patients often develop lymphadenopathy, including preauricular node involvement. The lids may become ulcerated, and enlarged lymph nodes may lead to ectropion and corneal ulcers. Tuberculous abscesses may rarely appear in the conjunctiva and develop a Parinaud-like syndrome, in which patients have unilateral chronic granulomatous conjunctivitis and visible ipsilateral preauricular and submandibular adenopathy. Patients with scleritis present with pain, photophobia, ocular hyperemia, and decreased vision (**Figure 39–5**); chronic ocular involvement can lead to glaucoma, cataract, macular edema, and phthisis bulbi. The differential diagnosis of tuberculous scleritis includes varicella zoster, syphilis, systemic vasculitis, and aspergillosis. Corneal ulcers, interstitial keratitis, and infiltrates can be immunologic manifestations of the disease (**Figure 39–6**).

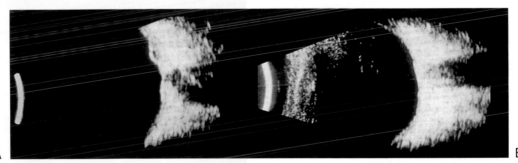

Figure 39–4   B-scan ultrasound shows choroidal thickening and serous retinal detachment (SRD) (*A*), and the fellow eye has choroidal thickening without SRD (*B*).

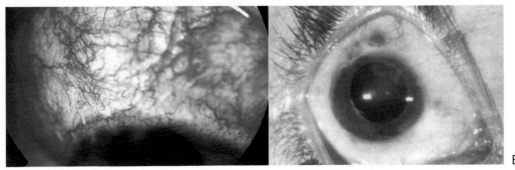

Figure 39–5   Tuberculous scleritis: before (*A*) and after (B) antituberculosis treatment.

Chapter 41

Fungal Infections

J. FERNANDO AREVALO, MD, FACS • CARLOS F. FERNÁNDEZ, MD • ARISTIDES J. MENDOZA, MD

41.1 Introduction

A large number of fungal species exist in nature, but only a relatively small number cause serious primary and opportunistic human diseases. Endogenous fungal infections of the choroid, retina, and vitreous cavity are complications of disseminated fungal infections. Ocular involvement occurs in 10% to 29% of patients with fungemia. Risk factors include bacterial sepsis, prolonged hyperalimentation, systemic antibiotic therapy corticosteroid therapy, recent abdominal surgery, alcoholism, diabetes, hemodialysis, intravenous drug abuse, immunosuppression due to acquired immuno-deficiency syndrome (AIDS), severe burns, malignancies, and chemotherapy. Exogenous fungal infections of the eye are usually complications of penetrating ocular trauma or intraocular surgery or direct extension from infected periocular and orbital tissues.

The most common organisms are from *Candida* species, followed by *Aspergillus*, and *Cryptococcus neoformans*. Other less commonly encountered fungi include *Sporothrix schenckii*, *Histoplasma capsulatum*, *Blastomyces dermatitidis*, and *Coccidioides immitis* (**Figure 41–1**).

41.2 Clinical Signs and Symptoms

Candida albicans is the most common cause of endogenous fungal endophthalmitis. The infection progresses slowly and may take days to weeks to produce damage. The patient may have no visual symptoms with extramacular or peripheral lesions. With progression of disease, patients will notice floaters due to early vitreous inflammation and blurred vision (**Figure 41–2**). Progression of the disease leads to visual loss, pain, and redness of one or both eyes. The typical *Candida* lesion is creamy white and round or oval measuring 1/8 to 1/4 disc diameter with overlying vitreous inflammation.

Lesions may be single or multiple and can increase in size and break into the vitreous, appearing as "cotton balls" or strand-like clusters of inflammatory cells. (**Figure 41–3**). Other signs include vitreous abscesses (**Figure 41–4**), intraretinal hemorrhages, and white-centered hemorrhages (Roth spots).

Aspergillus, a fungus with branching septate hyphae and long stalks or conidiophores, is the second most common cause of intraocular fungal infections. Intravenous drug abuse and systemic immunosuppression due to malignancy, chemotherapy, and the use of corticosteroids and immunosuppressive drugs are risk factors for *Aspergillus* endophthalmitis. Ocular symptoms include blurred vision, eye pain, hyperemia, eyelid edema, and chemosis. A large macular abscess and retinal pseudohypopyon are suggestive of the diagnosis (**Figure 41–5**). Intense reaction within the vitreous is common. Diffuse choroiditis with the formation of Roth spots within the retina, depigmented retinal lesions, or whitish-yellow chorioretinal opacities have been observed.

Cryptococcosis is a systemic infection caused by the round, encapsulated saprophytic fungus *C. neoformans*. An uncommon cause of human disease, it may infect healthy persons but has a special predilection for immunocompromised patients. Ocular symptoms are present in 36% to 40% of patients with cryptococcal meningitis. The most common intraocular manifestation is chorioretinitis that appears initially as a solitary, slightly elevated yellowish-white chorioretinal lesion (**Figure 41–6A** and **B**) often in a juxtapapillary location with minimal or no associated vitreitis. Secondary involvement of the retina may result in retinal whitening, retinal vasculitis, vitreitis, or rarely panophthalmitis or endophthalmitis. Multifocal *C. neoformans* choroiditis may occur in patients with AIDS (**Figure 41–6C** and **D**).

H. capsulatum is associated with two clinical presentations. One is due to the active proliferation of the

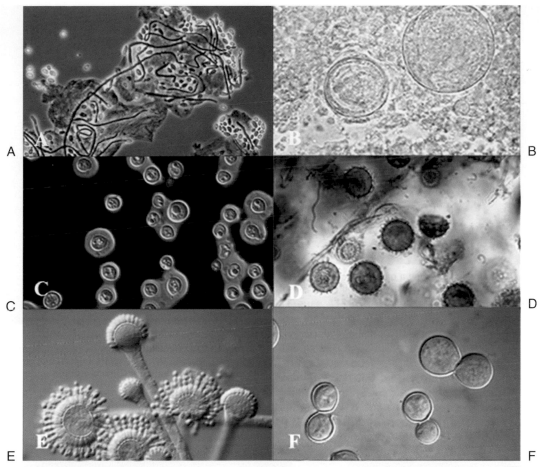

Figure 41–1 Differential interference contrast microscopy: *A: Candida albicans* (yeast cells and pseudohyphae, potassium hydroxide preparation). *B: Coccidioides immitis* (spherules, potassium hydroxide preparation). *C: Cryptococcus neoformans* (the round yeast cells are surrounded by polysaccharide capsules, India ink). *D: Histoplasma capsulatum* (rough-walled macroconidia, Sabouraud glucose agar). *E: Aspergillus* (stages in development of fruiting bodies). *F: Blastomyces dermatitidis* (broad-based budding, thickened cell walls, and globose shape). (Modified from http://www.doctorfungus.org.)

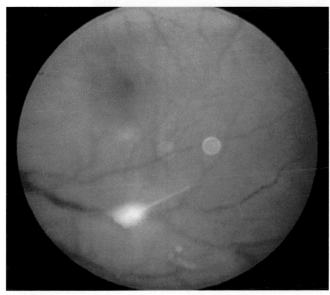

Figure 41–2 Candidiasis. Early vitreous inflammation with a focus of *Candida* chorioretinitis. (Courtesy of Dario Savino-Zari, MD.)

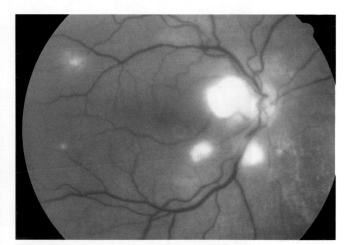

Figure 41–3 Several large and small *Candida* chorioretinal lesions with vitreous invasion are noted temporal to the optic nerve head in the right eye. In addition, healed cytomegalovirus retinitis is seen inferonasal to the optic nerve head in this patient with AIDS.

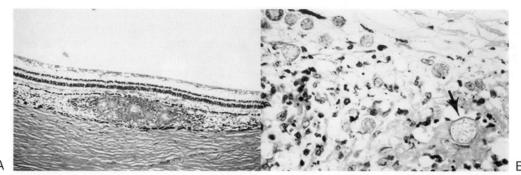

Figure 41–20 *A:* Focal granuloma in the fundus of a man who died of disseminated coccidioidomycosis. *B:* Multiple spherule-containing endospores (*arrow*). (Modified from Boyden BS, Yee D. Bilateral coccidioidal choroiditis: A clinicopathologic case report. Trans Am Acad Ophthalmol Otolaryngol. 1971;75:1006–1010.)

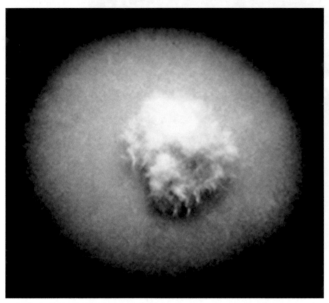

Figure 41–21 • Colony of *B. dermatitidis* on mold inhibitory agar. (Modified from http://www.doctorfungus.org.)

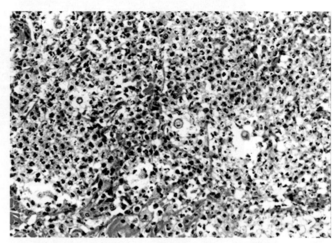

Figure 41–22 Granuloma containing *B. dermatitidis*. (Lewis H, Aaberg TM, Fary DRB, Stevens TS. Latent disseminated blastomycosis with choroidal involvement. Arch Ophthalmol. 1988;106:527–530.)

ACKNOWLEDGMENT

This work was supported in part by the Fundacion Arevalo-Coutinho para la Investigación en Oftalmología (FACO), Caracas, Venezuela.

SUGGESTED READINGS

Arevalo JF, Fuenmayor-Rivera D, Giral AE, Murcia E. Indocyanine green videoangiography of multifocal *Cryptococcus neoformans* choroiditis in a patient with acquired immunodeficiency syndrome. Retina. 2001;21:537–541.

Blumenkranz MS, Stevens DA. Endogenous coccidioidal endophthalmitis. Ophthalmology. 1980;87:974–984.

Brourman ND, Blumenkranz MS. Fungal disease. In: Guyer DR, Yannuzzi LA, Chang S, Shields JA, Green WR, eds. Retina-Vitreous-Macula. Philadelphia, Pa: Saunders, 1999:772–792.

Parke DW 2nd, Jones DB, Gentry LO. Endogenous endophthalmitis among patients with candidemia. Ophthalmology. 1982;89:789–796.

Singh G. Presumed ocular histoplasmosis syndrome. In: Foster CS, Vitale AT, eds. Diagnosis and Treatment of Uveitis. Philadelphia, Pa: Saunders, 2002:348–363.

granulomas may result by distribution of the endospores via the ophthalmic artery (**Figure 41–20**).

B. *dermatitidis* is dimorphic (septate mycelia and conidia). The organism grows almost exclusively in the yeast form, with a rare occurrence of hyphae (**Figure 41–21**). It produces a granulomatous reaction with choroidal and retinal involvement (**Figure 41–22**).

S. *schenckii* produces suppurative and granulomatous reactions, occasionally with caseating necrosis. The organism can be found in the anterior chamber, vitreous cavity, retina, subretinal space, retinal pigment epithelium, and choroid.

Chapter 42

Endophthalmitis

INGRID U. SCOTT, MD, MPH • HARRY W. FLYNN, JR., MD

42.1 Introduction

Endophthalmitis is a potentially devastating eye disease that can lead to severe and permanent visual loss (**Figure 42–1**). An estimated 1 in 1000 intraocular surgeries are complicated by endophthalmitis. Based on a survey at the Bascom Palmer Eye Institute, the overall incidence of postoperative endophthalmitis during a 7-year period (1995 through 2001) was 0.05% (**Table 42–1**). In comparison, the incidence of endophthalmitis after penetrating ocular trauma is much higher and ranges between 3.2% and 30% in reported series (**Figure 42–2**).

It has been reported that external ocular flora represent the most important source of the causative organism in postoperative endophthalmitis (**Figure 42–3**). In one study of endophthalmitis, molecular epidemiologic techniques demonstrated the genetic identity of bacteria from vitreous aspirates to be the same as those from eyelid or conjunctival isolates in 82% of 17

patients. Similarly, in an analysis of 105 eyes with coagulase-negative *Staphylococcus* endophthalmitis with paired isolates from each patient's eyelid and intraocular compartments, pulsed-field gel electrophoresis demonstrated genetically identical organisms in 67.7%.

TABLE 42–1

Incidence of Endophthalmitis in a 7-Year Study at the Bascom Palmer Eye Institute

Procedure	Incidence (%)
Cataract surgery with or without intraocular lens	0.04
Glaucoma filtering surgery	0.2
Penetrating keratoplasty	0.08
Pars plana vitrectomy	0.03
Secondary intraocular lens placement	0.2

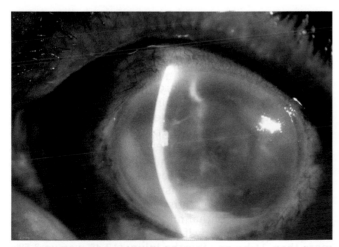

Figure 42–1   Patient with endophthalmitis after a clear corneal phacoemulsification and intraocular lens insertion.

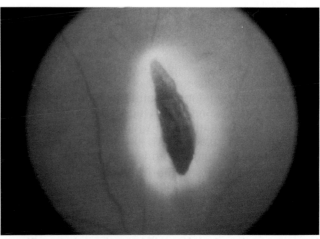

Figure 42–2   Retained intraocular foreign body with surrounding exudates after penetrating ocular trauma.

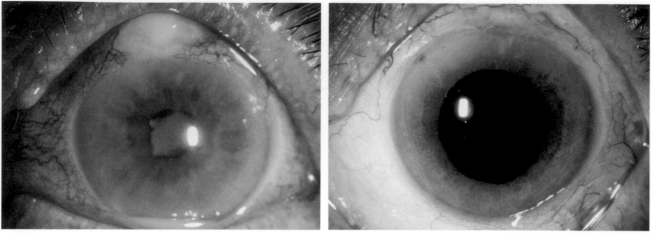

A   B

Figure 42–8 *A:* Bleb-associated endophthalmitis with a purulent bleb, hypopyon, miotic pupil, and dense vitreitis. Visual acuity was hand motions. *B:* After the use of iris hooks to dilate the miotic pupil, pars plana vitrectomy with injection of intravitreal antibiotics was performed and visual acuity improved to 20/40. *S. epidermidis* was cultured from the anterior chamber and vitreous. (From Flynn HW Jr, et al. Indigenous fungal endophthalmitis. In: Vitreo-Retinal and Uveitis Update: Proceedings of the 47th Annual Symposium of the New Orleans Academy of Ophthalmology, New Orleans, La, April 3–5, 1998. Kugler Publications. The Hague, the Netherlands, 1998: 298 [Figure 1].)

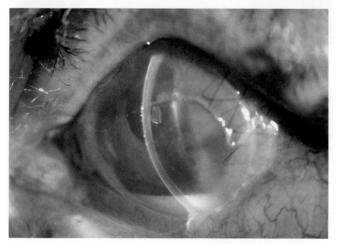

Figure 42–9 Hypopyon, fibrin in the anterior chamber, and marked visual loss after secondary intraocular lens implantation.

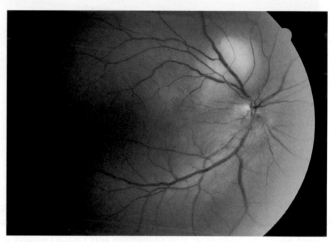

Figure 42–10 Patient with tuberculous choroiditis.

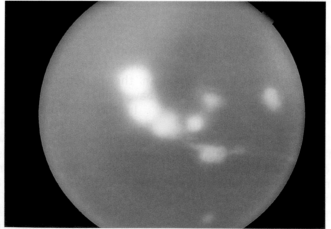

Figure 42–11 Endogenous endophthalmitis caused by *Candida albicans* may present with a "string of pearls" in the vitreous. (From Flynn HW Jr, et al. In: Vitreo-Retinal and Uveitis Update: Proceedings of the 47th Annual Symposium of the New Orleans Academy of Ophthalmology, New Orleans, La, April 3–5, 1998. The Hague, the Netherlands, 1998:297–305.)

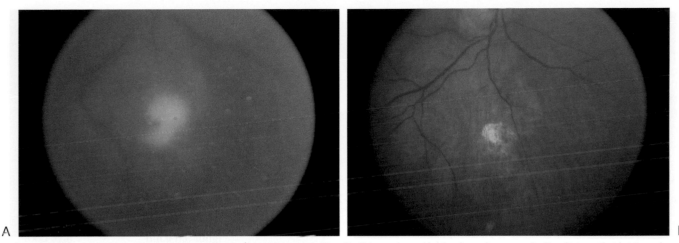

Figure 42–12 *A:* Patient with endogenous endophthalmitis caused by *C. albicans* 4 weeks after bowel surgery. *B:* Resolution of vitreitis and focal lesion after pars plana vitrectomy and intravitreal injection of amphotericin B.

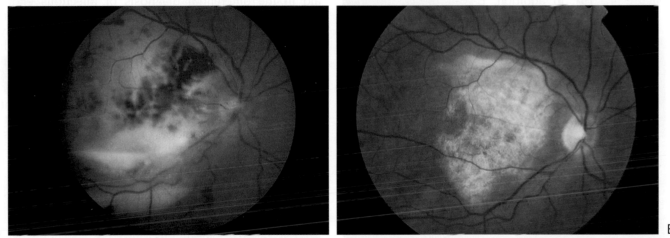

Figure 42–13 *A:* Mild vitreitis, a diffuse macular chorioretinal lesion with subretinal and subhyaloid hypopyon, intraretinal hemorrhages, and papillitis in a patient with endogenous endophthalmitis caused by *Aspergillus*. *B:* Two months after treatment, a macular scar, preserved overlying retinal vessels, and temporal disc pallor are seen. Final visual acuity was 20/400. (From Weishaar PD, Flynn HW Jr, Murray TG, et al. Endogenous *Aspergillus* endophthalmitis. Clinical features and treatment outcomes. Ophthalmology. 1998;105:57–65.)

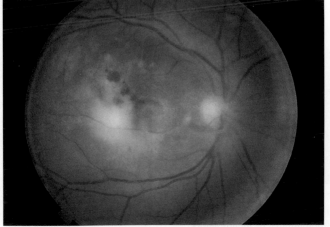

Figure 42–14 Patient with reactivation of toxoplasmosis chorioretinitis, which may resemble endogenous endophthalmitis.

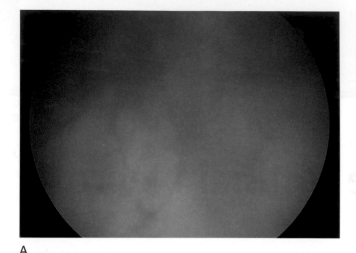

A

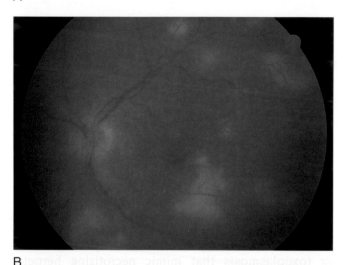

B

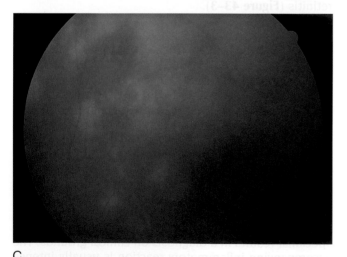

C

Figure 43–1 *A:* The left fundus of this 21-year-old man shows classic findings of peripheral confluent retinal whitening. The whitened retina is edematous with the appearance of venous stasis. *B:* The posterior pole of the same patient shows scattered retinal infiltrates. This degree of posterior involvement is somewhat unusual. *C:* Extensive confluent necrotizing retinitis was present for 360 degrees. Viral diagnostic studies (PCR) from the aqueous humor confirmed herpes simplex II infection.

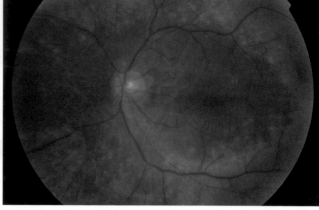

Figure 43–2 Progressive outer retinal necrosis variant. This HIV-infected patient displays extensive retinal necrosis with no vitreous cell or vascular inflammation or inflammatory optic neuropathy.

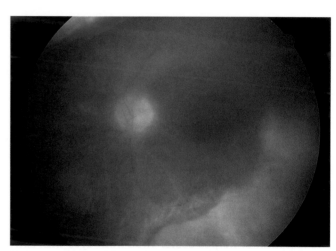

Figure 43–3 Toxoplasmic chorioretinitis mimicking ARN in a 77-year-old woman, who developed 6 clock hours of retinitis after reactivation of toxoplasmic chorioretinitis.

severity is the number of clock hours involved; another is the extent of posterior progression. Multifocal lesions that are not adjacent to the ora are not typical for ARNS and suggest other infectious etiologies. Isolated posterior lesions are more properly thought of as satellites than as distinct foci of disease (**Figure 43–1B**). Arteritis is often occlusive and can lead to permanent loss of vision (**Figure 43–4**). Optic nerve edema is common. Whether the profound optic atrophy that may occur is due more to widespread axonal loss or to residua of optic nerve edema is unclear (**Figure 43–5**). Retrobulbar optic neuropathy can lead to loss of the perception of light before the development of visible retinal lesions (**Figure 43–6**).

Immunocompromised individuals may lack the intense inflammatory reactions and present only with necrotizing retinitis. The lack of inflammation results in striking clinical images of the dying retina (**Figure 43–7**).

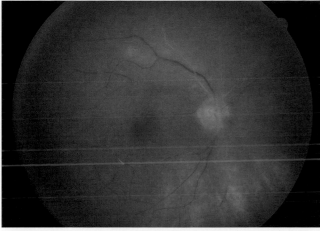

A

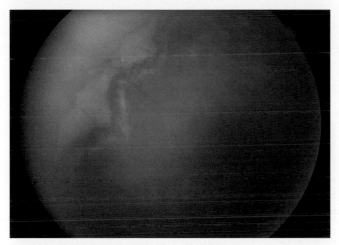
B

Figure 43–4 *A:* Superior arterioles appear sheathed and occluded in this elderly patient with necrotizing herpetic retinopathy. Vision was 20/400. *B:* Peripheral retinitis involved less than one quadrant, despite the severe vasculopathy. The lesion is in the process of healing. Addition of oral prednisone improved blood flow, and vision increased to 20/50.

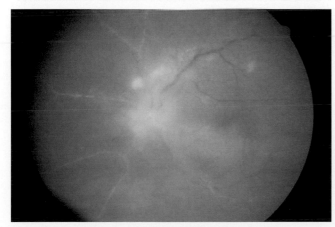

Figure 43–5 Intense inflammatory papillopathy culminated in optic nerve pallor and light perception vision. Arterioles are sclerotic. (Courtesy of Harry Flynn, MD.)

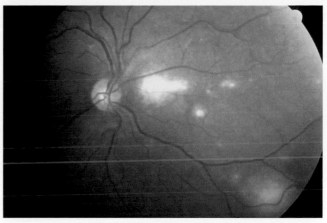

Figure 43–6 Vision was light perception due to retrobulbar optic neuropathy in this HIV-infected woman with sparse patches of retinal whitening.

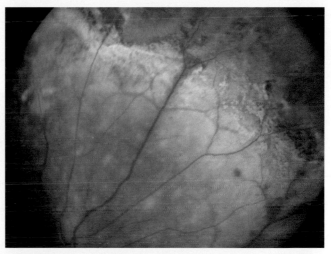

Figure 43–7 Rapid progression of herpetic retinitis in an HIV-infected man led to three distinct zones of retinal infection: peripheral detachment of gliotic retina, confluent retinal whitening, and a broad band of satellite lesions.

Disseminated varicella can cause multiple cutaneous lesions (**Figure 43–8**).

Treatment is typically administration of intravenous acyclovir 10 mg/kg every 8 hours for 7 to 10 days or longer, depending on the patient's response. Immuno-compromised individuals treated with acyclovir have a high rate of bilateral blindness. Combination antiviral treatment with ganciclovir and foscarnet reduces the risk of blindness. Intravitreal injection of ganciclovir, foscarnet, or combined ganciclovir and foscarnet is helpful in controlling severe, progressive disease. Corticosteroids are used to mitigate inflammatory damage to the optic nerve and retinal blood vessels. Although recurrences in the same eye are very rare, involvement in a previously uninvolved second eye can occur at any time. Risk is greatest in the first 14 weeks after involvement of the first eye, and oral antiviral therapy is recommended for 3 months after completion of intravenous treatment.

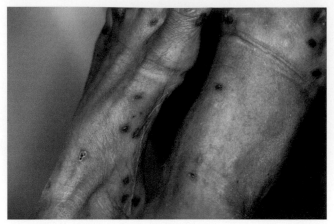

Figure 43–8 Diffuse verrucous skin lesions had been present for weeks before development of bilateral necrotizing herpetic retinopathy. Skin biopsy confirmed varicella zoster.

Effective treatment stops the posterior progression of lesions. As the retinitis heals, the borders first become atrophic or faintly pigmented (**Figure 43–4B**). The peripheral retinal whitening then recedes, leaving progressive chorioretinal scarring in its wake with variable degrees of hyperpigmentation, usually mild (**Figure 43–9A** and **B**). Optic nerve edema subsides slowly and may result in optic nerve atrophy. Retinal vessels are typically narrowed or occluded (**Figure 43–9C**).

Retinal detachment occurs in about 50% of patients, usually at 8 to 12 weeks after presentation (**Figure 43–10**) and is treated by vitrectomy, usually without scleral buckling. Silicone oil is commonly used in retinal detachment repair (**Figure 43–11**). Laser photocoagulation in areas of healthy retina to demarcate the necrotic areas may reduce that risk fourfold (**Figure 43–12**). Retinal detachment is felt to be a key determinant of poor visual prognosis in treated eyes.

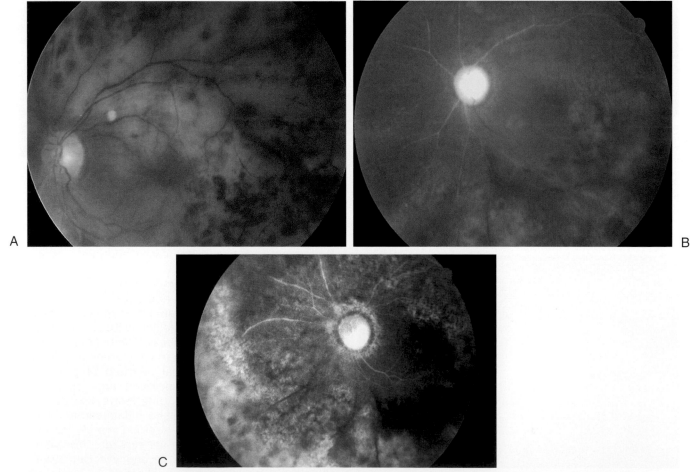

Figure 43–9 *A:* Fulminant necrotizing retinopathy in an HIV-infected patient. *B:* Healing occurred with combination antiviral therapy and intravitreal injections of ganciclovir and foscarnet. The patient retained 20/200 vision. *C:* Fluorescein angiography showed pigmentary scarring and vascular occlusion in the areas of retinitis.

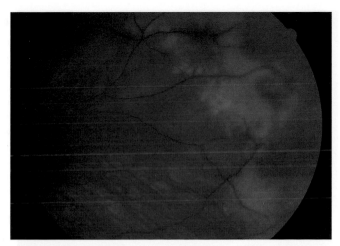

Figure 43–10 Retinal detachment is beginning in the area of confluent retinal infection in this iatrogenically immunosuppressed patient.

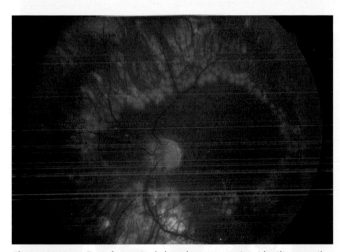

Figure 43–11 Eye after retinal detachment repair with silicone oil. There is peripheral scarring from prophylactic laser, posterior laser placed at surgery, and a large temporal retinal pigment epithelium rip. Vision is 20/40. (Same patient as in **Figure 43–1**.)

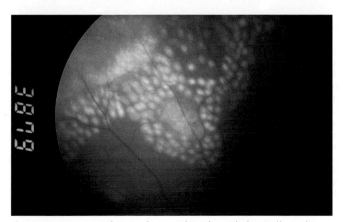

Figure 43–12 Laser barricade was placed prophylactically in this HIV-infected patient. Retinal detachment did not occur, and vision remained 20/30.

43.3 Imaging and Diagnostic Tests

43.3.1 FLUORESCEIN ANGIOGRAPHY

Diffuse leakage from retinal veins and the optic nerve is common in the presence of vitreous inflammation. Occlusive vasculopathy is prominent in some patients with ARNS (**Figure 43–13**). Angiographic signs of retinal vascular inflammation are helpful diagnostically in early occurrences without prominent retinal whitening (**Figure 43–14A** and **B**). After healing, there is complete closure of retinal vessels within the lesions (**Figure 43–9C**).

43.3.2 OPTICAL COHERENCE TOMOGRAPHY

Findings are consistent with a coagulative necrosis of inner retina, retinal thickening, and exudation of shallow subretinal fluid (**Figure 43–14C**).

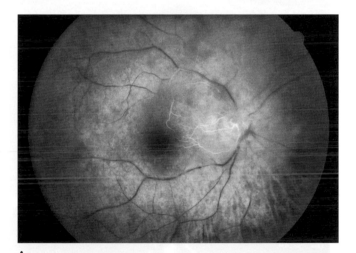

A

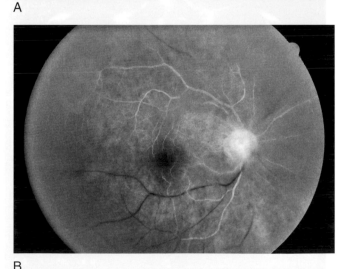

B

Figure 43–13 *A:* Early-phase angiogram of the patient in **Figure 43–4** shows marked arteriolar occlusion. *B:* Mid-phase angiogram shows persistent poor filling of arteries and veins. The patient recovered vision with prednisone treatment.

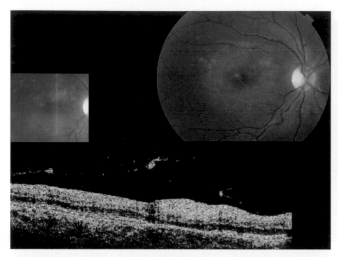

Figure 44–7 OCT image in active OT showing increased retinal thickness, disorganization, and superficial changes.

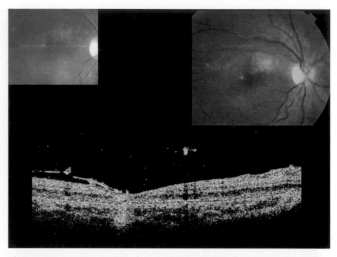

Figure 44–8 OCT image showing partial posterior vitreous detachment (PVD), vitreous attached to the toxoplasmic scar, and focal retinal thinning with atrophy.

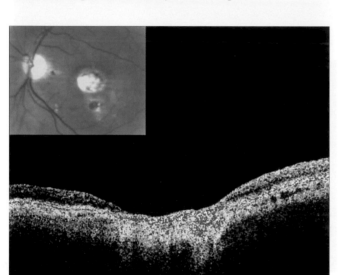

Figure 44–9 OCT image showing a chorioretinal scar and total disorganization within the retina.

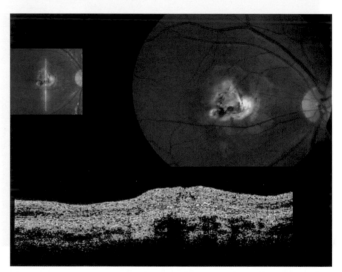

Figure 44–10 OCT image showing deep retinal involvement and partially preserved superficial retina.

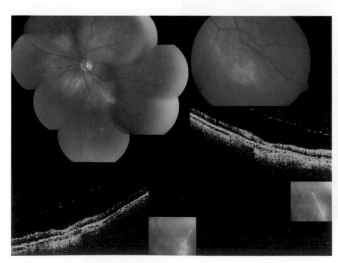

Figure 44–11 OCT image showing retinal thinning with atrophy in an acquired toxoplasmic lesion.

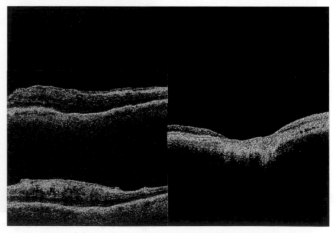

Figure 44–12 OCT image comparing active OT with intraretinal fluid and increased intraretinal backscattering *(left)* with a chorioretinal scar (inactive OT) with complete loss of neurosensory retinal tissue *(right).*

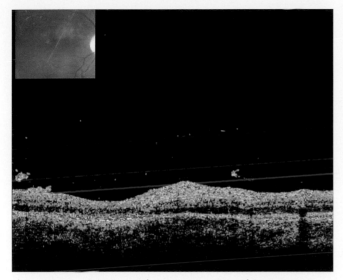

Figure 44–13   OCT image showing active OT with vitreous opacities, foveal depression, and focal retinal thickening.

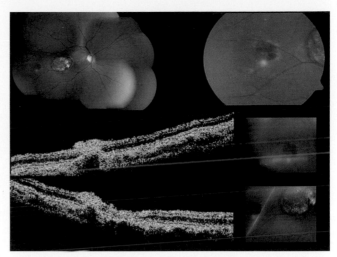

Figure 44–14   OCT image showing active OT recurrence, no vitreous cells, and retinal thickening.

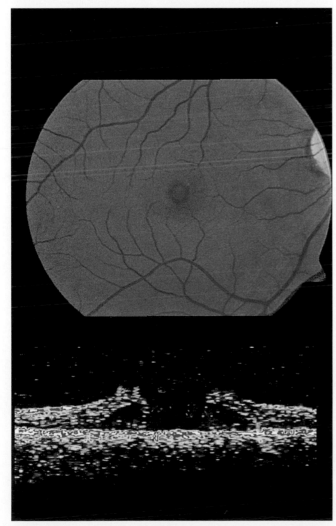

Figure 44–15   OCT image showing one complication from OT: a macular hole.

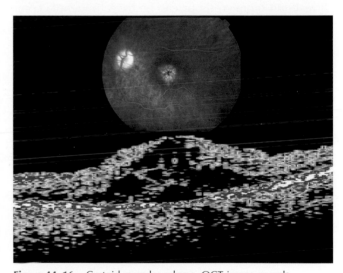

Figure 44–16   Cystoid macular edema. OCT image reveals intraretinal cysts.

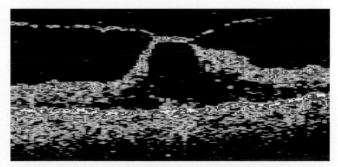

Figure 44–17   OCT image reveals epiretinal membrane with traction.

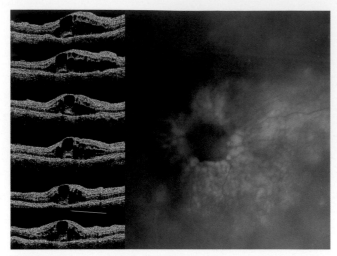

Figure 44–18   Cystoid macular edema. OCT images reveal intraretinal cysts.

44.3.4 ULTRASONOGRAPHY

Ultrasound biomicroscopy can be used to identify complications in the anterior portion of the eye including ciliary body detachment, intraocular lens displacement, angle-closure glaucoma, and others. B-scan ultrasound is used in patients in whom fundus examination is difficult or impossible due to the presence of posterior synechiae, cataract, or corneal opacification. B-scan ultrasound can identify complications such as retinal and choroidal detachment, vitreous hemorrhages or opacities, and vitreoretinal traction.

44.4 Pathology

OT in immunocompetent patients is characterized by foci of coagulative necrosis of the retina with sharply demarcated borders. Inflammatory changes can be widespread in the eye and may involve the choroid, iris, and trabecular meshwork. Cysts can be found in the retina with little disruption of the retinal architecture. Chorioretinal scars are characterized by gliosis, obliteration of vessels, and hyperpigmentation at the borders. Calcification can be present. Immunosuppressed patients with ocular toxoplasmosis may have both tachyzoites and cysts in areas of retinal necrosis and within retinal pigment epithelial cells. Parasites can occasionally be found in the choroid, vitreous, and optic nerve.

SUGGESTED READINGS

Gilbert RE, See SE, Jones LV, Stanford MS. Antibiotics Versus Control for Toxoplasma Retinochoroiditis (Cochrane Review). The Cochrane Library, Issue 1. Oxford, England: Update Software, 2002.

Holland GN. Ocular toxoplasmosis in the immunocompromised host. Int Ophthalmol. 1989;13:399–402.

Holland GN, Lewis KG. An update on current practices in the management of ocular toxoplasmosis. Am J Ophthalmol. 2002; 134:102–114.

Holland GN, O'Connor GR, Belfort R Jr, Remington JS. Toxoplasmosis. In: Pepose JS, Holland GN, Wilhelmus KR, eds. Ocular Infection and Immunity. St. Louis, Mo: Mosby-Year Book, 1996:1183–1223.

Silveira C, Belfort R Jr, Muccioli C, et al. The effect of long-term intermittent trimethoprim/sulfamethoxazole treatment on recurrences of toxoplasmic retinochoroiditis. Am J Ophthalmol. 2002;134:41–46.

Chapter 45

Toxocariasis

HAROLDO VIEIRA DE MORAES, JR., MD, PhD

45.1 Introduction

Toxocariasis is an infection usually caused by *Toxocara canis*, a canine intestinal parasite and less often by another nematode, *Toxocara cati*.

T. *canis* was first identified in human beings by Beaver in 1952. After that, several authors described the disease in many different countries. Wilder (1950) found nematode larvae in histologic specimens of 24 of 46 enucleated eyes with differential diagnosis of retinoblastoma, and Nichols in 1956 identified those larvae as *Toxocara* in its second stage. Many cases of endophthalmitis (first type) caused by nematodes have been described ever since. Ashton published a different presentation of ocular involvement with granulomatous lesions located on the posterior pole (second type), and Hogan et al. in 1965 described the third form of ocular manifestation, which includes a sole retinal granuloma. Finally, Gass in 1978 reported on a fourth type called *diffuse unilateral subacute neuroretinitis* (DUSN).

An enzyme-linked immunosorbent assay (ELISA) is used in epidemiologic studies to determine the prevalence of *Toxocara*. Sensitivity and specificity are 75% and 95%, respectively, for a sera titer of 1:32. Results showed a wide range of prevalence from 1% in Canada to 92.8% in The Reunion Islands in the Indian Ocean. Maetz et al. in 1987 found 1 positive case in 1000 inhabitants in Alabama in the United States. Some studies relate the prevalence of human infection to a direct rate of soil contamination caused by canine feces.

45.2 Clinical Signs and Symptoms

Ocular involvement by T. *canis*, often unilateral, usually occurs in children between 4 and 6 years of age (**Figure 45–1**). Bilateral involvement and adult manifestations are rarely found. Visual complaints include a decrease in visual acuity, strabismus, and leukocoria. Orefice et al. reported 100% incidence of vitreitis and 73% of anterior

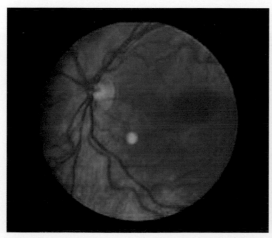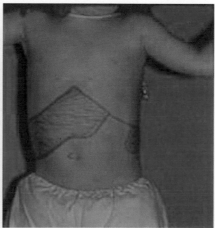

Figure 45–1 Acute phase of visceral larva migrans in a child with hepatosplenomegaly and a granuloma in his left eye. (Courtesy of Fernando Orefice, MD.)

chamber inflammation in 30 patients examined. Based on a literature review in 1984, Shields found nine types of clinical presentation for ocular toxocariasis: endophthalmitis, posterior pole granuloma, peripheral granuloma, DUSN, subretinal mobile larvae, optic neuritis, keratitis, conjunctivitis, and lens involvement. The first three types are the ones found most often.

Endophthalmitis is the most common form, manifested by severe vitreous inflammation, exudative retinal detachment, posterior synechiae, granulomatous keratic precipitates, flare, cells, and hypopyon. Hyperemia, photophobia, and pain are not prominent. After the initial episode, a membrane posterior to the lens, iris seclusion, and cataract can be found (**Figure 45–2**).

A *posterior pole granuloma* is characterized by a sole granulomatous lesion located in the posterior segment, usually between the optic disc and macula (**Figure 45–3**). A whitish mass surrounded with a black halo (blood) and perilesional edema can be seen. A mild anterior chamber inflammatory reaction and moderate vitreous reaction occur. During the chronic phase, an elevated white lesion without hemorrhage can be found. In some eyes, a traction overlying the retina from the lesion to the optic disc or macula is seen (**Figures 45–4** to **45–6**).

A *peripheral granuloma* is a large, white mass located between the equator and periphery of the retina, near the posterior lens, usually associated with retina folds and presenting a "tail" headed toward the retina (**Figures 45–6** and **45–7**). Some patients have a vitreoretinal traction, which leads to macular heterotopia and decreased vision. Differential diagnosis includes retinoblastoma.

DUSN can affect children and young adults, with progressive vision loss and funduscopy changes. The initial phase has nummular lesions (evanescent crops of grayish white dots) that scar in weeks with adjacent lesions appearing. Mild vitreitis and retinal vasculitis are followed by arteriolar attenuation and optic disc atrophy ("wipe-out" phase), which occurs with about 2 years of evolution. The only treatment is to find the helminth moving on the retina through careful ophthalmoscopic examination and perform laser photocoagulation on it to destroy the worm (**Figures 45–8**). Recently, some cases of bilateral involvement have been described.

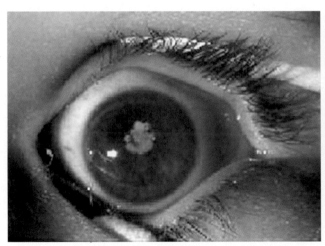
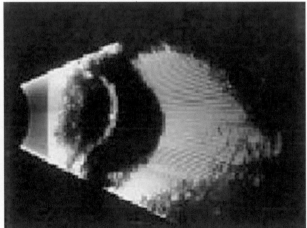

Figure 45–2 Sequelae of endophthalmitis form: cataract and iris seclusion with correspondent B-scan ultrasound. (Courtesy of Fernando Orefice, MD.)

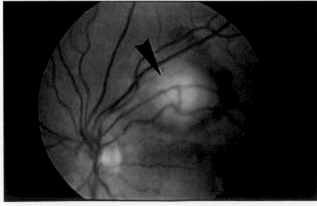
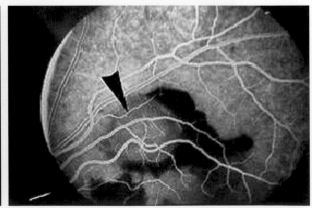

Figure 45–3 Posterior pole granuloma form: active lesion surrounded by edema and hemorrhage; fluorescein angiography shows blockage with arteriovenous shunt.

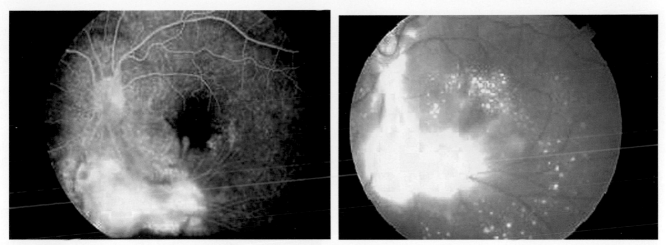

Figure 45–4 Active lesion with traction between the granuloma and optic nerve; fluorescein angiography reveals the extent of the exudative lesion.

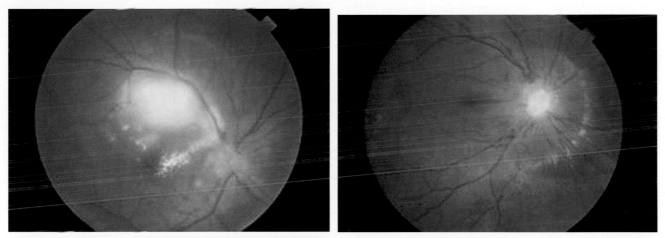

Figure 45–5 Posterior pole granuloma peripapillary lesion with severe exudation surrounding the lesion. (Courtesy of Fernando Orefice, MD.)

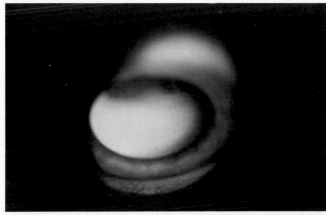

Figure 45–6 Peripheral granuloma. (Courtesy of Fernando Orefice, MD.)

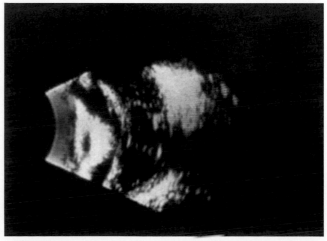

Figure 45–7 B scan ultrasound shows mass posterior to the lens.

Figure 45–8 Subretinal mobile larva. (Courtesy of Carlos Garcia, MD.)

45.3 Imaging and Diagnostic Tests

Confirming toxocariasis by biopsy is rare because of the difficulty in getting a sample for examination.

Clinical and epidemiologic data are of utmost importance for a correct assessment. These include the child's age (4 to 6 years), the history of contact with dogs (puppies younger than 6 months of age), geophagia, and unilateral ocular involvement.

Serum anti-toxocara antibodies (ELISA) which detect immunoglobulin G antibody, have 75% sensitivity and 95% specificity for titers equal to 1:32 (sometimes titers from the aqueous humor can be measured); cross-reactions can occur with other helminths, rheumatoid factor, and reactive protein C tests. A titer of 1:8 in the serum is usually taken as evidence of a positive test result for ocular toxocariasis.

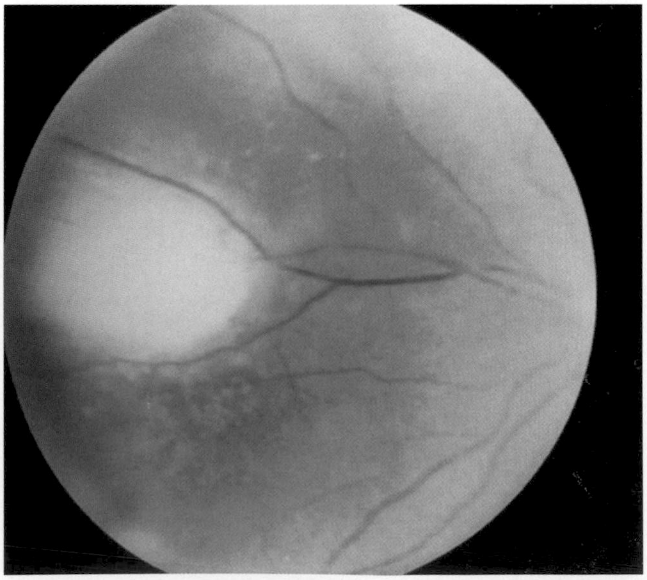

A blood eosinophilia rate higher than 30% of the total leukocyte count occurs in 35% of positive patients. Stool analysis in ocular toxocariasis is always negative.

Fluorescein angiography may show hemorrhagic blockage, arteriovenous shunts, macular edema, and the extension of the exudative process. Early phases may show hypofluorescence determined by blockage of visible intralesional vessels. Late phases may reveal a hyperfluorescent area (fluorescein surrounding the lesion) with a progressive increase, leading to enlargement of the hyperfluorescence; the retina is impregnated and a discrete leakage can occur (**Figures 45–9** to **45–11**).

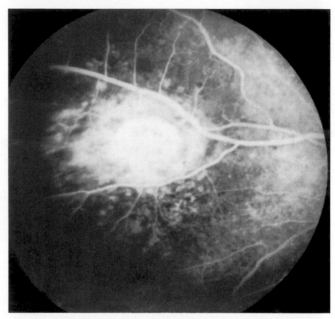

Figure 45–10 Fluorescein angiography shows hyperfluorescent area and dye impregnation, surrounding the lesion (late phase).

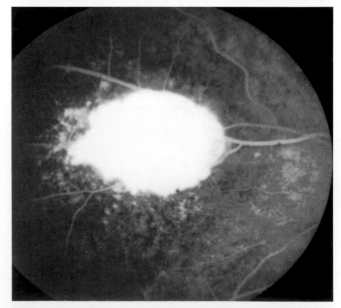

Figure 45–9 Posterior pole granuloma. (Courtesy of Fernando Orefice, MD.)

Figure 45–11 Fluorescein angiography (late phase) reveals more impregnation and discrete leakage to the vitreous (same patient as in **Figure 45–10**).

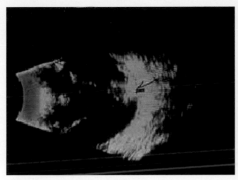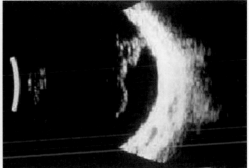

Figure 45–12 B-scan ultrasound reveals two different presentations of a posterior polar granuloma.

Indocyanine green angiography is not useful in the diagnosis or management of the disease.

B-scan ultrasound can reveal an inflammatory mass (granuloma) (**Figure 45–12**) and retinal detachment; it is an important examination for the differential diagnosis of retinoblastoma. Although there are no pathognomonic echographic criteria for toxocariasis, three characteristics are common in eyes with either clear media or with endophthalmitis: an elevated granuloma that may be calcified, a vitreous membrane extending from the granuloma to the posterior pole, and posterior traction retinal detachment or a retinal fold

Ultrasound biomicroscopy seems to be specific and sensitive in patients with a presumed diagnosis of peripheral toxocariasis.

Orbit x-rays and orbit computed tomography can disclose calcium inside the affected eye.

On optical coherence tomography, a macular granuloma initially appears as a highly reflective mass protruding above the retinal pigment epithelium and shows dye leakage by fluorescein angiography. After treatment, the lesion is no longer exudative, and it is less elevated and covered by retinal pigment epithelium,

with a presentation similar to that of idiopathic choroidal neovascularization.

The following should be considered in the differential diagnosis, on the basis of the clinical and funduscopic findings: Coats' disease (**Figure 45–13**), retinoblastoma, ocular toxoplasmosis, pars planitis (**Figure 45–14**), persistent hyperplastic primary vitreous, and retinopathy of prematurity.

45.4 Pathology

Manifestations of ocular toxocariasis vary according to the clinical presentation and lesion localization. Granulomas consist of eosinophils surrounded by epithelioid cells in the retina; helminthic fragments can also be found in the center of the granuloma.

ACKNOWLEDGMENT

The author is indebted to Fernando Orefice, MD, and wishes to acknowledge his contribution and figures for this chapter.

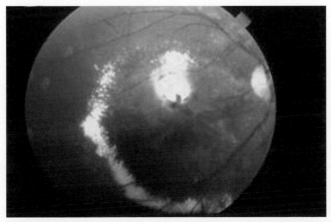

Figure 45–13 Polar granuloma mimicking Coats' disease. (Courtesy of Fernando Orefice, MD.)

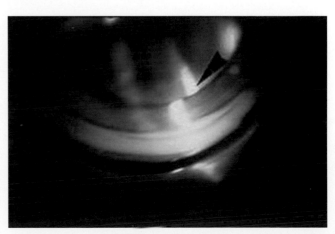

Figure 45–14 Pars planitis.

SUGGESTED READINGS

Mets MB, Noble AG, Basti S, et al. Eye findings of diffuse unilateral subacute neuroretinitis and multiple choroidal infiltrates associated with neural larva migrans due to *Baylisascaris procyonis*. Am J Ophthalmol. 2003;135:888–900.

Orefice F. Toxocariasis. In: Uveitis: Clinical and Surgical. Textbook and Atlas. Rio de Janeiro, Brazil: Cultura Medica, 2000:717–730.

Sabrosa NA, de Souza EC. Nematode infections of the eye: Toxocariasis and diffuse unilateral subacute neuroretinitis (review). Curr Opin Ophthalmol. 2001;12:450–454.

Shields JA. Ocular toxocariasis. A review. Surv Ophthalmol. 1984;28:361–381.

Taylor MR. The epidemiology of ocular toxocariasis (review). J Helminthol. 2001;75:109–118.

Chapter 46

Cysticercosis

LOURDES ARELLANES-GARCÍA, MD

46.1 Introduction

Cysticercosis is caused by the encystment of the larvae of the tapeworm *Taenia solium*; it is the most common ocular platyhelminth infestation in humans. Pigs are the intermediate hosts and humans are the definitive hosts for T. *solium*. In cysticercosis, humans become the intermediate host by ingesting eggs of T. *solium* from contaminated pork meat, vegetables, polluted water, or other material contaminated with human feces. After penetrating the intestinal wall, the embryo invades the bloodstream and can disseminate to the skin, brain, eye, and other tissues. Human helminthiasis and porcine cysticercosis have been known as long as medical records have been recorded; in fact, they were noted in the Ebers Papyrus (ca. 1500 BC) in Egypt and in the writings of Hippocrates. T. *solium* has a worldwide distribution, with higher incidence in Mexico, Africa, Southeast Asia, Eastern Europe, and South America. Some risk factors for human infestation have been described: older age groups, absence of sanitary facilities, poor formal education, poverty, and the inability to recognize infected pork. The age incidence for ocular involvement is preferentially the first four decades of life. Earlier reports failed to reveal a sex predilection, but recently a male preponderance of 3:1 was reported in 44 Indian patients. Bilateral involvement has rarely been found. Neurocysticercosis and ocular cysticercosis seem to be more common in Latin America, whereas skin disease is relatively more common in India.

The ocular cysticercus can be localized in any part of the eye, such as the anterior chamber (**Figure 46–1**), subconjunctival space, optic disc, subretinal space, and vitreous cavity.

46.2 Clinical Signs and Symptoms

Of more than 500 reported cases of ocular cysticercosis, approximately 20% were located subconjunctivally, 8% involved the anterior segment, and 68% were located in the posterior segment.

In the eye, the life cycle of the cysticercus is at least 2 years, and symptoms may be absent in the early stages while the parasite is small. As it grows, the parasite can cause progressive and painless loss of vision. The patient may describe a dark, round, and mobile spot in the visual field. If the cysticercus is located in the macular subretinal space or at the optic disc, there is an acute decrease in visual acuity, along with nonspecific defects in the visual field. When the parasite dies, the secondary inflammatory response is responsible for symptoms such as ocular pain, photophobia, and decreased visual acuity. Sometimes a severe inflammatory reaction may simulate an acute endophthalmitis. Neurologic manifestations such as seizures, intracranial hypertension with papilledema, visual field defects, mental changes, and cranial nerve palsies suggest concurrent central nervous system involvement.

The parasite reaches the globe through the posterior ciliary arteries and enters the subretinal space; in about

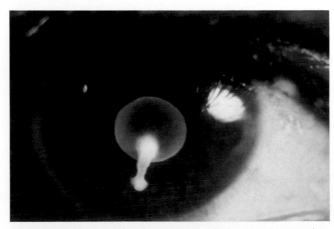

Figure 46–1 Anterior chamber cysticercus with a prominent scolex and an intact cyst.

80% of patients, the macular area is affected (**Figures 46–2** and **46–3**). The cysticercus may perforate the retina (**Figures 46–4** and **46–5**) and present in the vitreous humor as a free-floating cyst (**Figure 46–6**). The living parasite may show contraction, expansion, and undulation movements that can be elicited by light.

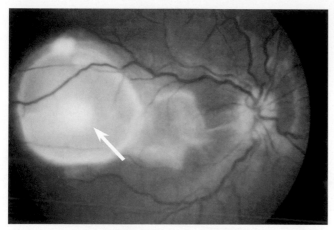

Figure 46–2   Subretinal temporal cysticercus with subretinal fibrosis. The scolex appears as a white spot in the center of the cyst (*arrow*).

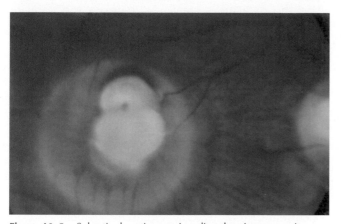

Figure 46–3   Subretinal cysticercus invading the vitreous cavity through a retinal hole with surrounding serous retinal detachment. (Courtesy of Magin Puig-Solanes, MD, and Rafael Sánchez-Fontan, MD.)

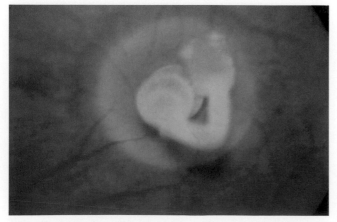

Figure 46–4   Scolex migration into the vitreous cavity. (Courtesy of Magin Puig-Solanes, MD, and Rafael Sánchez-Fontan, MD.)

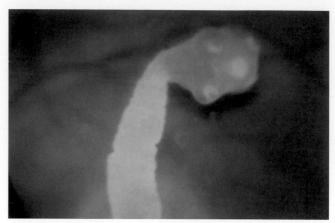

Figure 46–5   Close-up of the scolex head in the vitreous cavity. (Courtesy of Magin Puig-Solanes, MD, and Rafael Sánchez-Fontan, MD.)

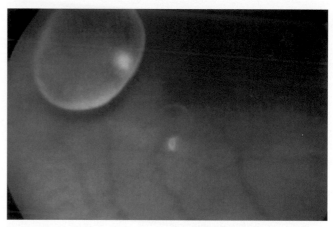

Figure 46–6   Free cysticercus cyst floating in the vitreous cavity. (Courtesy of Magin Puig-Solanes, MD, and Rafael Sánchez-Fontan, MD.)

Tractional, rhegmatogenous, and exudative retinal detachments have been reported in about half of patients. A recent report registered a high incidence of proliferative vitreoretinopathy (60%). If the parasite is not surgically removed, a severe exudative choroiditis and vitreitis that can lead to disorganization of the globe may develop.

46.3 Imaging and Diagnostic Tests

With A-scan ultrasonography, two highly reflective spikes showing the anterior and posterior walls of the cyst can be seen (**Figure 46–7**). 100% reflectivity can be seen inside the cyst, representing the scolex, which usually has an eccentric position. Mode B reveals a cystic mass with a highly reflective eccentric opacity, which may show undulation movements (**Figure 46–8**).

An enzyme-linked immunosorbent assay (ELISA) test for *T. solium* is not useful in the diagnosis of ocular cysticercosis.

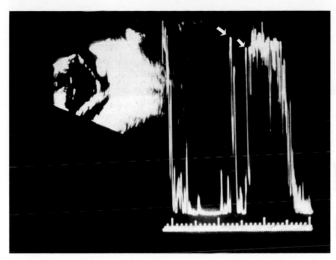

Figure 46–7 Ocular mode A ultrasound: two high-reflectivity spikes showing the anterior and posterior walls of the cyst (*arrows*). Mode B ultrasound: cystic mass with highly reflective eccentric opacity. (Courtesy of Eduardo Moragrega, MD.)

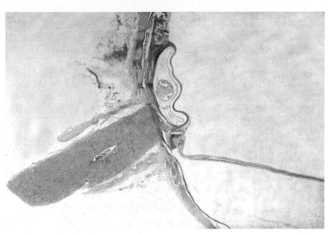

Figure 46–9 Subretinal cysticercus adjacent to the optic nerve head. Hematoxylin and eosin, original amplification ×2. (Courtesy of Abelardo Rodríguez, MD.)

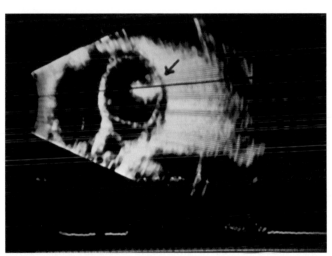

Figure 46–8 Ocular mode B ultrasound: subretinal cysticercus. The *arrow* points to the scolex inside the cyst. (Courtesy of Eduardo Moragrega, MD.)

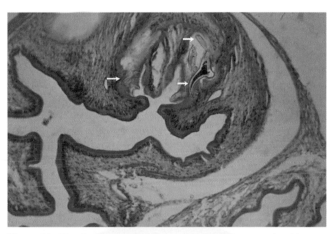

Figure 46–10 Scolex with sucker system and numerous hooklets (*arrows*). There is also a branched cavity that corresponds to the parasite's intestinal tube. Hematoxylin and eosin, original amplification ×10. (Courtesy of Abelardo Rodríguez, MD.)

46.4 Pathology

Late-stage histopathologic studies show the presence of a central eosinophilic mass with some parasite fragments, surrounded by a polymorphonuclear infiltrate. Eosinophils, neutrophils, and macrophages surround the dying organism. Lymphocytes and plasma cells infiltrate the choroid. The cyst contains fluid and a single invaginated scolex. The scolex has four large suckers and rostellum armed with a double row of large and small hooklets, numbering 22 to 32. The hooklets are acid-fast and birefringent (**Figures 46–9** to **46–11**).

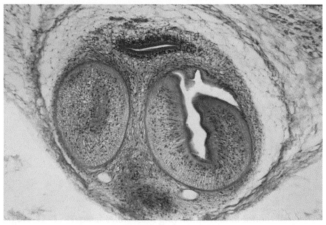

Figure 46–11 Transversal view of the internal structures of a cysticercus. Hematoxylin and eosin, original amplification ×10. (Courtesy of Abelardo Rodríguez, MD.)

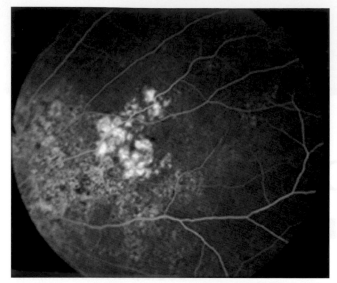

Figure 47–2 Subtle RPE tracks are well demonstrated with fluorescein angiography.

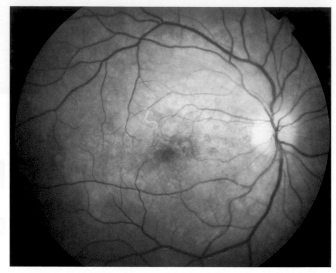

Figure 47–4 Parasite beneath the macula. The size of the organism is consistent with *B. procyonis*. (Courtesy of Mark Law, MD.)

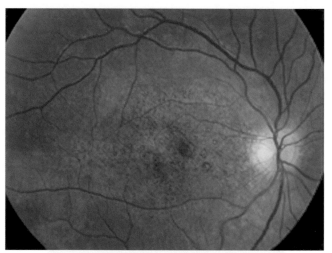

Figure 47–3 Late DUSN demonstrates vascular attenuation, widespread RPE disruption, and optic atrophy.

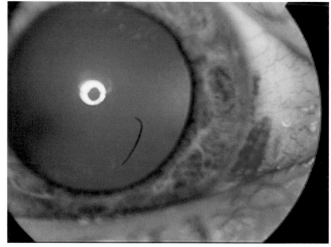

Figure 47–5 If a retinal tear or hole is present, the worm can migrate into the vitreous.

Later in the disease, visual function decreases. Although the macula may appear to be relatively uninvolved, the visual acuity can be poor and a relative afferent papillary defect is often present. As the process continues, there is progressive disruption of the RPE accompanied by optic atrophy and retinal vascular attenuation. Visual loss is irreversible and probably results from two mechanisms. First, the nematode causes destruction of photoreceptors and retinal pigment epithelial cells. Second, visual loss may be the result of a toxic effect on the retina and optic nerve.

The worm is usually difficult to visualize. Accurate diagnosis requires a high index of suspicion sometimes coupled with multiple patient visits to search for the organism. The organism is usually located in the subretinal space (**Figure 47–4**). Peripheral retinal damage can lead to rhegmatogenous retinal detachment. When

a retinal tear or hole is present, the organism can travel into the vitreous (**Figure 47–5**). Intraocular larvae can become encysted in the vitreous (**Figure 47–6**).

The differential diagnosis includes toxoplasmosis, syphilis, tuberculosis, sarcoidosis, acute posterior multifocal placoid pigment epitheliopathy, multiple evanescent white dot syndrome, serpiginous choroidopathy, ocular histoplasmosis syndrome, unilateral retinitis pigmentosa, traumatic choroidopathy, and neuroretinitis of another cause such as cat scratch disease. The diagnosis is established by ophthalmoscopic examination because laboratory tests are usually unrevealing. Mild eosinophilia may be noted in the peripheral blood. If hepatic involvement is present, serum lactate dehydrogenase and aspartate aminotransferase levels can be elevated. *Toxocara* titers are typically negative. A serum immunofluorescence assay

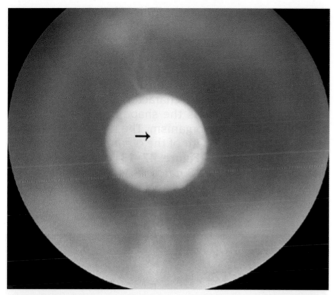

Figure 47–6 Vitreous cyst around *A. mesocercaria*. The organism is visible within the cyst (*arrow*) (Courtesy of H. Richard McDonald, MD.)

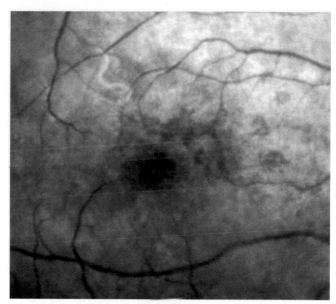

Figure 47–8 Red-free photographs may improve contrast, aiding visualization of the subretinal worm.

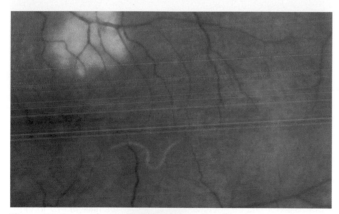

Figure 47–7 A subretinal worm that survived laser photocoagulation and continued to migrate. Note the fresh white laser burn in the superior macula and the organism in the temporal macula. (Courtesy of Barrett Katz, MD.)

47.3 Imaging and Diagnostic Tests

47.3.1 FUNDUS PHOTOGRAPHY

Given the difficulty in locating a subretinal nematode, color fundus photography may be helpful in searching for the worm. A series of photos is recommended, providing overlapping coverage of as much of the fundus as possible. Photographs can be especially helpful in evaluating patients who are photophobic and are unable to tolerate a lengthy ophthalmoscopic examination. Ideally, both color photos and red-free photos should be obtained. Red-free photos may provide improved contrast, which can better demonstrate the organism (**Figure 47–8**).

47.3.2 FLUORESCEIN ANGIOGRAPHY

Active inflammatory lesions typically appear hypofluorescent early and exhibit hyperfluorescent staining late in the angiogram. Leakage from the optic nerve head produces optic disc hyperfluorescence in the middle and late phases of the study (**Figure 47–9**). Perivascular leakage, when present, usually involves the retinal venules. Advanced disease is characterized by widespread mottled hyperfluorescence consistent with window defects from the diseased retinal pigment epithelium. Fluorescein angiography is not helpful in locating the worm.

47.3.3 ELECTRORETINGRAM

Electroretinogram studies usually demonstrate decreased retinal function which may be extinguished late in the course of the disease. The b wave is typically more reduced than the a wave.

for B. procyonis is available but may be negative if there is little systemic involvement.

The treatment of choice is laser photodestruction of the worm. Once the organism is identified, treatment should be performed immediately because there is a risk that the motile worm will be difficult to locate later. The patient should be followed closely after treatment to verify the success of the treatment. The larva sometimes survives laser treatment and continues to migrate (**Figure 47–7**). There is little or no inflammation induced by the destruction of the worm. Successful treatment stabilizes the disease and prevents future visual loss. Consequently, the prognosis is correlated with the timeliness of treatment.

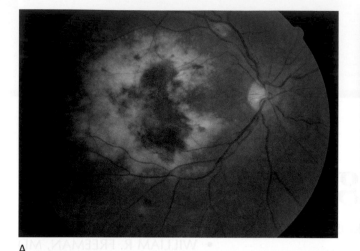

A

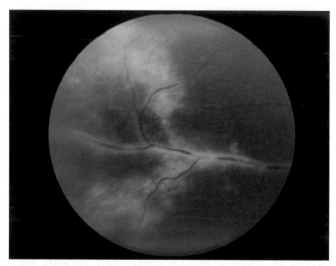

Figure 48–3   Granular form of CMV retinitis.

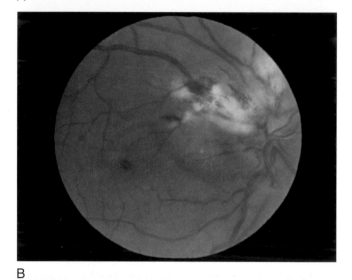

B

Figure 48–1   *A and B:* Yellow-white fulminant/edematous CMV retinitis lesion with prominent retinal hemorrhages.

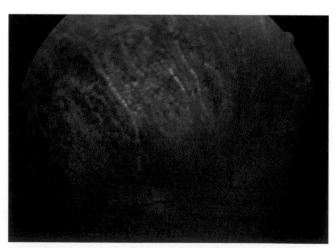

Figure 48–4   Frosted branch angiitis in a patient with CMV retinitis.

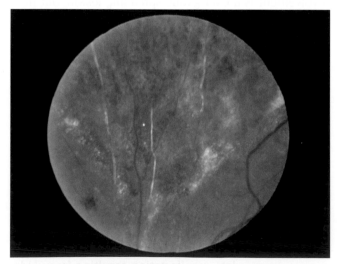

Figure 48–2   Healing lesion with atrophic center and active borders.

Figure 48–5   Avascular retina with RPE atrophy after resolution of retinitis (same patient as in **Figure 48–3**).

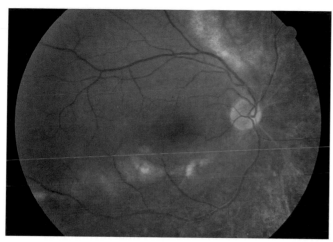

Figure 48–6 Recurrence of CMV retinitis. Note the active white borders at the edges of previously healed retinitis in the inferior temporal and nasal retina of the right eye.

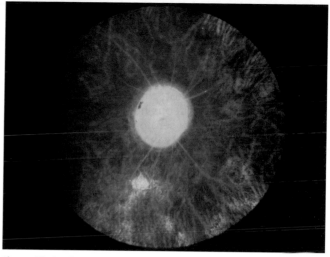

Figure 48–9 In contrast to patients with AIDS, immunosuppressed patients due to organ transplantation have moderate-to-severe vitreitis in association with CMV retinitis.

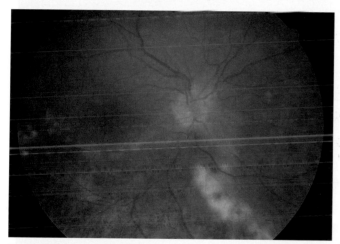

Figure 48–7 The active border is sparing the fovea whereas the other active border is advancing toward the nasal retina.

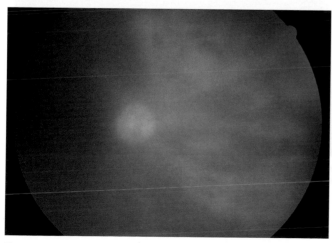

Figure 48–8 Optic atrophy and widespread retinal destruction after CMV retinitis.

rarely seen. The most common anterior segment finding in a patient with CMV retinitis and AIDS is the presence of fine stellate keratic precipitates on the corneal endothelium.

Treatment for CMV retinitis may be systemic or local or a combination of the two. There are currently five medications approved by the U.S. Food and Drug Administration (FDA) for the treatment of CMV retinitis: ganciclovir, valganciclovir, cidofovir, foscarnet, and fomivirsen.

Since the advent of HAART, many patients with AIDS have had a dramatic restoration of immune system function. This has also been associated with a sustained drop in the plasma human deficiency viral load to low or undetectable levels. With the prevalent use of HAART, the incidence of CMV retinitis has decreased approximately 75%. Patients who have a sustained CD4$^+$ count elevation of more than 100 cells/μL in response to HAART for at least 3 to 6 months can discontinue anti-CMV treatment but should be carefully monitored for re-activation, which can occur if the CD4$^+$ count diminishes despite HAART.

Immune recovery uveitis (IRU) only occurs in eyes with healed CMV lesions in patients who responded to HAART with immune reconstitution. The incidence rate of this phenomenon has varied, with reports ranging from 0.11 to 0.83 per person-year. Prevalence rates have varied between 15.5% and 37.5%. Eyes in which CMV retinitis lesions involve large surface areas of retina seem to be at higher risk for development of IRU. Patients with IRU exhibit signs of inflammation such as iritis, vitreitis, macular edema, and epiretinal membrane formation. Cataract, vitreomacular traction, proliferative vitreoretinopathy, optic disc and retinal neovascularization, panuveitis with hypopyon, and uveitic angle-closure glaucoma with posterior synechiae have also been reported in IRU. Vision loss from these inflammatory sequelae is usually associated with macular edema and associated macular surface changes or cataract in most patients.

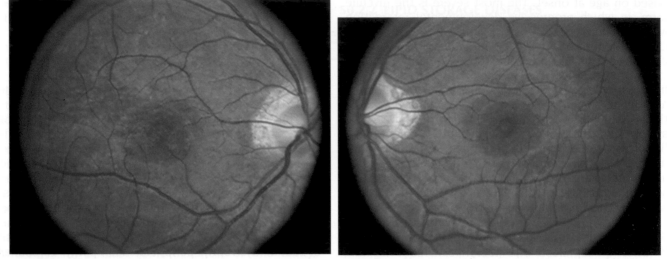

Figure 50–3 *A* and *B:* A 35-year-old patient with adult Refsum's syndrome. Note the mild posterior pole retinal pigment mottling. The ERG was nonrecordable.

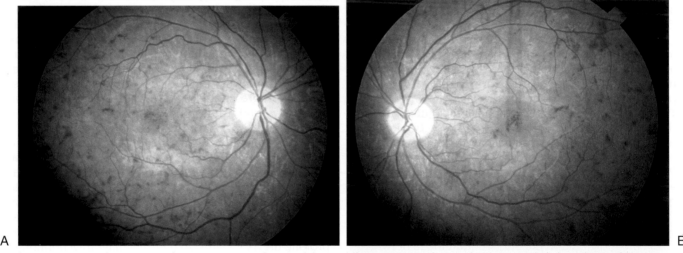

Figure 50–4 *A* and *B:* Patient with Kearns-Sayre syndrome exhibiting diffuse posterior pole retinal pigment epithelial mottling and clumping.

50.2.4 PROTEIN STORAGE DISEASES

The two most important protein storage diseases (aminoacidurias) for the ophthalmologist are cystinosis and gyrate atrophy. Both are inherited in AR fashion. Some authors group cystinosis with the oculorenal syndromes (see later).

Cystinosis is characterized by toxic accumulation of cystine, an oxidation product of the amino acid cysteine. Similar to NCL, cystinosis is divided into three types, based on age at onset. The gene responsible for infantile nephropathic cystinosis (Fanconi's syndrome) is cystinosin, a lysosomal membrane protein. The syndrome consists of crystalline renal failure and growth retardation. Ocular complications include crystalline deposition in the cornea and conjunctiva, with pigmentary retinopathy but a normal ERG (**Figure 50–5**). Juvenile cystinosis is a milder disease, with nephropathy, corneal crystals, and mild retinopathy, and adult cystinosis lacks

retinal findings. The genes responsible for most juvenile cystinosis and all adult cystinosis have not yet been identified. Treatment is with cysteamine (Cystagon, Mylan, Morgantown, WV), which reduces cystine levels, and, when necessary, renal transplantation. Topical cysteamine reduces crystals on the ocular surface, but does not improve retinopathy.

Gyrate atrophy is associated with deficient ornithine aminotransferase (OAT), leading to toxic accumulation of the amino acid ornithine. The defective gene is OAT. Most reported patients are Finnish. Systemic findings are highly variable and may include mild intellectual deterioration or neurologic signs. Ocular findings are striking and include nummular atrophy of the RPE and choroid with a characteristic scalloped appearance (**Figure 50–6**). The atrophy begins peripherally and moves centripetally, involving the macula late in the disease course. The ERG progressively becomes extinguished. Disease progression may be slowed by

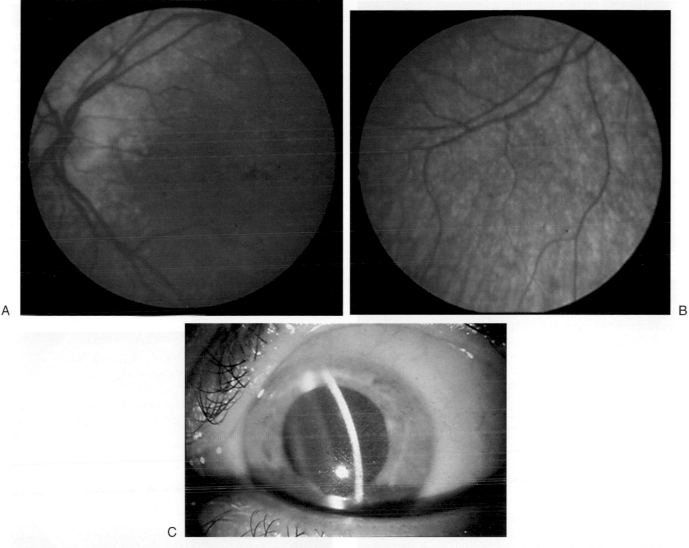

Figure 50–5 *A* and *B:* Patient with infantile nephritic cystinosis exhibiting diffuse retinal pigment epithelial mottling with mild posterior pole clumping. There are no retinal crystals. *C:* Corneal crystals.

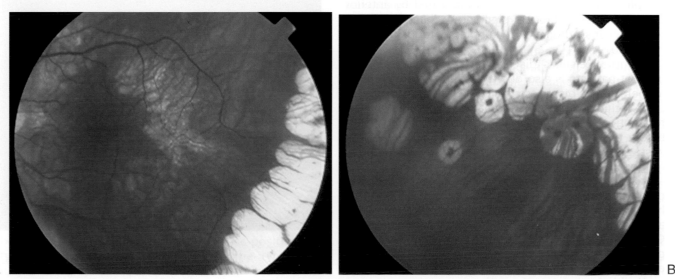

Figure 50–6 *A* and *B:* A 38-year-old patient with gyrate atrophy exhibiting peripheral scalloped areas of RPE and choroid loss, with relative sparing of the posterior pole.

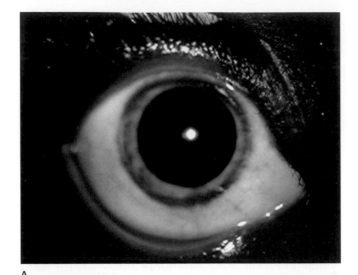

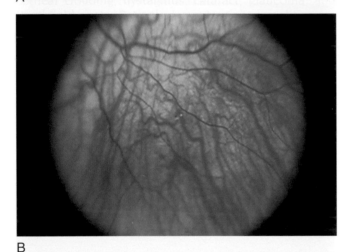

Figure 50–9 Patient with OCA1, revealing (*A*) blue irides with transillumination defects and (*B*) diffuse retinal pigment attenuation posteriorly and throughout the entire periphery. Posteriorly there is absence of a foveal depression.

skin, hair, and irides with age. Visual acuity is typically in the 20/40 to 20/200 range, but may improve slightly as pigmentation develops.

There are several named variants of OCA, but two are particularly important because they are associated with life-threatening systemic abnormalities. Hermansky-Pudlak syndrome, concentrated in the Arecibo region of Puerto Rico, consists of OCA with platelet dysfunction, bleeding diathesis, and restrictive lung disease. Chediak-Higashi syndrome consists of OCA with immunodeficiency, leading to bacterial infections and malignancies.

OA is typically inherited in an XL fashion (Nettleship-Falls OA, OA1), although AR pedigrees occur. Patients have normal skin and hair pigmentation but ocular findings similar to those in OCA. An exception occurs in African-American patients, who may have apparently normal irides and fundi (ocular albinism cum pigmento), complicating the diagnosis in a child with congenital nystagmus. Because of the XLR inheritance pattern,

female heterozygotes may have irregular and variable pigmentary disturbances in the retina.

Treatment of all forms of albinism is generally supportive. Referral to a genetic counselor is warranted, as is a hematologic consultation in the rare but life-threatening Hermansky-Pudlak and Chediak-Higashi subtypes.

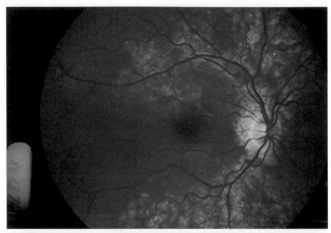

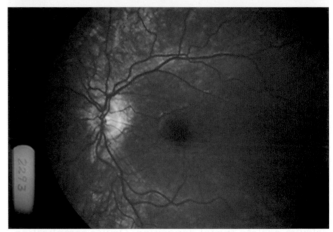

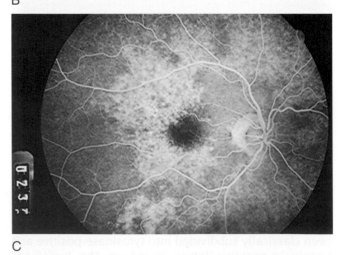

Figure 50–10 *A* and *B:* Patient with abetalipoproteinemia, exhibiting diffuse retinal pigment mottling throughout the posterior pole and periphery and (*C*) exemplified as transmission defects on a fluorescein angiogram.

50.3.4 ABETALIPOPROTEINEMIA (BASSEN-KORNZWEIG DISEASE)

Abetalipoproteinemia (Bassen-Kornzweig disease) is an AR syndrome consisting of fat malabsorption, ataxia, neuropathy, and abnormal erythrocyte morphology (acanthocytosis). The responsible gene is microsomal triglyceride transfer protein. Ocular findings include pigmentary retinal dystrophy, optic atrophy, strabismus, and nystagmus (**Figure 50–10**). A related AD syndrome, familial hypobetalipoproteinemia, is caused by mutations in the apolipoprotein B gene. Supplementation with vitamins A and E is beneficial.

50.4 Nutritional Anomalies

In general, nutritional deficiencies are more common in the developing world than in the United States. When these diseases occur in industrialized nations, they are typically related to malabsorption syndromes or bizarre dietary practices. In most cases, these deficiencies are effectively treated by supplementation of the deficient vitamin(s).

Vitamin A deficiency causes increased mortality in children, typically due to pneumonia and enterocolitis and is the leading cause of childhood blindness in the developing world. In the United States, this disease may occur as a complication of gastrointestinal bypass surgery. Ocular manifestations of vitamin A deficiency are numerous and include xerophthalmia with keratomalacia and corneal ulceration, conjunctival Bitot's spots, and retinal changes. Nyctalopia is often a presenting symptom, and ERG abnormalities occur. In advanced disease, the xerophthalmic fundus may develop, characterized by small, peripheral areas of RPE atrophy, similar to a salt-and-pepper pattern, or, alternatively, similar to fundus albipunctatus (**Figure 50–11**). Conversely, high intake of vitamin A is a risk factor for pseudotumor cerebri.

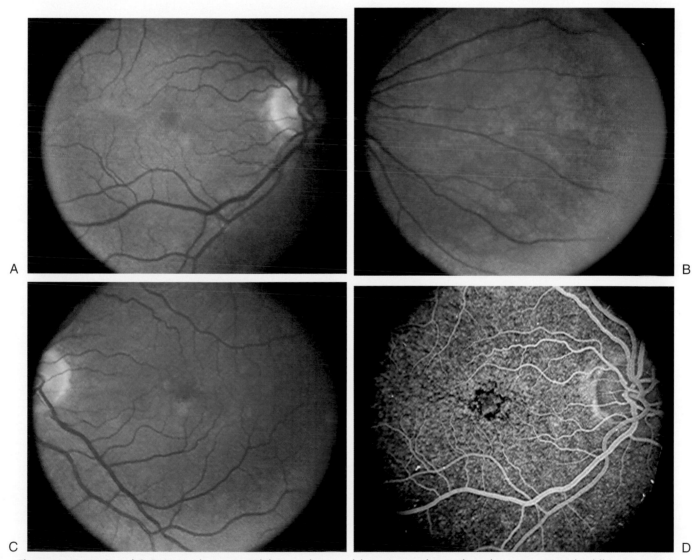

Figure 50–11   A, B, and C: Patient with vitamin A deficiency due to malabsorption syndrome after colon surgery. Note the diffuse pigment mottling with a slight degree of macular pigment clumping. *D:* This pattern of retinal pigment mottling is nicely highlighted on a fluorescein angiogram.

Vitamin B$_1$ (thiamine) deficiency may cause beriberi, which results in a range of clinical manifestations, including cardiovascular disease (wet beriberi) and neurologic disease (dry beriberi and Wernicke-Korsakoff syndrome). In the United States, this is typically a disease of alcoholics. Ocular complications include nystagmus, ophthalmoplegia, optic atrophy, and perhaps alcohol amblyopia.

Vitamin B$_3$ (niacin) deficiency may cause pellagra, characterized by dermatitis, dementia, and diarrhea. Ocular complications include loss of the foveal reflex, vascular abnormalities, pigmentary changes, and optic atrophy. Conversely, pharmacologic niacin supplemen-tation to lower serum lipids may lead to a characteristic and reversible pseudo-cystoid macular edema without fluorescein leakage.

The main systemic complication of iron deficiency is anemia. Ocular complications primarily include retinal hemorrhages and cotton-wool spots.

ACKNOWLEDGMENTS

This work was partially supported by National Institutes of Health Center Grant P30-EY014801 and by an un-restricted grant to the University of Miami from Research to Prevent Blindness, New York, NY.

Chapter 51

Medications and Retinal Toxicity

STEPHEN G. SCHWARTZ, MD • WILLIAM F. MIELER, MD •
ROBERT A. MITTRA, MD

51.1 Introduction

Pharmaceutical damage to the retina and its supporting structures has been recognized for at least 200 years. Toxic effects may cause permanent vision loss or herald life-threatening medication overdoses. Prompt recognition may prevent significant morbidity and even mortality in some cases.

In this chapter we provide an overview of medications known to damage the retina. The medications are organized according to mechanisms of deleterious effect: pan-retinal toxicity, vasculopathy, maculopathy, uveitis, and multiple toxic effects (**Table 51–1**).

51.2 Drugs Causing Pan-Retinal Toxicity

Although the initial findings may be confined to the macula, these agents eventually may cause generalized retinal degeneration, with abnormal recordings on electrophysiologic tests such as electroretinograms (ERGs). They are subdivided here into drugs causing pigmentary disturbances, crystalline deposition, retinal edema, retinal necrosis, and no apparent fundus changes.

51.2.1 PIGMENTARY DISTURBANCES

Quinolines

In the United States, the synthetic quinoline antimalarials chloroquine (Aralen, Sanofi Winthrop Pharmaceuticals, New York, NY) and hydroxychloroquine (HCQ, Plaquenil, Sanofi Winthrop Pharmaceuticals, New York,

NY) are more commonly used to treat rheumatologic disorders. Their toxic effects are similar.

Initially noted is an asymptomatic blunting of the foveal light reflex with incidental verticillata-like changes in the cornea. Macular stippling ensues, progressing to the classic bull's-eye lesion (**Figure 51–1**) and finally to a generalized retinal degeneration with diffuse pigmentary alterations, arteriolar attenuation, and optic atrophy (**Figure 51–2**).

Automated perimetry of the central 10 degrees is quite sensitive, particularly with a red test object. There may be an emerging role for multifocal electroretinography (mfERG) in early diagnosis.

The precise mechanism of toxicity remains unclear. Histopathologic examination and electron microscopy demonstrate disorganization of the photoreceptors with pigment-laden cells in the retina. The quinolines bind melanin granules and concentrate in the retinal pigment epithelium (RPE) and choroidal melanocytes, which may potentiate toxicity.

With discontinuation of the agent, early retinopathy may resolve, but advanced cases may progress. These medications have an exceptionally long clearance time, and some patients first develop toxicity years after discontinuation (**Figure 51–3**).

Toxicity from hydroxychloroquine (HCQ) is much less common than toxicity from chloroquine—in the range of 1 case per 1000 patient-years. The reason for the relative safety of HCQ is unknown. Nevertheless, toxicity may occur below the generally accepted "safe" dosage levels and despite appropriate screening.

One reason for this discrepancy may be related to the patient's weight (**Figure 51–4**). Quinolines are stored to a greater degree in lean body tissues than in fat.

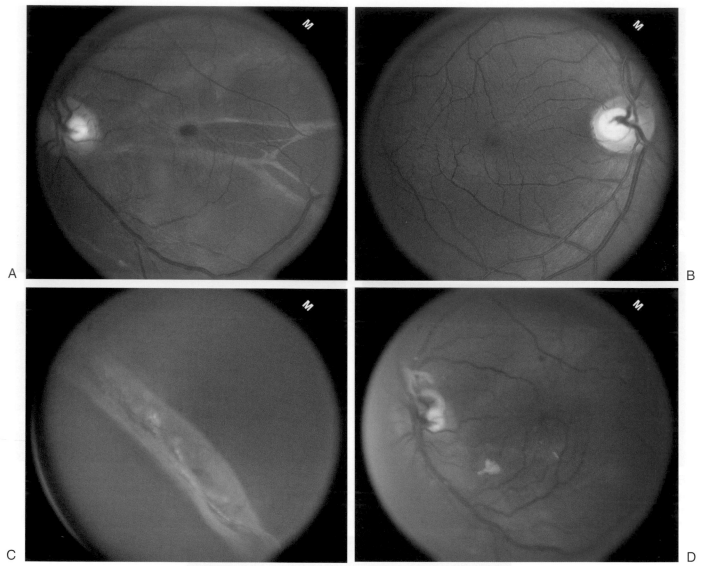

Figure 52–10   Patient presented with reduced vision after repair of retinal dialysis with retinal detachment. *A:* Recurrent detachment present with epiretinal and subretinal membranes in the macula. A pseudo-macular hole is present centrally. *B:* The fellow eye shows crystal deposits in the retina. *C:* Peripheral examination reveals a chronic, large retinal dialysis. The retina is detached and folded with RPE hyperplasia along the posterior edge. *D:* After vitrectomy, retinectomy, and subretinal membrane removal, the retina is reattached under silicone oil.

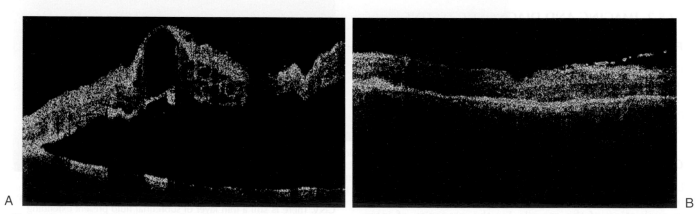

Figure 52–11   *A:* OCT image reveals neurosensory retinal detachment in the macular with the presence of subretinal fibrous bands and intraretinal cystic changes. *B:* OCT image demonstrates reattachment of the neurosensory retina with marked resolution of intraretinal cystic changes after surgical repair. Residual epiretinal membrane is present under silicone oil.

diagnosing the presence of persistent subretinal fluid after successful retinal reattachment.

Ultrasonography

When media opacity precludes the diagnosis of a retinal tear or detachment, ultrasonography is indicated. Retinal breaks are often difficult to identify with ultrasound unless the break is large and associated with significant vitreous traction. Retinal detachment is identified because it produces a bright linear signal with variable mobility on B-scan testing. If the detachment extends to the optic nerve, the retina should insert into the nerve. The overall configuration of the detachment is quite variable. Early on, the retina is often shallow-flat progressing to a smooth-bullous configuration. Retinal detachment associated with proliferative vitreoretinopathy may have a folded or corrugated appearance. With time, the retina exhibits a funnel or V shape that is open initially but closes as proliferation progresses. Standardized A-scan testing should produce a 100% spike when the probe is perpendicular to the detached retina. When significant vitreous hemorrhage is present, it may be difficult to differentiate a posterior vitreous detachment from a retinal detachment. Characteristics that suggest a PVD rather than a retinal detachment are the following:

- The membrane does not insert in the optic nerve head but rather inserts in a peripapillary location.

- The membrane has less than a 100% spike on A-scan testing or the spike is less than 100% in the periphery.
- The membrane is very mobile.
- When two separate membranes are present, one will generally represent the retina, whereas the other represents the vitreous separation.

SUGGESTED READINGS

Aaberg TM. Macular holes. Surv Ophthalmol. 1970;15:139–162.

Akman A, Kadayifcilar S, Oto S, Aydin P. Indocyanine green angiographic features of traumatic choroidal ruptures. Eye. 1998;12(Pt 4):646–650.

Arend O, Remky A, Elsner AE, Wolf S, Rein M. Indocyanine green angiography in traumatic choroidal rupture: Clinicoangiographic case reports. Ger J Ophthalmol. 1995;4:257–263.

Goffstein R, Burton TC. Differentiating traumatic from nontraumatic retinal detachment. Ophthalmology. 1982;89:361–368.

Haimann MH, Burton TC, Brown CK. Epidemiology of retinal detachment. Arch Ophthalmol 1982;100:289–292.

Johnson RN, McDonald HR, Lewis H, et al. Traumatic macular holes: Observations, pathogenesis and results of vitrectomy surgery. Ophthalmology. 2001;108:853–857.

Kennedy CJ, Parker CE, McAllister IL. Retinal detachment caused by retinal dialysis. Aust NZ J Ophthalmol. 1997;25:25–30.

Kohno T, Miki T, Shiraki K, Kano K, Hirabayashi-Matsushita M. Indocyanine green angiographic features of choroidal rupture and choroidal vascular injury after contusion ocular injury. Am J Ophthalmol. 2000;129:38–46.

Secretan M, Sickenberg M, Zografos L, Piguet B. Morphometric characteristics of traumatic choroidal rupture associated with neovascularization. Retina. 1998,18:62–66.

Yanagia N, Akiba J, Takahashi M, et al. Clinical characteristics of traumatic macular holes. Jpn J Ophthalmol. 1996;40:544–547.

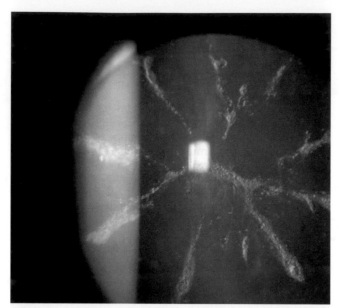

Figure 53–5 Retroillumination view of lens in a patient with Stickler's syndrome reveals posterior subcapsular cataractous changes in a branching pattern.

Prophylactic treatment of retinal tears or breaks should be considered. Associated systemic findings, not found in Wagner's syndrome (see later), include orofacial and skeletal anomalies stemming from underlying collagen abnormalities.

53.3.3 ANCILLARY TESTING

Ring scotomas and restriction of peripheral visual fields have been reported. ERG tracings are usually normal.

53.4 Snowflake Degeneration

53.4.1 GENETICS

Inheritance: autosomal dominant
OMIM number: 193230
Symbol: none
Gene and gene locus: unknown

53.4.2 CLINICAL SIGNS AND SYMPTOMS

Snowflake degeneration is characterized by small, yellow-white, superficial opacities in the mid-peripheral or peripheral retina, associated with overlying vitreous condensation. Anterior segment findings vary from cataracts to superficial opacities of the lens. Vascular sheathing or obliteration and even retinal neovascularization may be present in the posterior segment. The disorder may be stationary or may run a progressive course with possible rhegmatogenous retinal detachment that responds poorly to surgical treatment.

53.4.3 ANCILLARY TESTING

Areas of capillary nonperfusion that border areas of abnormal retinal vessels are noted on fluorescein angiography. Retinal function may become progressively abnormal, with decreased amplitudes in the scotopic b wave of the ERG. Goldmann perimetry may show peripheral visual field defects not corresponding to visible pathologic changes.

53.5 Autosomal Dominant Vitreoretinochoroidopathy

53.5.1 GENETICS

Inheritance: autosomal dominant
OMIM number: 193220
Symbol: VRCP, ADVIRC
Gene and gene locus: unknown

53.5.2 CLINICAL SIGNS AND SYMPTOMS

Clinical findings have been described in patients aged 7 to 88. This is a very slowly progressive disorder, and signs and symptoms may only be prominent in older individuals. Some patients are slightly myopic or have mild nyctalopia. Visual acuity is generally very good. A crescent-shaped area of choroidal atrophy accompanied by progressively increasing pigmentary changes and a discrete posterior border is highly characteristic of this disorder (**Figures 53–6** and **53–7**). All adults with this

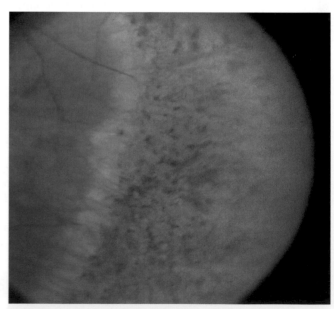

Figure 53–6 Transition between normal posterior retina and peripheral fundus with heavy pigmentary changes in a patient with autosomal dominant vitreoretinochoroidopathy (ADVIRC). (From Kaufman SJ, Goldberg MF, Fishman GA, et al. Autosomal dominant vitreoretinochoroidopathy. Arch Ophthalmol. 1982;100:272–278.)

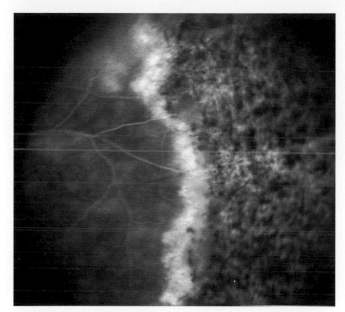

Figure 53–7 Angiogram of peripheral fundus in a patient with ADVIRC shows staining of the area of demarcation between the posterior normal fundus and the more peripheral avascular zone.

condition have developed cataracts in their 30s and 40s. There is mild fibrillary degeneration of the vitreous.

53.5.3 ANCILLARY TESTING

Cystoid macular edema with dilation of posterior pole capillaries and breakdown of the blood-retina barrier has been reported in occasional patients. ERG tracings are essentially normal in younger patients and mildly reduced in older patients. The EOG Arden ratio has been reported to be markedly decreased.

53.5.4 HISTOPATHOLOGY

Specimens from two patients demonstrate disorganization of the peripheral retina with altered retinal pigment epithelial cells surrounding retinal vessels and loss of photoreceptor cells in the equator. An extensive membrane of condensed vitreous, cellular debris, and Müller cells was found on the surface of the retina.

53.6 Wagner's Syndrome

53.6.1 GENETICS

Inheritance: autosomal dominant

OMIM number: 143200

Symbol: WGN1, ERVR

Gene and gene locus: unknown/5q13–14 and 12q13.11-q13.2

53.6.2 CLINICAL SIGNS AND SYMPTOMS

Optically empty vitreous, peripheral vascular sheathing with attenuation of retinal arterioles, perivascular pigmentary clumping (**Figures 53–8** and **53–9**), and lenticular changes are the hallmark features of Wagner's syndrome. Neovascular glaucoma and peripheral retinal detachment, typically occurring in older patients,

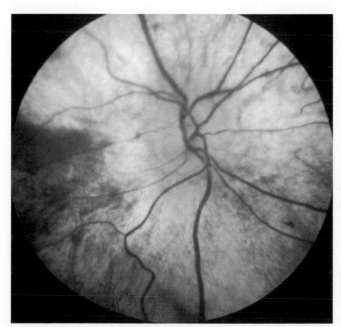

Figure 53–8 Peripapillary area of choroidal sclerosis and some vascular attenuation and pigmentary changes in a patient from the original Wagner's syndrome pedigree (Courtesy of Irene H. Maumenee, MD.)

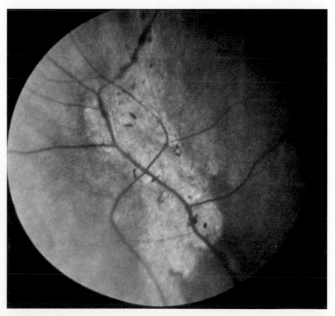

Figure 53–9 Peripheral perivascular patch of chorioretinal atrophy and clumped pigmentation in a patient from the original Wagner's syndrome pedigree. (Courtesy of Irene H. Maumenee, MD.)

may lead to a decline in visual acuity. Unlike Stickler's syndrome, there are no associated systemic or skeletal abnormalities in Wagner's syndrome.

53.6.3 ANCILLARY TESTING

The EOG is reduced in some patients, even in early stages of the disease. The ERG, however, is normal early, but evidence of rod and cone dysfunction occurs with time. This is an indication of a true underlying retinal dystrophy in Wagner's syndrome.

53.6.4 HISTOPATHOLOGY

Retinoschisis at the level of the outer plexiform layer, isolated areas of chorioretinal atrophy, and vitreous membranes consisting of cells of glial origin have been described in one patient.

53.7 Knobloch Syndrome

53.7.1 GENETICS

Inheritance: autosomal recessive
OMIM number: 267750
Symbol: KNO
Gene and gene locus: COL18A1/21q22.3

53.7.2 CLINICAL SIGNS AND SYMPTOMS

High myopia, vitreoretinal degeneration, macular abnormalities, and a high incidence of retinal detachment are the important ocular manifestations of this disease. The distinguishing characteristic of Knobloch syndrome is the presence of an occipital encephalocele. The skull defect may be subtle, so careful examination for a soft spot over the occiput is essential in making the diagnosis.

53.8 Syndrome of Myelinated Nerve Fibers, Vitreoretinopathy, and Skeletal Malformations

53.8.1 GENETICS

Inheritance: autosomal dominant/X-linked dominant
OMIM number: none
Symbol: none
Gene and gene locus: unknown

53.8.2 CLINICAL SIGNS AND SYMPTOMS

High myopia, poor visual acuity, and nyctalopia are seen in this extremely rare disorder. The distinguishing

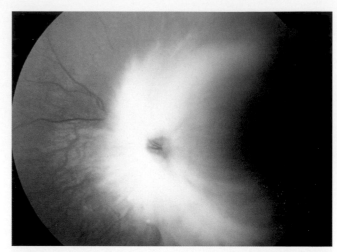

Figure 53–10 Extensive myelination of the nerve fiber layer in the mother reported by Traboulsi et al. with the syndrome of myelinated nerve fibers, vitreoretinopathy, and skeletal malformations.

features are extensive myelination of the retinal nerve fiber layer bilaterally from the optic nerves along the temporal vascular arcades involving the macula (**Figure 53–10**), as well as severe vitreous liquefaction and peripheral chorioretinal atrophy.

53.8.3 ANCILLARY TESTING

An ERG performed on one patient revealed severely diminished photopic and scotopic responses. Goldmann visual field testing showed generalized constriction of the peripheral visual field and centrocecal scotomas.

SUGGESTED READINGS

Blair NP, Goldberg MF, Fishman GA, et al. Autosomal dominant vitreoretinochoroidopathy (ADVIRC). Br J Ophthalmol. 1984;68:2–9.

Hirose T, Lee KY, Schepens CL. Snowflake degeneration in hereditary vitreoretinal degeneration. Am J Ophthalmol. 1974;77:143–153.

Kaufman SJ, Goldberg MF, Orth DH, Fishman GA, Tessler H, Mizuno K. Autosomal dominant vitreoretinochoroidopathy. Arch Ophthalmol. 1982;100:272–278.

Knobloch WH, Layer JM. Retinal detachment and encephalocele. J Pediat Ophthalmol. 1971;8:181–184.

Niffenegger JH, Topping TM, Mukai S. Stickler's syndrome. Int Ophthalmol Clin. 1993;33:271–280.

Robitaille J, MacDonald MLE, Kaykas A, et al. Mutant frizzled-4 disrupts retinal angiogenesis in familial exudative vitreoretinopathy. Nat Genet. 2002;32:326–330.

Rosberger DF, Goldberg MF. Hereditary vitreoretinopathies. In: Traboulsi, EI, ed. Genetic diseases of the eye. Oxford, England: Oxford University Press; 1999.

Sertie, AL, Quimby M, Moreira ES, et al. A gene which causes severe ocular alterations and occipital encephalocele (Knobloch syndrome) is mapped to 21q22.3. Hum Mol Genet. 1996;5:843–847.

Traboulsi EI, Lim JI, Pyeritz R, et al. A new syndrome of myelinated nerve fibers, vitreoretinopathy, and skeletal malformations. Arch Ophthalmol. 1993;111:1543–1545.

Traboulsi EI, Payne JW. Autosomal dominant vitreoretinochoroidopathy: Report of the third family. Arch Ophthalmol. 1993;111:194–196.

Chapter 54

Retinitis Pigmentosa and Allied Disorders

ALEX MELAMUD, MA, MD • QING WANG, PhD • ELIAS I. TRABOULSI, MD

54.1 Introduction

Retinitis pigmentosa (RP) is a term used to describe a heterogeneous group of hereditary retinal dystrophies with certain common clinical and pathologic characteristics that include night blindness, contraction of the peripheral visual field, and photoreceptor abnormalities as measured by an electroretinogram (ERG). RP is one of the most common hereditary forms of blindness, affecting 1 in 4000 people, and is responsible for visual morbidity in 1.5 million individuals worldwide. Typical (with bony spicule pigmentary changes, optic nerve head pallor, and retinal vascular attenuation) and atypical (with other ophthalmoscopic characteristics) forms for RP have been described as isolated ocular traits or in association with a large number of systemic diseases such as Usher's and Bardet-Biedl syndromes.

Most cases are not associated with extraocular manifestations and can be classified according to the pattern of familial inheritance or more recently according to the defective gene (**Tables 54–1** and **54–2**).

54.2 Clinical Signs and Symptoms

Patients notice progressive onset and worsening of night blindness at various ages, as a result of rod-photoreceptor abnormalities. As the disease progresses, cones become involved and central vision abnormalities are added to peripheral field loss. Pigment migrates from the retinal pigment epithelium (RPE) into the retina, resulting in pigment clumping, usually in the mid-peripheral retina. The pigment often surrounds the retinal vessels, resulting in "bone spicule" formation

TABLE 54–1

Genetic Loci and Disease Genes for Autosomal Dominant RP

Disease Category	Mapped Genes (Not Cloned)	Mapped and Cloned Genes	Total Number of Genes
Autosomal dominant retinitis pigmentosa	RP17	CRX, FSCN2, HPRP3, IMPDH1, NRL, PRPF8, PRPF31, RDS, RHO, ROM1, RP1, RP9	12
Autosomal recessive retinitis pigmentosa	RP22, RP25, RP28, RP29	ABCA4, CERKL, CNGA1, CNGB1, CRB1, LRAT, MERTK, NR2E3, PDE6A, PDE6B, RGR, RHO, RLBP1, RPE65, SAG, TULP1, USH2A	15
X-linked retinitis pigmentosa	RP6, RP23, RP24	RP2, RPGR	5

Adapted from RetNet: Daiger SP, Sullivan LS, Rossiter BJF. Online Retinal Information Network. Houston, Tx: University of Texas-Houston Science Center, 1996–2004. Available at: http://www.sph.uth.tmc.edu/Retnet/.

TABLE 54–2
Functional Grouping of Known RP Genes

Functional Group	Genes
Visual cascade (Figure 54-1)	RHO, PDE6A, PDE6B, CNGA1, arrestin (SAG)
Visual cycle	RPE65, RLBP1, RGR, ABCA4
Structural protein	RDS, ROM1
Transcriptional factor	NRL, CRX, NR2E3
Extracellular protein	CRB1, USH2A
Protein kinase	MERTK, RP1, PRKCG
Unknown function (intracellular trafficking?)	RP2, RPGR, TULP1

From Wang Q, Chen Q, Zhao K, et al. Update on the molecular genetics of retinitis pigmentosa. Ophthalmic Genet. 2001;22:133–154.

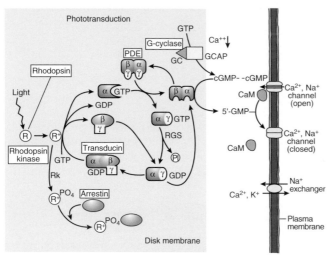

Figure 54–1   Major reactions in vertebrate phototransduction. Light triggers the isomerization of 11-cis-retinol to all-trans-retinol, which leads to activation of rhodopsin (R*) through a series of conformational changes. R* binds to transducin and then activates its α subunit (Tα) by catalyzing the exchanges of guanosine diphosphate (GDP) for guanosine triphosphate (GTP) on transducin and the dissociation of Tα from the β subunits (Tβ). The Tα then stimulates phosphodiesterase (PDE) by binding to the inhibitory subunit of PDE and releasing it from the α and β subunits of PDE. The activated PDE α and β subunits catalyze the hydrolysis of cyclic guanosine monophosphate (cGMP) to 5'-GMP. The decrease in intracellular cGMP concentration causes the cGMP-gated Na$^+$/Ca^{2+} channels in the plasma membrane to close and the photoreceptor cell to hyperpolarize. As the Na/Ca-K exchanger in the plasma membrane continues to extrude Ca^{2+}, intracellular Ca^{2+} levels decrease. The resulting drop in Ca^{2+} concentration leads to the reduction in the synaptic release of neurotransmitter glutamate. Photorecovery begins by the shut-off of the visual transduction cascade and cGMP resynthesis. Inactivation of the visual cascade includes the phosphorylation of R* by rhodopsin kinase (Rk) and the subsequent binding to arrestin and the hydrolysis of GTP to GDP on Tα and the subsequent reassociations of Tα to Tβ and the subunit of the PDE to the α and β subunits of PDE to form the inactivated transducin and PDE. The drop in the intracellular Ca^{2+} levels stimulates the guanylyl cyclase (GC) through the calcium binding protein (GCAP) to resynthesize cGMP. The Na$^+$/Ca^{2+} channels reopen as the intracellular cGMP concentration increases and the sensitivity of the channels to cGMP increases because of the dissociation of calmodulin (CaM) from the channels. The photoreceptor cell returns to its depolarized state. The *shaded area* represents the disk membrane in the photoreceptor outer segment. (From Wang Q, Chen Q, Zhao K, Wang L, Wang L, Traboulsi EI. Update on the molecular genetics of retinitis pigmentosa. Ophthal Genet. 2001;22:133–154.)

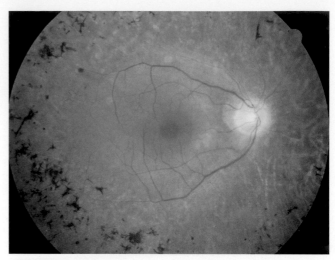

Figure 54–2   Typical appearance of the fundus in RP. The optic nerve head is pale, the retinal vessels are attenuated, and there is formation of bony spicule pigmentation in the mid-periphery. Fine atrophic and pigmentary changes are present in the macula.

(**Figure 54–2**). Pigmentation is variable, however, and may be absent altogether (retinitis pigmentosa sine pigmento). White dots can be observed deep in the retina in some patients. If the white dots are present in significant amounts, the phenotype is known as *retinitis punctata albescens.*

Vessels are often attenuated and narrowed. Early in the disease a grey-green discoloration of the RPE may be noticed, giving a tapetal-like reflex. Some heterozygous carriers of X-linked RP may have a similar fundus discoloration. Other findings on examination of the fundus include areas of RPE atrophy (**Figure 54–3**), waxy pallor of the optic disk, cystoid macular edema, and epiretinal membranes. Vitreous cells and posterior subcapsular cataracts are variably present.

Autosomal dominant RP has been divided by some into diffuse and regional categories based on the pattern of visual loss. The diffuse disease variety is typified by widespread loss of rod function with sparing of cone function at some stage in its evolution. Night blindness is the earliest reported finding, with symptoms of peripheral visual field constriction by day following some 20 years later. Mid-peripheral pigmentation builds gradually and is often sparse until late in the disease. In contrast, the regional form of autosomal dominant RP affects both rods and cones early in the disease process. Sharply demarcated areas of atrophy and severe visual loss occur next to regions of near normal function. Pigmentation occurs early in the disease process.

RP can also rarely be associated with Coats' disease–like vascular and exudative changes. In these patients, pigment clumping and photoreceptor dysfunction are found in association with vessel telangiectasia, venous dilation, microaneurysms, and areas of capillary non-perfusion (**Figures 54–4** and **54–5**). As the disease progresses, patients often develop massive intraretinal and subretinal exudates.

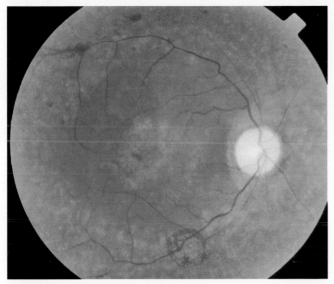

Figure 54–3 Fundus of a patient with X-linked RP. There are small deep depigmented lesions along and outside the arcades in addition to pigmentary changes, some of which are in a circular pattern along the inferior arcade. The optic nerve is waxy pale and the retinal blood vessels are attenuated.

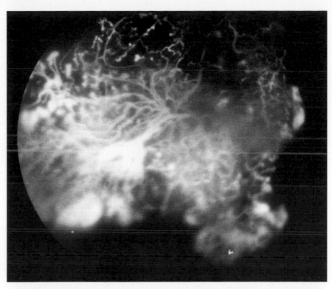

Figure 54–5 Angiogram of the fundus shown in **Figure 54.4**. There are extensive areas of capillary non-perfusion as well as telangiectatic vessels.

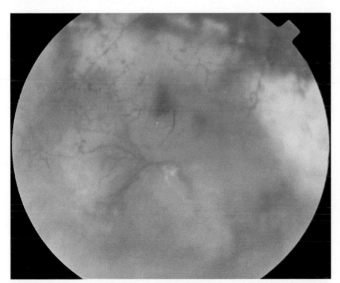

Figure 54–4 Coats' disease–like response in a patient with RP. There are extensive subretinal exudates and areas of vascular dilatation. (Courtesy of Rachel Kuchtey, MD, and Jonathan Sears, MD.)

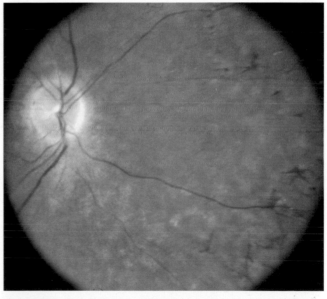

Figure 54–6 Nasal retinal periphery of a patient with LCA. There are deep, irregular depigmented lesions in addition to bony spicules. The optic nerve head is of relatively normal color. Some of the arterioles are attenuated.

54.3 Infantile Retinitis Pigmentosa (Includes Leber Congenital Amaurosis)

A number of inherited retinal dystrophies have their onset at birth or very early in childhood. The majority are associated with severe visual loss. Leber congenital amaurosis (LCA) is a genetically heterogeneous condition that presents in infancy with severe visual loss, nystagmus, sluggish pupillary responses, variable ophthalmoscopic appearance, and an extinguished ERG. The retina may appear normal, or varying degrees of pigmentary disturbance (**Figures 54–6** and **54–7**) or macular atrophy or "colobomas" may be evident. Additional ocular features include high degrees of hypermetropia or less commonly myopia, cataracts, and keratoconus. The diagnosis of LCA is made on the basis of clinical findings and severely attenuated or absent scotopic and photopic electroretinographic responses.

Five causative genes and two loci have been identified to date in patients with LCA. The genes include the retinal guanylyl cyclase gene (GUCY2D; for LCA1 [OMIM number 204000]) or RETGC-1 involved in the phototransduction cascade; the RPE65 gene essential to

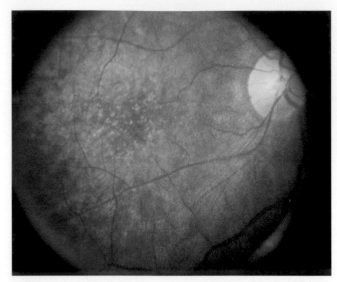

Figure 54–7 Posterior pole of a patient with LCA. There is fine pigment mottling in the macular area. The optic nerve head and retinal vasculature appear normal.

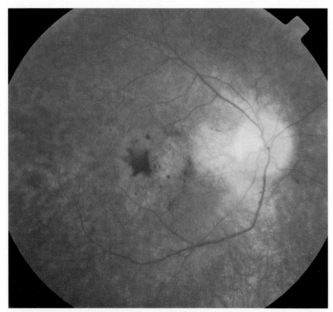

Figure 54–8 Right fundus of a 35-year-old woman with *RPE65*-related retinal degeneration. There is a central hyperpigmented spot, optic nerve pallor, attenuation of retinal blood vessels, and peripapillary and perimacular retinal and RPE atrophy.

vitamin A metabolism (LCA2 [OMIM number 204100]) (**Figure 54–8**); CRX, a homeobox gene encoding a transcription factor associated with LCA4 (OMIM number 604393); AIPL1 (OMIM number 604392), an aryl hydrocarbon protein-like gene expressed in photoreceptors and the pineal gland; and guanylate cyclase activating protein GCAP3 involved in phototransduction on chromosome 3q13.1. The loci at which the genes have not been identified are on chromosome 14q24 (LCA3 [OMIM number *604232]) and on chromosome 6q11-q16 (LCA5).

An LCA phenotype has been associated with polycystic kidney disease (Senior-Loken syndrome) and cone-shaped epiphyses (Saldino-Mainzer disease).

54.4 Retinitis Pigmentosa Associated With Systemic Diseases

The number of systemic conditions associated with a retinal degeneration that mimics RP is large and cannot be covered in this atlas. The reader is referred to other texts in which this subject is covered in detail. We will give two examples that illustrate diseases for which patients may initially present to the ophthalmologist (**Table 54–3**).

Usher's syndrome is an autosomal recessive disorder characterized by RP associated with sensorineural hearing loss. It is the most common cause of combined visual and hearing impairment in the United States. Several types of Usher's syndrome have been described. Type I disease presents with severe sensorineural hearing loss early in life, ataxia due to vestibular dysfunction, and a severely diminished or absent ERG. Visual decline is typically noted by early adolescence and progresses to severe visual dysfunction by early adulthood. Patients with type II Usher's disease present with moderate to severe nonprogressive hearing loss, normal vestibular function, and a recordable ERG. Visual dysfunction is noted by late adolescence and declines at a slower rate.

Bardet-Biedl syndrome is an autosomal recessive disease characterized by mental retardation, obesity, polydactyly, hypogenitalism, and pigmentary retinopathy (**Figure 54–9**). Macular pigment mottling is characteristic although there is usually minimal bone spicule clumping (**Figures 54–10 and 54–11**). The ERG is consistent with a rod-cone dystrophy. *Laurence-Moon syndrome* is distinguished from Bardet-Biedl syndrome by

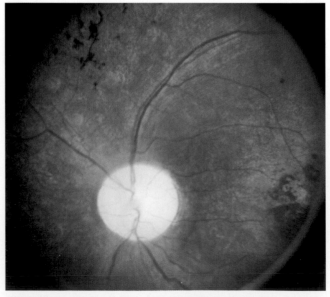

Figure 54–9 Pale optic nerve head and dense pigmentary changes in the macular area of a patient with Bardet-Biedl syndrome.

TABLE 54–3
Systemic Syndromes Associated with Pigmentary Retinopathy

Disorders of amino acid, protein, and lipoprotein metabolism	Hallervorden-Spatz syndrome
Gyrate atrophy of the choroid and retina	Friedreich's ataxia
Cystinosis	Retinitis pigmentosa with pallidal degeneration
Cobalamin-C defects (methylmalonic aciduria with homocystinuria)	Saldino-Mainzer syndrome
Imidazole aminoaciduria	Charcot-Marie-Tooth disease
Abetalipoproteinemia (Bassen-Kornzweig syndrome)	Marinesco-Sjögren syndrome
Hypobetalipoproteinemia	Joubert's syndrome

Disorders of amino acid, protein, and lipoprotein
  metabolism
  Gyrate atrophy of the choroid and retina
  Cystinosis
  Cobalamin-C defects (methylmalonic aciduria with
    homocystinuria)
  Imidazole aminoaciduria
  Abetalipoproteinemia (Bassen-Kornzweig syndrome)
  Hypobetalipoproteinemia
Lysosomal storage diseases
  Mucopolysaccharidoses I-H (Hurler's syndrome); I-S
    (Scheie's syndrome); I-HS (Hurler-Scheie syndrome); III
    A and B (Sanfilippo's syndrome)
Peroxisomal disorders
  Cerebrohepatorenal syndrome (Zellweger syndrome)
  Neonatal adrenoleukodystrophy
  Infantile Refsum disease
  Acyl-CoA oxidase deficiency
  Peroxisomal thiolase deficiency
  Primary hyperoxaluria
Neurologic disorders
  Neuronal ceroid lipofuscinoses
  Olivopontocerebellar atrophy with retinal degeneration
    (spinocerebellar ataxia type 7; SCA7)
  Kearns-Sayre syndrome
  Myotonic dystrophy

Hallervorden-Spatz syndrome
Friedreich's ataxia
Retinitis pigmentosa with pallidal degeneration
Saldino-Mainzer syndrome
Charcot-Marie-Tooth disease
Marinesco-Sjögren syndrome
Joubert's syndrome
Dermatologic disorders
  Darier's disease
  Incontinentia pigmenti (Bloch-Sulzberger disease)
  Rud's syndrome
  Sjögren-Larsson syndrome (fatty alcohol oxidoreductase
    deficiency)
Renal disease
  Renal-retinal dysplasia (Senior-Loken syndrome)
  Hereditary hemorrhagic nephritis (Alport's syndrome)
Skeletal anomalies/dwarfism
  Asphyxiating thoracic dystrophy (Jeune's syndrome)
  Cockayne's syndrome
  Osteopetrosis
Other multisystem disorders
  Bardet-Biedl syndrome
  Cohen's syndrome
Retinitis pigmentosa and deafness
  Usher's syndrome
  Flynn-Aird syndrome

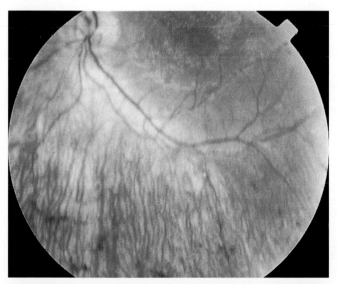

Figure 54–10 Inferior fundus of another patient with Bardet-Biedl syndrome. There is a circular area of atrophy around the fovea, optic atrophy, and peripheral bony spicules.

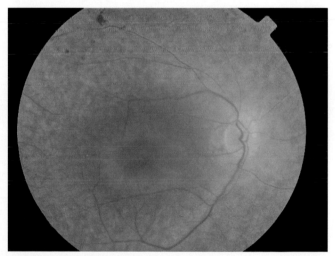

Figure 54–11 Macular bulls'-eye lesion and peripheral pigmentary changes in another patient with Bardet-Biedl syndrome.

the lack of polydactyly and obesity and by the presence of spastic paresis.

54.5 Imaging and Diagnostic Tests

Visual field testing, particularly using the Goldmann apparatus, is useful in assessing visual function and monitoring the progression of the disease in patients with RP. It is common to find bilateral symmetric loss of the mid-peripheral visual fields that gradually encroaches on central vision (**Figure 54–12**). Color vision is variably affected. Screening with pseudo-isochromatic plates followed by more extensive diagnostic testing with Farnsworth-Munsell arrangement tests can reveal decreased color vision associated with photoreceptor dysfunction.

Intravenous fluorescein angiography (IVFA) may help identify areas of RPE atrophy and cystoid macular

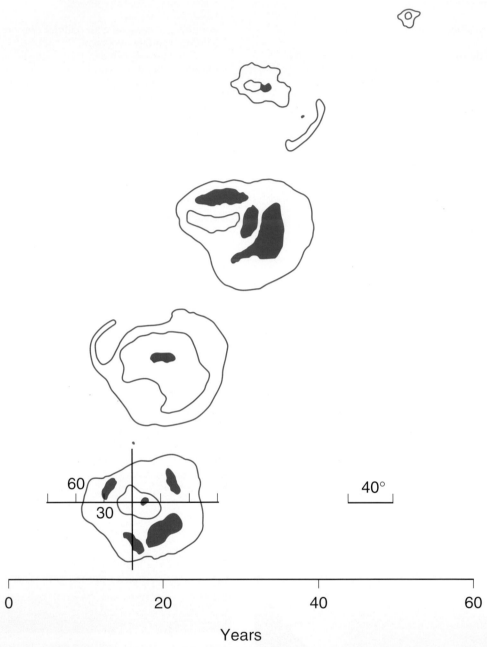

60

30

40°

0   20   40   60

Years

Figure 54–12 Progressive loss of field of vision in a patient with autosomal dominant RP over the course of several decades.

edema that are not clinical obvious. Cystoid edema in RP may be clinically indistinguishable from that found in inflammatory disorders and responds in some patients to oral acetazolamide treatment. In RP associated with Coats' disease, IVFA demonstrates telangiectatic vessels, leakage, and areas of capillary nonperfusion.

Optical coherence tomography provides a high-resolution cross-sectional view of the vitreoretinal interface and retina. This modality may aid in the evaluation of subtle epiretinal membranes, cystoid edema, and macular holes associated with RP. Epiretinal membrane

proliferation generally occurs in the macular area, particularly over or adjacent to the fovea. A pseudohole may appear if the membrane has a gap or hole.

The ERG is useful in measuring photoreceptor dysfunction. On scotopic testing, photoreceptor cells are dark adapted and then stimulated with a brief flash of light. This allows measurement of rod response. Photopic testing is similar, but cells are first light adapted, allowing measurement of cone response. In typical RP, initial changes include alterations in the scotopic waveform. As the disease progresses, the photopic response also becomes abnormal. By the end stages, the ERG responses are almost completely extinguished. Allied retinal disorders may show different patterns of ERG response. In cone-rod dystrophy, for example, initial weakening of the photopic response is seen, followed by diminution of the scotopic waveform. In cone dystrophy, only the photopic response is affected.

54.6 Pathology

Histologic evaluation of the retina in RP reveals atrophy of the photoreceptor layer, RPE hyperplasia, and migration of pigment into the retina.

SUGGESTED READINGS

Bird AC. Retinitis pigmentosa. In: Traboulsi EI, ed. Genetic Diseases of the Eye. New York, NY: Oxford University Press, 1998.

Grover S, Fishman GA, Alexander KR, et al. Visual acuity impairment in patients with retinitis pigmentosa. Ophthalmology. 1996; 103:1593–1600.

Kimura AE, Drack AV, Stone EM. Retinitis pigmentosa and associated disorders. In: Wright KW, ed. Pediatric Ophthalmology and Strabismus. St Louis, Mo: Mosby, 1995.

Van Soest S, Westerveld A, de Jong PT, et al. Retinitis pigmentosa: Defined from a molecular point of view. Surv Ophthalmol. 1999; 43:321–334.

Wang Q, Chen Q, Zhao K, Wang L, Wang L, Traboulsi EI. Update on the molecular genetics of retinitis pigmentosa. Ophthalmic Genet. 2001;22:133–154.

Tumors

Chapter 55

Retinoblastoma

AUDINA M. BERROCAL, MD • ELIAS C. MAVROFRIDES, MD • TIMOTHY G. MURRAY, MD

55.1 Introduction

Retinoblastoma is the most common intraocular malignancy in childhood and the third most common cancer overall affecting children. The incidence of retinoblastoma has increased over the past 60 years from 1 of 34,000 live births to 1 of every 15,000 live births. There is no sex or race predilection, and in 90% of the patients retinoblastoma is diagnosed by the age of 3 years. The retinoblastoma gene is a tumor suppressor gene located on the long arm of chromosome 13 (13q14). Sixty percent of the mutations are somatic, and 40% are germline. Somatic mutations tend to form a solitary tumor with a later, unilateral presentation (mean age, 24 months). Germline mutations tend to form bilateral, multifocal disease, which presents earlier (mean age, 13 to 15 months). Only 5% to 8% of patients have a family history of retinoblastoma with an autosomal dominant inheritance pattern, whereas the remainder of the tumors represent sporadic mutations (new germline or somatic mutation). In recent studies, sporadic retinoblastoma has been associated with the human papilloma virus.

55.2 Clinical Signs and Symptoms

Small intraretinal tumors are most commonly identified in infants with a family history of retinoblastoma in which screening begins at an early age. These tumors have a whitish-grey appearance within the retina (**Figure 55–1**) and are easily treated with local therapy (**Figure 55–2**). Because only 5% to 8% of patients have a positive family history, most patients with retinoblastoma present with more advanced disease. The most common presenting sign is leukocoria (54% to 62%) (**Figure 55–3**) followed by strabismus (18% to 22%) and a red, painful eye (7%). Less common presenting signs include anisocoria, hyphema, iris heterochromia, pseudohypopyon (**Figure 55–4**), orbital cellulitis, and cataract.

Larger tumors have two distinct growth patterns: endophytic and exophytic. Endophytic growth extends from the retina into the vitreous cavity (**Figures 55–5 and 55–6**). These tumors have a chalky-white, irregular surface and are often associated with vitreous seeding (**Figures 55–7 and 55–8**). Exophytic growth is seen in tumors that grow under the retina, and this growth pattern is more commonly associated with serous retinal detachments and choroidal invasion (**Figure 55–9**). Occasionally, tumors may exhibit characteristics of both growth patterns (**Figure 55–10**).

A rare presentation is seen with diffuse infiltrating retinoblastoma tumors (**Figure 55–11**). These unilateral and nonfamilial tumors expand along the surface of the

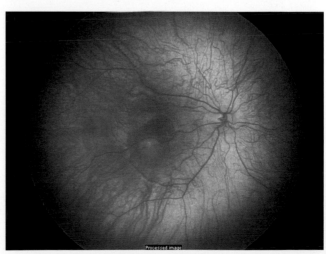

Figure 55–1 Small intraretinal retinoblastoma in the macula showing slight thickening and grayish coloration.

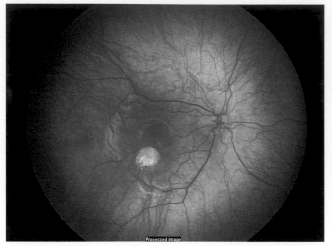

Figure 55–2   Area of chorioretinal scarring after treatment of tumor with diode laser photocoagulation.

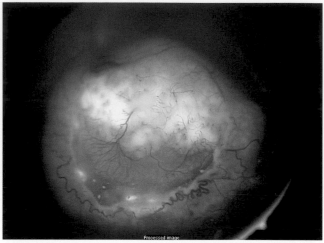

Figure 55–5   Tumor with endophytic growth pattern and overlying vitreous seeds.

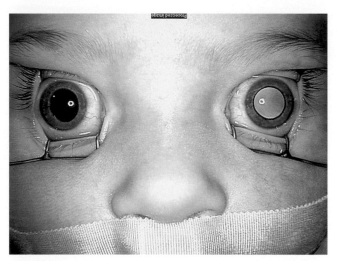

Figure 55–3   Leukocoria of the left eye in an infant with retinoblastoma.

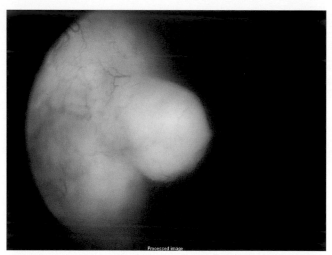

Figure 55–6   Large endophytic tumor extending into the vitreous cavity.

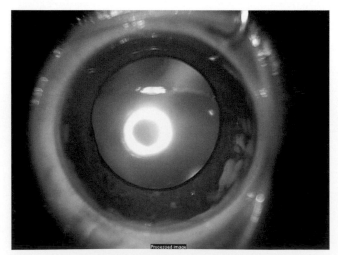

Figure 55–4   Pseudohypopyon in a patient with advanced retinoblastoma involving the anterior chamber and angle.

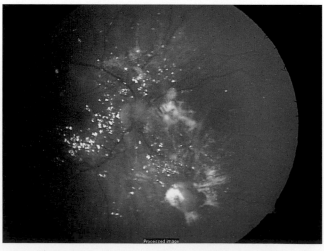

Figure 55–7   Regression of vitreous seeds after EBRT.

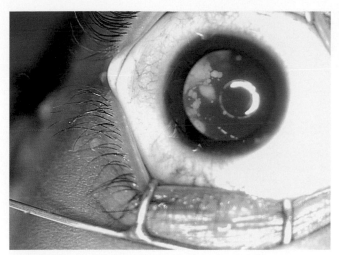

Figure 55–8 External photograph showing an endophytic tumor with large vitreous seeds in the retrolental space.

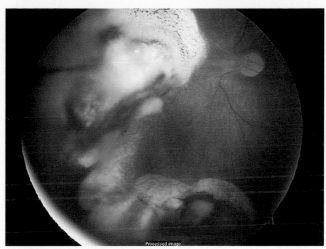

Figure 55–11 Patient with diffuse retinoblastoma after treatment with EBRT.

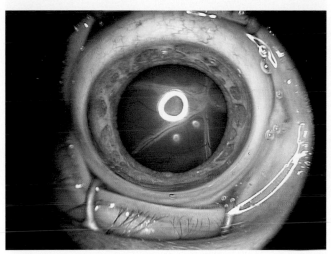

Figure 55–9 External photograph showing total exudative retinal detachment associated with a large exophytic tumor.

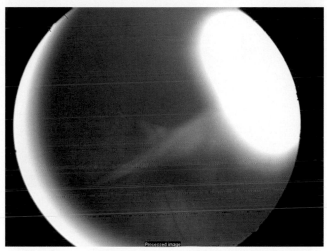

Figure 55–12 Persistent fetal vasculature showing insertion of the stalk into the posterior lens surface.

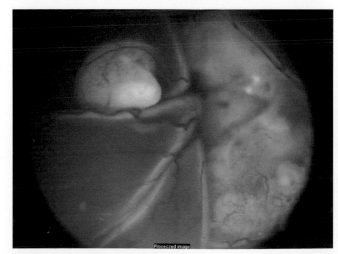

Figure 55–10 Advanced retinoblastoma showing both endophytic and exophytic growth patterns.

retina and have a later presentation (5 to 10 years of age). Calcification is not common, but iris nodules, hyphema, and pseudohypopyon are often seen. Misdiagnosis or delay in diagnosis often occurs.

The top three diseases in the differential diagnosis of retinoblastoma are persistent fetal vasculature, also known as *persistent hyperplastic primary vitreous* (**Figure 55–12**), Coats' disease (**Figures 55–13** to **55–15**), and ocular toxocariasis (**Figures 55–16** and **55–17**). Other conditions that must be distinguished from retinoblastoma include familial exudative vitreoretinopathy (FEVR) (**Figure 55–18**), retinopathy of prematurity (ROP) (**Figures 55–19** and **55–20**), and tuberous sclerosis (**Figure 55–21**).

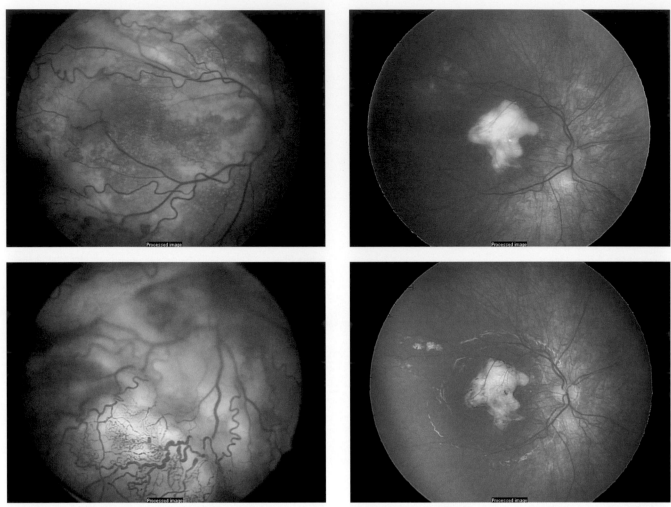

Figures 55–13 and 55–14 Exudative retinal detachment with evidence of telangiectatic retinal vessels in Coats' disease.

Figures 55–16 and 55–17 Macular granuloma in a child with ocular toxocariasis. Lesion shows chorioretinal scarring 5 years after presentation.

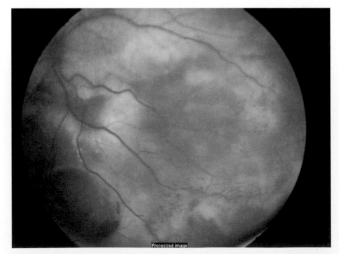

Figure 55–15 Coats' disease with extensive subretinal exudates and a retinal macrocyst.

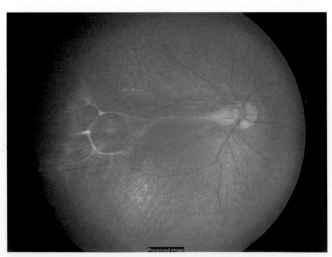

Figure 55–18 Macular dragging with fold formation in a patient with FEVR.

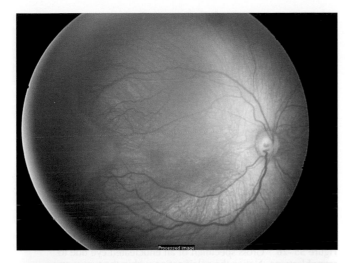

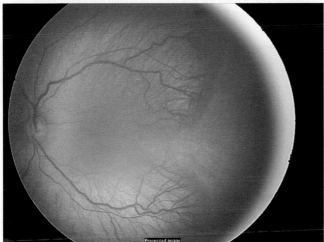

Figures 55–19 and 55–20 ROP showing stage 3 and mild plus disease in both eyes.

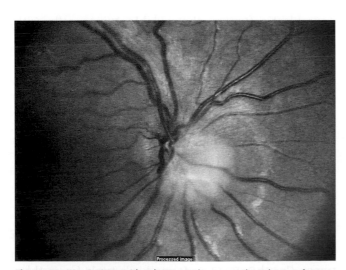

Figure 55–21 Patient with tuberous sclerosis and evidence of a peripapillary astrocytic hamartoma.

55.3 Imaging and Diagnostic Tests

55.3.1 ULTRASONOGRAPHY

B-scan ultrasound can be diagnostic and can aid in the assessment of the tumor size. Calcification within the retinoblastoma can be seen as highly reflective areas with associated orbital shadowing (**Figures 55–22** and **55–23**). High-resolution ultrasound has also been used to look at eyes with tumor in the anterior chamber (**Figures 55–24** and **55–25**).

55.3.2 COMPUTED TOMOGRAPHY

Computed tomography imaging can detect calcifications within the tumor and may also be useful in identifying optic nerve and/or orbital extension.

55.3.3 MAGNETIC RESONANCE IMAGING

Magnetic resonance imaging (MRI) is a better test to detect soft tissue invasion, especially when contrast

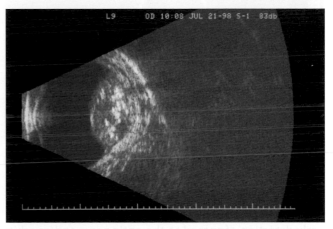

Figure 55–22 B-scan showing a large retinoblastoma tumor. Areas of high reflectivity within the tumor represent calcification.

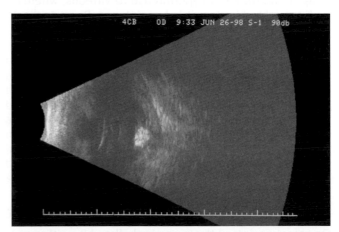

Figure 55–23 Small retinoblastoma showing orbital shadowing as a result of the tumor's calcification.

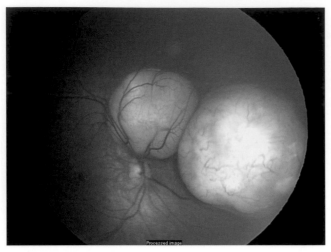
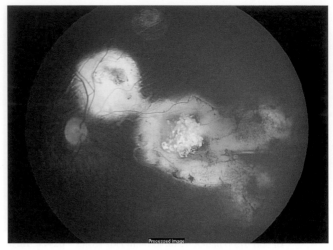

Figures 55–32 and 55–33 Multifocal tumor involvement in a child with familial retinoblastoma. Total regression is evident after treatment with chemoreduction and laser ablation.

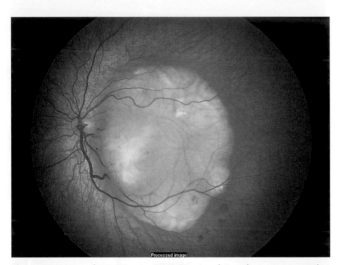
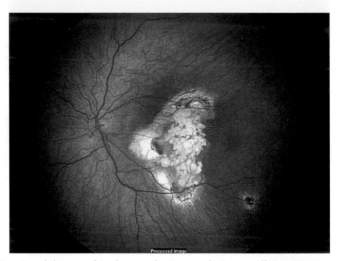

Figures 55–34 and 55–35 Large tumor involving the entire macular region. Local therapy after chemoreduction results in a smaller chorioretinal scar.

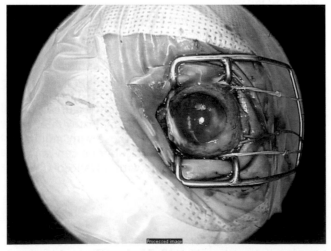
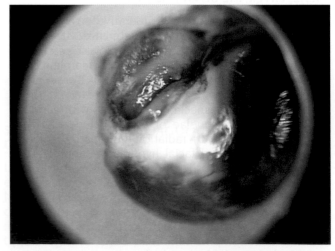

Figures 55–36 and 55–37 External photographs showing tumor invasion in the anterior chamber and protrusion through the nasal sclera.

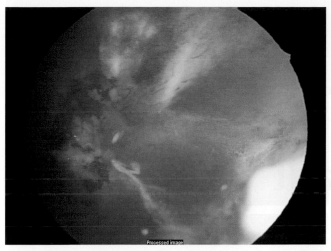 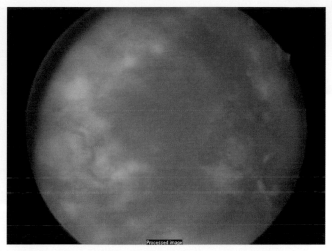

Figures 55–38 and 55–39 Vitreous hemorrhage after trauma in a patient with retinoblastoma. Enucleation was performed.

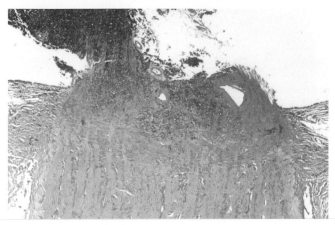

Figure 55–40 Histopathologic specimen showing retrolaminar invasion. (Courtesy of Sander R. Dubovy, MD.)

(**Figures 55–36** to **55–39**). Because retinoblastoma can invade the central nervous system through the optic nerve, it is critical to obtain a long section of the nerve at the time of resection (**Figure 55–40**).

SUGGESTED READINGS

Benz MS, Scott IU, Murray TG, Kramer D, Toledano S. Complications of systemic chemotherapy as treatment of retinoblastoma. Arch Ophthalmol. 2000;118:567–568.

Duncan JL, Scott IU, Murray TG, Gombos DS, van Quill K, O'Brien JM. Routine neuroimaging in retinoblastoma for the detection of intracranial tumors. Arch Ophthalmol. 2001;119:450–452.

Roth DB, Scott IU, Murray TG, et al. Echography of retinoblastoma histopathologic correlation and serial evaluation after globe-conserving radiotherapy or chemotherapy. J Pediatr Ophthalmol Strabismus. 2001;38:136–143.

Sussman DA, Escalona-Benz E, et al. Comparison of retinoblastoma reduction for chemotherapy vs external beam radiotherapy. Arch Ophthalmol. 2003;121:979–984.

Uusitalo MS, Van Quill KR, Scott IU, Matthay KK, Murray TG, O'Brien JM. Evaluation of chemoprophylaxis in patients with unilateral retinoblastoma with high-risk features on histopathologic examination. Arch Ophthalmol. 2001;119:41–48.

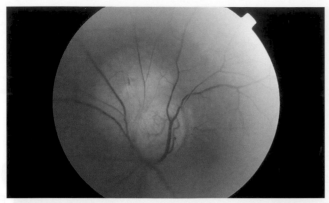

Figure 56–4   Amelanotic melanoma involving the peripapillary area.

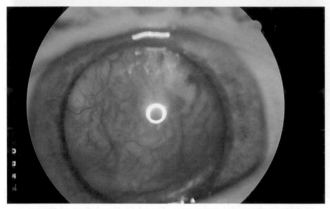

Figure 56–5   Amelanotic melanoma occupying the entire vitreous cavity.

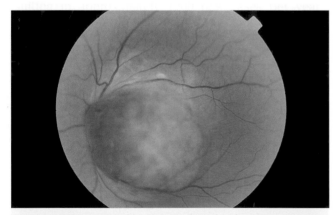

Figure 56–6   Mushroom-shaped melanoma.

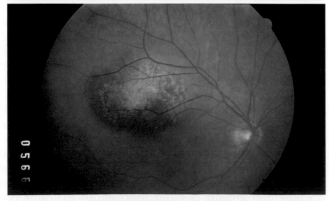

Figure 56–7   Melanoma with orange pigment on the surface.

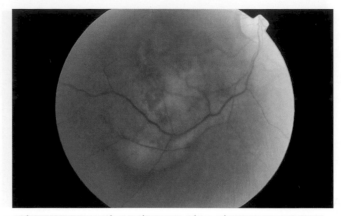

Figure 56–8   Another melanoma with overlying orange pigment.

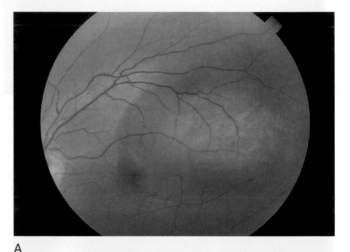

A

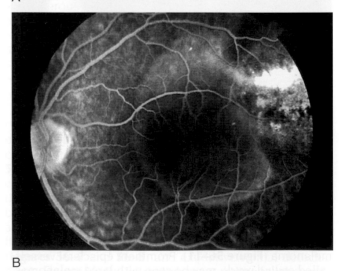

B

Figure 56–9   *A:* Choroidal melanoma with associated serous retinal detachment into the fovea. *B:* Fluorescein angiogram performed 1 week later, showing extension of the serous detachment.

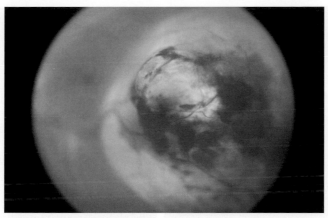

Figure 56–10 Hemorrhage associated with large melanoma that has broken through Bruch's membrane.

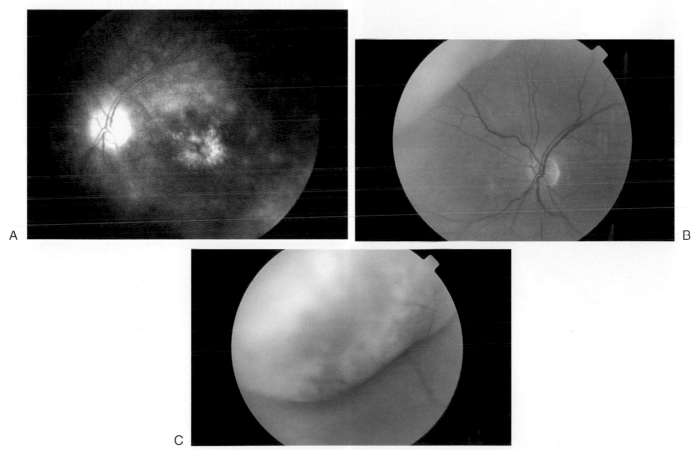

Figure 56–11 *A:* Late-frame fluorescein angiogram revealing cystoid macular edema. *B* and *C:* Fundus photographs of the same patient demonstrating a peripheral choroidal melanoma.

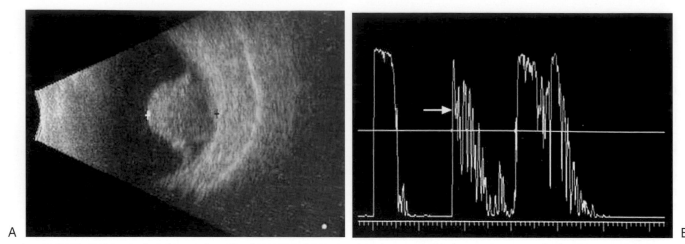

Figure 56–16   *A:* B-scan of mushroom-shaped melanoma with associated serous retinal detachment. *B:* Nonstandardized A-scan of the same lesion (*arrow*) demonstrating medium to low reflectivity with smooth attenuation. (Courtesy of Lois Hart, RDMS.)

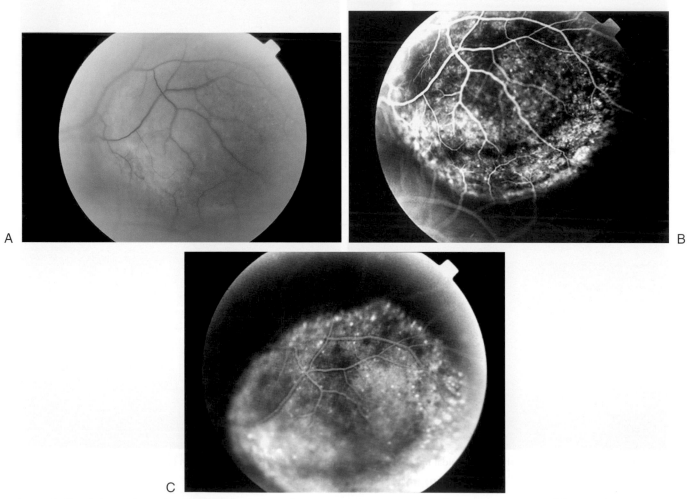

Figure 56–17   *A:* Large, dome-shaped melanoma with overlying orange pigment. *B* and *C:* Fluorescein angiogram of the same lesion revealing areas of early pinpoint hyperfluorescence with late staining.

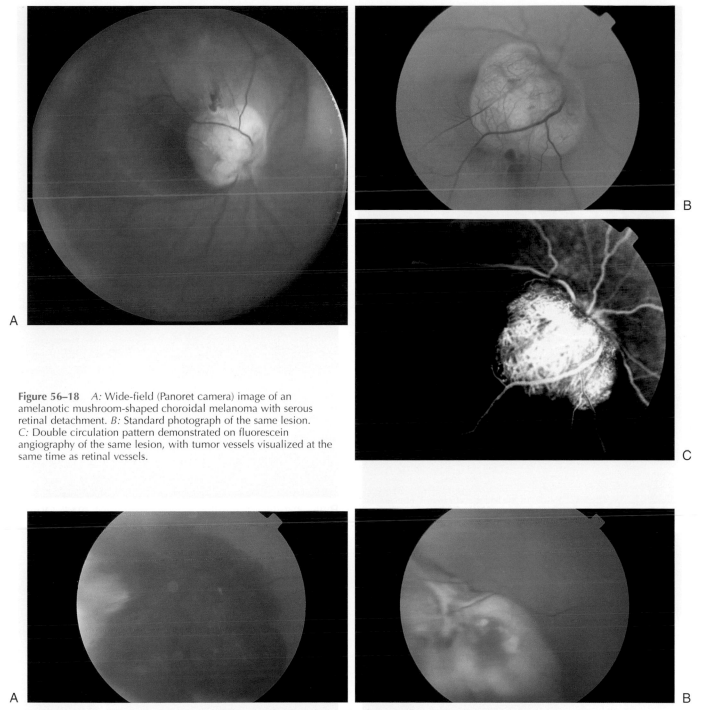

Figure 56–18 *A:* Wide-field (Panoret camera) image of an amelanotic mushroom-shaped choroidal melanoma with serous retinal detachment. *B:* Standard photograph of the same lesion. *C:* Double circulation pattern demonstrated on fluorescein angiography of the same lesion, with tumor vessels visualized at the same time as retinal vessels.

Figure 56–19 *A:* Hemorrhagic extramacular disciform lesion simulating a choroidal melanoma. *B:* Same lesion 3 months later.

clear advantage over ultrasonography in the diagnosis and management of uveal melanoma.

56.3.5 MAGNETIC RESONANCE IMAGING

Uveal melanomas typically appear hyperintense to vitreous on T1-weighted images and hypointense to vitreous with T2 weighting. They enhance brightly with gadolinium, which can help in differentiating tumor from subretinal fluid. Extraocular extension can also be

evaluated by magnetic resonance imaging (MRI). However, the role of MRI in the diagnosis and management of uveal melanoma has yet to be fully determined.

56.3.6 FINE-NEEDLE ASPIRATION BIOPSY

Occasionally, needle biopsy for cytologic analysis may be indicated when the diagnosis is particularly difficult. Concerns include possible seeding of the needle tract and false-negative results due to insufficient sampling.

Chapter 57

Choroidal Nevus

IVANA K. KIM, MD • EVANGELOS S. GRAGOUDAS, MD

57.1 Introduction

A choroidal nevus is a benign tumor composed of uveal melanocytes. The reported prevalence of choroidal nevi ranges widely from 0.2% to 30%, with the higher rates mostly derived from histopathologic studies. Nevi are extremely rare in children and seem to develop or become more pigmented around puberty. Approximately 90% of these lesions occur posterior to the equator with the majority of these located in the posterior one-third of the globe. Although there is still controversy over whether all choroidal melanomas arise from nevi, there certainly are patients in whom nevi do transform into malignant tumors. It has been estimated that 21 of 100,000 choroidal nevi will become malignant melanomas over 10 years.

57.2 Clinical Signs and Symptoms

A typical choroidal nevus is a flat or slightly elevated slate-gray lesion with fairly well-defined borders (**Figure 57–1**). Some clinicians make the distinction between choroidal nevi and choroidal freckles, which are always flat and represent a pronounced area of normal choroidal pigmentation with no malignant potential. The majority of nevi measure between 1.5 and 5 mm in diameter, but they can range from 0.5 to 10 mm. Although most nevi are flat, some may reach a height of 2 mm or more. Variations in pigmentation within and among nevi are also seen. Some lesions may be amelanotic (**Figure 57–2**), whereas others may be partially pigmented (**Figure 57–3**). The *halo nevus* is a variant in which the pigmented lesion is surrounded

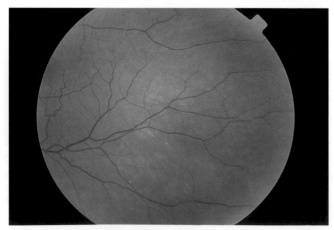

Figure 57–1 Typical choroidal nevus: flat, slate-gray lesion with fairly well-defined borders.

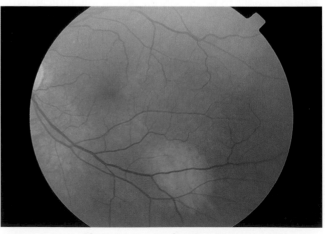

Figure 57–2 Amelanotic nevus.

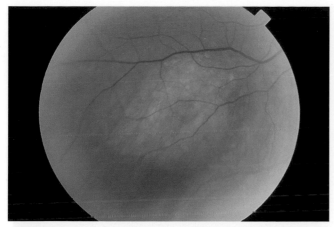

Figure 57–3   Nevus with a mixture of heavy and light pigmentation.

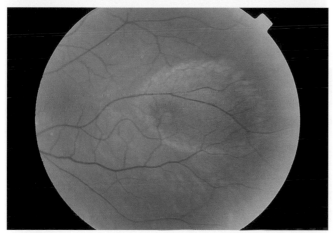

Figure 57–4   Halo nevus.

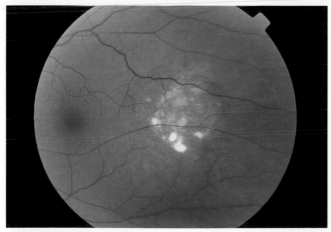

Figure 57–5   Choroidal nevus with drusen and overlying RPE changes.

by a yellow ring, which may represent balloon cell degeneration (**Figure 57–4**).

Changes in the retinal pigment epithelium overlying nevi are common (**Figures 57–5** and **57–6A–C**). Drusen are the most common finding, and clumping and

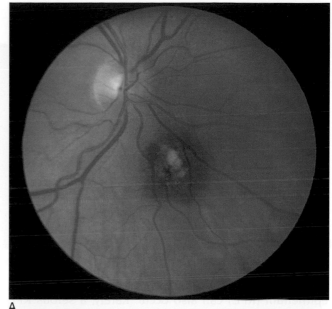

A

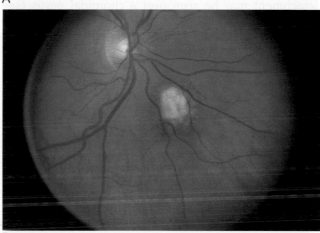

B

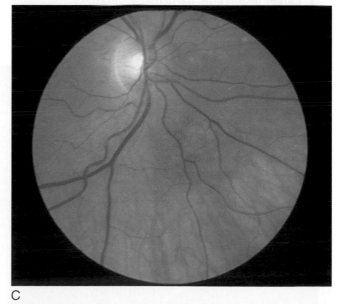

C

Figure 57–6   Variations in a nevus over time. *A:* Nevus with overlying RPE changes. *B:* Same nevus 8 years later. *C:* Same nevus 16 years later.

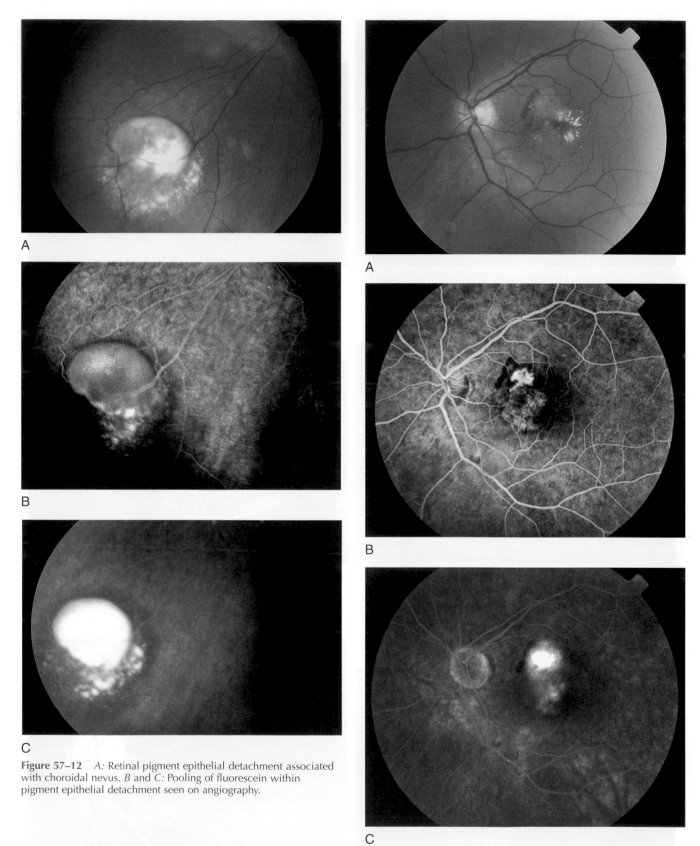

A

B

C

Figure 57–12 *A:* Retinal pigment epithelial detachment associated with choroidal nevus. *B* and *C:* Pooling of fluorescein within pigment epithelial detachment seen on angiography.

A

B

C

Figure 57–13 *A:* Choroidal nevus with associated subretinal fluid, hemorrhage, and exudates. *B* and *C:* Fluorescein angiography reveals choroidal neovascularization.

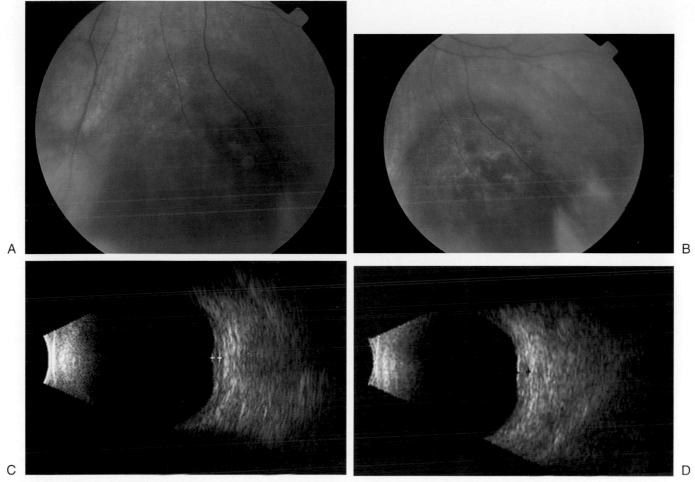

Figure 57–14 *A:* Choroidal nevus. *B:* Same nevus 5 years later, with minimal change on ophthalmoscopy. *C:* Ultrasound of nevus in *A*, showing a thickness of 1.2 mm. (Courtesy of Karen Capaccioli, RDMS.) *D:* Five years later, the same nevus measured 1.9 mm in thickness on ultrasound and was treated as a melanoma. (Courtesy of Lois Hart, RDMS.)

57.3.2 ULTRASONOGRAPHY

Ultrasound cannot distinguish between elevated nevi and small melanomas, but remains important in the evaluation of these lesions. Serial measurement of lesion elevation by ultrasonography is a key element in monitoring for growth (**Figure 57–14**).

57.4 Pathology

Four types of uveal nevus cells have been identified:

1. Plump, polyhedral: These deeply pigmented cells are the most common type of nevus cells. A melanocytoma is a nevus composed entirely of these cells.

2. Slender, spindle: These cells are the second most common cell type and contain little or no pigment.

3. Plump, fusiform, and dendritic: These cells are intermediate in pigmentation between plump, polyhedral and slender, spindle cells.

4. Balloon: These are large cells with abundant, foamy cytoplasm; they are less common than the other types and are similar to cells founding cutaneous and conjunctival nevi.

SUGGESTED READINGS

Augsburger JJ, Schroeder R, Territo C, Gamel JW, Shields JA. Clinical parameters predictive of enlargement of melanocytic lesions. Br J Ophthalmol. 1989;73:911–917.

Ganley JP, Comstock GW. Benign nevi and malignant melanomas of the choroid. Am J Ophthalmol. 1973;76:19–25.

Naumann G, Yanoff M, Zimmerman LE. Histogenesis of malignant melanomas of the uvea: I. Histopathologic characteristics of nevi of the choroid and ciliary body. Arch Ophthalmol. 1966;76:784–796.

Shields JA, Shields CL. Choroidal nevus. In: Intraocular Tumors: A Text and Atlas. Philadelphia, Pa: WB Saunders, 1992:85–100.

Yanoff M, Fine BS. Melanotic tumors of the uvea: Ciliary body and choroid. In: Ocular Pathology. 5th ed. Philadelphia, Pa: Mosby, 2002:667–672.

Chapter 58

Cavernous Hemangioma of the Retina

ARUN D. SINGH, MD • ELIAS I. TRABOULSI, MD

58.1 Introduction

Cavernous hemangioma of the retina (CHR) is a rare benign vascular tumor. Clinically, two forms are recognized: sporadic and syndromic. CHR is associated with cerebral cavernous malformations (CCMs) in the context of an autosomal dominant syndrome with high penetrance and variable expressivity. It has been suggested that the CCM syndromes should be included with the neuro-oculo-cutaneous (phakomatoses) syndromes, but the association of cerebral and cutaneous hemangiomas is inconsistent.

The association of retinal and cerebral hemangiomas in an individual family necessitates that all patients in whom CHR is diagnosed and their first-degree relatives undergo detailed ophthalmoscopic examinations and neuroimaging studies even if they are asymptomatic. The diagnosis of familial CCMs requires histopathologic or imaging documentation of cavernous hemangiomas in at least two family members. Familial CCMs have been linked to three loci on chromosomes 3q, 7p, and 7q (**Table 58–1**).

TABLE 58–1
Genetic Subtypes of CCMs

Subtype	Locus	Protein	Frequency (%)
CCM1	7q11.2-q21	Krev interaction trapped 1	40
CCM2	7p15-p13	Malcavernin	20
CCM3	3q25.2-q27	Unknown	40

58.2 Clinical Signs and Symptoms

Cavernous malformations may involve any part of the central nervous system but are found three times more often in the supratentorial regions than in the infratentorial regions. The tumors can occasionally involve the spinal cord. About 25% of patients with cavernous malformation syndrome are asymptomatic. Seizures, hemorrhage, or progressive focal neurologic deficits are common manifestations. Intracranial hemorrhage occurs in 12% to 48% of patients. Central cavernous hemangiomas are best visualized by magnetic resonance imaging (MRI) and have a central enhancing core and a dark ring from previous hemorrhages (**Figure 58–1**). Because these lesions are venous in origin, they may be difficult to detect on angiography.

CHRs are believed to be congenital hamartomas that may not be detected in childhood. The age of presentation in a series of nine patients ranged from 1 to 55 years. Patients with CHRs may be asymptomatic or may present with reduced vision from a macular location of the hemangioma, macular fibrosis, or rarely, vitreous hemorrhage. Retinal lesions appear as grape-like clusters of blood-filled saccular spaces in the inner layers of the retina or on the surface of the optic disc (**Figure 58–2**). The size and location of the hemangiomas are variable, but epiretinal membranes are usually present. There are no prominent feeder vessels, and there is a lack of subretinal or intraretinal exudation. In general, CHRs are nonprogressive, may undergo spontaneous thrombosis, and rarely cause vitreous hemorrhage. No effective treatment is known, although laser photocoagulation has been attempted in a few patients.

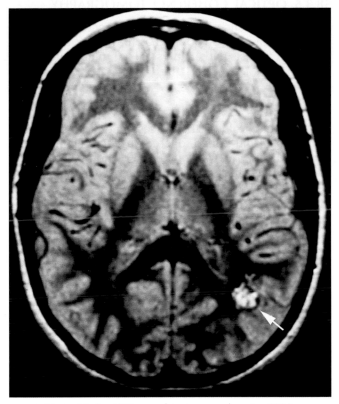

Figure 58–1   MRI scan showing an enhancing CCM.

The ophthalmoscopic features and fluorescein angiographic findings of CHR are characteristic, but this lesion should be differentiated from other vascular disorders such as Coats' disease, retinal capillary hemangioma, retinal arteriovenous communications, and retinal vasoproliferative tumors. The presence of retinal exudation argues against the diagnosis of CHR, and the absence of feeder vessels supports its diagnosis.

58.3   Imaging and Diagnostic Tests

58.3.1   FUNDUS PHOTOGRAPHY

The diagnosis of CHR is usually suspected on ophthalmoscopic examination. Fundus photographs can be used to document and monitor the lesion over prolonged periods of time.

58.3.2   FLUORESCEIN ANGIOGRAPHY

This test demonstrates the retinal origin of the hemangioma. The CHR is a low-flow system with delayed filling in the venous phase (**Figure 58–3**). The saccular dilatations in the hemangioma appear as fluorescein caps owing to sedimentation of erythrocytes and staining of supernatant plasma (**Figure 58–4**). The flow through the CHR is sluggish with relative isolation from the retinal circulation. Although cavernous hemangiomas are distributed randomly in the fundus, they tend to follow the course of a major vein, but feeder vessels are not prominent. There is characteristic absence of leakage.

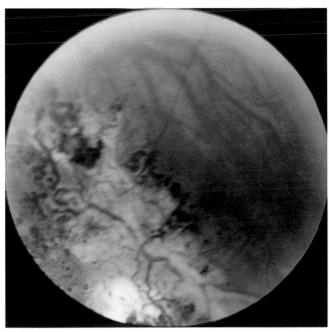

Figure 58–2   Fundus appearance of a cavernous hemangioma of the retina. Note the multiple clusters of saccular spaces in the inner layer of retina with an epiretinal membrane. There are no prominent feeder vessels and a lack of retinal exudation.

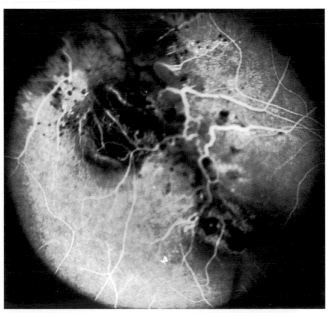

Figure 58–3   Fluorescein angiogram shows vascular communication of the cavernous hemangioma of the retina with the retinal circulation.

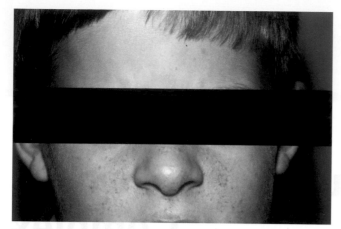

Figure 61–2 Angiofibroma appears like acne but has a characteristic butterfly facial distribution.

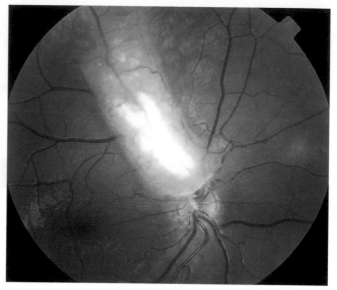

Figure 61–4 Fundus appearance of a typical retinal astrocytic hamartoma.

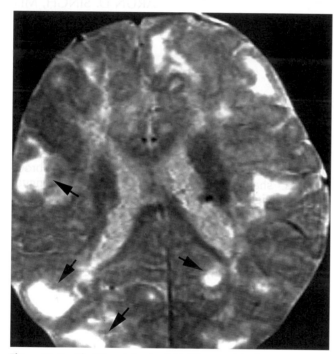

Figure 61–3 The T2-weighted axial MRI scan of the brain demonstrates multiple subcortical high-signal intensity areas consistent with subcortical tubers in a patient with TSC (*arrows*).

morbidity associated with TSC. About 50% of patients with TSC are mentally retarded, ranging from mild to profound retardation. The severity of neurologic disease directly correlates with the extent and number of cortical tubers detected on magnetic resonance imaging (MRI) scans (**Figure 61–3**).

61.2.3 VISCERAL MANIFESTATIONS

In addition to well-recognized hamartomatous involvement on brain, skin, and retina in TSC, hamartoma can also occur in viscera. Lung, kidney, and heart involvement in TSC manifests as pulmonary lymphangiomyomatosis, renal angiomyolipoma, and cardiac rhabdomyoma.

61.2.4 RETINAL ASTROCYTIC HAMARTOMA

Approximately 33% to 50% of patients with TSC have retinal or optic nerve hamartomas, and in half of these patients, the hamartomas are bilateral. The retinal hamartomas are located superficially in the retina and are usually situated near the optic disc in the posterior pole. Three morphologic types of retinal hamartomas have been described (**Figure 61–4**). The noncalcified type of retinal astrocytic hamartoma is a subtle, semi-transparent, and flat lesion. The calcified retinal astrocytic hamartoma appears as a white, elevated, and multi-nodular ("mulberry") lesion. A third type of lesion has a noncalcified portion peripherally with calcified central nodularity. Noncalcified regions may progressively calcify over many years.

A vast majority of astrocytic hamartomas remain stable; rare instances of aggressive astrocytic hamartomas have also been observed. Such unusual occurrences can lead to retinal exudation, vitreous seeding, and even extraocular extension (**Figure 61–5**). Although retinal hamartomas are vascularized, the feeding retinal blood vessels are of normal caliber in contrast to those for retinoblastoma from which retinal astrocytic hamartoma must be differentiated.

61.3 Imaging and Diagnostic Tests

The diagnosis of TSC is essentially clinical. There is no single sign that is present in all affected patients. According to the revised diagnostic criteria, the clinical and radiographic features of TSC have been divided into major and minor categories. For a definitive diagnosis of TSC, either two major features or one major feature plus two minor features should be present (**Table 61–1**).

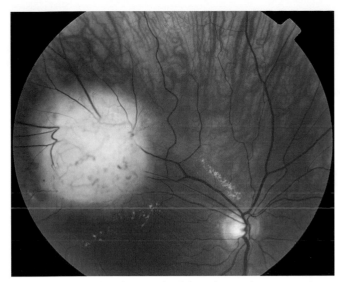

Figure 61–5 Fundus photograph of the right eye showing a circumscribed yellow-white retinal lesion. Note retinal exudation. (Reproduced with permission from Giles J, Singh AD, Rundle PA, et al.: Retinal astrocytic hamartoma with exudation. Eye. 2005;19:724–725.)

61.3.1 FUNDUS PHOTOGRAPHS

The diagnosis of astrocytic hamartoma can be made readily by ophthalmoscopy. Fundus photographs can be used to document the lesions and monitor them over prolonged periods of time.

61.3.2 FLUORESCEIN ANGIOGRAPHY

Fluorescein angiography demonstrates the retinal origin of the astrocytic hamartoma. The lesion appears hypofluorescent with a fine lacy network of intrinsic vessels that communicates with retinal circulation. Diffuse hyperfluorescence is seen in the late phases of the angiogram (**Figure 61–6**).

61.3.3 INDOCYANINE GREEN ANGIOGRAPHY

In the early phases of the angiogram, tumor intrinsic vascularity similar to the appearance on the fluorescein angiogram is observed (**Figure 61–7**).

61.3.4 ULTRASONOGRAPHY

B-scan ultrasonography is very helpful in establishing the diagnosis by detecting intrinsic calcification (**Figure 61–8**).

61.3.5 OPTICAL COHERENCE TOMOGRAPHY

Optical coherence tomography is not useful in establishing the diagnosis of astrocytic hamartoma.

TABLE 61–1

Revised Diagnostic Criteria for Tuberous Sclerosis Complex

Definite Diagnosis	Two major features
	One major feature plus two minor features
Probable Diagnosis	One major feature plus one minor feature
Possible Diagnosis	One major feature
	Two minor features

Major Features	Minor Features
Facial angiofibroma or forehead plaque	Multiple dental enamel pits
Ungual/periungual fibroma	Hamartomatous rectal polyps
Hypomelanotic macules (three or more)	Bone cysts
Shagreen patch	Cerebral white matter migration lines
Multiple retinal hamartomas	Gingival fibromas
Cortical tuber	Nonrenal hamartoma
Subependymal nodule	Retinal achromic patch
Subependymal giant cell astrocytoma	"Confetti" skin lesions
Cardiac rhabdomyoma (one or more)	Multiple renal cysts
Lymphangiomyomatosis	
Renal angiomyolipoma	

Criteria formulated by the Tuberous Sclerosis Complex Consensus Conference 1998. (Roach ES, Gomez MR, Northrup H. Tuberous Sclerosis Complex Consensus Conference: Revised clinical diagnostic criteria. J Child Neurol. 1998;13:624–628.)

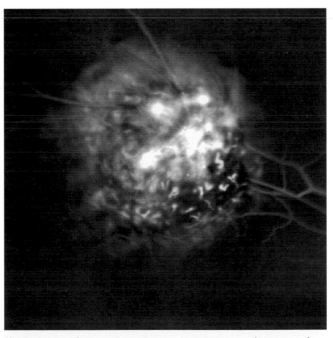

Figure 61–6 Fluorescein angiogram (arteriovenous phase) reveals fine intrinsic vessels. (Reproduced with permission from Giles J, Singh AD, Rundle PA, et al.: Retinal astrocytic hamartoma with exudation. Eye. 2005;19:724–725.)

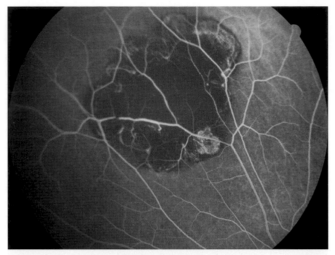

Figure 63–8 Fluorescein angiogram of the same patient as in **Figure 63–7**, demonstrating blockage in the area of the CHRPE.

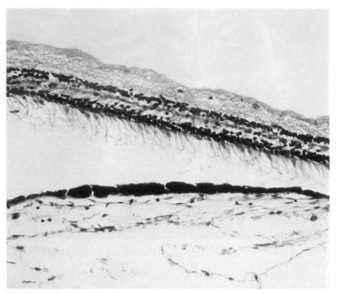

Figure 63–9 Photomicrograph showing hyperpigmented and hypertrophic RPE in a patient with Gardner's syndrome. (Courtesy of Richard Green, MD, and Elias Traboulsi, MD.)

63.3.3 INDOCYANINE GREEN ANGIOGRAPHY

Indocyanine green angiography is not useful in diagnosing CHRPE or related conditions.

63.3.4 OPTICAL COHERENCE TOMOGRAPHY

Optical coherence tomography is useful in demonstrating the hypertrophy of the RPE. The overlying retina is usually normal.

63.4 Pathology

Only a few reports on the histopathologic findings of CHRPE and its variants exist (**Table 63–2**). In solitary CHRPE, hypertrophic RPE cells with hyperpigmentation have been reported (**Figure 63–9**). Additional findings have included macromelanosomes and the absence of lipofuscin within the abnormal RPE cells. In contrast, the grouped CHPRE is composed of normal-sized RPE cells with hyperpigmentation. The CHRPE-like lesions seen in Gardner's syndrome show evidence of RPE hyperplasia and even hamartomatous changes in addition to RPE hypertrophy and hyperpigmentation (**Figure 63–10**).

The neoplastic lesions of the RPE are classified as *adenoma* or *adenocarcinoma*. The tumor is composed of pigment containing solid or vacuolated polygonal cells arranged in tubule-like groups with vascularized connective tissue septae and prominent basement membrane (**Figure 63–11**). Tumors demonstrating nuclear atypia and local invasiveness are classified as adenocarcinoma.

TABLE 63–2

Histopathologic Findings in Variants of CHRPE

| Type | RPE Cells | Pigment Granules | | | Other Findings |
		Size	Density	Shape	
Solitary	Hypertrophy Hyperplasia	Large macromelanosomes	Increased	Spherical	Thickened Bruch's membrane Atrophic RPE (lacunae) Atrophic photoreceptors Absence of lipofuscin
Grouped	Normal	Large	Increased	Ellipsoid	Absent RPE hypertrophy Absent RPE hyperplasia Normal photoreceptors
Atypical	Hypertrophy Hyperplasia	Large	Increased	Spherical	RPE hamartoma Abnormal melanogenesis

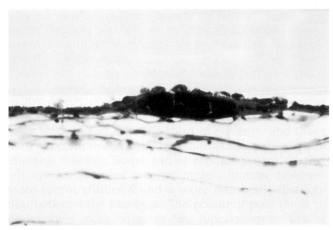

Figure 63–10   Photomicrograph showing hamartoma formation at the level of the RPE in a patient with Gardner's syndrome. (Courtesy of Richard Green, MD, and Elias Traboulsi, MD.)

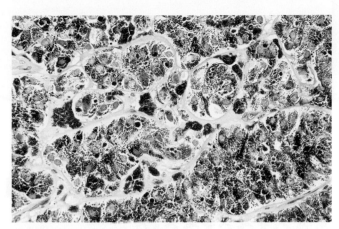

Figure 63–11   Photomicrograph showing tumor consisting of pigment containing polygonal cells arranged in tubule-like groups with vascularized connective tissue septae and a prominent basement membrane (hematoxylin and eosin, ×100).

SUGGESTED READINGS

Buettner H. Congenital hypertrophy of the retinal pigment epithelium. Am J Ophthalmol. 1975;79:177–189.

Gass JD. Focal congenital anomalies of the retinal pigment epithelium. Eye. 1989;3:1–18.

Regillo CD, Eagle RC Jr, Shields JA, Shields CL, Arbizo VV. Histopathologic findings in congenital grouped pigmentation of the retina. Ophthalmology. 1993;100:400–405.

Shields JA, Shields CL, Shah PG, Pastore DJ, Imperiale SM Jr. Lack of association among typical congenital hypertrophy of the retinal pigment epithelium, adenomatous polyposis, and Gardner syndrome. Ophthalmology. 1992;99:1709–1713.

Traboulsi EI, Maumenee IH, Krush AJ, Giardiello FM, Levin LS, Hamilton SR. Pigmented ocular fundus lesions in the inherited gastrointestinal polyposis syndromes and in hereditary non-polyposis colorectal cancer. Ophthalmology. 1988;95:964–969.

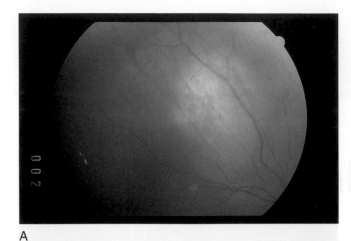

A

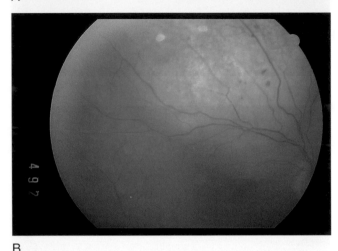

B

Figure 64–4 Lung cancer metastasis to the choroid can show rapid growth. *A:* At presentation, the choroidal lesion was yellow, mildly elevated, and associated with mild retinal pigment epithelial changes. *B:* Five weeks later, the lesion is substantially larger.

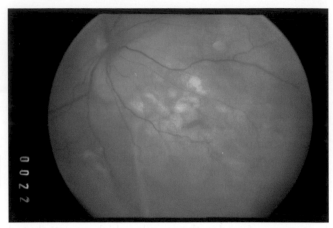

Figure 64–5 This choroidal metastasis had an associated bullous exudative retinal detachment. Note the irregular shape of the invasive choroidal lesion and retinal folds inferiorly.

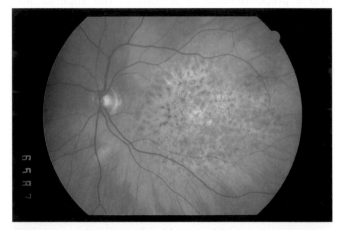

Figure 64–6 Clumping and proliferation of the retinal pigment epithelium is common for larger metastases.

or, rarely, contralateral choroidal melanoma or very large breast, lung, or gastrointestinal tumors. Orange metastases tended to be due to carcinoid tumor or renal cell carcinoma. In general, metastatic tumors were usually flatter than choroidal melanomas of comparable basal size, and lung metastases were flatter than breast metastases. Associated exudative retinal detachment (88% of patients) (**Figure 64–5**) or retinal pigment epithelial change (**Figure 64–6**) was common.

64.3 Imaging and Diagnostic Tests

The diagnostic evaluation is aided by a history of a known primary tumor, although the choroidal lesion is the presenting sign in 34% of patients. Bilateral or multifocal findings are also important clues. Lesions sometimes simulating choroidal metastases include the following: choroidal melanoma, osteoma, hemangioma, sequelae of choroidal neovascularization, posterior scleritis, cytomegalovirus retinitis, subretinal granuloma, ocular histoplasmosis syndrome, choroidal detachment,

retinal pigment epithelial detachment, or other rare lesions. Unlike true choroidal metastases that are typically creamy yellow in color, pseudo-metastases may be red-orange like choroidal hemangiomas (which are also almost always unilateral and unifocal) or white like amelanotic choroidal melanomas. Choroidal metastases are also usually plateau- or dome-shaped and rarely show the collar-button configuration characteristic of choroidal melanoma. Choroidal osteomas, which may also be bilateral and yellow, are rarely significantly elevated, commonly have associated choroidal neovascularization and show very high reflectivity by ultrasound and bone density on computed tomography. Inflammation and pain are sometimes seen with choroidal metastases, especially in the setting of choroidal detachment but should be distinguished from inflammatory conditions, including Harada's disease, uveal effusion syndrome, posterior scleritis, and similar diseases by diffuse choroidal thickening found in those entities. Choroidal neovascularization and cytomegalovirus retinitis rarely present with a confusing picture because of the prominent hemorrhage as a lesion component when these entities present as an elevated mass.

64.3.1 FLUORESCEIN ANGIOGRAPHY

Fluorescein angiography is not required to make a diagnosis but may be useful, for example, to demonstrate a reason for visual loss. Metastatic choroidal tumors usually show blocked choroidal fluorescence in the early phase and then show a combination of diffuse leaks, pinpoint leaks, and discrete large, round leaks from the retinal pigment epithelium in the late phase of the study (**Figure 64–7**). Although these fluorescein angiographic characteristics are nondiagnostic and do not permit differentiation from pseudo-metastases, choroidal hemangiomas characteristically show more prominent early choroidal filling than is usually seen with metastatic lesions, and choroidal neovascularization may show early choroidal filling and more leakage than is usually seen with metastatic lesions. If the diagnosis is relatively certain, fluorescein angiography may still be useful to assess basal lesion size and to monitor the effect of treatment. Although relatively flat areas of

choroidal metastases can be difficult to assess clinically, there is always some alteration of the retinal pigment epithelium, which is highlighted on the fluorescein angiogram (**Figure 64–8**).

64.3.2 INDOCYANINE GREEN ANGIOGRAPHY

Indocyanine green angiography of some choroidal metastases shows a smooth and regular hypofluorescence and may be useful in delineation of choroidal metastases with associated retinal detachment.

64.3.3 OPTICAL COHERENCE TOMOGRAPHY

Optical coherence tomography of a retinal breast metastasis shows high reflectivity with shadowing.

64.3.4 ULTRASONOGRAPHY

Standardized echography is the key ancillary test. B-scan ultrasonography is useful in evaluating patients with media opacity or retinal detachment when the choroidal lesion is suspected but cannot be clearly seen. The

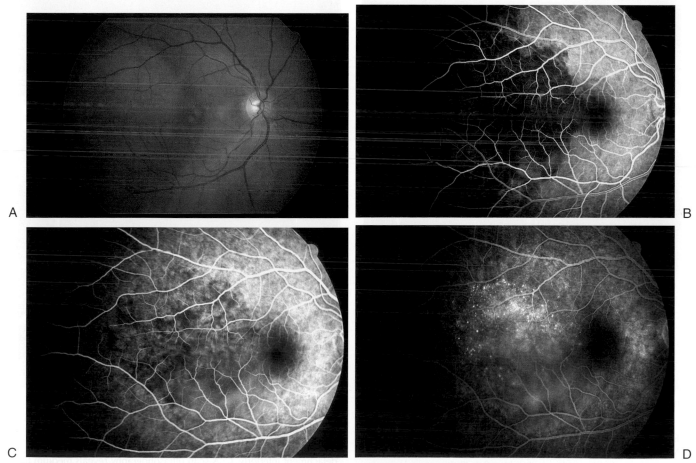

Figure 64–7   This breast cancer metastasis to the choroid shows typical fluorescein angiographic features. *A:* The large breast metastasis is somewhat brown in color, which is more common in larger lesions. *B:* The early phase of the fluorescein angiogram shows blocked fluorescence corresponding to the border of the choroidal mass. *C:* The transit phase of the angiogram showing abnormal pinpoint hyperfluorescence temporally and diffuse hyperfluorescence inferiorly. *D:* The late phase of the angiogram showing a combination of pinpoint and diffuse leakage from the pigment epithelium with pooling in the subretinal space inferiorly.

standardized ultrasonography. The value of CT and or MRI may be in the detection and delineation of associated intracranial lesions. Perhaps 25% of patients with a choroidal metastasis have concomitant central nervous system lesions.

64.3.6 FINE-NEEDLE ASPIRATION BIOPSY

A fine-needle aspiration biopsy (FNAB) should be considered only under special circumstances, such as an unknown primary tumor after extensive systemic evaluation in a patient with a characteristically appearing choroidal lesion, lesions that present major diagnostic uncertainty, or patients who refuse treatment without histopathologic verification of the tumor. The standard of care before radiation therapy for most tumor locations is to obtain a tissue diagnosis. Given the risks of FNAB (potential biopsy-related tumor seeding or vision-threatening complications), biopsy of choroidal tumors is *not* the norm. The ophthalmologist is encouraged to discuss the rationale for treatment without biopsy with the radiation oncologist. Steps that might be taken in advance to improve specimen collection for cytologic diagnosis include the following: use of an aspiration pistol and relatively large syringe, use of a needle of sufficient caliber (25-gauge), biopsy of the tumor directly, and arranging in advance for appropriate

processing and pathologic review of the aspirate. Steps that might be taken to minimize risk of tumor cell dissemination and of visual complications include the following: use of an indirect transvitreal route, use of as fine a needle as possible, use of an instrument trocar in the pars plana, use of a connector tubing between needle and aspirating device to avoid "jiggling" of the needle at the time of aspiration, maintenance of secure fixation on the globe during biopsy, and avoidance of large-caliber retinal and tumor vessels (**Figures 64–12** and **64–13**). When the treating oncologist requires histologic diagnosis for treatment, nonocular sites are favored and additional consultations may be obtained.

64.3.7 MISCELLANEOUS LABORATORY TESTS

When a new intraocular metastasis is recognized, coordination with the primary medical doctor or oncologist is essential. In patients with a known primary tumor site, systemic evaluation to provide repeat tumor staging would be indicated. If the primary tumor site is unknown, the patient should receive a careful history, physical examination, and systemic evaluation, which may include chest radiograph, abdominal and pelvic CT scans, liver function tests, fecal occult blood testing, brain MRI scans, and mammograms in women or prostate-specific antigen measurement in men.

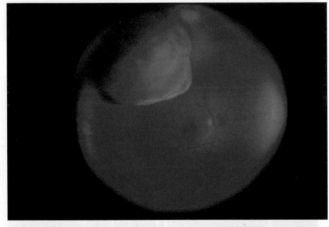

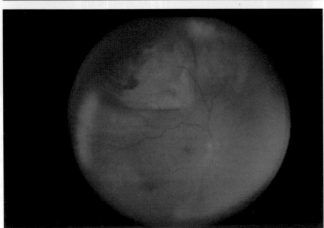

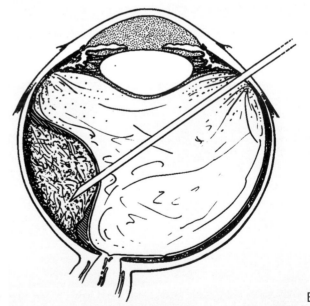

Figure 64–12 FNAB. *A:* This patient had a choroidal melanoma but insisted on a tissue diagnosis before treatment. (From Shields JA, Perez N, Shields CL, Singh AD, Eagle RC Jr. Orbital melanoma metastatic from contralateral choroid: Management by complete surgical resection. Ophthalmic Surg Lasers. 2002;33:416–420.) *B:* Schematic diagram of the biopsy procedure showing the preferred indirect transvitreal route to limit potential tumor cell dissemination. *C:* Appearance of the mass immediately after withdrawal of the 25-gauge needle. The cytologic specimen was consistent with a choroidal malignant melanoma. (Clinical photos courtesy of Ocular Oncology Service, Wills Hospital.)

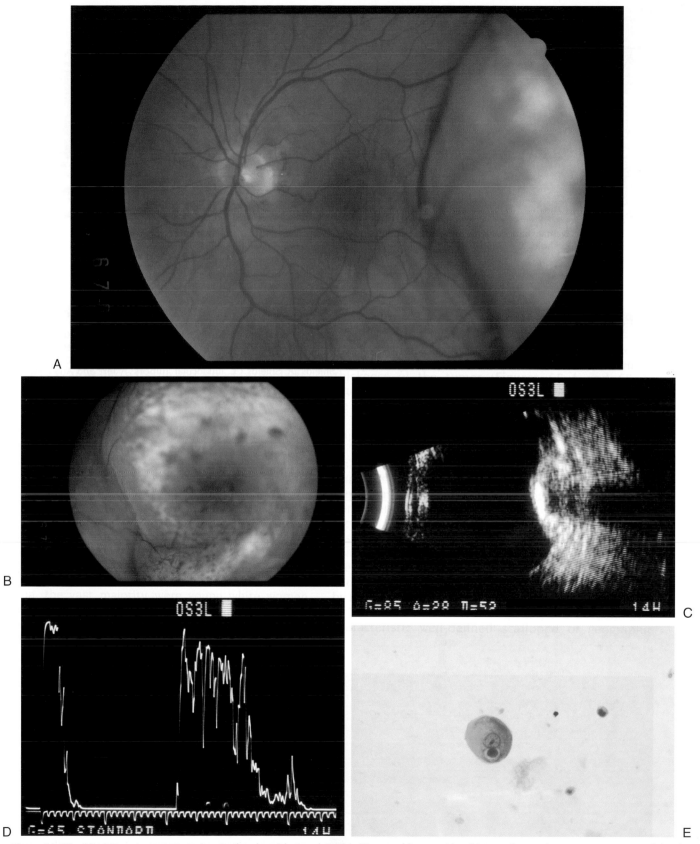

Figure 64–13 Prostate cancer metastasizes to the choroid. *A and B:* This 58 year-old man with a history of treated prostate cancer complained of gradually worsening vision in the left eye for 1 year and presented with this irregularly shaped white-yellow choroidal mass. *C:* B-scan ultrasonography showed a solid mass with shadowing, an irregular internal structure, and no internal vascularity. *D:* A-scan ultrasonography revealed medium to high internal reflectivity. *E:* After a fruitless extensive workup for other metastatic disease, an FNAB was performed, but cytologic analysis revealed only inflammatory cells and epithelial cells.

Continued

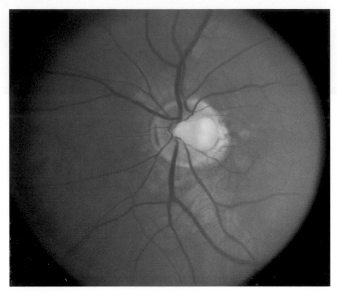

Figure 67–1 Large temporal pit in this left eye. There is no accompanying serous retinal detachment.

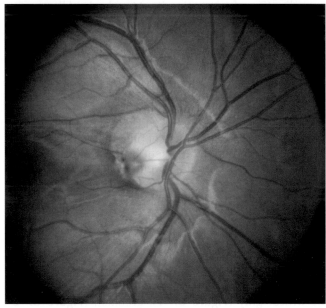

Figure 67–2 Small greenish temporal optic pit. Reflexes in the temporal bundle area indicate the possible presence of a serous macular detachment. (Courtesy of Froncie Gutman, MD.)

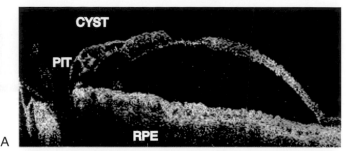

A

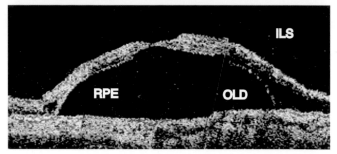

B

Figure 67–3 *A:* OCT horizontal section through the macula and disc of a patient with a pit and serous detachment demonstrating outer layer detachment (OLD). The OLD is in close approximation to the inner layer separation (ILS) except at its margins. Nasally the ILS is cystic. *B:* Vertical section through the macula of another patient better delineates the OLD and ILS as separate layers. RPE, retinal pigment epithelium. (From Lincoff H, Kreissig I. Optical coherence tomography of pneumatic displacement of optic disc pit maculopathy. Br J Ophthalmol. 1998;82:367–372.)

67.3.3 ULTRASONOGRAPHY

There is no specific role for ultrasonography in the diagnosis of optic pits or the associated macular detachment. B-scan ultrasonography will show separation of the sensory retina with or without a schisis cavity in eyes in which these abnormalities are present.

67.3.4 OPTICAL COHERENCE TOMOGRAPHY

There is a typical macular schisis pattern on optical coherence tomography (OCT) in patients with an optic pit with serous maculopathy that helps differentiate this condition from other macular elevations. In patients with associated maculopathy, OCT demonstrates a retinal detachment with a typical convex schisis of the outer retinal layer in most patients. In addition, OCT demonstrates the associated neurosensory detachment with or without intraretinal cyst formation. Communication between a schisis cavity or subretinal space and the optic nerve pit can be imaged in all eyes with associated serous macular detachment, whereas it cannot be in eyes with evidence of resolved detachment or in those without clinical macular pathologic lesions. Cystic degeneration and schisis are usually imaged in the peripapillary retina, macula, or both in most eyes with optic pits. Lincoff et al. used OCT to demonstrate a separation between the inner and outer layers of the retina that connected with the optic disc pit, confirming the two-layer structure of optic disc pit maculopathy

hypofluorescence and late staining of the optic pit on fluorescein angiography. All 17 eyes presented a delineated late hyperfluorescence corresponding to the area of macular elevation on both ICG angiography and fluorescein angiography. The intensity of the hyperfluorescence was milder in patients with long-standing maculopathy. The increased hyperfluorescence in the late phases of the macular elevation in the studied eyes could be attributed to leakage of indocyanine or fluorescein dye into the schisis cavity and the subretinal fluid.

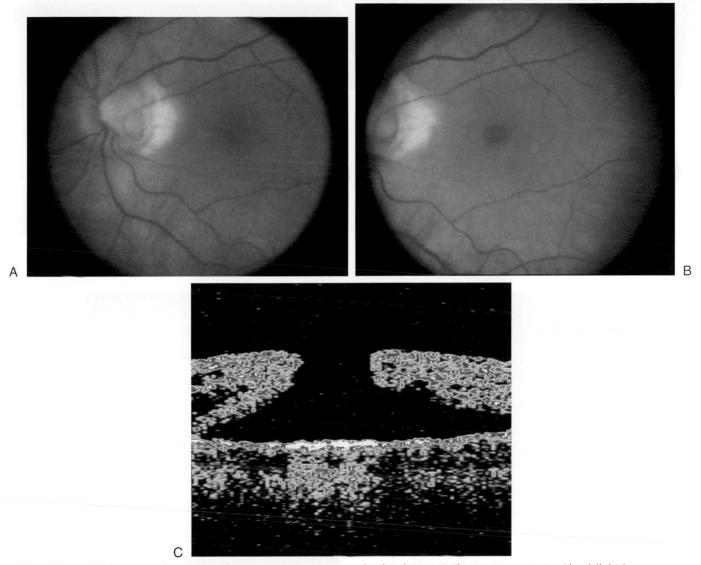

Figure 67–4 *A:* Inferotemporal optic pit with accompanying serous macular detachment. *B:* The same eye as in *A*, with a full-thickness macular hole, also shown on OCT in *C.* (Courtesy of Hilel Lewis, MD.)

(**Figure 67–3**). OCT is useful in following up patients after surgical intervention.

SUGGESTED READINGS

Borodic GE, Gragoudas ES, Edward WO, Brockhurst RJ. Peripapillary subretinal neovascularization and serous macular detachment: Association with congenital optic nerve pits. Arch Ophthalmol. 1984;102:229-.

Brown GC, Shields JA, Goldberg RE. Congenital pits of the optic nerve head. II. Clinical studies in humans. Ophthalmology. 1980;87:51–65.

Gass JDM. Serous detachment of the macula secondary to congenital pit of the optic nervehead. Am J Ophthalmol. 1969;67:821–841.

Hassenstein A, Richard G. Optical coherence tomography in optic pit and associated maculopathy. Ophthalmologe. 2004;101:170–176.

Irvine AR, Crawford JB, Sullivan JH. The pathogenesis of retinal detachment with morning glory and optic pit. Retina. 1986;6:146–150.

Lincoff H, Kreissig I. Optical coherence tomography of pneumatic displacement of optic disc pit maculopathy. Br J Ophthalmol. 1998;82:367–372.

Lincoff H, Lopez R, Kreissig I. Retinoschisis associated with optic nerve pits. Arch Ophthalmol. 1988;106:61–67.

Lincoff H, Schiff W, Krivoy D, Ritch R. Optic coherence tomography of optic disk pit maculopathy. Am J Ophthalmol. 1996;122:264-266.

Slusher MM, Weaver RG Jr, Greven CM, Mundorf TK, Cashwell LF. The spectrum of cavitary optic disc anomalies in a family. Ophthalmology. 1989;96:342.

Sobol WM, Blodi CF, Folk JC, Weingeist TA. Long-term visual outcome in patients with optic nerve pit and serous retinal detachment of the macula. Ophthalmology. 1990;97:1539.

Stefko ST, Campochiaro P, Wang P, Li Y, Zhu D, Traboulsi EI. Dominant inheritance of optic pits. Am J Ophthalmol. 1997;124:112–113.

Theodossiadis GP, Ladas ID, Panagiotidis DN, Kollia AC, Voudouri AN, Theodossiadis PG. Fluorescein and indocyanine green angiographic findings in congenital optic disk pit associated with macular detachment. Retina. 1999;19:6–11.

supply, predisposing the nerve to disc hemorrhages and ischemic optic neuropathy. Once ONHD become clinically visible, thinning of the nerve fiber layer (NFL) can be observed through several modalities. The level of NFL loss detected is correlated with the degree of ONHD visible on examination and often precedes any visual field loss. Deep or buried drusen tend not to demonstrate NFL thinning; however, calcification can be detected with B-scan ultrasound or computed tomography. Unfortunately, ONHD enlarge with age, and both thinning of the NFL and field loss are slowly progressive over time.

68.3 Imaging and Diagnostic Tests

68.3.1 ULTRASONOGRAPHY

B-scan ultrasound can reveal an ovoid echogenic lesion at the junction of the retina and optic nerve (**Figure 68–5**). The degree of acoustic shadowing is proportional to the size of the echogenic focus.

68.3.2 RED-FREE PHOTOGRAPHY

Red-free photography may reveal autofluorescence of the drusen without the administration of fluorescein (**Figure 68–6**). Alterations in the peripapillary retinal nerve fiber layer may include varying degrees of regional thinning, especially nasally, or diffuse loss of NFL. Deep or buried ONHD tend not to show any NFL changes on red-free photography.

68.3.3 FLUORESCEIN ANGIOGRAPHY

Late phases of the fluorescein angiogram may show late focal hyperfluorescence and fluorescein staining of the peripapillary vessel wall (**Figure 68–7**).

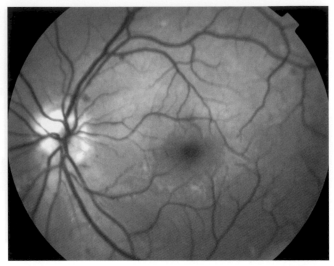

Figure 68–6 Red-free photograph demonstrating autofluorescence of optic disc drusen.

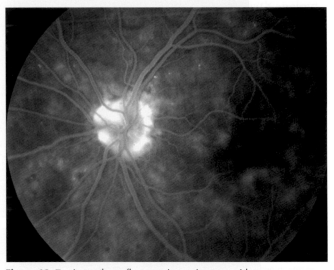

Figure 68–7 Late-phase fluorescein angiogram with hyperfluorescence of the peripapillary region.

68.3.4 COMPUTED TOMOGRAPHY

Often an incidental finding, intraorbital calcifications at the level of the optic nerve head may be revealed on high-resolution head or orbital scans. These are especially well visualized with bone windows (**Figure 68–8**).

68.3.5 OPTICAL COHERENCE TOMOGRAPHY

Circular scans around the optic nerve reveal varying levels of NFL loss. The amount of thinning appears to be proportional to clinically visible excrescences of the optic disc. Localized thinning is seen in quadrants in which drusen are most aggregated (**Figures 68–9** and **68–10**). In eyes with generalized dense drusen of the entire disc, diffuse NFL loss is observed. A radial scan of

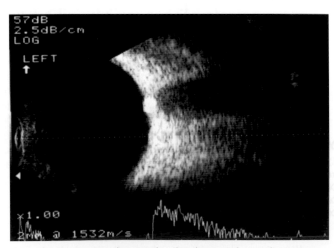

Figure 68–5 B-scan ultrasound with echogenic foci at the optic nerve head. Same patient as shown in **Figure 68–4.**

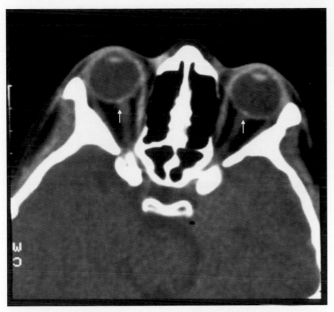

Figure 68–8 Intraorbital calcifications at the level of the optic nerve head on a computed tomography scan.

the optic nerve performed through the drusen can illustrate elevation within the nerve head and obscuration of the physiologic cup (**Figure 68–11**).

68.3.6 POLARIMETRIC NERVE FIBER ANALYSIS

Scanning laser polarimetry is capable of detecting loss of the nerve fiber layer. In eyes with dense drusen obscuring the cup, retinal nerve fiber layer (RNFL) thickness change may be observed (**Figure 68–12**).

68.3.7 HEIDELBERG RETINA TOMOGRAPHY

Heidelberg retina tomography (HRT) allows a three-dimensional topometric analysis of the optic nerve head (**Figure 68–13**). Elevation of the disc surface is best seen on profiles of surface height. HRT measures peripapillary RNFL height, which may correlate with visual field abnormalities.

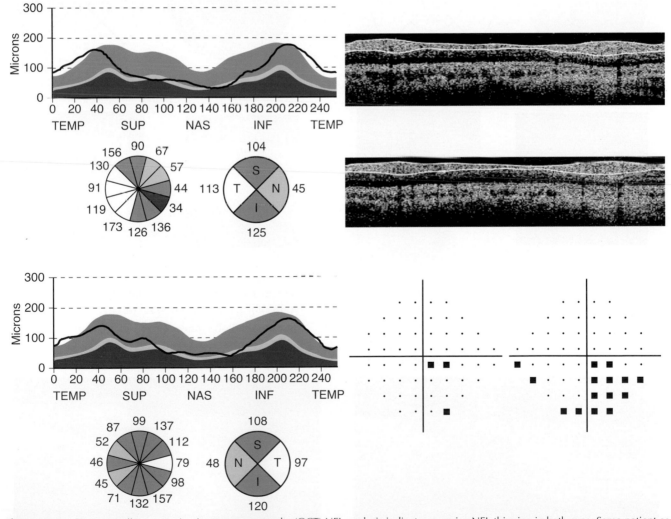

Figure 68–9 Circumpapillary optical coherence tomography (OCT) NFL analysis indicates superior NFL thinning in both eyes. Same patient as in **Figures 68–4** and **68–5**.

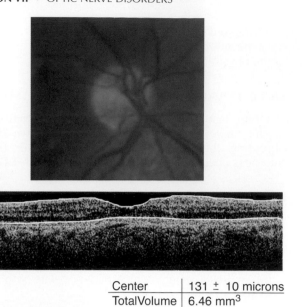

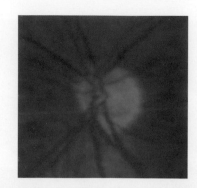

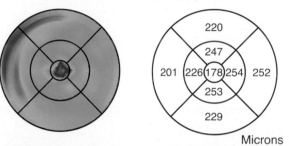

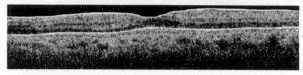

Center	131 ± 10 microns
TotalVolume	6.46 mm^3

Center	128 ± 8 microns
TotalVolume	6.27 mm^3

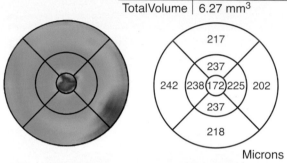

Microns

Microns

Figure 68–10 OCT macular thickness analysis correlates with NFL loss in both eyes. Same patient as in **Figures 68–4** and **68–5**.

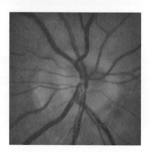

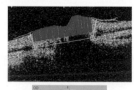

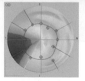

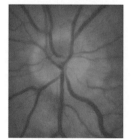

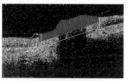

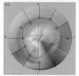

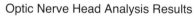

Optic Nerve Head Analysis Results
Vertical integrated rim area (volume)   1.864 mm^2
Horizontal integrated rim width (area)   2.4 mm^2

Disk area:	2.799 mm^2	Cup/Disk area ratio:	1
Cup area:	2.799 mm^2	Cup/Disk horizontal ratio:	1
Rim area:	0 mm^2	Cup/Disk vertical ratio:	1

Optic Nerve Head Analysis Results
Vertical integrated rim area (volume)   2.444 mm^2
Horizontal integrated rim width (area)   2.583 mm^2

Disk area:	3.403 mm^2	Cup/Disk area ratio:	1
Cup area:	3.403 mm^2	Cup/Disk horizontal ratio:	1
Rim area:	0 mm^2	Cup/Disk vertical ratio:	1

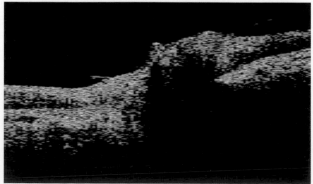

Figure 68–11   Radial OCT scan demonstrates elevation of the optic nerve head.

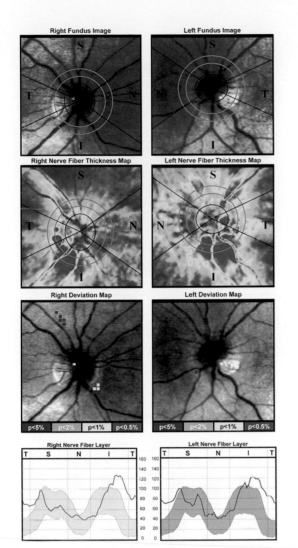

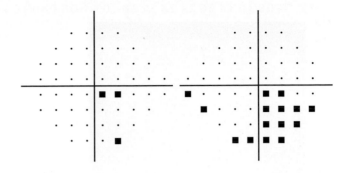

TSNIT Parameters	OD Actual Val.	OS Actual Val.
TSNIT Average	74	79
Superior Average	71	79
Inferior Average	92	99
TSNIT Std. Dev.	24	23
Inter-Eye Symmetry	0.91	
NFI	8	5

p>=5%	p<5%	p<2%	p<1%	p<0.5%

Thickness Map Legend (microns)

0   20   40   60   80   100   120   140   160   180   200

Figure 68–12   Scanning laser polarimetry analysis by the GD system in the same patient as in **Figures 68–4** and **68–5** indicates relative NFL thinning superiorly.

68.4 Pathology

Optic drusen are collections of two to three small nodules, up to 40 or 50 colloid bodies ranging from 5 to 1000 microns in diameter (**Figure 68–14**). Histologically, they consist of needle-like calcium depositions in the mitochondria of axons, disruption of the plasmalemma, leakage of axoplasmic components into the interstitial space, and heavy deposition of calcium crystal in extracellular mitochondria.

ACKNOWLEDGMENT

This work was supported in part by National Institutes of Health Grants R01-EY13178-4 and RO1-EY11289-16.

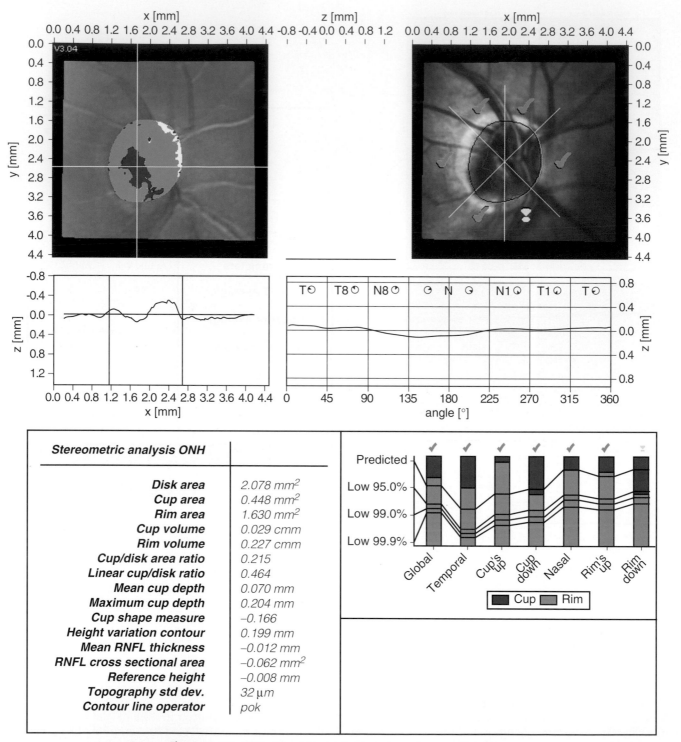

Stereometric analysis ONH	
Disk area	2.078 mm²
Cup area	0.448 mm²
Rim area	1.630 mm²
Cup volume	0.029 cmm
Rim volume	0.227 cmm
Cup/disk area ratio	0.215
Linear cup/disk ratio	0.464
Mean cup depth	0.070 mm
Maximum cup depth	0.204 mm
Cup shape measure	−0.166
Height variation contour	0.199 mm
Mean RNFL thickness	−0.012 mm
RNFL cross sectional area	−0.062 mm²
Reference height	−0.008 mm
Topography std dev.	32 µm
Contour line operator	pok

Figure 68–13   HRT of the right eye demonstrates optic nerve elevation.

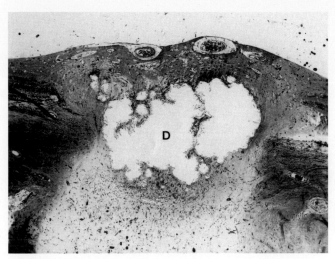

Figure 68–14 Multilobulated drusen filling the optic nerve head cup. (From Tso MO: Pathology and pathogenesis of drusen of the optic nerve head. Ophthalmology. 1981;88:1068.)

SUGGESTED READINGS

Kurz-Levin M, Landau K. A comparison of imaging techniques for diagnosing drusen of the optic nerve head. Arch Ophthalmol. 1999; 117:1045–1049.

Lorentzen S. Drusen of the optic disk. A clinical and genetic study. Acta Ophthalmol Suppl. 1996;90:1–180.

Mustonen E, Nieminen H. Optic disc drusen-a photographic study. II. Retinal nerve fibre layer photography. Acta Ophthalmol. 1982; 60:859–72.

Roh S, Noecker AR, Schuman J, Hedges TR 3rd, Weiter JJ, Mattox C. Effect of optic nerve head drusen on nerve fiber layer thickness. Ophthalmology. 1998;105:878–885.

Tso M. Pathology and pathogenesis of drusen of the optic nervehead. Ophthalmology. 1981;88:1066–1080.

Chapter 69

Melanocytoma of the Optic Disc

ARUN D. SINGH, MD

69.1 Introduction

Melanocytoma is a benign pigmented ocular tumor that predominantly involves the optic disc and uvea. Optic disc melanocytoma is considered to be a congenital hamartoma, arising from dendritic uveal melanocytes normally present in the lamina chordalis. The term *melanocytoma* was proposed by Zimmerman and Garron because they observed a resemblance between cells that comprise this tumor and those of ocular melanocytosis (melanosis oculi). The alternative term *magnocellular nevus* emphasizes the fact that melanocytoma is a nevus variant and that it is composed of large pigmented cells of neural crest origin. Other descriptive terms such as *benign melanoma of the optic nerve head* are no longer used. It is important to recognize this entity and to differentiate it from optic nerve melanoma and juxtapapillary choroidal melanoma.

69.2 Clinical Signs and Symptoms

Although optic disc melanocytoma is congenital, it is rarely observed in the pediatric population. The mean age at diagnosis is 50 years. Optic disc melanocytoma is more commonly seen in blacks and other darker-skinned races than in whites. These tumors are typically unilateral, sporadic, and not associated with other ocular or systemic anomalies. Rare bilateral tumors may be associated with optic nerve hypoplasia and central nervous system abnormalities. The majority of patients are asymptomatic, and the tumors are diagnosed on a routine examination. Optic disc melanocytoma has the characteristic ophthalmoscopic appearance of a dark black, flat, or slightly elevated mass that occupies the inferotemporal aspect of the optic disc (**Figure 69–1**).

It is associated with an adjacent deep choroidal component in 50% of patients and a superficial retinal component in about 75% of patients. The retinal portion is usually darker than the choroidal component and has feathery margins due to extensions into the nerve fiber layer (**Figure 69–2**). Larger melanocytomas can completely obscure the optic disc and lead to pigment dispersion in the vitreous cavity (**Figure 69–3**). Prominent intrinsic vasculature, subretinal fluid, and retinal exudation are not typically associated with optic disc melanocytoma.

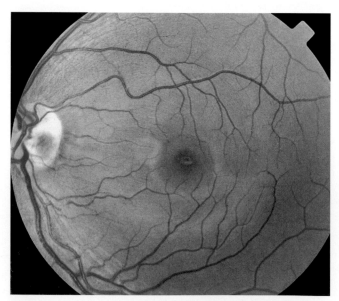

Figure 69–1 Fundus photograph of the left eye showing a small, black, flat melanocytoma occupying the inferotemporal aspect of the optic disc.

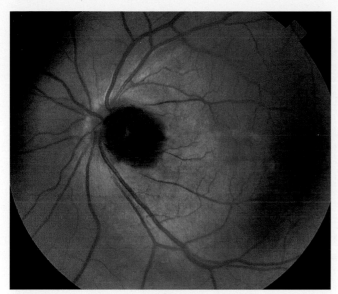

Figure 69–2 Characteristic ophthalmoscopic appearance of an optic disc melanocytoma. Note the adjacent deep choroidal component and a dark black superficial retinal component.

An afferent pupillary defect and nerve fiber bundle defects are present on visual field testing, even in the presence of normal visual acuity, suggesting subclinical optic nerve dysfunction. Rapid deterioration of vision due to ischemic necrosis within an optic disc melanocytoma manifesting as papillitis, neuroretinitis, and central retinal artery or vein occlusion can occur.

Optic disc melanocytoma is a benign tumor and therefore remains stable over many years in the majority of patients. Subtle growth over several years can be observed in about 15% of tumors. In general, rapid progressive enlargement is indicative of malignant transformation into a melanoma. However, such growth without malignant transformation has also been observed. Nevertheless, the majority of eyes demonstrating a rapid increase in the size of the optic disc melanocytoma undergo enucleation because of concerns of malignant transformation. Otherwise, once documented, the majority of optic disc melanocytomas are kept under periodic observation.

Optic disc melanocytoma should be differentiated from optic disc melanoma, adenoma of the juxtapapillary retinal pigment epithelium, and combined hamartoma of the retinal pigment epithelium and retina. Optic disc melanoma usually arises from the juxtapapillary choroid and extends over the optic nerve, causing significant visual symptoms, unlike an optic disc melanocytoma. In addition, a melanoma is brown in color and does not infiltrate the nerve fiber layer, and its intrinsic vasculature is evident on angiographic studies. Adenoma of the retinal pigment epithelium may be difficult to differentiate from an optic disc melanocytoma on the basis of clinical findings alone. Combined hamartoma of the retinal pigment epithelium and retina is generally diagnosed in a younger age group and has prominent vascular and gliotic components.

69.3 Imaging and Diagnostic Tests

69.3.1 FUNDUS PHOTOGRAPHY

The diagnosis of optic disc melanocytoma is usually suspected on ophthalmoscopic examination. Fundus photographs are used to document and monitor the lesion over prolonged periods of time.

69.3.2 FLUORESCEIN ANGIOGRAPHY

An optic disc melanocytoma appears as an area of dense hypofluorescence that persists through all phases of the angiogram (**Figure 69–3**). There is a characteristic absence of intrinsic vasculature and leakage.

69.3.3 INDOCYANINE GREEN ANGIOGRAPHY

Similar findings are noted on this test with persistent hypofluorescence and the absence of intrinsic vasculature.

69.3.4 ULTRASONOGRAPHY

B-scan ultrasonography detects an acoustically solid optic disc mass. With A-scan ultrasonography there is a high initial spike and low to medium internal reflectivity.

69.3.5 OPTICAL COHERENCE TOMOGRAPHY

Optical coherence tomography shows a high reflectance signal anteriorly, which is continuous with the retinal nerve fiber layer. Optical shadowing is observed posteriorly.

69.3.6 MAGNETIC RESONANCE IMAGING

T1-weighted image with the fat suppression technique shows an enlargement of the optic nerve and may demarcate the posterior extension. The melanocytoma appears hyperintense with respect to the vitreous due to paramagnetic properties of melanin. Enhancement with gadolinium may also be present.

69.4 Pathology

Histopathologically, optic disc melanocytoma is a variant of a nevus. The dark-pigmented mass within the substance of the optic nerve has extensions to the surrounding choroid and superficial retina. The tumor cells are deeply pigmented because of numerous macromelanosomes, and cellular details are not evident until bleaching is performed. The majority of cells are plump, round, or polyhedral. A smaller population of lightly pigmented spindle-shaped melanocytoma cells are also present. The nuclei are bland, uniformly small, and normochromic.

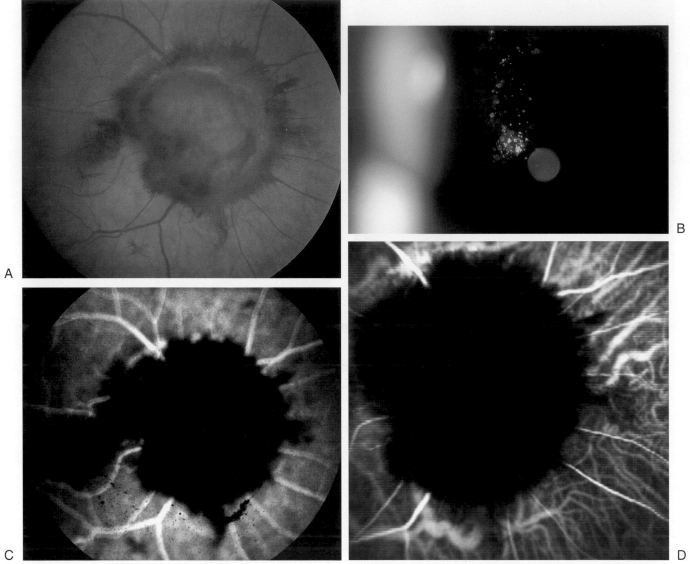

Figure 69–3 Fundus photograph of the right eye showing a large melanocytoma completely obscuring the optic disc. Note its feathery margins (*A*). The tumor was associated with pigment dispersion in the vitreous cavity (*B*). Fluorescein angiography showing an area of dense hypofluorescence that persists through all the phases of the angiogram corresponding to the location of the tumor (*C*). Similar findings are noted on the indocyanine green angiogram with a characteristic absence of intrinsic vasculature (*D*).

SUGGESTED READINGS

Antcliff RJ, ffytche TJ, Shilling JS, Marshall J. Optical coherence tomography of melanocytoma. Am J Ophthalmol. 2000;130:845–847.

Apple DJ, Craythorn JM, Reidy JJ, Steinmetz RL, Brady SE, Bohart WA. Malignant transformation of an optic nerve melanocytoma. Can J Ophthalmol. 1984;19:320–325.

Brodsky MC, Phillips PH. Optic nerve hypoplasia and congenital hypopituitarism. J Pediatr. 2000;136:850.

Cogan DG. Discussion-pigmented ocular tumors. In: Boniuk M, ed. Ocular and Adnexal Tumors; New and Controversial Aspects. St. Louis, Mo: Mosby, 1964:385.

Howard GM, Forrest AW. Incidence and location of melanocytomas. Arch Ophthalmol. 1967;77:61–66.

Joffe L, Shields JA, Osher RH, Gass JD. Clinical and follow-up studies of melanocytomas of the optic disc. Ophthalmology. 1979;86:1067–1083.

Juarez CP, Tso MO. An ultrastructural study of melanocytomas (magnocellular nevi) of the optic disk and uvea. Am J Ophthalmol. 1980;90:48–62.

Loeffler KU, Tecklenborg H. Melanocytoma-like growth of a juxtapapillary malignant melanoma. Retina. 1992;12:29–34.

Mansour AM, Zimmerman L, La Piana FG, Beauchamp GR. Clinico-pathological findings in a growing optic nerve melanocytoma. Br J Ophthalmol. 1989;73:410–415.

Meyer D, Ge J, Blinder KJ, Sinard J, Xu S. Malignant transformation of an optic disk melanocytoma. Am J Ophthalmol. 1999;127:710–714.

Reese AB. Congenital melanomas. Am J Ophthalmol. 1974;77:789–808.

Reidy JJ, Apple DJ, Steinmetz RL, Craythorn JM, Loftfield K, Gieser SC, Brady SE. Melanocytoma: nomenclature, pathogenesis, natural history and treatment. Surv Ophthalmol. 1985;29:319–327.

Shields JA, Eagle RC Jr, Shields CL, De Potter P. Pigmented adenoma of the optic nerve head simulating a melanocytoma. Ophthalmology. 1992;99:1705–1708.

Zimmerman LE. Melanocytes, melanocytic nevi, and melanocytomas. Invest Ophthalmol. 1965;34:11–41.

Zimmerman LE, Garron LK. Melanocytoma of the optic disc. Int Ophthalmol Clin. 1962;2:431–440.

Chapter 70

Papilledema

MARK BORCHERT, MD

70.1 Introduction

Papilledema is swelling of the optic nerve head (optic disc) that occurs only with elevated intracranial pressure (ICP). It can be seen with an ophthalmoscope and does not usually result in loss of vision unless it has been present for weeks or months. Papilledema only occurs when the normal communications between the subarachnoid spaces of the optic nerve and brain are patent, so that intracranial pressure can be transmitted to the optic nerve. The subarachnoid pressure of the optic nerve is very nearly equal to that of the brain.

The elevation of pressure within the subarachnoid space of the optic nerve results in stasis of axoplasmic transport at the optic nerve head with consequent swelling of axons. In experimental animal models of papilledema, using labeled amino acids injected into the vitreous cavity, axoplasmic transport is blocked at the scleral canal (lamina cribrosa) as the axons pass from the intraocular to the extraocular space on their way to the brain. Histologically, the axons become swollen, but there is no increase in extracellular fluid, and no swelling of supporting tissue. In other words, true edema is not necessarily present in papilledema. Obstruction of retinal venous outflow by swollen axons at the lamina cribrosa may result in dilation and tortuosity of retinal veins with consequent true retinal edema, exudates, and peripapillary hemorrhages.

Papilledema is clearly due to elevation of the subarachnoid pressure of the optic nerve. Surgical relief of this optic nerve pressure by creating a window in the optic nerve sheath results in resolution of optic nerve axon swelling despite persistently elevated ICP. This technique has become the primary treatment for optic nerve damage from papilledema in patients with chronic intracranial hypertension.

Because blockage of axoplasmic transport identical to papilledema can be produced by reducing the intraocular pressure (IOP) and because the IOP is higher than the ICP under normal circumstances (IOP: 12–20 mm Hg; supine ICP: 7 to 14 mm Hg; standing ICP: 0 to 2 mm Hg), stasis of axoplasmic flow can be presumed to result from a relative increase in the retrolaminar optic nerve pressure compared with the IOP. This presumably causes an inward bowing of the lamina cribrosa with sufficient deformation of its trabecular structure to block axoplasmic flow but not impair transmission of electrical impulses from the retina to the brain. The susceptibility of the lamina cribrosa to such deformation has been demonstrated by varying the IOP alone.

Alternatively, just the tissue pressure gradient between the prelaminar optic nerve and the retrolaminar optic nerve may be sufficient to cause stasis of axoplasmic flow independent of shifts in the position of the lamina cribrosa. In vitro, this can occur with pressure gradients of at least 30 mm Hg, which is considerably higher than that encountered in most clinical circumstances.

70.2 Clinical Signs and Symptoms

Papilledema is indistinguishable in appearance from other causes of optic disc swelling. Other causes of disc swelling (e.g., ischemia and inflammation) result in stasis of axoplasmic flow at the site of injury, but differ from papilledema in that they also block impulse transmission by direct injury to axons and result in acutely or subacutely decreased vision. Persistent vision loss with papilledema usually occurs gradually in patients with chronic disease. On the other hand, transient obscuration of vision in one or both eyes lasting a few seconds is common with papilledema. This usually occurs when the patient changes position from supine to sitting from or sitting to standing. The mechanism for this phenomenon is uncertain.

Papilledema is nearly always bilateral, although it may be quite asymmetric. Disc swelling due to other causes is usually unilateral, but it may be bilateral. Consequently, one must probe for symptoms of elevated ICP if the optic discs are bilaterally swollen and vision is normal or indeterminate.

The major symptom of elevated ICP is headache that tends to worsen while patients are supine or awaken them at night. Headaches may be focal or diffuse or pounding or pressure-like, depending on the cause of the elevated pressure. Nausea or vomiting may be present, but unlike migraines, vomiting does not usually alleviate the headache.

Headaches due to elevated ICP are often accompanied by sixth cranial nerve palsies and occasionally by fourth cranial nerve palsies. Finally, a subjective bruit or whooshing sound is common in intracranial hypertension.

70.3 Imaging and Diagnostic Tests

Swelling of the optic nerve axons can develop quickly with intracranial hypertension. Papilledema can be clearly seen in humans within 2 to 4 hours after an acute intracranial hemorrhage. The earliest visible manifestations of papilledema are disputed. Most neuro-ophthalmologists agree that loss of the superficial light reflections from the retina immediately surrounding the optic nerve is an early sign. This can be most easily seen using red-free light and can be ascribed to the fact that the most superficial axons of the optic nerve head are the earliest and most significantly affected, sometimes swelling to 10 to 20 times their normal size.

However, in an animal model of papilledema, the earliest manifestation was elevation of the disc that could only be appreciated with stereoscopic photography. Unfortunately, this can only be identified if prior stereoscopic photographs from the patient are available for comparison because many persons have normally elevated optic discs (pseudopapilledema).

70.3.1 OPHTHALMOSCOPY

Funduscopy with a direct ophthalmoscope or indirect slit-lamp ophthalmoscope remains the easiest and most sensitive means of detecting papilledema. In its full-blown form, papilledema has all the manifestations of axoplasmic constipation and peripapillary venous obstruction (**Figure 70–1**). These include hyperemia and elevation of the optic disc with obscuration of the disc margins, dilation and tortuosity of the retinal veins, peripapillary nerve fiber hemorrhages and cotton-wool spots, macular exudates, and circumferential peripapillary wrinkles of the retina (Paton's lines).

Less florid papilledema may be difficult to distinguish from pseudopapilledema (due to buried optic disc drusen or congenital optic disc elevation). Mild to moderate papilledema is characterized by elevation of the optic disc with obscuration of the disc margins and loss of peripapillary superficial light reflections (**Figure 70–2**). The retinal vessels course through the nerve fiber layer and are consequently obscured by

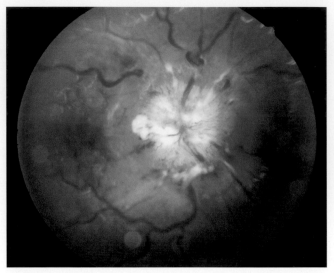

Figure 70–1 In florid papilledema, the veins are dilated and tortuous. Peripapillary cotton-wool spots and nerve fiber layer hemorrhages are common.

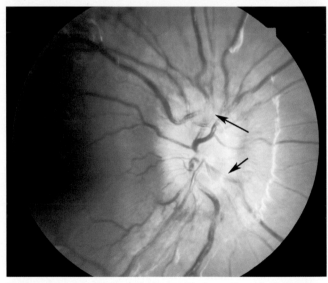

Figure 70–2 In mild to moderate papilledema, the retinal vessels are obscured by overlying swollen axons (*arrows*), and there is loss of surface retinal reflections, especially temporally.

the swollen axons as well. Resolution of papilledema occurs within days to weeks after normalization of ICP, depending on the severity of the disc swelling and whether or not there was associated true retinal edema (**Figure 70–3**). If there has been no permanent nerve damage, the disc returns to its normal appearance including reappearance of normal reflections off the internal limiting membrane. In pseudopapilledema, the optic disc is elevated and the margins are indistinct, but the blood vessels are not obscured by swollen axons, and the veins are not swollen (**Figure 70–4**). Retinal venous and/or arterial tortuosity is common in congenital pseudopapilledema. Arterial tortuosity is not a feature of true papilledema.

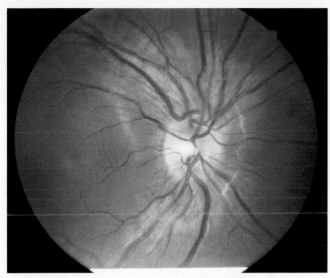

Figure 70–3 With resolution of papilledema, the disc margins and vessels become more visible and surface reflections return temporal to the disc.

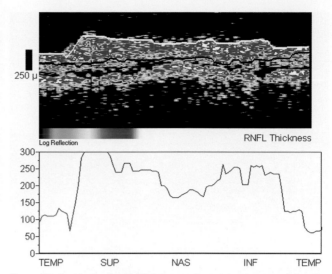

Figure 70–5 A circular OCT 5.5-mm diameter scan around the disc reveals nerve fiber layer swelling especially superiorly and inferiorly that often exceeds the measurement limits of OCT.

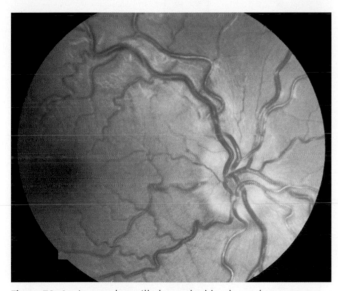

Figure 70–4 In pseudopapilledema, the blood vessels are not obscured, whereas the disc margins are obscured. Retinal arteries as well as veins may be tortuous.

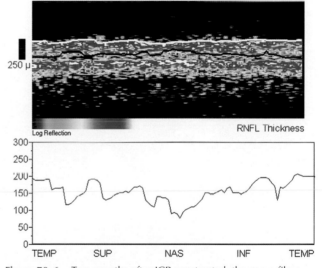

Figure 70–6 Two months after ICP was treated, the nerve fiber thickness measured from an identical 5.5-mm diameter scan has returned to nearly normal.

70.3.2 FLUORESCEIN ANGIOGRAPHY

There may be late staining of the disc due to venous or capillary leakage in true papilledema that distinguishes it from pseudopapilledema. This is often not present in mild papilledema. In addition, autofluorescence of buried disc drusen may be visible in pseudopapilledema. Otherwise, fluorescein angiography has little value in the evaluation of papilledema.

70.3.3 OPTICAL COHERENCE TOMOGRAPHY

Optical coherence tomography (OCT) has tremendous theoretical benefit in the monitoring of papilledema because it can detect swelling of the peripapillary nerve fiber layer that is not visible ophthalmoscopically. This is most pronounced superiorly and inferiorly on circular scans (**Figures 70–5** and **70–6**). In addition, it can be used to monitor the effects of treatment on disc elevation with radial scans (**Figures 70–7** and **70–8**).

Nerve fiber layer maps generated with OCT clearly show thickening of this layer with elevated ICP (**Figures 70–9** to **70–11**). Swelling is greater closer to the optic disc. The distance from the disc to which nerve fiber layer the swelling extends may correlate with the severity or duration of intracranial hypertension. Unfortunately, the current segmentation software for measuring nerve fiber layer thickness has not been

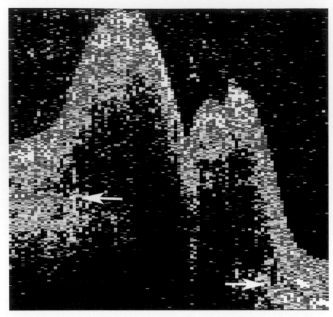

Figure 70–7 A radial OCT scan across a swollen optic disc reveals marked elevation of the disc and separation of the peripapillary retina from the retinal pigment epithelium.

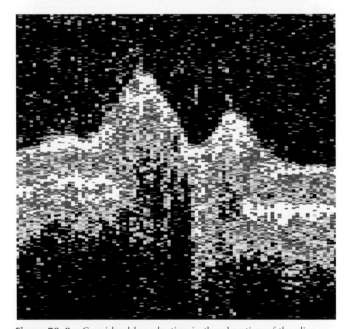

Figure 70–8 Considerable reduction in the elevation of the disc occurs shortly after ICP is reduced.

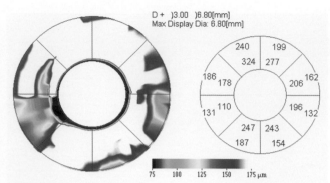

Figure 70–9 A nerve fiber layer map of the peripapillary retina in **Figure 70–2** shows nerve fiber layer swelling superiorly and inferiorly.

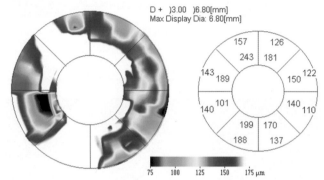

Figure 70–10 A nerve fiber layer map of the peripapillary retina in **Figure 70–3** shows improvement of the extent of nerve fiber layer swelling.

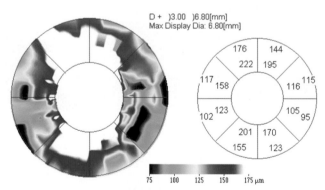

Figure 70–11 An age-matched normal peripapillary nerve fiber layer map.

validated in papilledema, and the limit of thickness measurement is 350 microns. Nerve fiber layer thickness in papilledema often exceeds 350 microns.

70.3.4 MAGNETIC RESONANCE IMAGING

Magnetic resonance imaging (MRI) or computed tomography (CT) scans of the brain should be obtained for all patients with suspected papilledema to rule out a tumor or other mass effect before lumbar puncture is performed for confirmation of elevated ICP. There are no abnormalities of the brain on MRI specific for elevated ICP. However, on orbital MRI scans one may see dilation of the optic nerve sheath and flattening of the posterior portion of the globe due to the increased pressure in the subarachnoid space of the optic nerve.

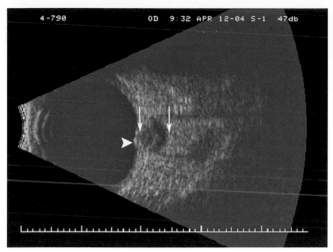

Figure 70–12 The optic nerve sheath in cross-section (*arrows*) can be seen behind the swollen nerve fibers (*arrowhead*) of papilledema with the eye in primary position on B-scan ultrasonography.

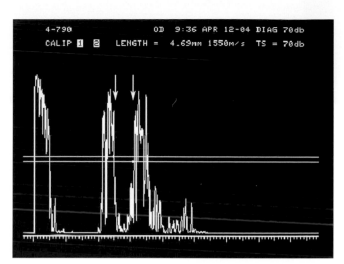

Figure 70–14 Cross-sectional diameter (*arrows*) of the swollen optic nerve sheath can be measured by A-scan ultrasonography with the eye in primary position. (Courtesy of Cathy Dibernardo.)

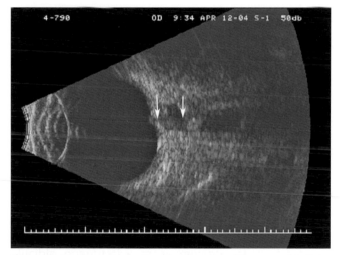

Figure 70–13 Upon abduction, the diameter of the nerve sheath in cross-section diminishes (*arrows*). (Courtesy of Cathy Dibernardo.)

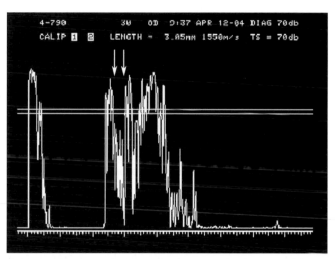

Figure 70–15 More than a 10% reduction in the diameter of the optic nerve sheath (*arrows*) upon 30-degree abduction of the eye suggests intracranial hypertension.

70.3.5 ULTRASONOGRAPHY

Dilation of the optic nerve sheath immediately behind the globe can also be detected with orbital ultrasonography by experienced practitioners. Dilation of the sheath due to elevated ICP measurably diminishes as the patient shifts his or her gaze from a primary position to 30 degrees abduction (**Figures 70–12** and **70–13**). This indicates that dilation of the sheath is due to fluid that can be forced posteriorly with stretching of the nerve. A decrease in optic nerve sheath diameter of 10% on A-scan ultrasonography with the "30-degree test" indicates that optic disc swelling is due to elevated ICP (**Figures 70–14** and **70–15**). In addition, ultrasound can distinguish pseudopapilledema due to buried disc drusen.

SUGGESTED READINGS

Burgoyne CF, Quigley HA, Thompson HW, Vitale S, Varma R. Measurement of optic disc compliance by digitized image analysis in the normal monkey eye. Ophthalmology. 1995;102:1790–1799.

Ernest JT, Potts AM. Pathophysiology of the distal portion of the optic nerve: I. Tissue pressure relationships. Am J Ophthalmol. 1968;66:372–387.

Hahnenburger RW. Effect of pressure barrier on fast axoplasmic flow: An in vitro study in the vagus nerve of rabbits. Acta Physiol Scand. 1978;104:299–308.

Hayreh SS, Hayreh MS. Optic disc edema in raised intracranial pressure: II. Early detection with fluorescein fundus angiography and stereoscopic color photography. Arch Ophthalmol. 1977; 95:1245–1254.

Hoyt WF, Knight CL. Comparison of congenital disc blurring and incipient papilledema in red-free light—A photographic study. Invest Ophthalmol Vis Sci. 1972;12:241–247.

Kilpatrick CJ, Kaufman DV, Galbraith JE, King KO. Optic nerve

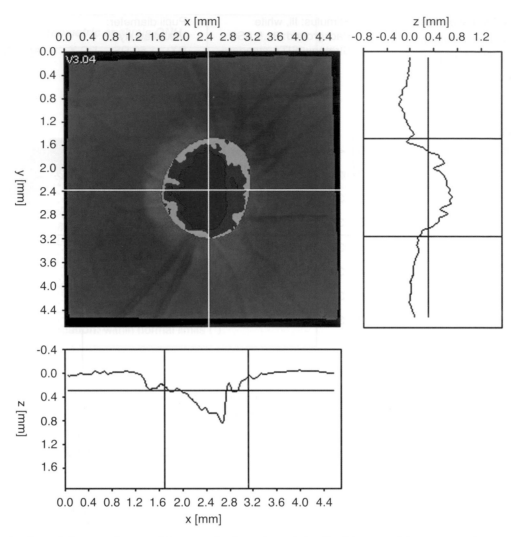

Figure 71–8 HRT: color-coded topography map (OD); generalized cupping with localized thinning of the neuroretinal rim in the temporal inferior region.

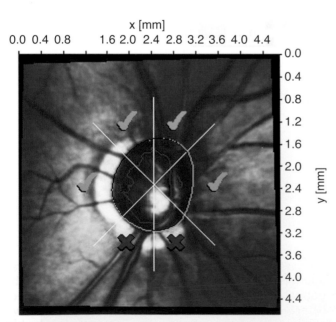

Figure 71–9 HRT: pseudocolor reflectance map with MRA (OD); abnormal temporal inferior and nasal inferior sectors.

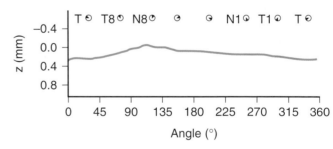

Figure 71–10 HRT: height contour graph (OD); attenuation of the inferior component of the typical "double hump" contour.

disclose an average disc area with reduced rim area, rim volume, height variation contour, and mean RNFL thickness, based on manufacturer-provided normative data (**Figure 71–11**). Breakdown of the MRA shows the two abnormal inferior sectors, especially in the nasal inferior region, and reveals an overall borderline global value (**Figure 71–12**).

Stereometric analysis ONH	
Disk area	1.937 mm²
Cup area	0.860 mm²
Rim area	1.076 mm²
Cup volume	0.165 cmm
Rim volume	0.159 cmm
Cup/disk area ratio	0.444
Linear cup/disk ratio	0.667
Mean cup depth	0.229 mm
Maximum cup depth	0.600 mm
Cup shape measure	−0.140
Height variation contour	0.278 mm
Mean RNFL thickness	0.162 mm
RNFL cross sectional area	0.802 mm²
Reference height	0.293 mm
Topography std dev.	33 μm
Contour line operator	pok

Classification: outside normal limits (*)

Figure 71–11 HRT: stereometric parameters (OD); average disc area with reduced rim area, rim volume, height variation contour, and mean RNFL thickness compared with manufacturer-provided normative data.

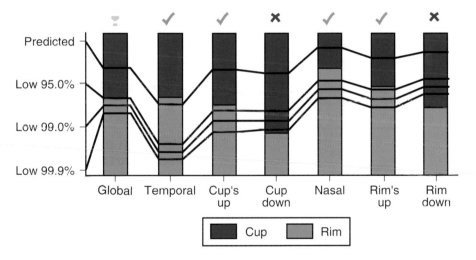

Figure 71–12 HRT: MRA bar presentation (OD); abnormal inferior sectors and an overall borderline global value.

Advanced Glaucomatous Damage (Left Eye)

This left eye (OS) of a 69-year-old woman with POAG demonstrates extensive generalized cupping (**Figure 71–13**). VF analysis shows a dense inferior hemifield defect and a superior paracentral defect (**Figure 71–14**).

The topographic image shows obvious rim thinning in the superior, temporal, and inferior regions, and the vertical and horizontal height profile graphs show elongation of the cup in both directions (**Figure 71–15**). MRA shows abnormal superior and inferior sectors corresponding well with the VF defects and a borderline temporal region (**Figure 71–16**). The height contour graph shows attenuation of the characteristic superior hump and a less attenuated inferior region (**Figure 71–17**). Stereometric analysis demonstrates decreased rim area and rim volume and a significantly increased cup shape measure compared with the normative data provided by the manufacturer (**Figure 71–18**). The

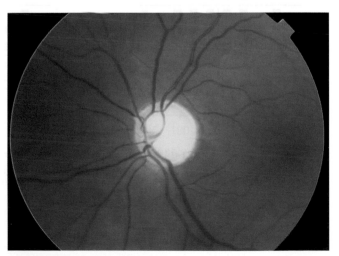

Figure 71–13 Fundus photograph (OS): extensive generalized cupping.

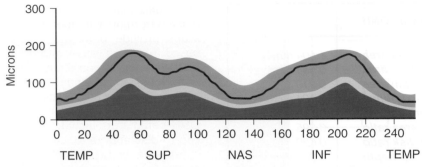

Figure 71–27   OCT: RNFL thickness average graph (OD); normal eye.

thickness may be useful as a surrogate indicator of glaucomatous damage to the ganglion cell layer. There are limited data on ONH analysis and its ability to discriminate normal from glaucomatous eyes, although ONH analysis has been shown to be associated with glaucoma disease status.

A limiting factor of OCT technology is related to the transverse sampling density of the scans. Although the axial resolution of OCT scans is high, the transverse resolution is limited by the number of sampled points along each scan. Even more apparent is the amount of surface area that goes unexamined with the macular and ONH scans. The spoke-wheel pattern of the scans leaves gaps between scans that are filled with interpolation. It is possible that increasing the number of scans or the use of scanning patterns other than the spoke-wheel could lead to more complete data on glaucoma status from macular and ONH scans.

The following are case examples of OCT scans of eyes showing varying degrees and patterns of glaucomatous damage.

Normal Eye (Right Eye)

This eye, the same eye as evaluated previously by the HRT, is presented to illustrate a normal scan for comparison with the subsequent abnormal scans. The RNFL thickness average analysis graphs, shown in **Figure 71–27**, demonstrate the peripapillary thickness (*black line*) well within the normal boundaries derived from the built-in normative database (*green shaded area*; the *yellow area* represents borderline measurements |between 1% and 5% of normal distribution percentile|, and the *red area* represents abnormal measurements |less than 1% of normal distribution percentile|). A single peripapillary scan demonstrates the various structures of the retina, with the various layers visible as different colored layers in the scan (**Figure 71–28**). The upper layer, outlined by the *two white lines*, represents the NFL, with characteristic thickening in the superior and inferior regions. The lower layer, consisting of primarily red pixels, represents the retinal pigment epithelium (RPE)/choriocapillaris layer. **Figure 71–29** shows the average RNFL thickness for the various clock hours (*left*) and quadrants (*right*). These are all colored *green* in this subject, indicating that the values are within the normal

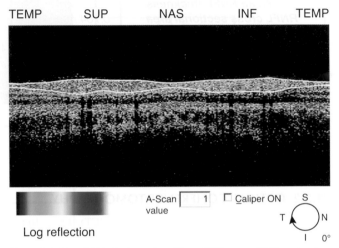

Figure 71–28   OCT: single peripapillary RNFL scan (OD); normal eye.

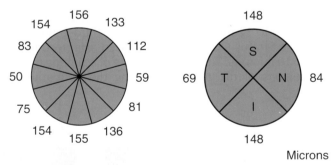

Figure 71–29   OCT: clock hour and quadrant-based average RNFL thickness charts (OD); normal eye.

range. **Figure 71–30** is a table of the various OCT RNFL parameters and their values for this normal subject in both eyes, and the inter-eye difference is calculated for each parameter. The NFL average thickness in this normal eye is 112 microns.

The macula scan of this normal subject is shown in **Figure 71–31**. The scan is vertically oriented through the fovea (central thinning) with the inferior macula on the left side of the scan and the superior to the right. The map created from all six linear scans contains a

	OD (N=3)	OS (N=3)	OD–OS
Imax/Smax	0.96	1.13	–0.18
Smax/Imax	1.04	0.88	0.16
Smax/Tavg	2.61	1.98	0.63
Imax/Tavg	2.50	2.25	0.25
Smax/Navg	2.16	2.34	–0.18
Max–min	137.00	136.00	1.00
Smax	181.00	158.00	23.00
Imax	174.00	180.00	–6.00
Savg	148.00	132.00	16.00
Iavg	148.00	145.00	3.00
Avg. thickness	112.36	105.96	6.40

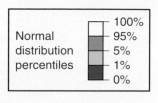

Normal distribution percentiles
- 100%
- 95%
- 5%
- 1%
- 0%

Figure 71–30   OCT: RNFL parameters table (both eyes [OU]); normal eyes.

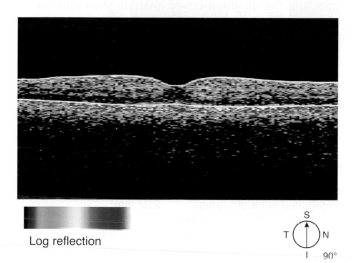

Log reflection

S
T — N
I — 90°

Figure 71–31   OCT: single macula scan, centered at the fovea (OD); normal eye.

central foveal depression (*blue-green color*) and a typical doughnut-shaped (can often be C-shaped in normal eyes) configuration representing normal parafoveal thickening (**Figure 71–32**). Normal papillomacular thickening is also seen as the *yellow color* in the nasal region of the macula. A sectoral thickness map shows that numerical values of thickness measurements are almost identical for the corresponding regions across the horizontal midline. The total macular volume is 7.79 mm^3.

Figure 71–33 demonstrates the ONH analysis of this normal eye. This is an inferior (*left*) to superior (*right*) vertical section of the ONH region. The edges of the RPE/choriocapillaris are demarcated by the *two blue crosshairs*, and the line anterior and parallel to the line connecting these two markers differentiates the rim (located above the line) from the cup (below the line). Six such cross-sections are used to construct the ONH map (**Figure 71–34**). On this map, the cup and rim area is automatically defined (cup within the *green circle* and rim within the *red circle*).

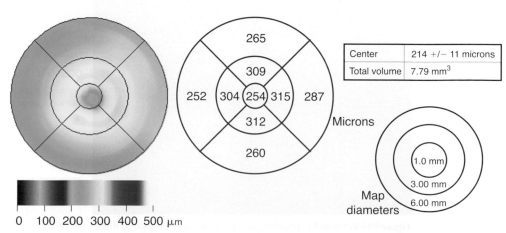

265
309
252   304 (254) 315   287
312
260

Microns

Center	214 +/– 11 microns
Total volume	7.79 mm^3

1.0 mm
3.00 mm
6.00 mm

Map diameters

0   100 200 300 400 500 μm

Figure 71–32   OCT: macula map, created from six linear scans (OD); normal eye.

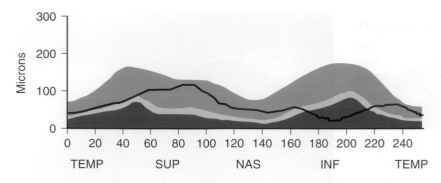

Figure 71–39 OCT: RNFL thickness average graph (OD); borderline values in the temporal superior region and abnormal values in the inferior region.

The OCT analysis of this eye confirms the VF and HRT findings and also adds more information that may be important in evaluating the glaucomatous status in this patient. The RNFL thickness of this eye varies from the normative database in two regions (**Figure 71–39**). The *black line*, representing this patient's RNFL thickness, falls within the *yellow shaded region* in the temporal superior region and it dips into the *red region* in the inferior region of the circular scan. This can be observed clearly in the cross-sectional image where the inferior region of the RNFL is markedly thinned (*arrow*), indicated by the proximity of the anterior and posterior boundaries of this layer as demarcated by the *two white lines* (**Figure 71–40**). The clock hour and quadrant-based charts summarize these findings (**Figure 71–41**). Note that the abnormal clock hours in the superior temporal region (10- and 11-o'clock) correspond with the inferior nasal finding. In the quadrant-based chart, the superior and temporal regions appear normal; although there is probably some damage in this area as seen in the clock hour presentation, the damage is spread over the two quadrants and thus is not reflected in the quadrant-based view. This finding highlights the importance of evaluating both the clock hours and quadrant analysis to obtain maximal information. Several of the OCT parameters of this eye were abnormal compared with

the normative database, and the overall RNFL average thickness was 60.64 microns (**Figure 71–42**).

Although the interpretation of the OCT macula scan is limited owing to the lack of normative values, this inferior (*left*) to superior (*right*) vertical scan shows an attenuation of the retinal thickness in the inferior region (**Figure 71–43**). The macular map shows widespread retinal thinning (*blue region*) in the parafoveal area, mostly pronounced in the inferior and the temporal regions. This finding can be quantitatively appreciated by noting how considerably lower each of the sectoral thickness values is in comparison to those of the normal eye presented earlier. Total macular volume is 5.4 mm³.

Advanced Glaucomatous Damage (Left Eye)

This eye was presented earlier in the HRT section: the left eye of a 69-year-old woman with POAG with extensive generalized cupping (**Figure 71–13**) and VF analysis with a dense inferior hemifield defect and a superior paracentral defect (**Figure 71–14**).

The circular peripapillary scan shows a remarkably flattened RNFL thickness graph. The superior and inferior regions of this patient's RNFL thickness values (*black line*) dip well into the abnormal (*red*) zone (**Figure 71–44**). An individual RNFL scan illustrates these

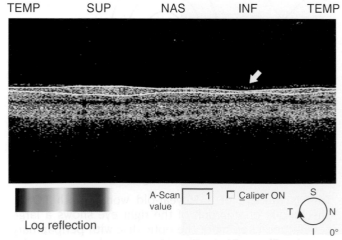

Figure 71–40 OCT: single peripapillary RNFL scan (OD); markedly thinned inferior region (*arrow*).

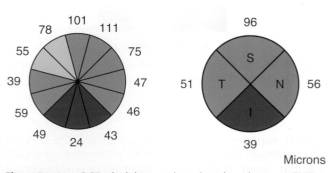

Figure 71–41 OCT: clock hour and quadrant-based average RNFL thickness charts (OD); abnormal inferior (clock hours 5-, 6-, and 7-o'clock) regions in both charts, and borderline clock hours 10- and 11-o'clock.

	OD (N=3)	OS (N=3)	OD–OS
Imax/Smax	0.50	0.94	–0.44
Smax/Imax	2.00	1.06	0.93
Smax/Tavg	2.25	2.41	–0.16
Imax/Tavg	1.13	2.27	–1.15
Smax/Navg	2.04	1.78	0.27
Max–min	94.00	87.00	7.00
Smax	115.00	120.00	–5.00
Imax	58.00	113.00	–55.00
Savg	96.00	104.00	–8.00
Iavg	39.00	93.00	–54.00
Avg. thickness	60.64	78.36	–17.72

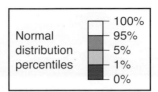

Normal distribution percentiles
- 100%
- 95%
- 5%
- 1%
- 0%

Figure 71–42 OCT: RNFL parameters table (OU); the right eye shows several abnormal and borderline values, including a low average RNFL thickness.

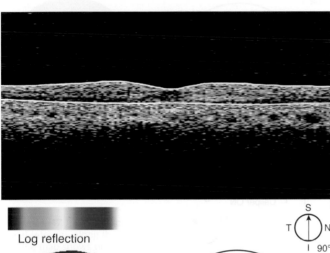

Log reflection

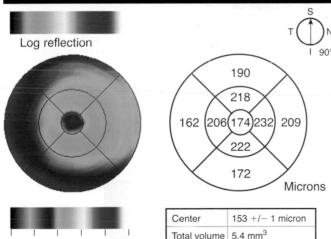

0 100 200 300 400 500 μm

190
218
162 | 206 (174) 232 | 209
222
172
Microns

S
T ⊕ N
90°

Center	153 +/– 1 micron
Total volume	5.4 mm³

Figure 71–43 OCT: macula scan and macula map (OD); vertically oriented macular scan through the fovea shows attenuation of the retinal thickness in the inferior (*left*) region, and the map shows widespread thinning that is most pronounced in the interior and temporal regions.

findings, showing marked, generalized thinning of the RNFL, especially in the superior and inferior regions of the scan (**Figure 71–45**). These areas of abnormality correspond with the superior and inferior VF defects. Beyond the obvious superior and inferior abnormalities, the clock hour analysis suggests some abnormalities in the temporal (2- and 4-o'clock) and nasal (10-o'clock)

regions, and the quadrant analysis shows that these regions are overall borderline (*yellow*) in thickness compared with the normative database (**Figure 71–46**). All but three of the OCT RNFL parameters are labeled as abnormal and the overall mean RNFL thickness was 46 microns (**Figure 71–46**).

The inferior (*left*) to superior (*right*) vertical macular scan shows diminished signal intensity (*decreased bright pixels*) in the retina along the entire scan despite a strong, continuous RPE/choriocapillaris layer suggesting thinning of these regions (**Figure 71–47**). The macular map composite shows an overall substantial diminished retinal thickness, because "cooler" colors (*blue/green*) predominate, especially in the normally thickened parafoveal and papillomacular regions, and the total retinal volume is diminished to 4.95 mm³ (**Figure 71–47**).

Central Scotoma (Left Eye)

This is the same eye that was presented previously in the HRT section: the left eye of an 88-year-old woman with bilateral normal tension glaucoma showing temporal inferior neuroretinal rim thinning (**Figure 71–20**) and a superior paracentral and nasal scotoma (**Figure 71–21**).

The circular RNFL thickness scan shows this subject's thickness values (**Figure 71–48**) falling into the abnormal range (*red area*) in the inferotemporal region, corresponding well with the HRT scan and the superior paracentral scotoma. The abnormality is shown clearly as a thinning of the RNFL in the inferotemporal (*right side* of the scan) region of the individual RNFL thickness scan (**Figure 71–49**). Clock hour and quadrant-based analysis of the RNFL scan shows an overall borderline inferior quadrant, with the most damage concentrated at 4- and 5-o'clock (**Figure 71–50**). The OCT parameter of "inferior average" is at a borderline value, and the overall average RNFL thickness is 76 microns (**Figure 71–50**).

The macula scan shows a marked reduction of the retinal thickness mainly in the inferior (*left side* of the scan) region (**Figure 71–51**). The pseudocolor macular map and sectoral macula thickness map show pronounced retinal thinning with *darker blue areas* mainly in the inferior region and lower thickness values in the inferior sectors (**Figure 71–51**). It should be noted

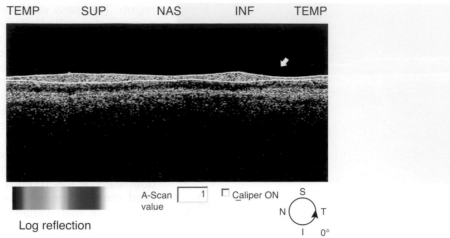

Figure 71–49 OCT: single peripapillary RNFL scan (OS); demonstrates thinning of the inferotemporal region (*arrow*).

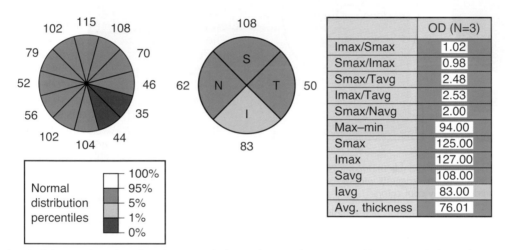

	OD (N=3)
Imax/Smax	1.02
Smax/Imax	0.98
Smax/Tavg	2.48
Imax/Tavg	2.53
Smax/Navg	2.00
Max–min	94.00
Smax	125.00
Imax	127.00
Savg	108.00
Iavg	83.00
Avg. thickness	76.01

Figure 71–50 OCT: clock hour and quadrant-based average thickness charts and parameter table (OS); borderline inferior quadrant with the most damage in clock hours 4- and 5-o'clock, and a borderline value for the inferior average parameter.

to falsely increase mean RNFL thickness values. The need to use the macula as an intraocular polarimeter to determine the necessary corneal compensation introduces a new limitation to this imaging modality because pathologic changes or anatomic abnormality of the macula could lead to difficulties in deriving the corneal compensation factor.

The following are case examples of GDx-VCC scans of eyes showing varying degrees and patterns of glaucomatous damage.

Normal Eye (Right Eye)

This is the same eye as presented previously in the HRT and OCT sections to illustrate a normal scan, so that the subsequent abnormal results can be compared. **Figure 71–52,** *left*, shows the reflectance image of the scanned area. The retardance-derived nerve fiber thickness map shows the normally thicker regions (*brighter colors*) in the superior and inferior regions (**Figure 71–52**, *center*).

The deviation map demonstrates only a few, sparse, areas (*dark blue squares*) in which measurements were aberrant from the normative database (**Figure 71–52**, *right*). The NFL chart shown in **Figure 71–53**, *left*, presents this subject's values (*dark green line*) lying within the normal distribution of thickness values (*light green band*). GDx-derived parameters are all within the normal range (**Figure 71–53**, *right*).

Preperimetric Glaucomatous Damage (Left Eye)

This is the same eye as that presented previously in the OCT section: a 55-year-old woman with POAG. The VF and HRT studies of the left eye appear normal; however, there is generalized cupping in the fundus photo (**Figure 71–35**) and the OCT reveals preperimetric damage as outlined previously.

Weak birefringence is seen in the inferior region of the nerve fiber thickness map indicating loss of inferior NFL tissue in this region (**Figure 71–54**, *center*). The deviation

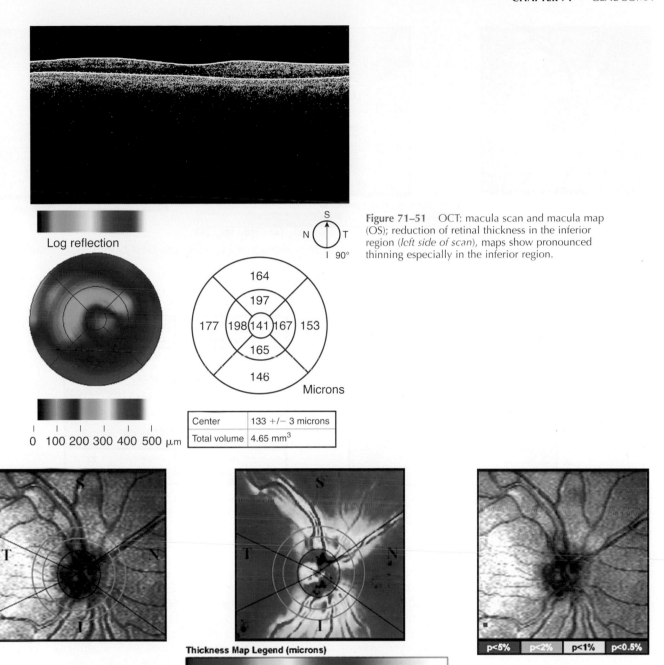

Figure 71–51 OCT: macula scan and macula map (OS); reduction of retinal thickness in the inferior region (*left side of scan*), maps show pronounced thinning especially in the inferior region.

Log reflection

164
197
177 198 141 167 153
165
146

Microns

Center	133 +/− 3 microns
Total volume	4.65 mm³

Figure 71–52 GDx-VCC: reflectance image (*left*), retardance map (*center*), and deviation map (*right*) (OD); normal eye.

Thickness Map Legend (microns)
0 20 40 60 80 100 120 140 160 180 200

p<5% p<2% p<1% p<0.5%

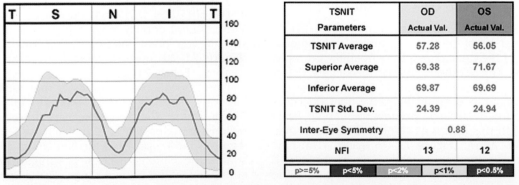

TSNIT Parameters	OD Actual Val.	OS Actual Val.
TSNIT Average	57.28	56.05
Superior Average	69.38	71.67
Inferior Average	69.87	69.69
TSNIT Std. Dev.	24.39	24.94
Inter-Eye Symmetry	0.88	
NFI	13	12

p>=5% p<5% p<2% p<1% p<0.5%

Figure 71–53 GDx-VCC: NFL thickness graph (*left*) and GDx parameters (*right*) (OD); normal eye.

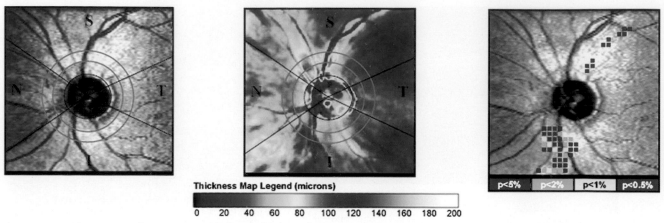

Figure 71–54 GDx-VCC: reflectance image (*left*), retardance map (*center*), and deviation map (*right*) (OS); weak birefringence inferiorly with corresponding abnormalities in the deviation map.

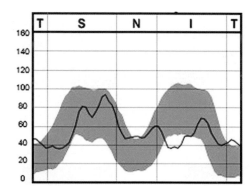

TSNIT	OD	OS
Parameters	Actual Val.	Actual Val.
TSNIT Average	54.16	54.12
Superior Average	66.07	65.80
Inferior Average	53.04	49.02
TSNIT Std. Dev.	12.21	15.37
Inter-Eye Symmetry	0.66	
NFI	28	22

p>=5%	p<5%	p<2%	p<1%	p<0.5%

Figure 71–55 GDx-VCC: NFL thickness graph (*left*) and GDx parameters (*right*) (OS); thickness values fall below the normal range (*purple area*) in the inferior region, with abnormal values for inferior average, TSNIT standard deviation, and intereye symmetry in the left eye.

map for this eye (**Figure 71–54**, *right*) and NFL graph (**Figure 71–55**, *left*) show inferior thinning and borderline superior temporal deviation, which confirm this loss and agree with the OCT findings of early damage in this eye, which is not yet apparent by VF testing. GDx parameters demonstrate abnormal values for inferior average, temporal, superior, nasal, inferior, temporal (TSNIT) standard deviation, and intereye symmetry measurements (**Figure 71–55,** *right*).

Moderate Glaucomatous Damage (Right Eye)

This is the eye of a 55-year-old woman with POAG. Fundus photograph of the right eye shows large generalized cupping of the optic disc with peripapillary atrophy (**Figure 71–6**). The VF shows a superior arcuate defect (**Figure 71–7**).

Inferior damage is seen in the nerve fiber thickness map; the area has decreased thickness (more blue, fewer bright colors) in this region as compared to the normal case described above (**Figure 71–56**, *center*). The high retardance in the temporal region is compatible with the peripapillary atrophy seen in the fundus photo. The deviation map shows a temporal inferior abnormality

and a localized superior temporal thinning, which corresponds to the superior arcuate and inferior nasal VF defects (**Figure 71–56**, *right*). The NFL graph of this eye shows thickness values at or above the normal levels (**Figure 71–57**, *left*). GDx parameters show an abnormal TSNIT standard deviation and significant intereye asymmetry in this eye (**Figure 71–57**, *right*).

Central Scotoma (Left Eye)

This is the same eye as that was presented previously in the HRT and OCT sections: an 88-year-old woman with bilateral normal tension glaucoma with a left eye showing temporal inferior neuroretinal rim thinning (**Figure 71–20**) and a superior paracentral and nasal scotoma (**Figure 71–21**).

The GDx-VCC NFL thickness map shows thinning inferiorly, especially in the inferotemporal region (**Figure 71–58**, *center*). The deviation map shows *yellow* and *red* regions denoting highly significant values in this area (**Figure 71–58**, *right*), and the NFL graph clearly demonstrates the patient's thickness values (*dark purple line*) falling below the normal range (*light purple band*) in the inferotemporal region (**Figure 71–59**, *left*). The inferior

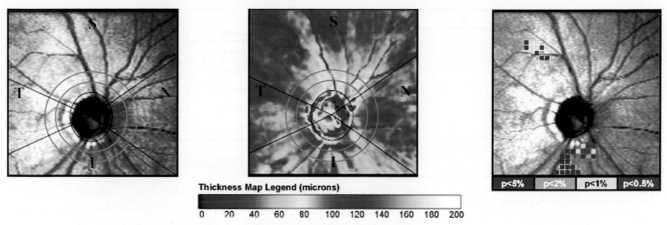

Figure 71–56 GDx-VCC: reflectance image (*left*), retardance map (*center*), and deviation map (*right*) (OD); inferior damage is seen in the retardance map, which corresponds with the deviation pattern that also shows a localized superior temporal abnormality.

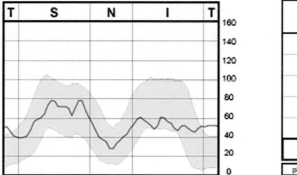

TSNIT	OD	OS
Parameters	**Actual Val.**	**Actual Val.**
TSNIT Average	54.16	54.12
Superior Average	66.07	65.80
Inferior Average	53.04	49.02
TSNIT Std. Dev.	12.21	15.37
Inter-Eye Symmetry	0.66	
NFI	28	22

p>=5%	p<5%	p<2%	p<1%	p<0.5%

Figure 71–57 GDx-VCC: NFL thickness graph (*left*) and GDx parameters (*right*) (OD); thickness values fall within the normal range (*green area*), the right eye demonstrates abnormal TSNIT standard deviation and significant intereye asymmetry.

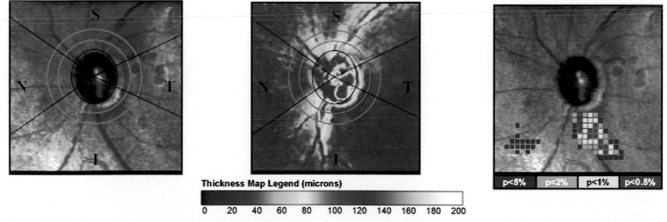

Figure 71–58 GDx-VCC: reflectance image (*left*), retardance map (*center*), and deviation map (*right*) (OS); inferior/inferotemporal thinning is seen in both the retardance and deviation maps.

average and TSNIT standard deviation parameters are flagged as abnormal in this eye (**Figure 71–59**, *right*). The damage seen with this imaging modality corresponds well with the superior paracentral scotoma seen on VF testing and also with the OCT and HRT findings of inferotemporal damage.

71.4 Pathology

Glaucoma is defined as a characteristic optic neuropathy, typically in the setting of measurable VF loss, and a primary risk factor for this disease is elevated IOP. IOP is regulated by the mechanisms of aqueous production

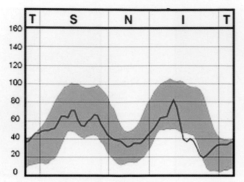

TSNIT Parameters	OD Actual Val.	OS Actual Val.
TSNIT Average	53.43	47.54
Superior Average	66.76	59.79
Inferior Average	57.73	45.39
TSNIT Std. Dev.	19.08	14.54
Inter-Eye Symmetry	0.79	
NFI	20	41

p>=5%	p<5%	p<2%	p<1%	p<0.5%

Figure 71–59 GDx-VCC: NFL thickness graph (*left*) and GDx parameters (*right*) (OS); the NFL thickness falls below the normal range in the inferotemporal region, with abnormal inferior average and TSNIT standard deviation in the left eye.

and outflow. Aqueous is produced in the ciliary processes and the nonpigmented ciliary epithelium. The aqueous passes from the posterior chamber through the pupil and into the anterior chamber and ultimately to the trabecular meshwork in the anterior chamber angle. Outflow obstruction is classically divided into open-angle and angle-closure mechanisms. In open-angle glaucoma, aqueous outflow resistance is localized to the trabecular meshwork and the inner wall of Schlemm's canal, although no anatomic obstruction can be observed clinically. In angle-closure glaucoma, a physical mechanism of angle blockage is often clinically observable. This is a key difference from open-angle glaucoma and because there is usually a simple mechanical reason for outflow obstruction, treatment methods are quite different.

The mechanism leading to the increased resistance to aqueous outflow and that of the resultant optic neuropathy associated with glaucoma are thought to be multifactorial. Mechanical theories have been proposed, suggesting that axonal fibers undergo pressure-induced compression against the openings of the sieve-like structure of the lamina cribrosa, interrupting axonal transport processes and ultimately leading to ganglion cell death. Possible ischemic mechanisms include those involving vasoactive substances, disturbances of blood-flow autoregulatory processes, and IOP effects on vascular flow. A number of other systems have been implicated in propagating glaucomatous damage, such as autoimmune processes, neurotoxicity, and the apoptotic pathway.

Regardless of the causative mechanism, the final pathway of all varieties of glaucoma appears to be a common one, consisting of optic neuropathy charac-terized by cupping of the optic disc, death of retinal ganglion cells, changes in the NFL, and ultimately VF loss. Although damage occurs both in the ONH and in the regions of the retina serving that area (the ganglion cells and the axons that lead to that specific region of the ONH), it is unclear where the damage occurs first.

The pathologic changes that occur in glaucoma can be often be detected by the various imaging modalities described in this chapter. If a VF defect is present, the results of the diagnostic imaging tests should correspond anatomically as they do in the cases presented in this chapter.

SUGGESTED READINGS

Ford BA, Artes PH, McCormick TA, et al. Comparison of data analysis tools for detection of glaucoma with the Heidelberg Retina Tomograph. Ophthalmology. 2003;110:1145–1150.

Greenfield DS, Bagga H, Knighton RW. Macular thickness changes in glaucomatous optic neuropathy detected using optical coherence tomography. Arch Ophthalmol. 2003;121:41–46.

Guedes V, Schuman JS, Hertzmark E, et al. Optical coherence tomography measurement of macular and nerve fiber layer thickness in normal and glaucomatous human eyes. Ophthalmology. 2003;110:177–189.

Mistlberger A, Liebmann JM, Greenfield DS, et al. Heidelberg retina tomography and optical coherence tomography in normal, ocular-hypertensive, and glaucomatous eyes. Ophthalmology 1999;106:2027–2032.

Schuman JS, Wollstein G, Farra T, et al. Comparison of optic nerve head measurements obtained by optical coherence tomography and confocal scanning laser ophthalmoscopy. Am J Ophthalmol. 2003;135:504–512.

Stein DM, Wollstein G, Schuman JS. Imaging in glaucoma. Ophthalmol Clin North Am. 2004;17:33–52.

Weinreb RN, Bowd C, Zangwill LM. Glaucoma detection using scanning laser polarimetry with variable corneal polarization compensation. Arch Ophthalmol. 2003;121:218–224.

Chapter 72

Optic Nerve Malformations

ELIAS I. TRABOULSI, MD

72.1 Introduction

The appearance of normal optic nerve heads varies depending on the size of the scleral canal, the tilting of the nerve as it exits from the globe, the pigmentation at the edge of the disc, the error of refraction, the size of the optic cup, and the pattern of branching of the retinal vasculature and their point of exit from the papilla. Differentiating normal optic nerve head variants from malformations may sometimes be difficult but is imperative and so is the specific characterization of individual malformations so that significant associated brain or other systemic defects are detected and precise genetic counseling is given. In this chapter, we will give examples of common optic nerve malformations and briefly review associated clinical abnormalities. The reader is reminded to obtain photographs and review them for patients in whom the appearance of the nerve head is not characteristic of a particular class of malformations. Such a review allows another objective evaluation of the nerve head size in relationship to posterior pole landmarks and an easier overview of the pattern of retinal vascular branching.

72.2 Clinical Signs and Symptoms

Decreased visual acuity and visual field defects are the main symptoms and signs associated with optic nerve head malformations. Although congenital absence of retinal and/or optic nerve tissue is an evident cause for vision loss, acquired causes such as strabismic or anisometropic amblyopia or retinal detachment are often encountered. Readers are cautioned about trying to predict the level of eventual vision in infants and very young children with optic nerve head malformations.

Some apparently severe defects may be compatible with moderately good vision, whereas other not so striking malformations may result in significant visual deficits. Exudative retinal detachment occurs in up to one-third of eyes with morning glory discs, and rhegmatogenous detachments have been well described in eyes with typical colobomas.

72.2.1 OPTIC NERVE HYPOPLASIA

Optic nerve hypoplasia (ONH) is a nonprogressive, segmental or diffuse, congenital abnormality of one or both optic nerves characterized by a decreased number of axons in the presence of otherwise normal glial and supportive mesodermal tissue. It is the most common ocular malformation. Males are affected as often as females, and bilateral occurrences are more common than unilateral ones. Strabismus is a common presenting sign in patients with unilateral or asymmetric disease, whereas poor vision and nystagmus are more common presentations of bilateral disease. Visual acuity varies from normal to very poor and depends at least in part on the preservation of the papillomacular bundle. Treatment of associated amblyopia can be rewarding. A variety of visual field defects may be present. Bitemporal defects and generalized constriction are most common in severe hypoplasia, whereas inferior altitudinal field defects that spare fixation predominate in segmental hypoplasia. Bitemporal field defects may indicate the presence of midline defects of the central nervous system.

Ophthalmoscopically, the nerve head is reduced in size, and there may or may not be a surrounding hypopigmented halo, the so-called "double ring sign" that indicates a smaller optic nerve than a scleral canal (**Figures 72–1** and **72–2**). Mild disease may be difficult

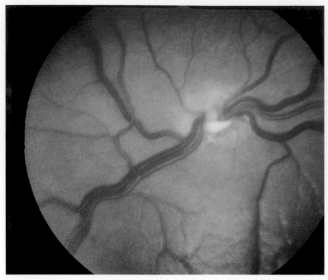

Figure 72–1 Severe ONH. There is little or no nerve tissue, and the blood vessels emerge from a small opening surrounded by a round depigmented area that simulates an optic nerve head.

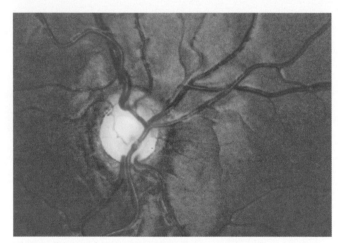

Figure 72–2 Another example of ONH in which there is a small rim of nerve tissue. There is a double ring sign most prominent inferiorly.

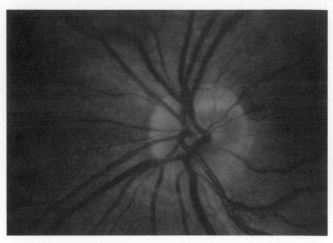

Figure 72–3 Sectoral ONH. The upper half of the nerve head is absent, and there appears to be a normal inferior complement of nerve fibers and nerve tissue.

to diagnose because of problems in assessing the optic nerve head diameter. Fundus photographs are helpful in obtaining absolute measurements or measurements relative to retinal arterial vessel diameter or to other retinal landmarks such as the distance from the center of the disc to the fovea. Retinal vessels are usually of normal caliber but are frequently tortuous. There may be a blunted foveal reflex because of the decrease in number of nerve fibers. Segmental ONH is much less common than the diffuse form and is often superior (**Figure 72–3**); it has been reported in children of insulin-dependent diabetic mothers.

ONH should be differentiated from the crowded disc in high hypermetropia. High errors of refraction are common, especially axial myopia and astigmatism. Hypoplastic discs have been incorrectly diagnosed as atrophic, although concomitant atrophy may be present.

Electroretinograms are abnormal in 35% of patients. The electro-oculogram is usually normal. Visual evoked responses are usually reduced in amplitude and correlate with the degree of visual acuity loss.

On histopathologic sections, the ganglion cells and optic nerve fibers are reduced in number, but the outer retinal layers are normal. The double ring sign results from an overgrowth of retinal pigment epithelial cells toward the center of the optic disc.

ONH is associated with a number of ocular and systemic conditions. Of most significance is the association with midline brain abnormalities; it occurs in 25% of patients with absence of the septum pellucidum, and 27% of patients with ONH have partial or complete absence of the septum pellucidum, so-called septo-optic dysplasia or DeMorsier syndrome, characterized by variable degrees of ONH and absence of the septum pellucidum or corpus callosum, mental retardation, spasticity, and impairment of taste and smell. Pituitary dysfunction and endocrinologic abnormalities may result from hypothalamic dysgenesis. Growth hormone deficiency is the most common endocrinologic abnormality in patients with septo-optic dysplasia. Pituitary dysfunction in patients with septo-optic dysplasia may lead to prolonged neonatal hyperbilirubinemia, hypotonia, or infantile hypoglycemia without hyperinsulinemia. Other associations include hydranencephaly, arrhinencephaly, aniridia, cyclopia, orbital encephalomeningocele, hypotelorism, and holoprosencephaly.

Magnetic resonance imaging (MRI) is indicated in all patients with ONH and allows visualization of the commonly associated central nervous system abnormalities, such as absence of the septum pellucidum (**Figure 72–4**), posterior pituitary ectopia, cerebral hemispheric migration anomalies (schizencephaly and cortical heterotopia), and perinatal hemispheric injury. MRI of the orbit may show a difference in the diameter of the optic nerve patients with unilateral conditions (**Figure 72–5**).

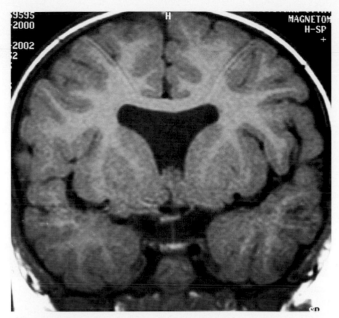

Figure 72–4 Coronal MRI section showing absence of the septum pellucidum in a patient with DeMorsier syndrome.

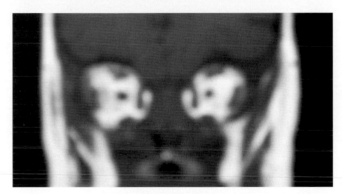

Figure 72–5 Coronal section of the orbits showing a smaller cross section of the right optic nerve compared with the left.

ONH results from failure of differentiation of the retinal ganglion cell layer between the 12- and 17-mm stages of retinal development. Excessive death (apoptosis) of ganglion cells after their excessive development may be another pathogenetic mechanism. Toxic agents taken during pregnancy as well as single gene defects may be operational. Nearly one half of patients with fetal alcohol syndrome have ONH.

72.2.2 MEGALOPAPILLA

Megalopapilla refers to an abnormally large optic disc without anatomic or physiologic defects (**Figure 72–6**). This condition is usually bilateral with a large cup and mimics low-tension glaucoma. The neuroretinal rim may appear pale because of the spreading out of axons, and megalopapilla has been confused with optic atrophy. Visual acuity is usually normal. There may be an enlarged blind spot. Neuroimaging is only recommended in patients with mid-facial anomalies such as

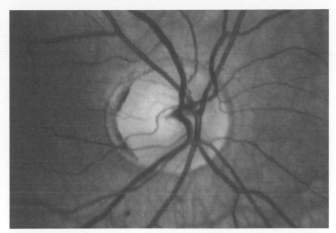

Figure 72–6 Megalopapilla. Note the large diameter of the optic nerve head and a large cup-to-disc ratio. All other ophthalmoscopic aspects are normal.

hypertelorism, cleft palate, cleft lip, and a depressed nasal bridge. Megalopapilla has been reported in patients with mandibulofacial dysostosis of the Franceschetti-Zwahlen type, Bannayan-Zonana syndrome, and retino-choroidal coloboma.

72.2.3 OPTIC DISC COLOBOMA

This congenital anomaly results from incomplete closure of the most posterior aspect of the embryonic fissure. It is part of a spectrum of defects ranging from small notches of the inferior iris or optic disc to large inferior retinochoroidal colobomas. Optic disc colobomas can be unilateral or bilateral. They may be sporadic or inherited in an autosomal dominant fashion. They may be associated with a large number of congenital malformation syndromes, the listing and discussion of which are beyond the scope of this book.

Ophthalmoscopically, the papilla is generally larger than normal; there is partial or total excavation with the deepest part located inferiorly (**Figure 72–7**). The surface of the coloboma may be glistening pearl white, and the retinal vessels course over the coloboma to exit at its borders. The coloboma may extend to involve the adjacent retina and choroid or may be accompanied by such defects. It is difficult to predict the level of visual acuity from the appearance of the coloboma, but vision depends chiefly on the involvement of the macular area and/optic nerve fibers. Complications include retinal and/or macular detachment.

It is imperative to distinguish a typical optic disc coloboma from the morning glory disc anomaly (MGDA) because the latter occurs sporadically whereas the former can be inherited, and patients have to be advised of the genetic implications of each.

72.2.4 MORNING GLORY DISC ANOMALY

The MGDA is characterized by an enlarged, excavated, and funnel-shaped optic papilla, with a central tuft

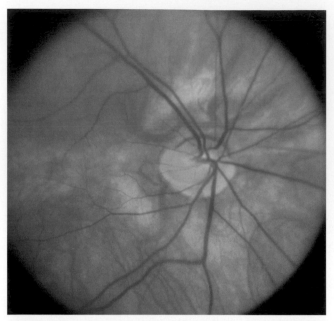

Figure 72–7   Typical inferior coloboma of the optic nerve head.

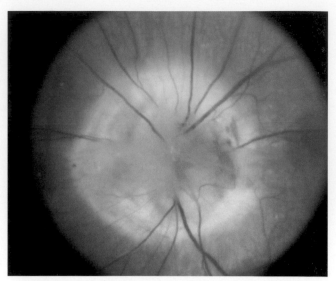

Figure 72–9   Another example of an MGDA with foveal luteal pigment at the edge of the papillary opening.

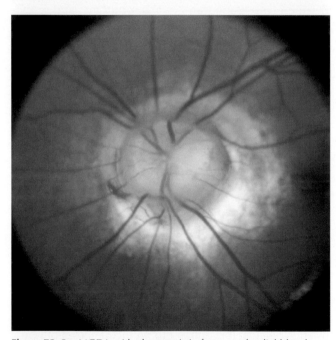

Figure 72–8   MGDA with characteristic features of radial blood vessels, enlarged scleral opening, rings of pigmentation and depigmentation, and a central tuft of glial tissue.

of white glial tissue and often a raised annulus of pigmentary chorioretinal changes (**Figure 72–8**). The descriptive term *morning glory disc anomaly* was coined because of the resemblance of the anomaly to the flower with that name.

The appearance of the nerve head varies with the degree of dysplasia, the size of the posterior scleral opening, the amount of surrounding chorioretinal pigmentation, the vascular pattern, and the amount of gliosis and remnants of the hyaloid system at the center of the disc. The macula can be dragged to the nasal edge of the disc, and the yellow macular xanthophyll pigment is often visible in that location (**Figure 72–9**). The retinal arterioles and venules emerge in a radial pattern from the enlarged scleral canal and are often bridged by vascular arcades close to the optic nerve head. Other straight arterioarterial bridging vessels can be seen more peripherally.

The majority of occurrences are unilateral and affect both sexes equally. One half of patients present with strabismus. MGDA is not a familial condition. There may be a white pupillary reflex. Up to 30% of patients develop a total, usually exudative retinal detachment, possibly from communication between the subarachnoid and subretinal spaces. Contractile movements have been described in the MGDA and may be due either to variation in the volume of the subretinal fluid or the presence of heterotopic smooth muscle fibers in the malformation. Amaurosis fugax can occur. Visual acuity ranges from 20/30 to poor light perception. Poor vision results from retinal and optic nerve dysplasia but may also be partly due to strabismic or anisometropic amblyopia. Associated ocular anomalies in the affected eye include strabismus, remnants of the pupillary membrane, cataract, aniridia, persistence of the hyaloid system, ciliary body cyst, vitreous cyst, retinal detachment, foveal dysplasia, epiretinal membranes, and microphthalmos. Retinal vascular tortuosity, optic pits, microphthalmos, anterior segment dysgenesis, Duane's retraction syndrome, and remnants of the pupillary membrane have been reported in the fellow eye. There is a well-documented association with basal encephaloceles. Agenesis of the corpus callosum and an absent chiasm has also been reported with MGDA. Congenital

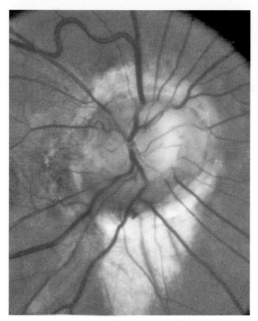

Figure 72–10 Optic nerve malformation with depigmented inferior "colobomas" and a small staphylomatous defect in which the optic nerve head is sunken.

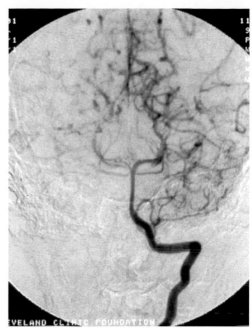

Figure 72–11 Cerebral angiogram of a patient whose optic nerve head photograph is shown in **Figure 72–10** revealing constriction of the internal carotid artery with distal capillary collateral formation in a puff-of-smoke pattern characteristic of moyamoya disease.

renal abnormalities can also occur. Narrowing of one or more of the branches of the internal carotid artery with formation of distal capillary network in a puff-of-smoke pattern, so called moyamoya disease, has recently been described in a number of patients with MGDA or with malformations of the disc that resemble an MGDA (**Figures 72–10** and **72–11**). These are potentially life-threatening abnormalities because of the associated cerebrovascular accidents. Computed tomography (CT) arteriography should be obtained in all patients with MGDA or similar malformations.

Ultrasonography, CT scans, and MRI can demonstrate the funnel-shaped junction of the optic nerve with the posterior aspect of the globe. Fluorescein angiography shows abnormal arteriovenous communications and reveals the origin of the retinal vasculature.

MGDA probably results from failure of the posterior sclera and the lamina cribrosa to form. This leads to herniation of intraocular contents through the defect and formation of the conical deformity. Remnants of the hyaloid system are often observed in the center of the MGDA. In peripapillary contractile staphyloma, myofibroblastic differentiation presumably leads to contractions of the papilla.

The great majority of occurrences of MGDA and optic pits, however, are isolated and the recurrence risk in siblings is negligible.

Visual prognosis is poor in patients who present with profound visual loss. Treatment of associated strabismic or anisometropic amblyopia may result in some regaining of vision. Treatment of the retinal detachment that occurs in about 30% of patients is indicated, but the visual outcome is guarded.

SUGGESTED READINGS

Aroichane M, Traboulsi EI. Congenital anomalies of the optic nerve head. In: Traboulsi EI, ed. Genetic Diseases of the Eye. New York, NY: Oxford University Press, 1999:115–142.

Bakri S, Siker D, Masaryk T, Luciano MG, Traboulsi EI. Moyamoya disease, ocular malformations and midline cranial defects: A distinct syndrome. Am J Ophthalmol. 1997;127:356–357.

Brodsky MC. Congenital optic disk anomalies. Surv Ophthalmol. 1994; 39:89–112.

Brodsky MC. Morning glory disc anomaly or optic disc coloboma? (Letter). Arch Ophthalmol. 1994;112:153.

Cennamo G, Sammartino A, Fioretti F. Morning glory syndrome with contractile peripapillary staphyloma. Br J Ophthalmol. 1983; 67:346–348.

Chang S, Haik BG, Ellsworth RM, St Louis L, Berrocal JA. Treatment of total retinal detachment in morning glory syndrome. Am J Ophthalmol. 1984;97:596–600.

Hellstrom A, Wiklund LM, Svenson E. The clinical and morphologic spectrum of optic nerve hypoplasia. J AAPOS. 1999;3:212–220.

Lambert SR, Hoyt CS, Narahara MH. Optic nerve hypoplasia. Surv Ophthalmol. 1987;32:1–9.

Manschot WA. Morning glory syndrome: a histopathological study. Br J Ophthalmol. 1990;74:56–58.

Morioka M, Marubayashi T, Masumitsu T, Miura M, Ushio Y. Basal encephaloceles with morning glory syndrome, and progressive hormonal and visual disturbances: Case report and review of the literature. Brain Dev. 1995;17:196–201.

Phillips PH, Spear C, Brodsky MC. Magnetic resonance diagnosis of congenital hypopituitarism in children with optic nerve hypoplasia. J AAPOS. 2001;15:27–280.

Siatkowski RM, Sanchez J, Andrada R, Alvarez A. The clinical, neuro-radiographic and endocrinologic profile of patients with bilateral ONH. Ophthalmology 1997;104:493–496.

Skarf B, Hoyt CS. Optic nerve hypoplasia in children. Association with anomalies of the endocrine and CNS. Arch Ophthalmol. 1984; 102:62–67.

Traboulsi EI, ONeill JF. The spectrum in the morphology of the so-called "morning glory disc anomaly." J Pediatr Ophthalmol Strabismus 1988;25:93–98.